# DISEASES OF CHILDREN

# DISEASES OF CHILDREN

### HUGH JOLLY
M.A., M.D., F.R.C.P., D.C.H.

*Physician in charge of the Paediatric Department*
*Charing Cross Hospital, London*

THIRD EDITION
SECOND PRINTING

BLACKWELL SCIENTIFIC PUBLICATIONS
OXFORD LONDON EDINBURGH MELBOURNE

I S B N: 0 632 00388 X

First Published 1964
Reprinted 1966
Second Edition 1968
Reprinted 1971, 1973, 1974
Third Edition 1976
Reprinted 1979
E L B S Edition
First Published 1971
Reprinted 1974

Distributed in the U.S.A. by
Blackwell Mosby Book Distributors
11830 Westline Industrial Drive
St Louis, Missouri 63141,

*in Canada by*

Blackwell Mosby Book Distributors
86 Northline Road, Toronto
Ontario, M4B 3E5,

*and in Australia by*

Blackwell Scientific Book Distributors
214 Berkeley Street, Carlton
Victoria 3053

Printed in Great Britain at the Alden Press, Oxford
and bound at Kemp Hall Bindery

# CONTENTS

# PREFACE TO THE THIRD EDITION

In view of the advances in paediatrics since publication of the second edition, extensive revision has been necessary and large sections have been rewritten. Despite a great deal of hard pruning of previous material, this edition is just over 50 pages longer than its predecessor owing to new material.

In line with modern child care, more space is given to normal development and to the care of the child with a handicap. A major change is now recommended for babies born with spina bifida. Instead of surgery for all, careful selection on the basis of ultimate prognosis is recommended.

Still greater emphasis is placed on history taking. I am increasingly convinced that the medical history is much more difficult than the clinical examination; and that in the care of children it is, if possible, even more important than with adults because it sets the child in the context of his family to which his problems are so intimately bound. Much of the examination is obtained by watching the child when taking the history. Doctors who insist that the child is undressed before they see him, handicap themselves needlessly.

The section on glomerulonephritis has been rewritten entirely. Having been taught by Arthur Ellis and brought up on his classification of Type 1 and Type 2 nephritis which did so much to clarify the situation at the time, I am now forced to agree that it has no place in modern nephrology. The sections on small stature and child abuse are also entirely new. Much greater space is given to the problems of non-accidental injury, and to emotional as well as physical battering.

A new section on the clumsy child adjoins that on cerebral palsy. The classic features of cerebral palsy are now less common in the U.K. as a result of improved obstetric and perinatal care. However, the number of children being treated for abnormal clumsiness is increasing. This must be due either to improved care, causing a reduction in severely affected children and an increase in those less severely affected, or because there is now an increased awareness of the very special needs of these children.

The section on chronic functional constipation has been totally altered in line with my altered practice that there is no longer any need to treat such patients with laxatives and bowel washouts. Other rewritten sections are those on disorders of carbohydrate metabolism, disorders of lipid metabolism, infantile hypotonia and leukaemia.

The global approach to paediatrics is maintained and enlarged so that special aspects relevant to the care of children in developing countries are frequently included. The doctor beginning work in a developing country faces problems of adjustment which are discussed in this edition. A mother in a developing country is even more liable than her counterpart in the U.K. to believe that giving twice the recommended dose of a medicine is twice as effective. For her, there is a pictorial scheme (Fig. 7, p. 26) to assist her understanding of the time of day to give the medicine. The section on protein calorie malnutrition is enlarged and a section on the hazards of native medicines has been added to the chapter on poisoning. Leprosy has been included for the first time.

Authors tend to get attached to old illustrations but I had no difficulty in removing the photograph of a child illustrating restrainers to prevent scratching since I now never use such appliances. It was more difficult to give up the illustration of pink disease since this was such a vivid reminder of these very sick children, but the disorder has now been almost totally eradicated.

I considered very seriously the comment of one reviewer of the last edition that the only old-fashioned aspect of the book was its title; he felt this should incorporate 'child health' since this aspect was emphasized in the text. I considered 'Children in health and disease' but decided against it since a book with this title should give as much space to child health as to diseases, whereas this book contains more on diseases.

*London, November 1975*                                    HUGH JOLLY

# PREFACE TO THE FIRST EDITION

This book is intended for medical students and general practitioners. Emphasis has been laid on the common disorders of childhood, but rare conditions are included so that it can be used for reference. The care of sick children is essentially a matter of teamwork, therefore, the advice the doctor should give the nurse who is assisting him has been included. It is hoped that nursing tutors will also find this of value.

The steady improvement in the mortality rates for infants and children should not lead the student to spend less time learning about normal and sick children. Most paediatric centres now report increasing pressure on their beds and out-patient clinics. Amongst other reasons, this is related to a greater emphasis on special-care units and the needs of premature infants, a more active approach to the management of congenital malformations, and a wider recognition of the needs of the emotionally disturbed child. Further factors increasing the demand for hospital beds are the loosening of family ties, whereby a grandmother is no longer available to nurse the sick child at home, and the frequency with which mothers go out to work.

A wide knowledge of the child in health and disease is essential for the family doctor, a large proportion of whose patients will be children. An ability to look after children is one of the keys to successful general practice, reputations being made more rapidly by success with children than in any other way. The problems of sick children in general practice and the needs of the general practitioner have been largely derived from nine years' experience as a consultant paediatrician in a large provincial area where it is possible to achieve a closer relationship between consultant and general practitioner than in a teaching hospital.

Paediatrics is changing fast, so that there is now much greater emphasis on the neonatal period, this being reflected in the number of pages devoted to this age group. The pattern of disease is also changing in older children; for example, in children over one year of age accidents are the most frequent cause of death, while cancer, although rare, is now the most common natural cause of death.

The sick child must be studied within the context of medicine as a whole;

this book anticipates a knowledge of general medicine in its readers. Stress is laid on the frequent occasions when the child's reaction to disease differs from that of the adult. The fact that the temperature of a newborn baby with infection is as likely to fall as to rise is an example of such a difference.

There is no separate chapter on Tropical Diseases. Many of the diseases of the tropics are the same as those in temperate climates, but their pattern is different because of alterations in the environment or in the response of the individual to disease. Other diseases, which used to be confined to tropical areas, and were often, therefore, left out of textbooks designed for use in temperate climates, have been incorporated within the systems affected. Nowadays, immigration and the speed of travel requires that every practitioner should be competent to recognize and treat these disorders. For the same reason a geographical history is described as part of normal history taking.

The more frequent references to West Africa, particularly Nigeria, than to other tropical areas result from a year spent working there. For the same reason a number of illustrations are of African children. It is hoped that an approach to paediatrics through a study of sick children both in temperate and tropical countries will assist students and doctors in both areas.

*London, January 1964*                                                HUGH JOLLY

# ACKNOWLEDGEMENTS

In preparing the third edition I am indebted to many colleagues for their criticisms of the second edition, particularly to Dr Herbert Barrie, Dr Donald Bentley and Dr Trevor Edmonds. Miss P.M.Turnbull, head of the Department of Medical Illustration, Charing Cross Hospital, has undertaken the majority of the illustrations and has continued to advise. It is a pleasure to record that her work in the first edition was awarded the Lancet Trophy, given annually for the best medical illustrations published.

For other photographs I am indebted to Mr Frank Speed and the Department of Medical Illustration, University College, Ibadan, Nigeria, and to the House Governor, University College Hospital, Ibadan, for permission to publish; Dr Ned Waldron, Dr Homer Smith and the Department of Medical Photography, S. Devon and E. Cornwall Hospital, Plymouth; Mr Derek Martin and the Department of Medical Illustration, Hospital for Sick Children, Great Ormond Street, London; and Mr S.W.Briandt, head of the Department of Medical Photography, Ghana Medical School, Accra.

I am grateful to Mr Lipmann Kessel for Fig. 58, Professor Alex Russell for Fig. 94, Dr John Sutcliffe for Fig. 103, Dr M.Munz and Dr F.W.Engmann for Fig. 109, Dr Gerald Parsons-Smith for Figs. 110 and 112, Dr Pampiglione for Fig. 113, Dr T.L.Chester-Williams and Miss Pat Beaman for Fig. 115, Dr Colin McDougall for Figs. 121 and 122, Dr Edward Hart for Fig. 127, Sir Wilfrid Sheldon for Fig. 129, Professor Ralph Hendrickse for Fig. 133.

Fig. 17 is reproduced from an article by the author in *The Practitioner* (1956), **176,** 369.

Fig. 25 is reproduced from an article by the author in the *Proceedings of the Royal Society of Medicine* (1959), **52,** 300.

Fig. 44 is reproduced from *Urology of Childhood* by T.Twistington Higgins, D.Innes Williams and D.F.Ellison Nash, 1951, Butterworths.

Figs. 66 and 67 are charts prepared by J.M.Tanner and R.H.Whitehouse, and made by Creaseys of Hertford.

Figs. 95, 96 and 116 are reproduced from the author's book *Sexual Precocity*, 1955, Charles C.Thomas.

I would like to express my appreciation of the courtesy I have received from my publishers and particularly to Mr Per Saugman and Mr John Robson.

# CHAPTER 1

# HISTORY TAKING AND EXAMINATION

When the patient is a child the doctor's approach is of especial importance since diagnosis is more difficult if the child is upset. If both parents come with the child, both should be allowed to enter the consulting room so that a better picture of the family is obtained. This must be stressed to hospital nurses who still tend to allow one parent only to accompany the child. If a grandparent or close friend comes with the mother they also should be allowed into the consulting room since, if they feel it important enough to come, they are obviously of consequence in the child's life. Moreover, a wider picture of the family may be obtained by this means. One can be certain that if a grandmother argues with her daughter in front of the doctor, even more does she do so at home! When taking the history, the doctor must decide whether it would be better for the child to stay outside rather than hear himself discussed.

The child needs to be put at his ease and to feel welcome. I usually greet him first, provided I do not feel this will embarrass him. My greeting sometimes takes the form of a complimentary remark about his clothes or showing him one of my toys. It may be appropriate to tell the child your name and then to ask his. Alternatively, a question such as 'do you go to school' may be easier for him to answer. The aim is to become friends and to help the child to make contact with the doctor.

All this is helped by not wearing a white coat and by arranging the consulting room or surgery office so that it looks as much like a toy shop and as little like an operating theatre as possible. An array of chromium-plated instruments may impress the mother but only frightens the child.

The mother should be put at her ease so that she is able to describe her child's problems in her own words and without hurry. The 'question and answer' type of history fails to give a real picture of the child's illness and should be used only at the end in order to fill gaps in the story.

## HISTORY

In children (and perhaps in adults) the medical history often provides more information than the clinical examination. The importance of learning how to elicit physical signs has been over-emphasized to medical students in comparison with the time spent on learning to take a good history. More skill is required in the taking of a history than in carrying out a clinical examination. Above all it is essential to learn how to listen as opposed to how to question.

Symptoms of illness in babies are normally non-specific; loss of appetite is a major symptom of serious illness, especially infection. Severe diseases of the renal tract may cause failure to thrive only, in a baby, there being none of the symptoms characteristic of the adult with urinary disorders. Only as the child gets older does illness produce more specific symptoms.

The description which follows is intended for those who see children referred to them by family doctors,* whether they are seeing them in hospital or in consultative private practice. Under such conditions the consultant, registrar (resident), houseman (intern) or medical student is without the GP's advantage of knowing the family background and the child's social and home circumstances. The vital link for bridging this gap is the GP's letter or telephone call which should give the reason for referral, the results of any investigations performed and the treatment already prescribed. It is helpful to be told when it is the parents who have made the initial request for a second opinion. The letter need not give lengthy details about symptoms since the hospital doctor will check these himself but it should include intimate information, such as the fact that a mother is unmarried, which the doctor in hospital should be protected from stumbling on without warning.

Since the GP will already know much of the family background his history in the busy surgery can be very much shorter. But if, as a student, he has not been trained in the technique of taking a comprehensive history he will, when busy, fail to pick out those salient features which are needed for a proper understanding of his patients.

In taking a medical history students are usually taught to inquire about the main complaint first, and then to go into the previous history and family history. With children, it is an advantage to inquire about the family and previous history before coming to the chief complaint. The doctor should try to obtain a picture of the patient in his home setting and it is helpful if this has been built up before discussing the main illness. The elderly mother of an only child will have a very different outlook from the mother who has had many children. These are facts which should be learnt at an early stage in taking the history.

---

* The term 'family doctor' is regarded as the best description for those whose task is the primary care of family units of patients. It is considered as synonymous with the term 'general practitioner' but gives a clearer picture of the role of the doctor concerned. For ease of reading, the term general practitioner (GP) will be used in the text.

**Family history**

It should be the duty of the receptionist to record the father's occupation and the religion of the family in addition to the usual routine details. The religion may well be relevant to the child's problem, but if requested by the doctor it becomes a much more personal question than if recorded with other routine matters by the receptionist. She should also record the child's date of birth and his present age. These should be carefully checked as mothers are very apt to give the age at next birthday.

The child's place in the family is learnt, together with the names and ages of any other children and whether they have suffered from any notable complaints. For example, a recent history of measles in one of the other children is of importance when seeing a child with a rash. A family history of fits is particularly significant if the child is brought for the same reason. Under other circumstances it may be necessary to inquire about a family history of allergic disorders such as asthma, hay fever or eczema, or whether there is a history of diabetes, rheumatic fever or tuberculosis in the family.

Specific inquiry should be made as to whether any children have died and whether there have been any miscarriages. Consanguinity should be determined in view of the influence of genetic factors in disease.

While taking the family history it is always wise to ask the mother what work she did before marriage and whether she still goes out to work. This not only furthers the understanding of the child's social circumstances and gives useful information about the mother, but also prevents the mistake of talking to a mother who is a doctor or a nurse as though she was a layman. To know the ages of the parents is helpful; elderly parents or parents with widely differing ages each have their own problems. However, care must be taken to avoid embarrassing parents who dislike mentioning their ages in front of their children.

**Previous history**

This includes details of pregnancy and labour as well as the child's previous illnesses. It is useful to start by asking where the baby was born, since this helps a mother to recall more details of the birth. It also ensures that if the birth was in hospital its address is recorded should further obstetric information be required. The amount of time given to antenatal and birth history will depend on the child's age and the complaint. More detail will be required if the patient is brought for mental retardation, fits or congenital malformations which could be related to disease or drugs in pregnancy, or difficulty in labour. The birth weight must be recorded and whether birth was at term or preterm. Detailed information about feeding must be obtained for all infants but, even with older children, it is an advantage to know whether or not they were breast fed. The manner in which this question is answered, as well as the answer itself, will often give useful information about the mother. The duration of breast feeding should be asked since some mothers will state that they have breast fed their children, when in fact this was only while they were in the maternity hospital.

It is helpful to ask whether the child has had vitamin supplements, such as cod liver oil and orange juice. This question is not so much to look for the possibility of a vitamin deficiency as to discover whether the mother has a conscientious approach to the feeding of her baby.

*Developmental history.* The age at which the child passed the normal milestones of development is then determined, although mothers often find difficulty in recollecting these facts. In the case of a baby or a retarded child the information must be detailed, whereas in other children it may be necessary to check only that the patient walked and talked within the normal period. When trying to establish whether the child is likely to have suffered brain damage at the time of birth or immediately afterwards, a number of questions may assist. The mother may know that special resuscitation measures were required or that he was nursed in an incubator for the first few days. She should be asked when she was first permitted to handle him: was he immediately placed in a cot beside her bed or was he kept in a special nursery for the first few days? Were there any feeding difficulties such as vomiting or a reluctance to feed? Did he require to be tube-fed? Did he become jaundiced?

The age of the baby when discharged from the maternity hospital is a good indication of his early progress. The baby who had to be kept in hospital after his mother was discharged is sure to have had some complicating factors.

Immunization details should be recorded, particularly BCG, since this alters the significance of a positive tuberculin test. Checking that the child has been fully immunized should be a natural item in the medical history of every young child. No opportunity should be missed for gentle and unobtrusive health education.

Finally, an inquiry into previous illnesses should be made and, if necessary, a specific inquiry about the infectious fevers such as measles, rubella and others. These are so often forgotten by the mother or merely recorded by the doctor as 'usual childish complaints'. An absence of this detailed information is particularly irritating in the case of children in hospital when another patient in the ward develops an infectious fever. If this happens it is necessary to know at once which of the other patients are at risk and need to be isolated. A direct question should be asked as to whether the child has had any operations. Mothers often regard the removal of tonsils and adenoids as routine and forget to mention the fact.

**History of present complaint**

Detailed information should be obtained about the child's illness which is recorded systematically so as to give separate paragraphs and headings to each new dateline, rather than giving the whole history in essay form. Thus:

| | |
|---|---|
| *4 weeks ago* | Onset of cough ........................................... |
| *3 days ago* | Sore throat ............................................... |
| *Yesterday* | Rash ...................................................... |
| *Today* | Convulsion .............................................. |

On no account should days of the week be written in the history since they give no indication of the duration of the disease. A common oversight is to forget to record the date on which the examination is taking place. Care must be taken to go far enough back in the history to discover when the symptoms first began or whether similar attacks have occurred before. Related earlier illnesses, such as a recurrent sore throat in a child with nephritis, should be given in this part of the history, whereas if unrelated they should be recorded under previous illnesses.

Specific inquiry of a number of symptoms relating to general health should be made if these have not already come up during discussion of the main complaint. These relate to appetite, bowels, micturition, sleeping habits and energy. With children of school age it is often instructive to learn how they are getting on at school and whether the mother has discussed the problem with the teacher.

**Geographical history**

An inquiry should be made into the child's recent whereabouts. In these days of air travel and holidays abroad, failure to ask this simple question can lead to a deadly disease, like malaria, being overlooked. Even if the patient has not travelled in a tropical area he may have acquired a disease from contact with someone who has.

**Social history**

The information being sought under this heading covers every facet of the social and family circumstances which might have a bearing on the child's illness. Environment and family relationships and feelings play such a large part in moulding a child's behaviour that these must be understood if the child is to be helped to the full. Some of the information, such as the physical circumstances of the child's home, including the question of overcrowding, is the sort of knowledge to be discovered at a glance by a visit to the home. Details of the parents' financial status may be helpful, though much of this can be surmised from knowing the father's occupation and the home address.

Some aspects of the social history could equally well be taken under family history but since, for the reasons given, it is preferable to learn the basic facts about the family at an early stage, so it is desirable to leave these more personal questions to a later stage when the parents have gained greater confidence in the doctor and when the relevance of the social factors in relation to the child's illness will be more clear.

Some children, particularly those with functional symptoms, may lead the doctor to discover a number of emotional factors within the family to account for the child's symptoms, For example, a child's abdominal pain may turn out to be functional and closely related to the incompatibility of his parents or possibly to the recent loss of one of them. A mentally handicapped child causes severe stresses within his family and may thereby be the cause of the symptoms which take one of his siblings to the doctor. A child presenting with a minor illness may bring into the open some basic family problem, in fact the child's illness may be used as a pretext, whether conscious or subconscious, for asking advice about family illness. Sometimes it is the fear of a family illness such as tuberculosis which brings the child to the doctor (see p. 16). Clyne (1961) reviewed the reasons for night calls made by a group of GPs in London. He emphasized the frequency with which 'the child is the presenting symptom' of a disturbed family and that this call, although ostensibly for the child is really for some other member of the family wanting advice. Moreover, the calls, although very common during the day, occurred more frequently at night.

Hopkins (1959) described one family in which, over a period of 40 months, both physical and emotional disorders (asthma, eczema, enteritis, depression, anxiety state, sinusitis, migraine, abdominal pains, influenza, bronchitis and more) recurred in different forms, being linked inextricably so that chain reactions were set off between the several members of the family. Such a report emphasizes the need to study family illness as a whole in order to uncover its causes and shows how meaningless a single episode in one of the members of this family might seem to the doctor working in isolation in the hospital or office. It is this sort of information which should be included in the GP's letter when referring a patient to hospital.

Apley (1963) uses the term 'family patterning' for many disorders which run in families, pointing out that many genetic and environmental factors in disease are inseparable, both contributing to the moulding of the individual. Preventive paediatrics must be increasingly concerned with family carriers of illness, not only in the physical field but also in the emotional, intellectual and social fields. A mother who as a child was made to worry because she did not eat as much as expected, thereby being forced to eat more, is likely to have her personal computer set so that she pressurizes her child in the same way.

A follow-up of children who fail to keep their appointment with the doctor may unearth social as well as physical reasons for defaulting (Knox & Dugdale, 1966).

So far it has been assumed that the history has been taken from the mother or whoever is accompanying the child. But the doctor must not forget to ask the child himself about the symptoms; even the very young can give most valuable information.

With children whose diagnosis is not apparent on the first visit, especially those under investigation in hospital, it is always helpful if a repeat history is taken. The mother of a child in hospital can often give a much clearer history at the second attempt than when flustered and anxious at the time of the child's admission.

## EXAMINATION

Much of the examination of a child has been taking place while listening to a mother giving her story of the problem. A glance should tell whether the child looks well, mildly ill or seriously ill. By the time the history is finished the doctor should have formed a shrewd idea as to whether the child is developmentally normal, a routine part of every child's clinical examination. The time is also used for evaluating a mother's feelings for her child from the way she handles him.

Arrangements for routine measurements will vary with the preferences of individual doctors. It is usual for the nurse in an outpatient department to record the child's weight and height and to perform routine tests of the urine. If the child is frightened by being measured it is better to postpone the investigations until after he has been seen by the doctor. Mothers should be instructed to bring a specimen of the child's urine with them since many children are unwilling to pass urine in the unusual surroundings of a doctor's surgery or hospital outpatient department. Routine temperature taking is usually unnecessary, this being better left to the doctor to carry out during his examination.

In childhood, inspection plays a greater part in the examination than at any other age. This has been going on throughout the taking of the history, the child being encouraged to play with toys which should be plentifully supplied in the room.

I used to have children undressed before they came into my room, but I have now stopped this since I feel it is unnatural for a child to be waiting outside half clothed. I prefer him to be playing naturally, and for this reason play specialists (p. 21) have a role in the waiting area of the outpatient department as well as in the wards.

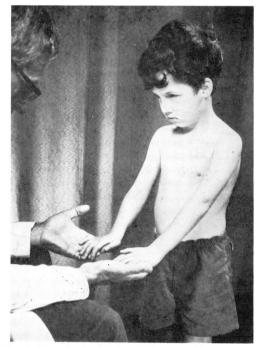

Fig. 1. Examination of the child starts with the hands.

Inside the consulting room I usually leave the mother to undress a young child since he is liable to be nervous of a stranger doing this. However, the clinging type of child will sometimes allow the doctor to help, even though he refuses to let his mother undress him. Asking a child if you can listen to his chest usually leads to his agreeing to letting you help him undress. I do not routinely have a nurse in my consulting room, but it is important that one should immediately be available for special occasions, such as helping with a hearing test.

The examination of a child cannot be systematically carried out from top to bottom as with an adult, since all those manoeuvres which are unpleasant and liable to upset the child, such as the examination of the ears or throat, must be left to the end. The doctor must be prepared to vary his routine to suit the child, and it may well be necessary to examine the back of the chest before the front, or the abdomen before the chest. This variable routine has the disadvantage that parts of the examination may be left out, but this can be prevented by a strictly systematic method of recording so that it is immediately obvious if any part of the examination has been overlooked.

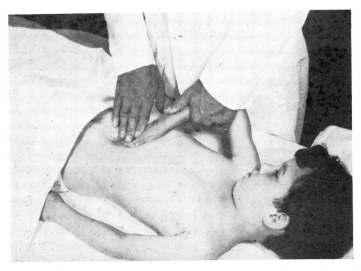

Fig. 2. A fretful child who refuses to stay quiet for ordinary abdominal examination will often permit palpation through his own hand.

Small children should, as far as possible, be examined on their mother's lap. The child can always be moved to the couch for further examination but, as this may make him cry, as much information as possible should be obtained beforehand while he is quiet on his mother's lap. If the child is asleep in his mother's arms much of the examination should be completed before he is woken up. The sleeping child may give the doctor the best chance to determine the type of respirations, the tension of the anterior fontanelle and to examine the abdomen and fundi. A crying baby can be quietened by being given a feed.

It is best to examine a child first standing up, since some will be frightened by being made to lie on a couch even though later they will agree to it. An examination of the hands makes a good starting point (Fig. 1). It is unlikely to upset the child who will already be used to seeing adults shake hands, and has the advantage of ensuring that this important examination is not forgotten. A great deal of information can be obtained from the hands, including simple observations such as whether they are unnecessarily dirty or whether the nails are bitten.

Babies and toddlers are easily upset and should not be stared at, since this causes them to lose confidence and cry. It is always wiser to look at the centre of a baby's forehead than to stare him in the eyes. A young child may be made to feel more at home if the doctor keeps up a 'running commentary' during his

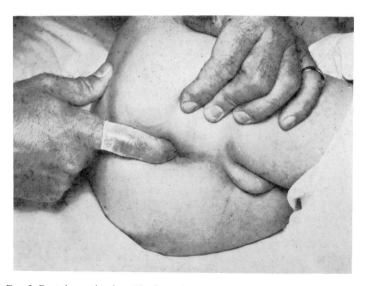

Fig. 3. Rectal examination. The finger is pressed flat against the posterior half of the sphincter before entering, rather than being inserted directly into the centre of the anus.

examination. The doctor asks questions as he goes along but if the child fails to answer one he should immediately pass on to another. A child can become acutely embarrassed by the silence after the doctor's question and start to cry, whereas he may be reassured by the doctor's ceaseless chatter, thereby being prevented from crying. A child who has been crying during the examination will usually stop when he is being dressed. If the manoeuvre of reclothing is drawn out, much valuable time, without crying, can be gained for further examination while his mother is slowly replacing his clothes.

In the examination of the chest, auscultation should precede percussion since the latter is more likely to upset a child. A diaphragm type of chest piece has the advantage that it can be slid from place to place more easily than the bell-end, thereby causing less disturbance, though there are occasions in listening to an abnormal heart when a bell-end is essential. If the child is fretful his confidence can often be gained by pretending to examine his mother's chest first. He is also more likely to accept the stethoscope if the end is first placed on his arm. If the end of the stethoscope is cold it should be warmed in the hand before use.

A mother will be watching every movement and facial expression that a doctor makes during his examination, in an attempt to sum up what he is thinking about her child. This is particularly true when it comes to the heart where a slight frown from the doctor may be misinterpreted. I suspect that most mothers immediately become aware when a doctor finds something wrong in her child's heart.

When a child is fretful and does not permit thorough palpation of the abdomen he can often be persuaded to co-operate if the doctor places the child's hand on the abdomen and then, covering it with his own hand, palpates through it (Fig. 2). During the first year of life the liver is relatively large and can be felt about two fingers breadth below the right costal margin. Examination of the genitalia includes, in the male, checking that the testicles are correctly situated (p. 644) and in the female that there are no labial adhesions (p. 194). Insufficient attention is paid to the routine examination of the genitalia in the female but this can be carried out without embarrassment to the child if performed with her lying on her side.

Rectal examination should always be left to last and, in carrying this out, the tip of the index finger should be pressed flat against the edge of the anus before insertion (Fig. 3). This method causes much less discomfort than insertion direct into the centre of the orifice.

In the examination of the central nervous system a great deal of time should be given to watching the child in action during spontaneous activity and play. It should be routine to check the development of every child being examined (for details see p. 250). Illness may prevent a proper assessment of development in which case the child must be rechecked when he is well. Much of this observation will have been accomplished while taking the history from the mother. In a child much more is learnt of neurological function by observation than by the use of the patella hammer, although this is still a necessary part of the examination. For example, if the legs are seen to perform normal reciprocal movement, spasticity can be excluded.

The more the child is made to feel that the examination is part of a game the more he will co-operate. Thus a formal examination for neck stiffness as in an adult is almost certainly doomed to failure and may give a false impression of rigidity as a result of the child's fear. However, a request that he should kiss his knee, an easy task for a normal child (Fig. 4), is much more likely to meet with success. If he does not co-operate in this manoeuvre you can try to get him to look at his teddy bear on the floor or to watch an object fall off his bed.

Hand movements and grasp are observed when small objects are picked up; for this a small sweet is likely to be an adequate bait! The repeated use of the same test material makes for accuracy of assessment, for example wooden spatulae are always at hand and young children enjoy being given them to play with. The newborn baby will grasp a spatula placed in the hand because of the normal grasp reflex (p. 272). At this age the infant takes no notice of the spatula and once the grasp reflex has disappeared, which happens about the third month of life, the spatula is soon dropped. However, by 4–5 months of age he will grasp it because he wishes to do so, though he is likely to use both hands together. At this age, when offered a second spatula, he is likely to drop the one he is holding in order to grasp the more enticing one which he is being offered. By 6 months he is beginning to grasp with one hand rather than with both. At 6–7 months of age, if he is offered a second spatula he will probably place the first spatula in the other hand, leaving the dominant hand free to take hold of the second one. He is also almost certain to try to get it into his mouth. When pushing the end into his mouth he may well cause himself discomfort and even pain without apparently associating his action with being the cause of the pain, so that he continues to perform the

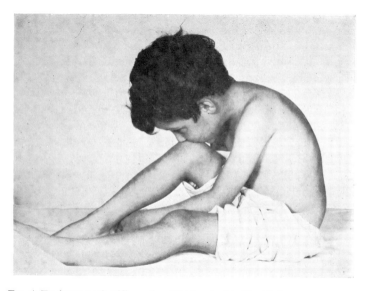

Fig. 4. To detect neck stiffness the child is asked to kiss his knee, a movement which is easily accomplished by the normal child.

action. By 9 months he finds that banging the two spatulae together makes an enjoyable noise. This not only indicates his advancing skills but is a positive demonstration of the fact that he can hear. In a young baby the observation that he enjoys making a noise is an excellent sign that he appreciates sound. More formal tests for hearing are discussed on p. 340.

**Cover test for squint**

An early onset type of squint (p. 223) should be discovered by the age of 6 months in order to initiate treatment to prevent blindness. This can be detected by the cover test which should be used routinely. Each eye is covered in turn while the child is attracted to fix on a target. This target may be a pencil of light or the examiner's finger. During the test the uncovered eye is closely observed to see if it makes any movement in order to take up fixation; this occurs if a squint is present. This test is also of value for detecting a latent squint. In this type the squint is normally held in check by the strength of the binocular reflexes but if these are dissociated by rapidly changing the covered eye the squint becomes manifest. Another test which has the advantage that it does not require the child's co-operation is to check the symmetry of the light reflex in both eyes. Provided there is no squint, the light reflex shows at exactly the same point on each pupil. It is important that the source of light should not be so close as to cause convergence.

### Visual acuity test

Since children do not complain of poor vision, routine eyesight tests should be performed at the age of 2 years and thereafter at yearly intervals. The most satisfactory methods for young children are the Stycar vision tests designed by Sheridan (1969). Two tests are available for children down to the age of 2 years. In one, matching Snellen letter cards are used, the child pointing on his sheet to the letter held by the examiner. In the other, miniature toys are used, such as a chair, car, plane and doll. The child gives the name of the toy to which the tester is pointing or matches it from his own duplicate set. Whichever method is used the child should use both eyes first in order to to gain confidence and learn the technique. Each eye should then be tested in turn, the other being very adequately covered by the tester.

A third test is available for children from 6 months to 2 years. It involves the use of white plastic balls of graded size which can either be rolled or used as fixtures mounted on black sticks. This test does not require speech, the tester watching the child's eyes as the balls move.

Examination of the fundi in children requires the utmost patience and it is sometimes necessary to dilate the pupils. In young babies, anaesthesia may be required for proper examination of the fundi. The optic disc in babies is paler than in the adult, sometimes causing a mistaken diagnosis of optic atrophy to be made. The disc margin is less distinct in children than in adults but differentiation from early papilloedema is made by the fact that all the vessels remain in focus since there is no swelling of the disc.

The size of the head should be noted and the head circumference measured (p. 248). Microcephaly (p. 217) or hydrocephalus (p. 215) may be present in children found to be mentally handicapped.

Palpation for the anterior fontanelle should always be included in the examination and, if present, its size should be noted (see p. 44). Normal fontanelle tension is one indication of health. This tension is reduced if the child is dehydrated, causing the fontanelle to become sunken. With raised intracranial pressure the tension increases and the normal pulsation of the fontanelle disappears. Uninstructed mothers are frequently alarmed by their discovery of the existence of the fontanelle; others are alarmed by its pulsation. This is just one aspect of the anatomy of a normal baby which requires to be taught to all mothers.

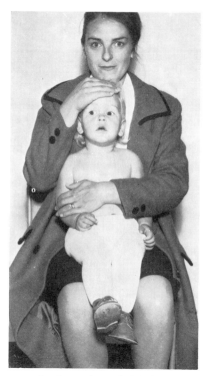

Fig. 5. The correct way for the mother to hold a fretful child for the examination of the throat. If necessary, the child's legs can be gripped firmly between the mother's knees.

Examination of the head should, under certain circumstances, include transillumination in a darkened room using a torch pressed closely to the scalp. In hydranencephaly (p. 217) and gross hydrocephalus (p. 215) the whole of the cranium may transilluminate. Large cysts (porencephaly) may also be shown up by this technique.

Examination of the mouth and ears is left to the end because it is likely to make the child cry. The ears should be seen first as this causes less upset to the child. A warm aural speculum is used but before it is inserted the pinna should be stretched and drawn a little backwards. By this means the auditory canal is straightened and the external meatus widened so that the speculum can more easily be inserted. An aural speculum with a very small aperture is useless, even in babies, because so little can be seen through it. The largest size possible should be used. Straightening the canal makes it unnecessary for the speculum to be inserted far.

Examination of the mouth and throat is likely to cause more difficulty than anything else in a fretful child, but this part of the examination must be thorough, even if it makes the child cry. If the child refuses to stay still he must be held correctly (Fig. 5). Whenever it is necessary to hold the child tight during the examination this should be undertaken by his mother rather than the nurse, as it is less frightening for him. Every doctor will acquire his own tricks to facilitate the examination; it should be remembered that many children can open their mouths so wide that, by protruding the tongue, a full view of the throat can be achieved without using a spatula. Some children gain the necessary confidence to open their mouths if they are allowed to hold the spatula themselves. Pretending to count the teeth will often hold a child's interest, allowing thorough examination of the teeth and gums at the same time. If a child refuses to open his mouth the spatula should be inserted into the side of the mouth and pressed against the gums. This always causes the

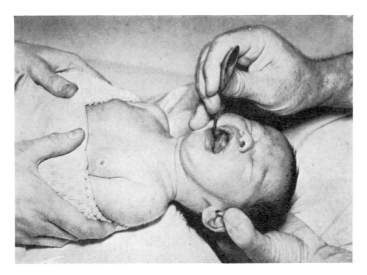

FIG. 6. A baby's throat can more easily be examined from above and for this age a teaspoon is a better size and shape than a spatula.

mouth to open so that the spatula can then be slipped over the back of the tongue. The spatula should never be forced against the clenched incisors since unnecessary pain is caused and the teeth may be damaged. In babies, full inspection of the throat is difficult because the tongue gets in the way, the throat seeming to be further back and lower down than in older children. This difficulty can be overcome by standing behind the baby so as to look into the mouth upside down; for this age group a teaspoon is a better size and shape than a spatula (Fig. 6).

Whenever a doctor or nurse carries out an examination or manoeuvre which might be painful, a careful watch must be kept on the child's face for evidence of pain. A patient may make no complaint when, for example, an excessive amount of enema fluid is being administered, but a glance at his face would show that the danger point had been reached. Children will permit a remarkable degree of discomfort if they are told beforehand what is going to happen. The statement that an injection is 'not going to hurt' is sheer stupidity and causes the child to lose trust, whereas the truth, that he will feel a prick, is usually accepted with equanimity.

At the end of the examination, or on completion of the investigations, the doctor should be able to answer the question: 'What is wrong with the patient.' But he should also be able to answer the question: 'Why was he brought now.' The answer to the second question may be less obvious and requires an understanding of the parents' real anxiety. For example, a mother may bring her child for a cough when her real fear is tuberculosis, but she is too frightened to say so. Sometimes the clue to this may come in the mother's final question, made just as she is leaving. Unless this second question can also be answered the visit to the doctor will have failed to achieve its object.

Do not forget to explain your findings to the child as well as to his parents. Sometimes it helps to talk to the child first, in front of his parents. If he understands and is satisfied by your explanation, his parents are likely to feel the same. Alternatively, it may be appropriate to talk alone with the parents first. Children are often helped to understand their body by the use of simple diagrams. This may also help the parents who often have a surprising ignorance of anatomy, though this need not be shown up if the diagrams are directed to their child. When describing an operation to a child, reference should be made to making an opening rather than cutting, which is much more alarming.

## BIBLIOGRAPHY*

APLEY J. (1963) Family patterning and childhood disorders. *Lancet*, **1**, 67.

*\* This bibliography and those that follow each chapter, list the references mentioned in the chapter, together with suggestions for further reading.*

APLEY J. (1966) The family unit of illness. *Lancet*, **1**, 810.

APLEY J. & MacKEITH R. (1962) *The Child and His Symptoms*. Blackwell Scientific Publications, Oxford.

CLYNE M.B. (1961) *Night Calls: A Study in General Practice*. p. 50. Tavistock Publications, London.

COURT S.D.M. (1963) *The Medical Care of Children*. Oxford University Press, London.

HOPKINS P. (1959) Health and happiness and the family. *Brit. J. clin. Pract.*, **13**, 311.

HOWELLS J.G. (1963) *Family psychiatry*. Oliver & Boyd, London.

KNOX E. & DUGDALE A.E. (1966) The child who did not attend. *Lancet*, **1**, 812.

MAEGRAITH B. (1963) Unde venis. *Lancet*, **1**, 401.

MAEGRAITH B. (1965) *Exotic Disease in Practice*. Heinemann Medical, London.

MILLER F.J.W., COURT S.D.M., WALTON W.S. & KNOX E.G. (1960) *Growing up in Newcastle-upon-Tyne*. Oxford University Press, London.

PAINE R.S. & OPPÉ T.E. (1966) Neurological examination of children. *Clinics in Developmental Medicine*, No. 20/21. Spastics Society/Heinemann Medical, London.

SHERIDAN M.D. (1969) The development of vision, hearing and communication in babies and young children. *Proc. roy. Soc. Med.*, **62**, 999.

SPENCE J., WALTON W.S., MILLER F.J.W. & COURT S.D.M. (1954) *A Thousand Families in Newcastle-upon-Tyne*. Oxford University Press, London.

YUDKIN S. (1961) Six children with coughs. *Lancet*, **2**, 561.

# CHAPTER 2

# GENERAL CARE OF THE CHILD IN HOME AND HOSPITAL

## Home care

The decision to nurse a sick child at home will depend on many factors but principally on the nature of his illness and the facilities available at home. The advantages to the child are obvious in that he is saved the emotional trauma resulting from separation from this parents. To his mother the advantage is not only that she is saved the distress caused by separation but she is given the chance of helping in nursing him back to recovery. Under these circumstances a mother will emerge at the end of her child's illness more competent and with a greater understanding of her child, while her confidence in her ability to deal with future illnesses in her children will increase.

In the United Kingdom the family doctor has the help of a District Nurse in looking after a sick child at home. Nurses should avoid doing everything themselves but should take time to teach the mother how to care for her sick child. This will not only help the mother but in the long run will save the nurse's time. Most mothers will soon learn how to keep temperature charts and intake and output fluid charts. Some mothers' intellect is such that they cannot grasp how to measure the daily intake and output. With such mothers, the nurse should ask that all urine is saved for her to measure. The fluid intake can be measured by the nurse if she instructs the mother to use only fluid from measured jugs; the amount the child has taken in a day can then be calculated by determining the amount left in the jugs.

Many mothers become alarmed if their sick child takes no solids but in most acute illnesses an adequate fluid intake is all that is required. Instruction will be needed on this point. Another common error is for mothers to overheat their sick children, having all the bedroom windows closed, in the false belief that if a child is feverish he must be kept warm. This mistake is often a factor in the production of febrile convulsions (p. 413).

It is the doctor's duty to instruct the nurse in the relevant danger signals to watch for in each case, so that she immediately reports these to him. For example, tachycardia as an early sign of heart failure, headache as a sign of rising intracranial pressure or oliguria as a sign of renal impairment.

The duration of bed rest should be discussed, remembering that there are very few occasions when a child who feels like getting up should be prevented from doing so. Children with acute nephritis used to be kept in bed until the urine was normal on microscopy but it is now realized that this is unnecessary (see p. 384). The presence of a rise in temperature or a raised sedimentation rate is not in itself sufficient reason for keeping a child in bed. The mistake of treating an investigation result rather than the whole child should be avoided. It is unfortunate that temperature charts have a thick line marked at 36·9° C (98·4° F) since this suggests that any deviation from this line, either above or below, is pathological. In practice, the normal temperature of many children is found to be above the figure of 36·9° C. Unless mothers are made aware of this and many other limitations of temperature recording, they are caused much needless anxiety which they are likely to pass on to their children. Most mothers believe they should call the doctor only if their child has a temperature. However, not only may the healthy child have a temperature above 'normal' but the sick child, particularly a young infant, may be below 36·9° C (see Neonatal cold injury, p. 132). These misconceptions about the meaning of a child's temperature frequently result from the attitude of the doctor. It is preferable that mothers should be instructed to call the doctor when they believe their child to be ill rather than that they should be expected, as so often now, to have taken the temperature, calling the doctor only if it is raised. The temperature level is an investigation and as such should be assessed by the doctor in the light of his clinical examination and other investigations. If a mother is expected to take her child's temperature why should she not also count his pulse? And if that, why not measure his blood pressure as well!

The best indication of health in a child is energy. Loss of energy or loss of appetite are definite indications for a medical opinion.

Mothers should be helped to maintain their maternal role and to avoid the role of doctor when their children are ill. This is particularly difficult if one parent is a doctor or nurse. Mothers sometimes ask that their child's tonsils be removed because they look big, but such mothers have no knowledge of the natural hypertrophy of lymphoid tissue around the age of 3 to 4 years. The variation and breadth of normal is possibly the most difficult aspect for parents to learn; for this reason, the child is expected to grow, develop and behave like his earlier siblings or like other children in the neighbourhood.

### Hospital care

When a young child has to be admitted to hospital his mother should ideally be provided with a bedroom in the children's ward. Opinions differ as to whether the child should share the same room, but the nursing staff may have more difficulty in getting to know the child and his needs if he is tucked away in his mother's room. It is probably best to be guided by the home pattern. If the child and his mother share a room at home, this should be repeated in hospital. But a child who has his own bedroom at home or shares it with his brothers or sisters can more easily be nursed in the main children's ward. Having his mother nearby means that she can easily be called if he needs her during the night, but having her own room gives her a better chance of rest. Mothers of very young babies would usually be expected to have their babies in the same room as themselves.

Not all hospitals will have facilities for mothers to live in separate rooms, but most should be able to provide collapsible beds which can be put up in a child's cubicle at night, or beside his bed in the main ward. Similar beds can be used to convert the play room into a mothers' dormitory at night.

UNRESTRICTED VISITING

This term indicates that parents can visit their sick child at any time of day or night. It should be adopted by all hospitals. This free and natural approach to visiting in hospital reduces one of the major disadvantages of hospital care when compared with home care and is a great relief to parents and children. Nurses on night duty must be trained in the correct way of handling the mother who arrives in the ward in the early hours of the morning because she is so worried about her child that she cannot sleep. A greeting indicating that he was asleep last time she looked but that they should go to his bed together will go far to allay her fears on future occasions.

It must be realized that unrestricted visiting places a considerable strain on the mother, who may feel she has to spend all day with her young child, since this is the situation when her child is at home. But at home a mother carries on with her housework, whereas in hospital it may be a matter of sitting all day beside her child's bed, a difficult situation to which to adjust. Mothers may also feel torn by the needs of their child in hospital and the opposing needs of their other children at home.

For nurses, unrestricted visiting brings a problem in that nursing procedures will be carried out in front of the parents. This may not be easy for young nurses in training but has the advantage that such nurses learn the care of the sick child within the family setting and not, as of old, in terms of an isolated child in a numbered cot. Doctors and nurses should not make the mistake of sending the mother out of the ward when they come to do some special procedure on the child. There are very few procedures which a mother cannot witness; if the mother is wisely handled her confidence in the staff will increase from knowing what is going on. At the same time the child is given greater security by having her mother with her on such occasions. If properly instructed a mother will be able to undertake much of the nursing required for her child. This will not only reduce the nurses' work but will also eliminate some of the risks of cross-infection which are such a hazard to young children in hospital (Pickerill & Pickerill, 1954).

Unrestricted visiting therefore has many advantages, particularly for the child between the ages of 1 and 4 years who is most likely to be disturbed by the deprivation caused by admission to hospital. But it also brings problems for the patient, parents and staff so that the subject requires a great deal of further study.

There are innumerable other ways by which the harmful impact of admission to hospital can be reduced for young children. As far as possible, children should not be admitted direct from the outpatient clinic unless for an emergency. It is preferable that the child should go home, returning for admission the next day, thereby giving his parents an opportunity to prepare him for his stay. It is an advantage to show the child the ward beforehand and to introduce both the child and his parents to the ward sister. A child managed in this way will not be frightened by attendance at the outpatient clinic after he is discharged from the ward, whereas one who has been admitted direct from the clinic will be likely to be frightened on each outpatient visit lest he is going to be kept in again.

Routine bathing of all children on admission to the ward should be eliminated. It is unnecessary and only adds to the fears of the child who, in any case, has probably already had an extra bath at home in preparation for coming to hospital. Children should be kept in bed only if there is a positive indication that this is required. It is very easy in hospital for a child to be put to bed or to be kept in bed because no one has considered whether or not he can be up. Children who are up should, as far as possible, be dressed in their own clothes so that they feel more at home. Many of them can be allowed to go for walks with their parents for part of the day, thereby also giving them an opportunity to meet their brothers and sisters who in some hospitals are not permitted to enter the ward for fear of increasing the risk of cross-infection. In actual practice, visiting by siblings has not been found to increase the amount of cross-infection, provided, of course, that children with coughs and colds are excluded, as well as those recently in contact with patients suffering from one of the infectious fevers. Sibling visiting is not only good for the patient but has the added advantage of preparing healthy children for what goes on in hospital, thereby removing fears.

PLAY SPECIALIST
For a long time hospitals have made use of voluntary helpers to amuse the

children and keep them occupied. The play specialist, however, is a trained ancillary worker whose role extends much further than simply amusing and occupying the children. Children in hospital are subjected to a large number of traumatic experiences in addition to separation from home. They are injected, X-rayed and operated on, but these and many other experiences can be made less frightening if a highly trained play specialist is part of the hospital team. Her work requires a deep understanding of children and a detailed knowledge of their development and psychology. She must also know a reasonable amount about children's illnesses and the practical aspect of investigations ordered.

The play specialist will study and play with the children individually and in groups, being assisted by the nursing and medical staff and by the parents. Her study of the children is undertaken by watching them at 'play' which for a child is a serious activity, the term having a much wider meaning than the narrower aspect of amusement with which it is often identified. In studying the children in this way the play specialist will be occupying and amusing them but, being trained, she will also be in a position to pass on essential information about each child's behaviour to the medical and nursing staff. She can reduce the degree of trauma by preparing the child for the new experiences to be encountered and should, whenever possible, accompany the child through them. Thus a play specialist can explain to a child what happens during the induction of anaesthesia, subsequently accompanying the child to the anaesthetic room and being present when he begins to come round from the anaesthetic. It must be emphasized that the play specialist does not displace the mother or the nurse but is complementary to both.

SCHOOL TEACHER

The hospital teacher has a therapeutic as well as an educative role. The child who has broken his leg but has exams ahead will be enormously relieved to find that he can continue his lessons in hospital. The hospital school teacher should contact the child's teacher at school in order to learn more about the child in general and to discuss what teaching should be continued in hospital. His parents should collect the relevant books from the school and bring them to the ward. School teachers should be encouraged to visit their pupils—many are unaware that most children's wards are delighted to see teachers as visitors.

Much of the ward teacher's time is spent not on formal lessons, but on working with the children on projects to enable them to learn more from all the new things they are experiencing in ward life.

GENERAL ASPECTS

Formal ward rounds are inappropriate to a children's ward where the majority of children, apart from babies, will be up and playing in playrooms. A child feels threatened by a group of adults clustered round his bed so it should only be necessary to have a child on his bed if he needs to be examined lying down. For the rest, the 'ward round' can take place in or near the playroom.

Staff must be particularly careful not to talk about a child's illness in his hearing. At the same time they must explain in simple language what is happening to him. There are some occasions when it is right to tell a child that he has a fatal illness. This depends on the questions he is asking and staff must be alert to their meaning and must provide the sympathetic atmosphere for parents to be able to talk out their feelings. Children are more frightened of the point of death than of no longer existing. Studies have shown that they believe death itself will be painful. Since a child has had honest answers from his parents to all previous questions, he has reason to expect an honest answer to the most crucial question of all—'am I dying?'. Parents may find it easier to leave the telling to the consultant or to a favourite nurse.

In talking to parents about lethal conditions such as leukaemia or cystic fibrosis it has to be realized that with many parents the death of their child begins when they are given the diagnosis. A medical social worker can provide immense support for such parents.

Frightening instruments should not be visible in a children's ward. A child is often unnecessarily frightened by seeing a tray of instruments for examination arrive beside his bed. It is better to carry these individually to his bedside. Supervised play with needles is safe and can go far to remove the fear of injections.

DAY CASES

Many children requiring cold surgery such as hernia repair or circumcision can be admitted for the day of operation only (Lawrie, 1964). Apart from the obvious advantage to the child and his parents there is the advantage to the hospital in the saving of beds. Much of the success of the method depends on careful selection of the mothers concerned who must be told beforehand that they will be expected to spend all day in the hospital with their child.

The natural fear of anaesthetists and surgeons that the mothers will not keep to their instructions to give no food or drink on the morning of the operation has not materialized. In fact it has been found that this risk is less with day cases than with those admitted to the ward in the ordinary way.

Admission as day cases can also be used for the investigation and management of certain medical problems (Smallpeice, 1958); for example, the infant who is failing to thrive or the baby with a feeding problem. The investigation of many of the handicapped children can also be undertaken as day cases (see p. 29).

The work of a children's unit should no longer be measured by its number of beds. By integrating its outpatient and inpatient departments a higher output of work can be achieved from a smaller number of beds.

LEAVING THE HOSPITAL

Before a child is discharged from the ward his parents must be told again exactly what has been wrong with him and what are his future needs. They must also be warned of possible behaviour problems resulting from being in hospital, such as a need to cling more to his mother or a temporary return to wetting or soiling. Some children become aggressive, others refuse to speak to their mothers. By understanding that these forms of behaviour indicate how much a child's feelings have been hurt and by sympathetic handling, a return to normal behaviour is hastened.

DEVELOPING COUNTRIES

The doctor trained in a western country who goes to work in a hospital in a developing country will find the change very difficult at first. He will be faced by vast numbers of patients attending the outpatient department, many of whom are acutely ill. The first step is to organize an emergency room where medical and nursing personnel can be concentrated so as to provide intensive care. Admission to the wards from the emergency room can take place in the early evening, thereby leaving the wards clear during the day to carry on with routine work unhampered by repeated interruptions to deal with new, acutely ill, children.

All mothers attending with children as outpatients should be given a numbered block of wood so that they know they will be seen in the order in which they have arrived. This prevents mothers from crowding round the entrance to the consulting room and encourages them to sit while they have to wait. It also makes it easier for the nurse to pick out those children who are acutely ill and requiring preferential treatment.

The new doctor may be surprised to find that apart from malaria, parasites are less often the cause of childhood illnesses than he had expected. He will spend more of his time treating disorders which, until recently, were common in the U.K.—malnutrition, anaemia and infection. Disorders which are largely preventable by a better understanding of health education—a subject which should occupy a large part of his time.

On many wards, parents will be permitted to visit for only a fixed 1–2 hour period during the day. It will be stated by those who support this regime that visitors in a hospital in a developing country will crowd the wards and prevent the staff from working. This is not my experience. Mothers in a developing country behave no differently from mothers in the U.K. if they are given free access to their children. It is only when they are kept from their children that they become aggressive and attack the staff. Permitting mothers free access to their children in hospital means that the children are happier and the mothers can share in their recovery. This is an opportunity for teaching mothers how to care for their children which should not be missed. I suspect that some of the abandoned children I have seen in hospitals in developing countries would not have been deserted by their mothers had they been allowed free access.

However, I do accept that in a developing country it is wise to permit unrestricted visiting to parents only, leaving the usual fixed daily period, which need not be more than one hour, for the numerous other relatives who will wish to visit.

Wherever he works, it is essential for the doctor to understand the cultural background of his patients in order to help them to the full. He must have a knowledge of the native medicines used locally and their dangers (see Accidents, p. 717).

He must strenuously avoid the common bad habit of doctors in developing countries of prescribing more than one drug at a time for no good reason. Polypharmacy is the disease of doctors working in developing countries and is just as unscientific as the practices performed by native healers.

He will find that the majority of his patients put more faith in a drug given by injection than by one given by mouth. But that is no reason for prescribing intramuscular therapy when oral therapy is as effective, particularly when the greater liability of provocation poliomyelitis (p. 411) is considered.

He will need to accept that some of his patients must leave hospital with a bottle of medicine when there is no pharmacological indication. Faith in medicine is such that lack of it may lead a mother straight to a native healer. Some Arab husbands require to see the bottle of medicine as evidence that their wife did attend the doctor.

However, if for these reasons a placebo is required it is better therapeutics to prescribe coloured water known in the pharmacy as 'Mist Placebo' rather than giving a vitamin or iron mixture which is more expensive and is not indicated pharmacologically. It will also be clear to subsequent doctors seeing that patient why the medicine was prescribed.

The ability of mothers to understand when the medicine is to be given must be carefully checked. Some mothers required to give a medicine three times a day will think their child will recover more quickly if a larger dose is given

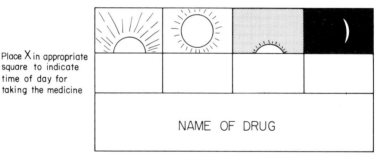

Place X in appropriate square to indicate time of day for taking the medicine

NAME OF DRUG

Fig. 7. A pictorial scheme to assist mothers in developing countries to understand when to give the dose of medicine.

more often than ordered. A simple diagram (Fig. 7) may help an illiterate mother to understand when to give the medicine.

*For more detailed advice on the care of sick children at home and in hospital, the reader is referred to chapters 28 and 29 of the author's 'Book of Child Care'.*

## BIBLIOGRAPHY

BROWSE N.L. (1965) *The Physiology and Pathology of Bed Rest.* Thomas, Springfield, Illinois.

HARDING V. & WALKER S. (1972) Let's make a game of it. *Nursing Mirror*, **135**, 14.

HARVEY S. & HALES-TOOKE A. (1972) *Play in Hospital.* Faber & Faber, London.

ILLINGWORTH R.S. (1963) Why put him to bed? *Clin. Pediat.*, **2**, 108.

JESSEL C. & JOLLY H. (1972) *Paul in Hospital.* Methuen, London.

JOLLY H. (1966) Put the child to bed. *Lancet*, **2**, 541.

JOLLY H. (1968) Play and the sick child. A comparative study of its role in a teaching hospital in London and one in Ghana. *Lancet*, **2**, 1286.

JOLLY H. (1969) Play is work. The role of play for sick and healthy children. *Lancet*, **2**, 487.

JOLLY H. (1975) *Book of Child Care.* George Allen & Unwin Ltd, London.

LAWRIE R. (1964) Operating on children as day cases. *Lancet*, **2**, 1289.

LINDHEIM R., GLASER H. H. & COFFIN C. (1972) Changing hospital environments for children. Harvard, Cambridge.

NOBLE E. (1967) *Play and the Sick Child.* Faber & Faber, London.

PICKERILL C.M. & PICKERILL H.P. (1954) Elimination of hospital cross-infection in children. Nursing by the mother. *Lancet*, **1**, 425.

SMALLPEICE V. (1958) Children as day patients. *Lancet*, **2**, 1364.

# CHAPTER 3

# THE CHILD WITH A HANDICAP

A handicapped child can be defined as one suffering from any continuing disability of body, intellect or personality which is likely to interfere with his normal growth, development or capacity to learn. About 5 per cent of children in the U.K. are handicapped. The disorders causing these handicaps are discussed in their appropriate sections. However, although their problems differ widely, handicapped children and their parents share certain aspects in common; for this reason it is relevant to consider the problem as a whole as well as in separate sections.

The majority of handicaps fall into the categories of physical, mental or emotional. Physical handicaps may be motor or sensory. The greater proportion of those with a motor handicap have either cerebral palsy (p. 425) or spinal palsy (p. 212), the latter being associated with spina bifida. Other motor defects result from congenital dislocation of the hip (p. 231), congenital or acquired limb deformities including those resulting from the administration of thalidomide during pregnancy (p. 144) and rare conditions such as arthrogryposis multiplex (p. 230). The principal sensory defects are visual or auditory. Mental handicap comprises those who are mentally retarded (p. 444). It also includes autism (p. 453) although such children may not be mentally retarded. Children with an emotional handicap may be physically and mentally normal, but very often children with either of these handicaps develop secondary emotional problems. The prevention of emotional problems is one of the major aims of therapy for children who are physically or mentally handicapped. This demands that the child's problems are studied as a whole instead of concentrating only on his handicap. He is a child with a handicap, not a handicapped child.

However, any chronic disorder may result in a handicap, for example, the child with epilepsy may be handicapped, though modern treatment should prevent this. Similarly, the child with severe heart disease, either congenital or acquired, may be handicapped. Chronic lung disease such as occurs in cystic fibrosis (mucoviscidosis) or severe bronchial asthma may also have this effect.

The early diagnosis and correct management of the handicapped child require the closest co-operation between the general practitioner, the paediatrician and the doctor working in the Public Health Service. One doctor must co-ordinate the available resources to ensure the child receives the best possible care. Such a doctor must be very experienced in the problems of the handicapped child, being on the alert for associated defects. Although many of the handicaps affect single organs or systems, the possibility of multiple handicaps must be considered. Otherwise, for example, a child might be receiving treatment for his cataracts but the associated deafness remain undetected. Probably about 30 per cent of handicapped children have more than one handicap.

In the past there have been unnecessary delays in diagnosis. Mothers of children whom they suspect to be deaf have been told the child is too young to test and asked to come back in six months or a year. Other mothers with babies who have developed a squint have been told that no treatment is available, thereby the baby being allowed to develop 'amblyopia of disuse' (p. 224). It is to prevent such calamities that the 'at risk' register (p. 91) has been developed (Sheridan, 1962) in order to increase the opportunities for early diagnosis. Early diagnosis may, in some disorders, prevent the development of a primary handicap as in the prevention of blindness by the treatment of a squint or the prevention of mental retardation by the early dietary treatment of phenylketonuria (p. 568) or galactosaemia (p. 572). Prevention of a secondary handicap is illustrated by the deaf child who if diagnosed early is prevented from deaf mutism. In other instances, as with congenital dislocation of the hip (p. 231), early diagnosis followed by correct treatment can result in cure. In the case of cerebral palsy early and correct management can do much to prevent deformity.

**Recognition of handicap**

Ideally, all children should be checked routinely for their developmental progress during their early years by a doctor who has been specially trained in the subject, i.e. developmental paediatrics. If everybody attended such a well-baby clinic there would be no need for a special clinic for those 'at risk' which in any case cannot hope to include all those babies who later turn out to be handicapped.

The doctor running such a clinic must know the breadth of variation in normal development and he must have a high index of suspicion. He has to be on the alert for any baby showing a lack of normal curiosity, or a delay in normal head control or normal vocalization. Any delay in the development of smiling is likely to be serious.

**Diagnosis**

Although the cause of the handicap can often not be pin-pointed, every handicapped child must be intensively investigated and every system checked.

In particular, full biochemical screening is essential in order not to miss a potentially treatable condition.

### Assessment

By this means the child is studied by a multidisciplinary team of experts working together. A paediatrician is usually the director of the team which comprises doctors from other disciplines such as orthopaedics, neurology, psychiatry, ophthalmology and audiology. In addition to the medical members there are physiotherapists, speech therapists, occupational therapists, psychologists and social workers.

At Charing Cross Hospital the children are studied on a daily basis for 3 weeks in association with normal children attending the hospital staff day nursery. The whole unit is termed the Child Development Centre, and it caters not only for the assessment of handicapped children, but also for their treatment. Some units are termed 'assessment centres', but this is only one part of their function. Moreover, the name is threatening to parents who are liable to regard 'assessment' as a form of exam which their child must 'pass'. The advantage of our type of unit is that the children can be observed playing in a group as well as being tested on an individual basis. By extending the period of observation to 3 weeks a much greater knowledge of the child's potential can be achieved compared with seeing him for only one or two days. Babies are studied on an individual basis since these are too young to be part of a nursery group.

### Treatment

At the end of the 3 week period a plan of treatment is worked out in association with the parents. This will involve the community services so that members of the community health team take part in the assessment of each child.

### Telling the Parents

The way in which the doctor breaks the news to parents that their child has a handicap is likely to influence their whole approach to their child. It will vary according to whether the handicap is visible at birth, such as spina bifida or a limb deformity or, as in the case of cerebral palsy, when it becomes obvious only later. It is essential to talk with both parents together though, if the abnormality is obvious at birth, it may be preferable to tell the father first and ask him whether he would like to be the one who actually breaks the news to his wife. On no account should the husband be asked not to tell his wife since this places an unnatural and intolerable burden on him at a time when mutual support of husband and wife is needed. Whether the doctor breaks the news to both parents together or leaves it to the husband to tell his wife, the doctor must then sit with the parents, explaining the situation and answering their questions.

With an abnormality which is obvious at birth the doctor should first expose the normal portion of the baby to the parents, slowly explaining the abnormality to them before it is exposed. When a child is born deformed it is almost always a mistake to suggest that the mother should not see the child. Her imagination of the deformity is likely to be worse than the real thing and if the child dies without her seeing him she may be left with feelings of guilt. Doctors sometimes advise that a child born deformed should be placed straight in a home but it is seldom that such a place is available at once. Moreover, if the parents never look after their child they are almost certain to have guilt feelings that they did not do all they might have done in caring for their child. It is preferable therefore that they should look after the child for a time. If after a trial they find the situation impossible, then every available step should be taken to get the child into a special home.

With a handicap such as cerebral palsy which does not become apparent until later, the reaction of the parents will be very different. They will already have accepted him and grown to love him, therefore they will be on his side in trying to do everything that is possible to help. The situation with some handicapped children, particularly mongols, is that the doctor is aware of the disorder before the parents. On p. 220 reasons are given for my belief that the parents of mongols should be told the facts at an early stage.

In talking to parents it is essential to be honest and to answer truthfully every question they pose. On the first visit they are unlikely to remember more than the fact that their child is handicapped because of the shock this gives. Doctors working with handicapped children must be extremely patient with their parents who will need to be seen frequently and for long discussions in the early years. Talking to parents is a matter of sharing all the information about their child.

Early diagnosis is essential so that the parents of a handicapped child can be told how best to help him, instead of being frustrated by not understanding why their child is not making normal progress. For example, a child with a motor handicap lacks the opportunity for normal visual exploration because lack of head control causes his head to bob up and down. By fixing his head, the parents can help him to look around.

Most parents of handicapped children, provided they are wisely handled and advised, adjust amazingly well to the particular needs of their child. A few will reject the child and others will over-protect. Some parents develop guilt feelings; in many cases marital problems result, particularly if there are differences of opinion over management. Fear of a similarly affected child in the next pregnancy causes much distress so that genetic counselling should always be offered.

The concept that a handicapped child causes the family from which he comes to be handicapped, broadens the understanding of the family's problems. It also helps to ensure that all the available social services are called in at an early stage in order that every aspect of the problem is studied and the best possible advice and help given. The family may qualify for financial support because extra expenses are involved in travel or because nappies are required for longer than with a normal child. Money can be supplied for alterations to a house so that a door is widened to allow space for a wheel-chair to pass or for the provision of a ramp instead of steps. Parents of a handicapped child who requires more than the normal amount of time spent in care may qualify for the Attendance Allowance.

The therapist needed for the individual child will be determined by his handicap. But in all cases the role of the therapist is to teach the mother (and father) how to treat her child. Treatment is not something which is carried out for set periods during the day, but involves her in understanding how to handle her child in every situation.

It helps if parents can meet other children and parents similarly involved. With many handicaps the parents of children with the same disability have organized themselves into groups to their mutual advantage. These parent groups have done much to stimulate interest both in their own problem and in that of their children. The group increases the moral support given to the parents though they should avoid attempting social work on each other or the giving of medical advice. Such groups have done much to stimulate research into the medical aspects of the disability though it is preferable that a separate body should handle any money raised for this object.

The handicapped child requires normal home surroundings in which to grow up, just as does the normal child. To be 'put away' in a long-stay hospital is a disaster for him and for his family. To achieve this the family must receive optimum support from the community services. The parents will have the difficult task of ensuring a correct balance within the family for its handicapped member and for its normal members.

The reactions of the child to the discovery that he is handicapped vary enormously and must be studied. He is likely to feel isolated from normal children of his own age, thereby becoming self-centred and easily taking offence; such tensions are liable to result in aggressive outbursts. To offset this, the handicapped child should be encouraged to move about by whatever means of locomotion available; parents must never make any movement for him, of which he is capable himself. To him, function is much more important than a good cosmetic appearance. This point is illustrated by some of the thalidomide children whose parents wanted them to have a nice looking artificial arm and hand whereas the child wanted a hook.

Objects for play for handicapped children should comprise common household items rather than old fashioned woolly toys. By this means the child's experience of everyday objects is widened.

## Schooling

Handicapped children can receive their education in ordinary schools or in 'special schools'. Special schools comprise those for the blind, the partially sighted, the deaf, those with partial hearing, the educationally sub-normal, the epileptic, the maladjusted, the physically handicapped, the 'delicate' and those with speech defects. The advantage of an ordinary school is that it provides a full range of educational opportunity whereas the special school limits the handicapped child's contacts with his normal contemporaries. Epileptic children used to be sent to special schools but today, due to a wider understanding of their problems and more sympathetic teachers, they are usually accommodated in normal schools.

The advantage of a special school is that it can provide more specialized management. Some special schools cater for one type of handicap only, for example cerebral palsy or mental retardation. Others take children with any type of motor handicap. The advantage to the child with cerebral palsy in going to a school dealing only with this disability is still greater specialism amongst those treating him. On the other hand, it is a help for him to mix closely with children with other disabilities including those acquired after birth, such as poliomyelitis. The advantage derived from mixing with children whose handicap differs and the frequency of more than one handicap in a child weigh in favour of special schools for multiple handicaps.

Probably the ideal schooling arrangement is the provision of one or more classes for handicapped children attached to an ordinary school. By this means the child can receive special training and other techniques, such as physiotherapy, but also mix with normal children.

Those in charge of the handicapped child should not be prejudiced either for or against a special school so that each child is managed according to his own particular problem. The decision will be influenced by the nature of the handicap, the personality of the child and his aptitude and ability. His social circumstances must also be considered together with his parents' philosophy and their approach to his handicap. The decision will also be affected by the particular normal schools and the particular special schools which are available.

The responsibility for correctly placing the child lies with the Local Authority. The Education Act of 1944 states that it is the duty of every Local

Education Authority to ascertain which children in their area require special educational treatment. To this end, the Local Authority is given the right to require the parent of any child who has reached the age of two years to submit him for medical examination to determine the presence and extent of any disability.

Having decided where to place the child in school this should not be regarded as final since each child should remain under continuous assessment, changes being made as and when they become necessary. The role of the special school should be to bring the child to the point at which the effect of his handicap, both from the physical and emotional aspects, is so reduced that he is capable of attending a normal school.

The education of the handicapped child, whether in a normal or a special school, must take care not only of his general education but also of his education within society. He must also be given vocational education so that he is trained for suitable employment according to his type of handicap. The choice of employment must also take into account the availability of occupation near his home since the handicapped child entering employment is usually better off if he is able to continue living at home. Hostel accommodation or lodgings puts an additional strain on the handicapped.

Education is possibly even more vital for the handicapped child than for one who is normal. For this reason, parents should be told that they should get him to school each day in order to be with his friends, however difficult this may be for them.

## BIBLIOGRAPHY

KERSHAW J. (1973) *Handicapped Children.* 3rd Ed. Heinemann Medical, London.
SHERIDAN M.D. (1962) Infants at risk of handicapping conditions. *Mth. Bull. Minist. Hlth. Lab. Serv.*, **21,** 238.

CHAPTER 4

# THE NEWBORN INFANT

As a consequence of improved results in the management of disease in older children, the emphasis in paediatrics has now swung towards the prevention and management of disease in infancy, particularly the newborn infant whose problems are now the subject of intensive research. Factors accounting for death in infancy are now being subjected to careful statistical analysis, for whose proper understanding certain definitions must be stated.

*Stillbirth.* A child born after the 28th week of pregnancy which, after being expelled from the mother, did not breathe or show other signs of life such as heart beat, umbilical pulsation or movement of muscles.

*Birth rate.* The number of births (both live and still) per 1000 of the population.

*Live birth rate.* The number of live births per 1000 of the population.

*Stillbirth rate.* The number of stillbirths per 1000 births (both live and still).

*Perinatal mortality rate.* The number of stillbirths and deaths during the first week of life per 1000 births (live and still).

*Neonatal period.* The first four weeks of life.

*Neonatal mortality rate.* The number of live-born infants who die under the age of 28 days per 1000 live births in the same year. Neonatal deaths are also divided into those occurring during the first week (early neonatal deaths) and those from 8–27 days of age (late neonatal deaths).

*Infant mortality rate.* The number of deaths during the first year of life per 1000 live births in the same year.

*Low birth weight.* A baby whose birth weight is 2·5 kg (5½ lb) or under. There are two varieties of low birth weight: preterm and small for dates. These are discussed on p. 47.

The figures for England and Wales in 1973 were as follows:

Live birth rate—13·7
Stillbirth rate—11·6
Infant mortality rate—16·9
Neonatal mortality rate—11·1

The extent of the fall in neonatal mortality during the past 60 years has

34

been disappointing in relation to the remarkable fall in infant mortality
during the same period.

TABLE 1. A comparison to show recent trends in
infant and neonatal mortality.

|          | Infant Mortality | Neonatal Mortality |
|----------|------------------|--------------------|
| 1906–10  | 117·1            | 40·2               |
| 1973     | 16·9             | 11·1               |

For the baby, the first day is the most dangerous, more deaths occurring on
that day than during the whole period from the age of 12 months to 25 years.
It is because the causes of stillbirths are closely associated with the causes of
death during the first week of life that the perinatal mortality is being investigated in great detail. In 1958 in Great Britain an intensive study of perinatal
mortality was carried out (Butler & Bonham, 1963; Butler & Alberman, 1969).
From these and subsequent studies have come a greater emphasis on the role
of obstetrics in the first week of life, together with a realization of the greatly
increased mortality for babies born prematurely or postmaturely. The mortality rate is also being reduced by intensive research on the prevention and
treatment of congenital malformations (see p. 137).

The much more rapid fall in mortality rates for infants from 1–12 months of
age results largely from improved methods of feeding together with better
prevention and treatment of infection. Neonatal mortality on the other hand
is concerned with the more complex problems of immaturity, postmaturity
and physiological failures together with birth injury, asphyxia, atelectasis and
congenital malformations.

## FACTORS INFLUENCING INFANT MORTALITY

### Social factors

Social factors are clearly involved in the improvement in infant mortality but
their influence on perinatal mortality has only recently come strongly to light.
As defined by the Office of Population Censuses and Surveys (1970) there are
five social classes, separation being based on the father's occupation (Table
2).

As one goes down the social scale there is a progressive increase in the
infantile, neonatal and perinatal mortality but, although these figures have

come down over the years, the social class difference persists despite a national tendency to level up the social classes. The infants born to the two lowest social classes are about twice as likely to die before their first birthday as those in the two highest social classes. This difference is partly nutritional but there is also evidence that mothers in the lower social classes take less advantage of the improved standard of medicine despite its greater availability. These mothers are likely to have less antenatal care because they are still working or because they have more children to look after or because, being less well educated, they do not realize its importance. Some of these factors also account for the higher mortality figures for illegitimate babies whose mothers are likely to hide the fact that they are pregnant as long as possible.

TABLE 2

| Social Class | Occupation | Example |
|---|---|---|
| I | Professional | Doctor, company director |
| II | Intermediate (Supervisory) | Farmer, teacher, shopkeeper |
| III | Skilled workers | Fitter, most clerks |
| IV | Semi-skilled workers | Machine minder, most agricultural workers |
| V | Unskilled workers | Porter, labourer |

To combat these effects, means must be found of bringing such mothers for antenatal care at an earlier stage, in fact as soon as they suspect they are pregnant. Experience has emphasized the difficulties in achieving this so that it will be necessary to set up some form of intelligence network to find the mothers and bring them for antenatal care. One technique used has been for a nurse to stay in a launderette, talking informally to the women arriving with their washing (Bain, 1965).

Poor social background is often associated with other adverse factors. Thus the mother from social class V is likely to have more babies than the mother from social class I and, therefore, to continue having pregnancies later into the child-bearing period. Being poor, her standard of nutrition will be lower so that she will be shorter than the average, yet she is likely to smoke more than her richer counterpart from social class I.

Somewhat surprisingly, social class also has an influence on the incidence of congenital malformations; major abnormalities of the central nervous system are more common in the lower social classes (see p. 144).

Other factors influencing perinatal mortality are as follows:

## Maternal age

Below the age of 20 the perinatal mortality is above the national average, especially for the very young multiparae. Between the ages of 20–30 it runs at a low level but after the age of 30 there is a steep and progressive rise.

## Parity

The risk is greatest for the first baby, lowest for the second and thereafter rises sharply with increasing parity. If it were possible to choose the optimum circumstances for both, the baby should be born the second child of a healthy married 23-year-old girl with no adverse family history of illness.

## Maternal height

Increasing height is a good indication of improved physique. Height potential is genetically determined but an individual may not attain her full stature if the environment during childhood and adolescence was unfavourable. Growth may be hindered by poor and overcrowded living conditions, by illness or by insufficient or poor quality food. Perinatal mortality increases with falling stature though this is correlated to some extent with social class, since the lower classes are shorter; however, the factor of height shows its influence within each social group. It appears therefore that poor environment in the growing years can so effect growth and development as to cause impairment in the efficiency of reproduction.

## Smoking

Butler & Alberman (1969) have shown that smoking after the fourth month of pregnancy significantly increased the risk of stillbirth and neonatal death. This increase is regardless of the age, parity, social class and height of the mother, or the presence or absence of severe pre-eclampsia.

## Geographical area

Perinatal death rates vary in different parts of the country. Mortality is lowest in the London and South-Eastern, Southern and Eastern regions. It increases in the Midlands reaching its highest in the North-Western regions of England and in Scotland and Wales. Although social factors are involved in these regional differences, the South of England, for example, being more prosperous than the North, the influence of the region itself has been shown to be effective. Thus, the perinatal mortality rates for professional groups in the North is more similar to that of skilled manual workers in the South; skilled workers in the North rank for mortality levels with semi-skilled workers in the South.

Maternal physique is also a factor in regional mortality differences since, for all social classes, women in the South are taller than those in the North.

### Influence of the number of mother's sibs

The Perinatal Mortality Survey indicates that the more brothers and sisters a woman grows up with the more likely she is to have a stillbirth, this holding good within each social class. This probably results from a greater scarcity of resources in a large family affecting the growth of the young girl.

### Sex of infant

Male infants have a smaller chance of survival than female infants, the male stillbirth rate and neonatal death rate being higher than the female. The ratio of male to female stillbirths increases with the age of the mother.

### Interval between births

There are indications that the interval between births may influence both the stillbirth and neonatal death rates. Very close and very distant spacing may be disadvantageous.

### Paternal age

The influence of paternal age is similar to that of maternal age and is independent of it. Thus the stillbirth and neonatal mortality rates are higher for the children of younger and older fathers when compared with fathers aged 25–34. These findings are independent of the relationship of the rates to the mother's age.

In summary, the major factors influencing perinatal mortality are poor socio-economic conditions, including illegitimacy. Maternal age, parity, height of mother, smoking in pregnancy, and the geographical area also influence the outcome. These are closely inter-related but also act independently. In general, age adjustment increases the difference between the social class figures whereas adjustment for parity decreases it. Improved socio-economic standards would be the best way to reduce the mortality rates; it is interesting that women who change their social class at marriage tend to have the characteristics of women in the class they have entered rather than those of the class from which they have come. Unfortunately, there is a considerable time lag before social improvements result in better health; many of the reasons for persisting social differences in mortality are poorly understood. The present gap between the mortality rates of the highest and the lowest social classes represents about 30 years of change. In other words social class V has only just reached the economic and social standards attained 30 years ago by class I.

Emphasis must also be placed on the effects of good antenatal care and the better results to be obtained when delivery is carried out in hospital.

## Physiological adjustments at birth

Modern experimental techniques have disproved the old ideas that the fetus, as term approaches, lives under conditions of oxygen deprivation, having only limited control over its oxygen supply. Although the oxygen environment of the fetus is less than that of the mother the difference between them is less than was supposed. Despite a relatively low arterial oxygen tension, adequate oxygenation of fetal tissues is maintained by an umbilical vein saturation of 80–85 per cent together with high cardiac output which ensures a large blood flow to the placenta and to fetal tissues. What is required is that enough fetal blood is exposed to enough maternal blood over a large enough area and for a sufficiently long period. Under these conditions the fetus has more than enough oxygen for its special conditions of life.

It has also been customary to think of renal function in the newborn as being very inadequate since it has been compared with the adult kidney. But tests of renal function suitable for adults cannot be applied to the newborn whose homoeostatic mechanisms are quite different. Homoeostasis in the newborn is maintained as much by its capacity for growth as by its kidneys, lungs and other integrated organs. The kidney of the newborn is well adapted to the needs of the infant (McCance & Widdowson, 1957).

In the fetus the two sides of the heart work in parallel, pumping blood from the great veins to the aorta and to the pulmonary trunk simultaneously. The right ventricle is almost as thick as the left. This route is possible because of the presence of the foramen ovale and the ductus arteriosus. The pressure in the pulmonary artery is higher than in the aorta so that much of the blood from the right heart flows through the ductus arteriosus.

During labour the fetus becomes increasingly acidotic since there is a reduction in the oxygen and $CO_2$ transport across the placenta. In healthy infants this acidosis is rapidly corrected after birth by the establishment of pulmonary function. The first breath results from asphyxia due to the tying of the umbilical cord. This acts on the brain through chemoreceptor reflexes from the aortic and carotid bodies. Cutaneous stimulation is an additional factor in the initiation of the first breath.

The changes which take place in the circulation at birth are dependent on two factors: the arrest of the umbilical circulation through the placenta and the increase in pulmonary blood following expansion of the lungs. Although these changes are abrupt in onset they are not completed at once; various adjustments continue to take place over a period of days or weeks. During this time there is a transitional circulation, intermediate between the fetal and the adult type.

Tying the umbilical cord causes the systemic resistance to rise while the first breath causes a lowering of pulmonary vascular resistance. The circulation then changes from the fetal route of right to left to the neonatal route of left to right, but during this transitional period before the foramen ovale and the ductus artereriosus are permanently closed, the circulation through both orifices may be right to left at times.

The ductus arteriosus constricts as a reaction of its smooth muscle to the raised arterial oxygen tension. Closure takes place in two stages: rapid constriction after birth, followed by anatomical obliteration over a period of weeks. If the pulmonary artery pressure rises before closure is complete the blood flow through the ductus is reversed. This occurs during periods of asphyxia, as in the respiratory distress syndrome (p. 64).

The foramen ovale closes because of the immediate fall in pressure in the inferior vena cava resulting from interruption of umbilical flow when the cord is tied, together with a rise in left atrial pressure from the increased pulmonary blood flow (Dawes, 1958).

### Management of newborn infant

As soon as the baby is born, the mouth should be sucked out. It is unnecessarily traumatic for the baby to be held upside down by the legs (Leboyer, 1975). The eyes should be cleaned with moist swabs, but prophylactic antibiotic eye-drops are no longer routinely given (p. 111).

The optimum time for cutting the cord and whether this should be 'early' or 'late' is still debated. In normal healthy full-term infants no harmful effects result either from early or late cord clamping. It has been suggested that delayed ligation may reduce the incidence of the respiratory distress syndrome (p. 64) but contradictory results have been obtained in this field. Delayed ligation increases the chance of hyperbilirubinaemia in preterm infants by permitting a greater red cell volume. A reasonable compromise is to clamp the cord about 30 seconds after delivery.

Ligation of the cord is most satisfactorily achieved by an elastic band since, unlike the standard umbilical tape, it maintains a constant pressure on the shrinking cord. This pressure reduces the risk of bleeding from the cord, particularly from a thick cord in which shrinkage is greatest. A special technique is used for the application of the elastic band (Neligan *et al.*, 1964). A short length of rubber or latex tubing can be used instead of the elastic band. This is slid over the end of the cord and pushed up for a short distance, thereby maintaining constant compression. The shorter the cord is cut, the greater its liability to bleed. To reduce the risk of umbilical infection,

Polybactrin spray (containing polymyxin, bacitracin and neomycin) can be applied daily to the cord until it separates.

The decision as to whether to leave the cord exposed or dressed depends on circumstances. In countries where the mother is likely to interfere with the cord, a dressing and binder must be used until the umbilical stump has healed, but otherwise binders should be avoided as they may interfere with abdominal respiration. Separation of the cord usually occurs by the end of the first week.

Routine bathing is unnecessary and possibly harmful, since the vernix forms a protective layer against skin infection. In the past, the bath immediately after delivery often caused chilling. The face and head should be cleaned; the hands should be washed as these may be covered with meconium which if then transferred to the eyes, causes chemical irritation. Large collections of vernix which sometimes accumulate in the axillae and groins are best removed, since in those sites they may cause local irritation. In hospital the baby need only be bathed once, shortly before discharge, unless more frequent bathing is required for instruction of the mother.

A fall in temperature is usual immediately after delivery so that steps should be taken to prevent chilling; at the same time the infant must not be over-clothed. Cotton is preferable to wool or nylon which may irritate the skin. Woollen mittens are particularly dangerous since a loose thread of wool may encircle a finger and even lead to gangrene. A window should always be open in the nursery and the baby may be taken outdoors when a week old in temperate climates and immediately after birth in tropical countries. No pillow is used since it is unnecessary and could be a factor in 'cot death' (p. 367). The baby should be nursed on his side to prevent inhalation of any vomit.

The application of 0·33 per cent hexachlorophane powder once daily for the first 10 days reduces the incidence of staphylococcal infections. There is no danger of toxicity when used in this strength.

EXAMINATION OF THE NEWBORN INFANT

A clinical examination should be carried out on all babies shortly after delivery. The immediate need is to exclude any obvious congenital malforma-tion, checking particularly that all orifices are patent. An imperforate anus is easily overlooked so that taking the rectal temperature as a routine is an additional safeguard.

It may be convenient to delay the full clinical examination until the morning after delivery but it should always be performed within the first 24 hours of life. The baby is placed on a flat surface (not in the cot), in a good light and at a convenient height for the comfort of the doctor. The best position for the examiner is to be seated. The mother should be present, since this gives her an opportunity to ask questions and to be assured that her baby is normal. Examining the baby on the mother's bed will give her this opportunity. If the mother cannot be present she should always be told the result of the examination. Many mothers are unaware that their newborn babies have been routinely checked.

The examination of the newborn infant follows the same principles described on p. 7. However, since exposure of the baby will always make a normal baby cry, the examination can be carried out methodically from head to toe. A great deal of time should be given to inspection. A normal baby is pink to red, preterm babies being more red than those born at term. A pale baby is an ill one.

Neurological examination of the newborn infant requires practice and skill (Prechtl & Beintema, 1964) but is an essential part of the investigation. It is necessary for the assessment of maturity and may also disclose transitory signs of underlying pathology. Such signs may be present for the first few days only, this being followed by a 'silent period' of apparent normality. The significance of abnormal neurological function appearing months or even years later will be appreciated only if it can be viewed in relation to the findings at birth.

Once the baby is exposed, the limbs move freely and asymmetrically owing to the righting reflexes. Reduced movement of a limb from paralysis is therefore obvious. For the first few days the baby tends to revert to the intrauterine position, normally one of flexion. An infant born by the breech with extended legs is obvious, since on removal of the covers the legs immediately rise. The reflexes described on p. 271 are elicited to ensure equality of movement on the two sides and to determine the state of maturity. They also comprise part of the examination for tone which in a normal baby is firm.

Three measurements should be made: the weight, length and head circumference. A flexible metal measuring tape is more satisfactory than a cloth tape since it does not stretch and can be sterilized. The full-term European baby weighs about 3·2 kg (7 lb) at birth, girls usually being a little lighter than boys. The weight falls during the first week but the birth weight should be regained by the tenth day. The fall in weight is about 5–10 per cent of the birth weight and is therefore greatest with the larger babies who should be given extra fluid to compensate. A full-term baby is 48–51 cm (19–20 inches) long with a head circumference of 33–35·5 cm (13–14 inches).

To examine the eyes an indirect method should be adopted in order to get them open since pulling down the lower lid, as in an older patient, encourages reflex closure and is likely to result in eversion of the lid (a difficult manoeuvre in adults but a very easy one in babies). If the baby is held upside down for a moment, he is almost certain to open his eyes when returned to the normal vertical position, provided the eyes are then away from the direct source of light. Alternatively, sucking on the nipple or a teat may encourage spontaneous opening of the eyelids.

A systolic murmur is commonly heard in normal newborn babies, due to the physiological adjustments taking place in the circulation immediately after birth. It also occurs in some pathological states such as asphyxia and the respiratory distress syndrome. Less often the murmur is due to congenital heart disease (see p. 179).

A single umbilical artery is associated with an increased incidence of congenital malformations. For this reason, the number of umbilical arteries should be recorded when the cord is cut. A single palmar crease also increases the likelihood of an associated congenital anomaly. Special attention is paid to the examination of the hips in all babies so as to exclude congenital dislocation (p. 231).

APGAR RATING

In addition to the routine examination, an assessment of the clinical state by a standard technique such as the Apgar (1962) scoring system is valuable. The assessment is made at the age of one minute, this being the average time for maximal depression, and is based on five objective signs (Table 3). A baby in perfect health scores ten marks while those who are less fit score progressively less.

This method ensures early evaluation of the clinical state, thereby preventing any unnecessary delay in resuscitation. It is of prognostic value in estimating the probable outcome in groups of babies since the lower the score the greater the liability of death or permanent cerebral damage. It will not predict the outcome for the individual baby.

Urine is normally passed shortly after birth but occasionally is not seen for the first 48 hours. In the majority of such cases it has been passed but the napkin has dried by the time it is changed. Complete obstruction to the flow of urine is almost unknown, but a normal stream of urine should always be witnessed in the first 2 weeks of life, before the newborn baby leaves the close care of the doctor or midwife. By this means partial urinary obstruction, such as occurs with an urethral valve (p. 200), can be excluded.

The first stool is normally passed during the first 24 hours and consists of meconium which is a sticky substance, dark green or black in colour. It is composed of the residue of mucous secretions from the bowel after digestion by proteolytic enzymes; its colour is due to biliverdin. After 3–4 days meconium is replaced by 'changing' stools which are yellow or brown from the residue of ingested milk. The passing of the first 'changing' stool is an important

TABLE 3. Apgar method of scoring for newborn infant at age of 1 minute.

| Sign | 0 | 1 | 2 | Score |
|---|---|---|---|---|
| Heart rate | Absent | Slow (<100) | >100 | |
| Respiratory effort | Absent | Weak cry Hypoventilation | Good Strong cry | |
| Muscle tone | Limp | Some flexion of extremities | Well flexed | |
| Reflex irritability (response of skin stimulation to feet) | No response | Some motion | Cry | |
| Colour | Blue/pale | Body pink Extremities blue | Completely pink | |

Apgar rating = Total =
(Score of 10 indicates infant in best possible condition)

milestone since it indicates patency of the whole intestinal tract; it must be recorded. The stools of a breast-fed baby are soft and golden-yellow in colour; they may be passed with every feed or at intervals of 1 or more days. A long interval of several days is equally normal, being due to the small residue from breast milk; the stool when passed is still soft. The stools of a baby fed on cow's milk are paler yellow, firmer and more offensive than the breast-fed stool. They should be passed at least once a day.

The fetal head may undergo considerable moulding during birth, oedema of the presenting part producing the *caput succedaneum*. This moulding is possible since the cranial bones have not yet united. The anterior fontanelle does not usually close until about the age of 12 months but may do so considerably earlier and yet be normal. The size of the fontanelle at birth varies from being only just palpable, to a breadth of 7·6–10 cm (3–4 inches). Mothers should be instructed to wash the infant's head regularly, as failure to do so increases the liability to seborrhoea of the scalp (p. 671). They should be told not to be frightened of damaging the anterior fontanelle, a fear which is widespread among inexperienced mothers.

*Craniotabes* is a condition in which areas of the vertex of the skull are unusually soft; these can sometimes be indented like a ping-pong ball. The condition may be found in newborn infants, particularly preterm babies who are otherwise normal, and results from delayed calcification. The skull

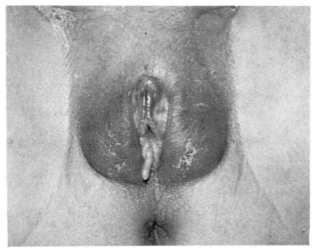

FIG. 8. Hymenal tag at birth due to maternal oestrogens causing epithelial overgrowth.

becomes normal as further calcification occurs. Craniotabes also occurs in rickets (p. 557).

Mothers should be told not to push back the foreskin as the prepuce and glans are united until the age of 9 months to 3 years (see p. 203). The external genitalia in the female are large at birth and the tissues may be so swollen that a tag from the hymen protrudes between the labia (Fig. 8). These changes result from the excess of maternal oestrogens. The genitalia remain large for the first month of life, although a protruding tag usually disappears before then. There is also an excess of vaginal mucus which may become blood-stained from endometrial bleeding about the fourth day of life. This bleeding probably results from the withdrawal of maternal oestrogens.

Engorgement of the breasts (neonatal mastitis) is common in full-term babies from the fourth to tenth days, occurring equally in either sex (Fig. 9). It is hormonal in origin and therefore the term mastitis, although used for the condition, is a misnomer. The exact hormonal cause is not clear; it is probably due to the interaction and withdrawal of oestrogens, progestogens and pituitary prolactin, derived partly from the mother and partly from the infant. Dis-appearance of engorgement is probably due to absence of mechanical stimu-lation; a number of cases have occurred where mothers have thought they should express the milk and in such cases secretion has continued for weeks, only ceasing when expression was stopped. Mothers should be told to leave the breasts strictly alone; infection of the breasts is usually the result of interference.

It is unusual for breast engorgement and endometrial bleeding to occur in the same infant, though the reason for this is not apparent. Breast engorgement does not occur in preterm babies, probably because their breast tissue is too immature to respond to the stimulus.

### Harlequin colour change

A transient colour change is often seen in babies, one half of the body becoming pale, the other half remaining the normal pink colour; a clear-cut

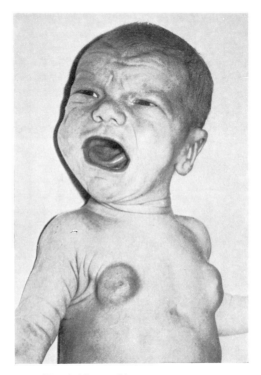

FIG. 9. Neonatal breast engorgement.

line of demarcation runs exactly down the middle of the body. This change, which occurs in attacks lasting 1–2 minutes, has been mainly seen in preterm babies but this is probably due to the fact that they are more often naked in incubators. The babies are otherwise normal and seem to be undisturbed by the attack. The side which is uppermost is always the paler so that the colour changes can be reversed by turning the body during an attack. It has no pathological significance and is probably due to a temporary imbalance of central vascular control. It is suggested that there are centres in the hypothalamus where the tone of the skin blood vessels in each half of the body is separately controlled.

## THE LOW BIRTH WEIGHT INFANT

### Definition

At one time all babies weighing 2500 g (5½ lb) or under were defined as 'premature'. This was unsatisfactory since there are two major causes of low birth weight: short gestation (i.e. preterm) and growth retardation. Infants are now defined as being of *low birth weight* (LBW) when the birth weight is 2500 g or less, irrespective of the duration of pregnancy.

The two varieties of LBW babies are separately defined:

*A preterm baby* is one who is born before the 37th week of pregnancy.

*A small for dates baby* is one whose growth has been so retarded that his birth weight is more than two standard deviations below the expected mean for the duration of gestation. As an approximation this means that the baby's birth weight is below the 3rd percentile. About 30 per cent of all babies

TABLE 4. Classification of newborn infants by birth weight and gestational age.

| Group | Birth weight (g) | Gestation (weeks) |
|-------|------------------|-------------------|
| I | 1500 or less | All gestations |
| II | 1501–2500 | Less than 37 |
| III | 1501–2500 | 37 or more |
| IV | 2501 or more | Less than 37 |
| V | 2501 or more | 37 or more |

This classification can be shown diagramatically (Table 5).

TABLE 5.

| g | 37th week | |
|------|-----|-----|
| | IV | V |
| 2500 | | |
| | II | III |
| 1500 | | |
| | I | |

weighing less than 2500 g are full-term infants (Lubchenco, 1970). On the other hand, some babies are of low birth weight due to a combination of both factors. The most important parameter is the duration of gestation or 'gestational age'. Although this is the usual term it, would be better described as the 'menstrual age' since it is calculated from the menstrual dates. The correct gestational age is two weeks more than the menstrual age.

A useful classification (Table 4) which combines birth weight and gestational age has been put forward by Yerushalmy (1970).

## Incidence

In Great Britain about 7 per cent of all live births fall within the definition of low birth weight. The incidence is higher in urban than rural areas.

## Aetiology

Many separate factors are involved, but these are so interdependent that careful statistical control is required for the individual assessment of each factor. For each low birth weight baby it is essential to determine whether this is due to being born preterm or small for dates, or a combination of both. The major causes of low birth weight are given in Table 6.

TABLE 6.

| Preterm | Small for dates |
|---|---|
| Antepartum haemorrhage | Pre-eclampsia |
| Premature rupture of membranes | Cigarette smoking by mother |
| Induced labour | Previous small for dates baby |
| Cervical incompetence | Intrauterine infection |
| Intrauterine infection | Multiple pregnancy |
| Pre-eclampsia | Poor socio-economic conditions |
| Multiple pregnancy | Short maternal height |
| Poor socio-economic conditions | Racial |
| Short interval between pregnancies | Severe congenital malformations |
| Maternal age $<16$ or $>35$ years | |

SOCIAL CLASS

The lower the social class (p. 35) the greater the incidence of low birth weight. Possibly this is the greatest single cause but it involves many different factors, particularly smoking, ignorance and less good antenatal care. A higher proportion of mothers of low birth weight babies work later in pregnancy, an aspect which also involves social class, since those from the lower social classes are more likely to have to work late.

Illegitimacy greatly increases the chance of low birth weight since the mothers of illegitimate children receive less antenatal care than those who are married.

MATERNAL ILLNESS

Of these, pre-eclampsia is the most important though antepartum haemorrhage, from placenta praevia or accidental haemorrhage, accounts for a number of cases. Any acute infection may precipitate premature birth but the role of infection is difficult to assess and has probably been over-emphasized. It is higher in those from the lower social classes so that other factors are involved. There is a higher incidence of low birth weight in women with bacteriuria, but in many instances this is due to underlying chronic renal disease. The role of accidents in the later months is equally difficult to assess since these are also more common in the lower social classes.

Maternal malnutrition and anaemia may be factors in the higher incidence of low birth weight in developing countries, but the part they play is difficult to assess since they are often associated with other aetiological factors. It appears that except under extreme conditions the nature and quantity of the maternal diet during pregnancy has little effect on fetal growth and therefore on birth weight. Probably this is due to maternal nutritional reserves buffering the fetus against deprivation. Maternal body fat is much increased around mid-pregnancy and may be used to meet extra needs during late pregnancy or lactation.

MATERNAL AGE

The lowest incidence of low birth weight is in the early twenties. After this age the incidence of low birth weight increases with rising maternal age. Under 20 years the incidence is higher but this may be an effect of social class since reproduction at an early age is predominantly found in the lower social classes.

MATERNAL HEIGHT

Mothers of low birth weight babies are shorter and lighter than their controls. This involves both social and genetic factors.

BIRTH ORDER

The birth weight is lower in the first pregnancy than in subsequent pregnancies.

SMOKING

Smoking during pregnancy has a deleterious effect on fetal growth. Lowe (1959) found the birth weight of infants born to mothers who smoked during pregnancy averaged 170 g less than those born to mothers who did not smoke. Similar results were obtained from the British Perinatal Mortality Survey of 1958 (Butler & Alberman, 1969). This difference persists when the effect of maternal age, height, parity and social class are taken into account. The cause is uncertain but it is probably due to reduced fetal oxygenation as a result of the action of nicotine and carboxyhaemoglobin. Nicotine reduces the blood supply to the fetus by constricting placental blood vessels. Carboxyhaemoglobin causes a shift to the left of the haemoglobin oxygen dissociation curve, so that for a given degree of oxygen saturation the $pO_2$ is lower.

Smoking in pregnancy increases the stillbirth and neonatal death rates (Butler et al., 1972). It can also cause educational backwardness in children (Davie et al., 1972). Smoking is heavier in mothers from the lower social groups and it rises with increasing parity, thereby adding yet one more adverse factor for the developing fetus. On the encouraging side is the fact that there is no carry-over into pregnancy of previous smoking habits; provided the mother does not smoke after the fourth month of pregnancy, earlier smoking habits have no effect on the fetus. These facts must be spelled out to pregnant women who are most likely to be influenced by the increased infant death rate and the long-term effect on intellect.

MULTIPLE PREGNANCIES

An important cause, particularly in areas such as West Africa where the incidence of twins and triplets is so much higher than in England.

CONGENITAL MALFORMATIONS

Intrauterine growth retardation occurs in almost all babies with chromosomal disorders. In addition, congenital anomalies are commoner in infants who are small for dates.

UNKNOWN CAUSES

The cause is unknown in about half the cases, particularly in those born after 37 weeks. In a proportion of these, labour has been initiated by premature rupture of the membranes; in such cases the possible role of an incompetent cervix is debated.

## Prevention

Improvement in social standards is the greatest requirement for the prevention of low birth weight births. The provision of good antenatal care is essential. Mothers must be warned to stop smoking during pregnancy. Family planning aids optimum spacing of births.

Ultrasound for measuring the size of the fetal head and examination of the amniotic fluid have been added to the methods available for determining fetal maturity in order to prevent a planned induction of labour from being undertaken prematurely. Staining of the fetal squames in the amniotic fluid determines their stage of development while the creatinine level in the fluid is related to the duration of pregnancy. A point-scoring system using these and other measurements from the amniotic fluid has been designed (Lind & Billewicz, 1971).

## Assessment of gestational age

An attempt should be made to determine the gestational age of all infants at birth. Not only is this essential for small infants but also for larger ones whose immature state may not be appreciated. An immature baby of 2·2–2·7 kg (5–6 lb) requires the availability of special care as do the smaller babies; if this is not provided the chances of survival are reduced.

If the infant is of low birth weight, assessment of the gestational age differentiates the preterm baby from one who is small for dates. This information is essential, since the management and prognosis for the two groups differ. For example, the preterm baby is liable to the respiratory distress syndrome (p. 64) and to intraventricular haemorrhage, whereas the small for dates baby is particularly susceptible to hypoglycaemia and to intrapulmonary haemorrhage.

Maturity is more important for survival than birth weight so that, in general, a twin of 1·5 kg has a better chance of survival than a single baby of the same weight, since the twin is likely to be the more mature. Conversely, intrauterine growth retardation may lead to intrauterine death.

One difficulty encountered in the assessment of maturity is that organs (and systems) mature at different rates. As the time for delivery approaches some organs are better adapted than others to withstand the change. At this point some tissues might benefit from a further few days of intrauterine existence whereas others have passed their peak. The optimum conditions for delivery therefore represent a state in which the organs have reached the best balance of maturity in relation to each other. In this sense, fetal maturity can be regarded as the point at which the fetus has gained the greatest possible benefit from intrauterine existence.

The most accurate measurement of gestational age is calculated from the date of the mother's last menstrual period, provided her cycles are regular and her memory accurate. Unfortunately, a large proportion of the world's women, particularly those in developing countries, keep no record of their periods so that this valuable information is unavailable in the very communities where the assessment of maturity is most difficult. Contraception by hormones which stop ovulation causes further difficulties since the return of ovulation after stopping the pill may be delayed. Consequently, if pregnancy occurs shortly after withdrawal of the pill and before normal menstruation has restarted, the date of ovulation is unknown.

Determination of the gestational age is therefore largely dependent on physical examination of the baby including an assessment of neurological maturity. By combining these findings with the pregnancy data, a reasonably accurate estimate of gestational age is obtained.

PHYSICAL CHARACTERISTICS

Three measurements of the baby should be made: birth weight, length and head circumference. If intrauterine growth has been normal, the weight and length are valuable for determining gestational age. If intrauterine growth has been retarded, the weight and length are less than normal for the gestational age. Head circumference is least affected by intrauterine growth retardation, but its normal variation is such that taken alone it does not give an accurate estimate of gestational age. At full term the average head circumference is 33–35·5 cm (13–14 inches); at 28 weeks it averages 25·4 cm (10 inches).

The more immature the baby the redder the skin. This colour is due to the skin being more translucent so that the blood in the capillaries is more easily visible. With increasing maturity this translucency disappears, being no longer apparent in the full-term infant. Negro babies are a light colour at birth, the most premature being the same red colour as those born to white mothers. The appearance of brown pigmentation in the premature Negro baby is evidence of good progress.

Preterm babies have little subcutaneous fat, this absence of insulation making heat regulation more difficult. As term approaches there is an increase in subcutaneous fat. Measurement of this increase, by skin calipers, has been used as an indication of maturity but at present there are no satisfactory comparative standards.

Vernix caseosa is absent in the most immature babies. Lanugo, the fine downy hair which covers the immature infant begins to disappear 2–3 weeks before term. The hair of the preterm infant is so fine that until about 38 weeks it feels like wool, individual strands being difficult to isolate. Thereafter, the hair thickens and becomes silky so that single strands, being coarser, can be picked up easily.

The nails are soft and short, not reaching the tip of the finger until term. Until 36 weeks the pinna of the ear is very soft and relatively shapeless. From then until full term it becomes increasingly stiffened by cartilage which makes its folds stand out prominently.

The size of the breast nodule has been correlated with gestation (Keitel & Chu, 1965). It cannot be felt until 33 weeks, and by term it measures 7 mm in diameter. Although underweight, full-term infants may have retarded breast development, large breast nodules always indicate full maturity.

Development of the skin creases on the sole of the foot is the single most reliable physical index of maturity (Usher *et al.*, 1966). Until 36 weeks there are only one or two transverse creases in the anterior part, the rest of the sole being smooth. By 38 weeks more creases have appeared, but the heel is still smooth. At term the whole sole is covered with creases, some forming deep clefts.

The external genitalia vary with the degree of maturity. At 36 weeks the scrotum is small and its rugae are limited to the area of the median raphe. The testicles may be seen at the top of the scrotum, having not yet fully descended. During the last 4 weeks of gestation the testes gradually descend so that the scrotum looks full and pendulous. By this time rugae cover the entire surface of the scrotum. In the female at 36 weeks the labia majora are still poorly developed so that the clitoris and labia minora are easily visible. By term, growth of the labia majora has hidden these organs.

Radiographic evidence from the appearance of the epiphysial centres in the knee and foot can be used to determine maturity provided modern protective measures, including the use of an image intensifier, are employed. The centre for the lower end of the femur appears about the 34th week and that for the upper end of the tibia and the cuboid about the 39th week.

The preterm baby cries less than the mature, the cry itself being more feeble. A continuous whimpering cry is of serious prognostic value. Preterm babies sleep most of the day; their cough and sucking reflexes are poorly developed, causing problems in feeding (p. 61).

*Neurological maturity.* Neurological assessment is valuable since the small for dates baby continues to mature neurologically despite a failure to gain weight at the normal rate. The immature infant is hypotonic, its attitude being mainly one of extension. As the baby matures its tone increases, flexion becoming predominant. By the time the baby is full term it has adopted the characteristic attitude of universal flexion. These changes are reflected in the baby's posture so that the limbs of the 28-week baby when supine are flat on the couch. By term the limbs, being strongly flexed, hardly touch the couch (Fig. 69(d)). When held in ventral suspension with the examiner's hand under the abdomen the 28-week baby is flaccid and all limbs are extended. At term the baby in this position has flexed limbs (Fig. 69(e)).

The 'scarf' sign is a manoeuvre in which one upper limb is made to wrap round the neck like a scarf. At 28 weeks lack of resistance permits the arm to be completely wrapped round. Thereafter the manoeuvre is limited by progressive increase in flexion of the baby so that at term the hand can only reach the opposite shoulder while the elbow does not quite reach the midline.

The 'window' sign involves flexion of the wrist. At 28 weeks, full flexion is impossible so that a window is left between the palm and the lower arm. At full term, the palm can be made to touch the lower arm, thereby removing the window.

Five reflexes are of particular value in assessing gestational age (Robinson, 1966). The pupil first reacts to light at 29–31 weeks. The glabellar tap reflex, consisting of a blink, appears at 32–34 weeks. The traction reflex appears at 33–36 weeks; in this manoeuvre the baby is pulled up by the wrists from the supine position, a positive response consisting of neck or arm flexion. The neck righting reflex, in which rotation of the head causes the trunk to follow, appears at 34–37 weeks. Head turning to a diffuse light appears at 32–36 weeks. Although the Moro reflex and the crossed exterior reflex depend on gestational age, they are unreliable for its assessment.

Maturity can also be assessed by motor nerve conduction which increases with gestational age. This is an indication of myelination and there is a direct relationship between the increase in velocity and the increase in gestational age.

### Small for dates

This condition was first called 'dysmaturity' (Sjöstedt et al., 1958), but this is unsatisfactory since maturity is least affected. Other terms which have been applied are 'intrauterine growth retardation' and 'pseudo-prematurity'.

It is due to intrauterine malnutrition, the fetus being starved of those substances necessary for its full growth. This starvation results from the causes listed on p. 48. When pre-eclampsia is the cause, the placenta is small and infarcted. In the case of twins, only the smaller one may have been starved in utero (p. 135).

The infant at birth is small, short and obviously undernourished, there being no subcutaneous fat (Fig. 10). Sometimes the skin is dry, cracked and meconium-stained as in the postmature infant (p. 56) because placental function has been disturbed in both conditions. Body temperature is poorly maintained, the babies being very liable to hypothermia. Respirations are often shallow and irregular, leading to periods of apnoea.

Head size is minimally affected compared with the rest of the body so that it appears proportionally large. This may be sufficient to lead to a suspicion of hydrocephalus when first seen. Studies of organ size have shown the brain

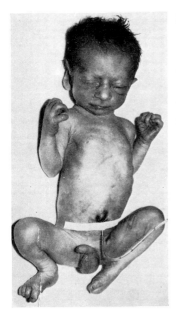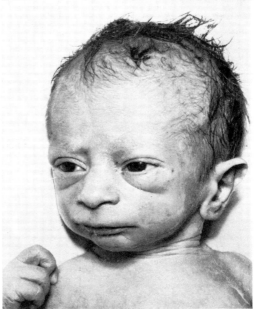

Fig. 10 Small for dates. Baby aged 2 days.
Although born at term this baby weighed 2·1 kg only. At birth there was
obvious evidence of malnutrition indicated by the lack of subcutaneous fat
and the dry parchment-like skin, especially of the hands. Convulsions caused
by hypoglycaemia occurred at the age of 24 hours. Intravenous glucose is
being administered through a catheter in the umbilical vein.
    The facial features are elfin-like; the forehead is prominent, the face tapering
down to a hypoplastic chin (see also Fig. 94, p. 280).

to be much larger than that of an immature infant of the same weight. Despite
this, the brain is still too small for the gestational age, but less so than any
other organ. On the other hand the liver and the thymus are very small. The
store of liver glycogen is very low and it is this which accounts for the greatest
immediate danger to these babies, namely hypoglycaemia (p. 641). These
babies are especially liable to disseminated intravascular coagulation (p. 601).
This may lead to another major cause of their death—massive pulmonary
haemorrhage (p. 130), the onset of which is so sudden as to suggest a cerebral
rather than a pulmonary cause for the symptoms.
    The babies also show a greater liability to neonatal jaundice which, no
doubt, is a further reflection of their poor hepatic function. For all these
reasons the mortality rate is high. Their care must therefore be even more
meticulous than that required by the simple immature infant. Their prognosis

carries the same problems as for other low birth weight babies (p. 69) but is even more hazardous. They are particularly liable to mental retardation and may be stunted in growth (p. 278).

## Postmaturity

Before discussing the special care required in the management of low birth weight babies it is relevant first to consider the postmature baby who also needs special care. In some respects the problem of postmaturity is closely related to that of small for dates, and it is not always possible to differentiate the two conditions. The reason for this is that in both states the infant is suffering as a result of placental insufficiency, though the cause of the placental disorder differs. As term approaches, placental growth wanes and uterine circulation decreases. When term is passed the placenta undergoes involution and infarction, the oxygen supply to the fetus being proportionately reduced. Anoxia is therefore the great hazard for the postmature infant, accounting for the sharp rise in perinatal mortality the longer the baby has remained undelivered after term.

The duration and the degree of placental insufficiency influences the type of 'distress' caused to the fetus. Gruenwald's concept (1963, 1964) of 'fetal distress' is helpful for a better understanding of the problem. He recognizes three types of fetal distress: acute, subacute and chronic. Acute fetal distress occurs during labour as a result of sudden interference with the placental blood supply; its duration can be measured in minutes. Subacute and chronic fetal distress are due to placental insufficiency before labour. The duration of subacute fetal distress is a matter of days and is commonly due to postmaturity. The duration of chronic fetal distress runs to weeks and is the condition of small for dates already described.

Whereas chronic fetal distress results in the baby being shorter than normal, subacute fetal distress does not affect the length since growth is normal until the condition develops a few days before birth. On the other hand, subacute fetal distress causes the baby to lose weight whereas in chronic fetal distress the baby does not lose weight because there is none to lose; he stops growing before he has any subcutaneous fat and before his muscle mass is great. The baby with chronic fetal distress is short and thin, the one with subacute fetal distress is long and thin.

The antenatal diagnosis of postmaturity requires an exact knowledge of the length of gestation but even then there is no sure guide to determine whether term has been reached in the individual mother. For this reason the risks of induction and the possibility of mistakenly inducing labour in a woman who has not yet reached term must be carefully judged against the dangers of postmaturity. The production of amniotic fluid slows down or ceases altogether after term so that a halt in the increase in maternal girth may be helpful. Even when the infant has been born the diagnosis may remain in doubt. Weight is of little use as a guide owing to the variation in normal. Length, on the other hand, is of greater value, a baby of 53 cm (21 inches) or more being likely to be postmature if there are other signs of the condition. Being a larger baby increases the chances of anoxia during delivery since labour is prolonged, particularly as the skull is more rigid and therefore less easily moulded. The nails are long, extending beyond the finger tips so that their ends are often broken. The skin becomes dry, cracked and meconium-stained as in the baby who is small for dates, though the changes are usually more severe. The skin is liable to peel and all these changes render it more liable to infection. The nails and cord are also often stained greenish-yellow by meconium. The feet often show a degree of talipes calcaneovalgus (p. 228); this is an exaggeration of normal dorsiflexion, probably resulting from the lack of amniotic fluid causing increased intrauterine compression.

Supporting evidence for the concept that postmature babies have suffered a recent loss of weight is the finding that their weight loss in the first few days of life is less than usual. In fact, there is commonly a rapid gain in weight once feeding is started.

The baby may seem more alert in behaviour than is usual for newborn infants and there may be radiographic evidence of advanced ossification. Careful watch must be kept for signs of hypoglycaemia, though the risk of this is less than with a baby who is small for dates.

## Management of the low birth weight baby

ANTENATAL CARE

From an early stage of pregnancy all mothers should be prepared for the possibility of premature labour, so that they are aware of the early signs of labour and have the material requirements at hand. The obstetric management required to prevent premature labour lies in the prevention and treatment of the causes discussed on p. 48.

CARE DURING LABOUR

Once the mother is in premature labour she should, if possible, be moved to hospital for the delivery since this increases the infant's chances of survival; it is safer for the baby to be transported *in utero* than in the ambulance. The attendant's problem will be to decide whether there is time for the mother to reach hospital, because delivery in the ambulance is more hazardous than delivery at home. A midwife skilled in the care of low birth weight babies should always accompany the mother on such journeys.

The hazards which exist for the preterm baby are the same as for the baby born at term but the risks are greater, particularly in the following respects:

### Intracranial birth injury

The small preterm head moves rapidly through the large bony pelvis and vagina without being moulded, immediately impinging on the perineum which has not had time to stretch as in a full-term delivery. It is this collision between the soft unmoulded head and the hard perineum that causes the intracranial damage to which preterm babies are particularly liable. This results in shearing strains and causes tears of the dura, especially of the tentorium. It must therefore be routine for an episiotomy to be performed for the delivery of all preterm babies. The additional measure of low forceps delivery to assist the head over the perineum is an added protection. Unfortunately, it is often mistakenly thought that forceps delivery is dangerous, but forceps correctly applied in the low cavity form a protective shield round the baby's head, thereby ensuring the safest delivery of a preterm baby. The incidence of breech delivery is increased in preterm babies and this increases the risk of intracranial injury.

### Asphyxia

The immature respiratory centre and poorly developed cough reflex renders the preterm baby more liable to asphyxia during labour and to cyanotic attacks at any time. Sedatives and anaesthetics for the mother should be avoided whenever possible and she must not be allowed to become cyanosed. Particular care must be taken in the clearing of the baby's air passages.

### Infection

The preterm baby is more liable to acquire infection so that the aseptic technique must be especially rigorous. Prophylactic antibiotics are not given as a routine but only for the same indications as for full-term babies (see p. 109).

### Loss of body heat

The baby loses heat easily because of the immature heat-regulating centre and the lack of insulation from the small amount of subcutaneous fat. The labour room should therefore be kept between 21 and 26° C (70–80° F). A heated cot or incubator should be ready, the baby being received into warmed towels with the minimum of exposure. In new units in tropical countries where labour rooms are air-conditioned, the optimal temperature for adults is too low for babies. Babies must therefore be moved from these as soon as they are born, in order to prevent chilling.

*Haemorrhage*

Haemorrhagic disease of the newborn (p. 129) is more common in preterm infants owing to immaturity of the liver. It is therefore wise to give them all prophylactic vitamin K. This is given intramuscularly shortly after birth, the dose not exceeding 1 mg since the drug increases the liability of preterm babies to hyperbilirubinaemia (p. 125). Vitamin $K_1$ should be given in preference to the water-soluble analogues of vitamin K since the risk of hyperbilirubinaemia is less with this preparation (Zinkham, 1963). It is possible that immature capillaries are more fragile, thus creating an additional cause for bleeding.

TREATMENT

The survival rate of low birth weight babies is directly related to the skill of the nursing staff who should have received special training in their care. Prematurity is one of the factors in the production of the cold injury syndrome (p. 132) so that extra heat must be provided day and night in the early days. This is gradually reduced when routine day and night temperatures show that the baby has become able to maintain normal body temperature. The temperature chart is an excellent guide to progress. At first there are wide fluctuations since the baby's temperature is determined by that of the environment, but as he matures these fluctuations disappear, a steadier chart resulting with variations only between 36·1 and 37·2° C (97–99° F). Extra heat by incubator, electric blanket or bottle should be provided for those who cannot maintain a body temperature of 36·1° C (97° F).

Studies (Silverman *et al.*, 1958; Jolly *et al.*, 1962) have shown that a higher survival rate is achieved by a policy aimed at keeping the baby's rectal temperature up to 36·1° C (97° F). This is related to the fact that a baby who is exposed to an environment below thermal neutrality increases his metabolic rate. This causes an extra consumption of oxygen and metabolic fuel, leading to a lowering of arterial oxygen tension.

The decision as to whether to nurse the baby naked in an incubator or clothed in a warm room depends on a number of factors. Observation of the naked baby is easier, making the nursing of very small babies safer. A room which is warm enough for small babies to be nursed in cots is uncomfortably hot for staff. However, if the ambient temperature is below the critical one the metabolic cost to a clothed baby is less than to a naked baby, and in hot conditions a cot-nursed baby can dissipate heat through his exposed face. In this sense the clothed baby in a cot is safer than the naked baby in an incubator in that his attendants need not control his environment so precisely (Hey & Katz, 1970; Hey & O'Connell, 1970).

High humidity is required for infants under 1·5 kg in order to reduce heat loss. Humidity itself has no beneficial effect so that if heat loss is prevented by nursing the baby in an incubator supplying radiant heat, then lower levels of humidity can be used. This is an advantage since infection is more likely to flourish in a very damp atmosphere. For babies not requiring incubator nursing who are being nursed in cots, there is no need to increase normal humidity unless the heating method is such as to dry the atmosphere excessively.

Oxygen should never be used routinely but only if the baby is cyanosed when enough must be given to ensure a good colour. Retrolental fibroplasia (p. 63) results from excessive oxygen therapy but fear of this disease has caused many low birth weight babies to be left anoxic. The condition cannot occur if the baby is cyanosed and such babies must be given 100 per cent

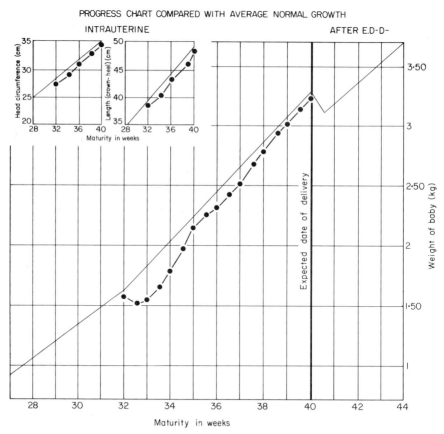

FIG. 11. Low birth weight baby progress chart with normal intrauterine growth curves for weight, length and head circumference for comparison.

oxygen if necessary, dropping to the safe level of 35 per cent when the colour improves.

The baby is nursed with the head on one side to prevent aspiration of vomit, the side being alternated at short regular intervals to prevent unequal compression of the soft structures. Particular attention must be paid to the external ear which being soft is easily bent forward on itself. Compression in this position between the mattress and the baby's head can lead to necrosis of the pinna. All procedures such as cleaning, weighing and changing must be carried out immediately before feeds, the child not being touched for 20 minutes after a feed, to reduce the risk of regurgitation.

The baby should be weighed twice weekly, the weight being plotted on a comparative scale which shows the normal weight curve for babies *in utero* (Fig. 11). A baby may be gaining weight but not at the correct rate; this will be obvious only if a comparative weight chart is used.

No routine bathing should take place but the skin may be cleaned with sterile liquid paraffin.

*Feeds*

Successful rearing of low birth weight babies is to a large extent a matter of calories. If adequate calories are supplied and not returned as vomit or diarrhoea, the baby should gain weight at the correct rate. For the average low birth weight baby, feeds should be gradually increased to at least 150 calories per kg daily and many will require larger quantities. The amount should be decided by the weight chart and not by any fixed formula. The interval between feeds is determined by the size of feed the infant can tolerate; 3-hourly is the usual routine but some babies require feeds more frequently, in which case an indwelling oesophageal catheter passed through the nose can be used, though not all babies will tolerate it. If an indwelling feeding catheter is used its end must be left open to permit the escape of swallowed air.

The best age at which to start feeding the low birth weight infant is still a matter of debate. At one time there was a vogue for delaying the first feed for up to 72 hours or even longer, but this is now regarded as dangerous owing to the increased risks of hypoglycaemia and hyperbilirubinaemia. These risks influenced Smallpeice & Davies (1964) to recommend 'immediate' feeding (within 2 hours of birth) with undiluted breast milk. Following their paper, Wharton & Bower (1965) carried out a controlled trial to compare 'immediate' feeding, as recommended, with later feeding (usually at 12 hours, using smaller volumes). Although they found hyperbilirubinaemia and hypoglycaemia to be less common in the 'immediate' group these babies had a higher mortality and there was a disturbingly high necropsy finding of inhalation of vomit among them.

Aspiration of feeds can now be eliminated by intravenous feeding. It is therefore recommended that all babies should be fed 4–8 hours after birth. Feeds should be given intravenously to those babies who are too immature to suck or swallow, especially those weighing less than 1250 g, and to those who are found to be liable to regurgitate. On no account should a pipette or Belcroy feeder be used since, if milk is injected into a baby who cannot swallow, it is very liable to enter the lungs.

The head must always be raised during feeds to reduce the risk of aspiration. Breast milk is ideal, but if not available, an evaporated milk or a high-protein half-cream dried milk can be substituted.

*Vitamin, iron and folic acid supplements*

Additional vitamins should be given from the age of 2 weeks and Abidec drops are a convenient multivitamin preparation. The daily dose of 0·6 ml (10 drops) contains:

| | | | |
|---|---|---|---|
| vitamin A | 5000 i.u. | vitamin B | 1 mg |
| vitamin C | 50 mg | vitamin $B_2$ | 0·4 mg |
| vitamin D | 400 i.u. | vitamin $B_6$ | 0·5 mg |
| | nicotinamide | 5 mg | |

The rate of fall of haemoglobin in preterm babies is considerably greater than that in full-term babies. This is largely due to dilution resulting from the relatively greater increase in blood volume in preterm infants. Lack of iron stores as the cause of the anaemia of prematurity has been exaggerated in the past and it is not the cause of the early and rapid fall in haemoglobin.

Iron supplements do not affect the course of the early anaemia but they do lessen the degree of the later anaemia. Ferrous sulphate is a suitable oral preparation of iron (p. 588) given after meals in a dose of 10 mg/kg (5 mg/lb) daily in divided doses. If the mother cannot be relied upon to give it, a useful alternative is a single intramuscular dose of 100 mg iron-dextran. The extra iron is started at the age of 4 weeks since there are always sufficient stores for the first month of life. However, if this delayed start is administratively difficult, for example, some mothers find it incomprehensible that a baby requires medicine at 4 weeks but not at 2 weeks, it can be started earlier. The iron should be continued until mixed feeding is established and at least until the age of 6 months.

Very low birth weight babies may later develop a megaloblastic anaemia from lack of folic acid. It is therefore advisable to give 0·5 mg daily to babies weighing less than 1·5 kg until mixed feeding is established.

## Care of the low birth weight baby in the home

An early problem is to decide whether or not to move the baby to hospital.

This will be decided by the state of the baby, the standard of the home, the intelligence of the mother and the availability of trained care. In general, all babies whose birth weight is under 2 kg should be sent to hospital.

The move to hospital is not an emergency and all resuscitation and immediate care should be carried out in the home. Low birth weight babies have sometimes died in transit because their move was regarded as an emergency and adequate resuscitation was not first carried out.

If the baby is to be nursed at home, the cot should be placed beside the mother's bed where she can see the baby. She must be instructed to watch for cyanotic attacks; if any occur the baby must be moved to hospital. The minimal amount of furniture is left in the room and, in order to reduce the amount of dust, vacuum cleaning and wet dusting should be used. The baby is removed to another warm room when visitors call.

Adequate fresh air should be insisted on as so many mothers think that the windows must not be opened. Draughts can be excluded by a blanket which passes under the mattress, over the cot sides, and is long enough to reach the floor. Heating must be provided day and night, the emphasis being placed on the night when so many parents forget to keep it going. A wall thermometer should be placed over the cot, the parents being instructed that the temperature must not drop below 18·5° C (65° F). Additional heat in the cot can be obtained from bottles. Extra humidity is not required unless the method of heating dries the atmosphere excessively, in which case a wet blanket over a radiator, or a slowly boiling kettle can be used. The baby who requires extra humidity should normally be in an incubator in hospital.

The weight at which a baby can be discharged from hospital depends on the same circumstances as those discussed in relation to transfer to hospital. As a guide, a baby should weigh 2·25 kg before he is sent home.

## Special problems affecting the low birth weight baby

INFECTION

The greater risks of infection have already been stressed; these particularly affect the lungs and skin. Thrush infection (p. 115) is common in special care baby units; this is partly a problem of overcrowded wards and insufficient staff, but is also due to its growth being favoured by the atmospheric conditions which must be maintained in the unit. Scrupulous attention must be paid to hand-washing and gown techniques.

DISORDERS OF THE EYE

*Retrolental fibroplasia*

This condition is due to excessive oxygen therapy and is largely confined to preterm babies; the more immature the baby the greater the risk. The earliest change is venous dilatation in the centre of the fundus. Following this the retinal arteries and veins at the periphery of the fundus develop angiomatous dilatations. The retina becomes oedematous and then detached; finally, an opaque white membrane fills the area behind the lens producing blindness.

Now that the relationship with excessive oxygen has been discovered the condition has been largely prevented.

*Myopia*

This is a recognized sequel of prematurity, occurring either alone or as a result of retrolental fibroplasia. It differs from the myopia of later childhood.

*Cataract*

There is an increased incidence of cataract in children of very low birth weight (McDonald, 1964; Harley & Hertzberg, 1965). Maternal toxaemia is one important factor but it is probable that any of the factors causing low birth weight can be involved.

HYPERBILIRUBINAEMIA

Owing to the immaturity of the liver, hyperbilirubinaemia is more liable to occur in preterm infants, particularly if the onset of feeding is delayed. The level of bilirubin may rise sufficiently high to require an exchange transfusion. This is discussed on p. 123.

RESPIRATORY DISTRESS SYNDROME (RDS)

*Infants at risk*

Most affected babies are preterm, this being the major problem facing such infants. It rarely occurs in full-term babies and the greatest incidence is the smallest preterm babies since immaturity is the main factor. In twins the frequency and severity of the condition is much greater in the second twin, probably because of the increased liability to asphyxia. Babies of poorly controlled diabetic mothers are at increased risk, and many of these will have been born before term. Caesarean section has been held responsible for some cases, but it seems likely that this association is due to the disorder requiring the Caesarean section rather than the operation itself.

*Aetiology*

Although the aetiology is still not clear much more is known than in the earlier days when the condition was wrongly ascribed to aspiration. The normal mature lung has alveoli lined by epithelial cells which secrete a substance called 'surfactant'. This substance, consisting of phospholipids, especially lecithin, is essential for normal lung stability since by lowering surface tension it prevents collapse of the air spaces. In RDS there is reduced surfactant activity which may or may not be due to an actual deficiency of the substance. Consequently, although the alveoli open with the first breath, the surface tension being high prevents them from remaining open, in fact it pushes all the air out again. The same thing happens with the next breath so that each breath is like a first breath because, between breaths, the lung returns to its previous airless state. RDS could therefore be called 'collapsing lung disease'. For a time the infant can open the alveoli with each breath, but later the air does not even reach the alveoli and the infant breathes through his bronchioles where air absorption is poor.

In the preterm baby surfactant activity is reduced because the lung is immature. Other conditions also may have the same effect, particularly intrauterine asphyxia. This causes a reduction in pulmonary blood flow, from pulmonary vasoconstriction, with consequent damage to the alveolar cells producing surfactant. In one fatal case of the disease one lobe of one lung was spared (Bozic, 1963). This lobe had a separate arterial supply from the aorta which presumably prevented the damage caused to the rest of the lung tissue from reduced pulmonary blood flow.

Clearly the syndrome results from prenatal factors. Once the infant is born the inadequate respirations cause a number of secondary effects, leading to a vicious circle. Hypoxia and fatigue cause a metabolic disturbance, meanwhile a transudate leaks into the alveolar air spaces. This transudate contains fibrin, leading to the formation of a hyaline membrane. The hyaline membrane is therefore a consequence of the disorder and not its cause as was supposed when the condition was first called 'hyaline membrane disease'.

At autopsy, the lungs are dull red; they contain very little air, thereby having the consistency of liver. No foam can be expressed from the lungs. Microscopically, the alveoli are collapsed but the bronchioles and alveolar ducts are distended. Since the alveoli were at one time expanded, their collapse has been termed 'resorption atelectasis'. But this term suggests the absorption of air distal to obstructed airways, whereas the actual mechanism of collapse already described would better fit the term 'expulsion atelectasis'. Hyaline membrane is seldom found in infants living only a few hours but it is common in those who have survived longer.

If the infant can survive the first 2–3 days there is an increase in surfactant activity so that recovery takes place. It is believed that the transudate and any hyaline membrane formed therefrom is absorbed. Extremely rarely, in cases of apparent recovery, death at a later age has shown organization of the hyaline membrane to have taken place (Wilson–Mikity syndrome, 1960). The incidence of this syndrome is increasing and it seems likely that it is iatrogenic.

It could be due to an irritant effect of high concentrations of oxygen or to the use of respirators with consequent difficulty in getting rid of secretions.

*Clinical features*

The clinical picture is one of increasing respiratory obstruction which usually dates from birth but may not be apparent until about 3 hours after birth. Respirations are rapid and laboured, and an expiratory grunt is audible. Grunting is a method of increasing the pulmonary inspiratory pressure so that the oxygen tension rises. This has been shown by passing an endotracheal tube into a grunting baby causing the grunt to stop and the oxygen tension to fall (Harrison *et al.*, 1968). The extra pull of the respiratory muscles on the soft thoracic cage causes retraction of the sternum (Fig. 12) and lower ribs. The degree of respiratory distress is such as to leave the baby unable to suck or even to cough. The air entry on auscultation is diminished, since even the violent respiratory movements are incapable of forcing as much air into the chest as normal. As a result the baby is cyanosed, and apnoeic spells with intense cyanosis are common. Crepitations are usually audible and oedema of the feet and hands an almost universal finding. A systolic murmur is common (p. 179).

As a consequence of anoxia these infants show signs of cerebral irritability and it is often very difficult to decide whether this irritability is primarily due

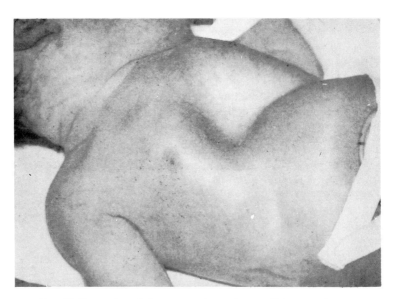

Fig. 12. Retraction of the sternum in respiratory distress syndrome.

to brain damage or to RDS. Moreover, cerebral bleeding—subarachnoid or intraventricular—is a relatively common post-mortem finding in RDS; this is thought to result from hypoxia and venous congestion.

Severely affected babies develop a solid feel to the cheeks, buttocks and thighs which is termed *sclerema*; cold is often a factor in its development (see p. 132). The chest X-ray is always abnormal, the changes sometimes occurring within 10 minutes of birth. The lung fields show a fine granular appearance, air being present in the bronchi (air bronchogram). A pneumothorax may result from alveolar rupture.

### Diagnosis

This is much the commonest cause of respiratory distress in preterm babies but other possibilities must always be excluded. Pneumonia (p. 114) can occur very early but seldom during the first day; on the other hand meconium aspiration (p. 114) can cause early severe respiratory difficulty. The X-ray changes in both are quite different from those in RDS in that if the lung pattern is altered it shows coarse irregular opacities. A diaphragmatic hernia (p. 154) causes immediate respiratory distress and is another reason for X-raying all such babies since an immediate diagnosis can then be made. Pneumothorax may occur in association with the respiratory distress syndrome but can occur separately, usually from over-vigorous attempts at resuscitation involving intubation and artificial respiration. Again, the diagnosis is made on X-ray which should include a lateral view in order not to miss an anterior mediastinal pneumothorax. Massive pulmonary haemorrhage (p. 130) causes similar respiratory distress and may be impossible to differentiate unless blood wells up the trachea a few hours after the onset, making the diagnosis obvious. Differentiation from cardiac failure is discussed on p. 181.

### Prevention

The main aim must be to prevent the onset of labour before term. Since the condition is liable to recur in succeeding pregnancies, particular attention must be paid to mothers with previously affected infants. In the case of an elective Caesarean section at term, the mother should, if possible, be allowed first to start natural labour. This reduces the risk of the section being carried out before term.

Amniocentesis to determine the level of lecithin and sphingomyelin can reduce the risk of induction before term. The mature lung secretes surfactant which contains these phospholipids, some of which enter the amniotic fluid. A high level of lecithin and particularly a high lecithin/sphingomyelin ratio indicates a low risk that the infant is immature and therefore liable to RDS (Gluck *et al.*, 1971).

The administration of steroids to mothers in premature labour may reduce the risk of RDS by inducing surfactant activity (Liggins and Howie, 1972).

*Treatment*

Once the condition has developed, treatment is largely supportive. A direct approach by providing surfactant has so far failed. The aim of therapy is therefore to maintain life and correct the secondary metabolic disorders, hoping the child will survive until his own surfactant activity takes over.

The single most important factor in survival is the maintenance of adequate arterial oxygenation. This can be satisfactorily determined only by sampling blood obtained from an artery since the colour of the baby is a poor guide. Moreover, the newborn baby may not become restless when anoxic. Oxygen is supplied through an incubator and, in severe cases, a respirator can be used. Continuous positive atmospheric pressure (CPAP) is now preferred to intermittent positive pressure ventilation (IPPV) since this prevents complete collapse of the alveoli, thereby increasing the absorption of oxygen. Results with hyperbaric oxygen have been disappointing.

Biochemical studies show a combined respiratory and metabolic acidosis. The respiratory acidosis results from inefficient pulmonary ventilation. The metabolic acidosis is due mainly to the accumulation of metabolites, such as pyruvic and lactic acids, resulting from incomplete carbohydrate metabolism. Consequent on the acidosis there is a rise in serum potassium which may produce typical changes in the electrocardiogram. The metabolic acidosis can be corrected by intravenous sodium bicarbonate given with glucose or fructose. To be effective, bicarbonate requires adequate ventilation; it does not deal with the respiratory component of the acidosis. For this reason an alkali, THAM (trishydroxymethylaminomethane), is sometimes used instead.

The baby's rectal temperature should be kept at 36·1–36·7° C (97–98° F). High humidity is used, its principal function being to enable the baby to maintain its heat in a slightly cooler atmosphere than otherwise. It reduces the loss of water from the skin and lungs, thereby cutting down heat loss from evaporation. Antibiotics have no direct influence on the condition; they should be used only if secondary infection is suspected.

Minimal handling of severely affected babies is essential since the least disturbance may cause sudden collapse. For this reason an indwelling oesophageal tube for feeding is preferable to the bottle if this causes any exhaustion. The Fulham score (Gomez *et al.*, 1969) is a guide to prognosis.

OEDEMA

This is sometimes regarded as a natural accompaniment of prematurity, but it does not occur in healthy preterm babies. It is seen particularly in the respiratory distress syndrome where it is an almost universal finding, and also in cold babies. It is not an indication for delayed feeding.

NEONATAL COLD INJURY (p. 132)

This condition is more liable to develop in low birth weight babies because of their lack of subcutaneous fat and an immature heat-regulating centre.

### Prognosis for low birth weight babies

The outcome for low birth weight infants can be accurately determined only by large studies involving carefully matched controls. Difficulties in the selection of controls account for some of the differences in follow-up studies. Many of the factors causing low birth weight are of a complex social nature which cannot be matched. The selected mothers must be of the same age and parity and come from the same social class. The babies must be of the same sex since the prognosis for boys is worse than that for girls.

The mortality amongst low birth weight babies is increased during the first 3 years, mainly from respiratory infections and to a lesser extent from congenital malformations. There is also an increased incidence of illness during the early years, especially from respiratory infections. This is partly the result of poor environment but comparisons within the same social group show a higher illness rate among low birth weight babies. Account must be taken of the fact that the mother of a low birth weight infant is more likely to call a doctor when the child is ill, because the special care she has been receiving for the baby may have conditioned her to be more anxious.

Drillien (1972) has separated three groups of low birth weight babies on the basis of their aetiology and prognosis. The group with the worst prognosis comprises those babies whose small size is due to a developmental abnormality of the fetus as a result of adverse factors early in pregnancy. Such babies have a high incidence of both minor and major congenital abnormalities. The babies may or may not be of appropriate size for the length of gestation, but are more often small for dates. The smaller the baby the greater the risk of mental handicap.

The second group is less severely affected; it comprises those babies who are small for dates as a result of hypoxia and malnutrition during the third trimester. Such babies seldom have major handicaps, but they are likely to show less serious impairments at a later age such as a mild degree of mental handicap and minor neurological abnormalities such as clumsiness (p. 434).

The last group comprises babies born before term of appropriate weight. With modern methods of care the outlook is good and this is likely to get still better as these methods are further improved.

In studying the outcome for height, strict attention must be paid to the height of the parents who, if small, can be expected to produce babies of low birth weight. When this is taken into account it is found that the babies of averaged sized parents usually reach average height by the age of 4 years.

Behaviour problems occur more often in those born with a low birth weight; this is partly due to brain damage and partly to parental overprotection. Considerable adjustments are necessary to achieve the right balance of parental care for a baby born small who may need nursing in an incubator and be separated from his mother for a long time.

Cerebral palsy from brain damage is much more common in low birth weight babies, the risk being greater the smaller the baby. Of children with cerebral palsy about 30 per cent are of low birth weight. There is a similar increase in the incidence of epilepsy and of deafness.

The increased risks for low birth weight infants of anaemia (p. 62), kernicterus (p. 129) and retrolental fibroplasia (p. 63) should be reduced by correct management.

## INFANT FEEDING

### BREAST FEEDING

The obvious reason for advocating breast feeding as opposed to artificial feeding is that breast milk is the natural food for human babies. But many mothers when given this reason will quite reasonably say they have seen many extremely healthy babies brought up entirely on cow's milk. The emphasis in the arguments in favour of breast feeding should be differently placed according to the mother with whom one is dealing. In Western communities, where the risk of gastroenteritis is now small, the emphasis should be placed on the close relationship between infant and mother achieved by breast feeding, whereby the mother feels a satisfaction which she never knows if the baby is

TABLE 7

|  | Human milk per cent | Cow's milk per cent |
|---|---|---|
| Protein | 1·5 | 3·5 |
| Casein | 1·1 | 3·0 |
| Lactalbumin | 0·4 | 0·5 |
| Fat | 3·5 | 4·0 |
| Sugar | 6·5 | 4·5 |

bottle fed. In developing countries, this close relationship is to a large extent obtained by having the baby on the mother's back all day and the emphasis to these mothers should be on the grave risk of gastroenteritis. There is at present a dangerous swing towards bottle feeding in developing countries, because of irresponsible advertising and because the bottle is often seen to be used by the educated members of their own community and by the white population. The result is a serious increase in gastroenteritis from lack of hygiene in the preparation of feeds.

A comparison between breast and cow's milk is shown in Table 7.

It will be noted that cow's milk has a higher percentage of protein and that this protein contains more casein. Casein is the least digestible part of the milk and for this reason the protein curds in the stomach of a baby fed on cow's milk are coarser so that they leave the stomach less easily than when the baby is breast fed. Occasionally these curds produce small intestinal obstruction if high calorie feeding with cow's milk has been introduced early (Cook & Rickham, 1969). One other disadvantage of the higher protein content of cow's milk is that if the function of the baby's kidneys is in any way impaired there will be a rise in blood urea.

Although the fat content of both milks is approximately the same, cow's milk fat is less easily absorbed because it contains more unsaturated and long-chained fatty acids. The higher percentage of sugar in breast milk provides an easily absorbed source of calories.

Breast milk contains more iron and copper than cow's milk but cow's milk contains more phosphorous, calcium and sodium. The mineral content of breast milk is ideally suited to the abilities of the neonatal kidney. For the bottle-fed baby the excessive phosphate load causes no problem provided he is well, but any situation in which the health of the baby is impaired reduces the ability of the kidneys to cope with the situation. Under these circumstances the excessive phosphate level causes depression of the serum calcium, leading to neonatal tetany. Similarly, the high sodium content of cow's milk puts the baby at risk of hypernatraemic dehydration (p. 722) if there is any renal impairment. For these reasons those preparations of cow's milk in which the manufacturers have reduced the electrolyte levels are safer.

Both milks contain sufficient vitamins A and B but insufficient vitamin D. The quality of vitamin C is adequate in breast milk but inadequate in cow's milk. The amount of vitamin C in cow's milk is only about one-quarter the amount in breast milk and this is destroyed by the boiling required for feed preparation.

Individual differences between mothers occur in the composition of breast milk though on the whole the content is relatively constant except for the amount of fat which may vary substantially (Hytten, 1954). Malnourished mothers produce a milk which is low in lipids and it is significant that this is an important constituent of brain tissue.

Weight for weight more calories are obtained from breast milk because the baby is unable to digest cow's milk completely.

Once breast feeding has been established it is easier, if the time taken in preparation of bottles is considered, and there are fewer feeding difficulties. It is also considerably cheaper.

Breast fed babies are less likely to develop eczema and they are less at risk of cot death (p. 367), possibly because they are not liable to hypernatraemia.

For all these reasons mothers should be encouraged to breast feed but they should never be forced to do so. Doctors and nurses must ensure that they do not make mothers feel guilty of failure when unable or unwilling to breast feed.

### Preparation for breast feeding

Preparation commences in the antenatal period; the first step is to explain the reasons for recommending breast feeding so as to enlist the mother's co-operation. If the baby's grandmother is likely to have an important influence in the matter of breast feeding her co-operation should also be sought at this stage. Some grandmothers persuade the mother to give up breast feeding because of a subconscious or even conscious desire to be able to feed and look after the baby themselves. If the mother has failed to feed any previous children the reasons for this should be determined, as it may well affect the handling of the present situation.

The breasts should then be examined. The skin should be as lax as the skin of the neck in order to accommodate the increase in size. If this is not so, engorgement may result; a special watch must therefore be kept on such patients. Obvious inversion of the nipple will be diagnosed without difficulty (Fig. 15) but it is important to pick out those which are potentially inverted. To do this the infant's jaws are simulated by pinching the nipple at the edge of the areola. The normal nipple then becomes more prominent (Fig. 13) but those which are potentially inverted recede into the breast tissue (Fig. 14), a situation which if it persisted would occur when the infant came to suck.

Both types of inversion can be treated with shields worn under the bra (Fig. 15) and by instructing the mother to pull out the nipples night and morning. Whether to give this treatment to all women with defective nipples is debated since some improve spontaneously during pregnancy. Hytten & Baird (1958) believe that the anatomical improvements claimed for treatment are probably due in most women to normal physiological changes during pregnancy. However, if a mother is keen to breast feed and has no objection to the treatment, it should be tried.

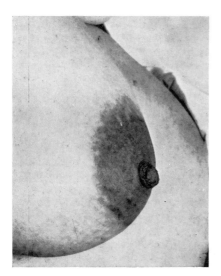
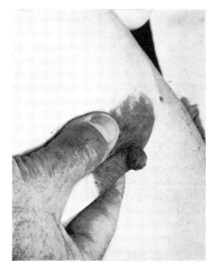

FIG. 13. Inversion test—the fingers pinch the edge of the areola to simulate the infant's jaws. The normal nipple then becomes more prominent.

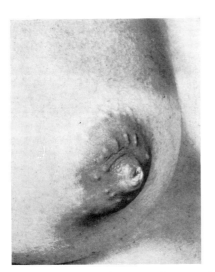
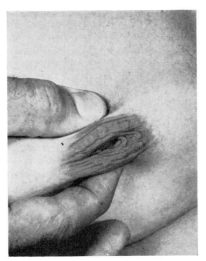

FIG. 14. Inversion test—the potentially inverted nipple recedes into the breast.

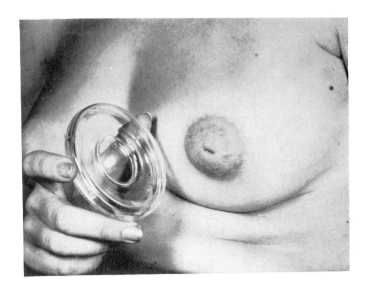

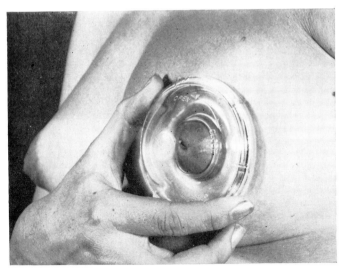

Fig. 15. Breast shield for use with inverted nipple (as illustrated) or for potentially inverted nipple.

*Above* Showing its inner surface.

*Below* Position when in use under the bra.

Daily manual expression of the breasts during the last three months of pregnancy has been shown to increase the chances of successful lactation (Waller, 1946). Mothers who are keen to breast feed can easily be taught the technique (Fig. 16) which also gives them the ability to ensure complete emptying of the breasts once feeding has been established. Moreover, if for any reason, such as prematurity, the baby cannot be put to the breast at once, the mother can still achieve a satisfactory supply of milk.

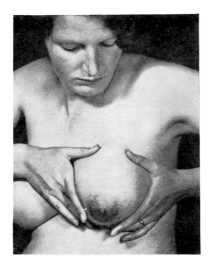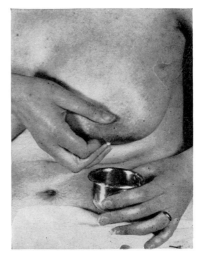

Fig. 16. The two steps in manual expression.

*Left* Gentle massage to initiate the 'let-down' reflex. The hands start flat on the chest wall and move towards the nipple.

*Right* The areola is rhythmically compressed between the thumb and index finger.

The physiology of lactation is incompletely understood but it is probable that its initiation results from the secretion of prolactin by the anterior pituitary. This secretion is related to changes in the levels of progesterone and oestrogen occurring at parturition.

The flow of milk from the breast is under the control of the draught or 'let-down' reflex. Sucking of the nipple causes afferent impulses to pass to the posterior pituitary which releases oxytocin. This passes by the blood stream to the breast where it acts on the smooth muscle fibres surrounding the alveoli so that milk is forced into the large ducts. Oxytocin also causes contraction of the smooth muscle of the uterus, thereby hastening involution. 'After-pains' may be severe for the first few days while breast feeding, so that their mechanism should be explained to all mothers.

The draught reflex is conditioned by the sight and handling of the baby. Dripping of milk from the breast not being sucked is due to the action of the draught reflex. Anxiety and embarrassment suppress the reflex by acting through the sympathetic nervous system. The mother should therefore handle her baby for a few minutes before putting him to the breast, every step possible being taken to put her at her ease. For this reason, babies should be nursed in cots adjoining their mothers' beds rather than in a nursery. The mother can then see her baby all the time and is relieved of much of the anxiety which results if her baby is out of sight. The baby should be removed to the nursery only at night if his crying disturbs his mother or others in the ward.

Milk is not secreted until the second or third day after birth. During the latter weeks of pregnancy and for the first two to three days after birth the breasts secrete colostrum. This is yellower than milk, so that the arrival of the more watery looking milk leads some mothers to believe 'their milk has turned to water' and, therefore, that it is no good. Colostrum has a higher protein and mineral content than breast milk. It also provides a considerable amount of IgA and some IgM, both of which have been unable to pass the placental barrier. Consequently, the newborn baby who is breast fed is better protected against infections, particularly *E. coli*.

Until the milk has arrived the baby should be put to the breast two or three times a day in order that mother and baby may begin to make close contact. It is ideal that the first occasion for the baby to be put to the breast is while waiting for the delivery of the placenta. The baby should not stay on the breast for long since vigorous sucking at an empty breast can cause the nipple to crack. The baby may require extra fluid during this time, in which case 5 per cent glucose can be given by bottle. Once the milk is in, the baby should be fed for about 10 minutes on each side every 3 or 4 hours depending on the baby's requirements. It should be left to the baby to decide the interval between feeds, not the nursing or medical staff.

A rigorous clock-controlled régime is no longer advocated; it should be made clear to mothers that if the baby wakes up for a feed before it is due, she should feed him without waiting the full interval. The term '*demand feeding*' is used to describe a régime where the baby is fed whenever he demands it, an application of the common-sense already given. However, it must be pointed out that some mothers practising demand feeding find the situation gets out of hand and become exhausted by being repeatedly disturbed. Such mothers sometimes respond better to a regular régime applied with common sense rather than to a timeless one.

The breast used first should be alternated at each feed. During the feed, care should be taken to ensure that the breast is kept away from the baby's nose so that breathing is not impeded.

### Insufficient breast milk

If there is insufficient milk the number of feeds should be increased, since the more the breast is stimulated the greater the flow of milk. Those on a 4-hourly régime should therefore be changed to 3-hourly. The breasts must be completely emptied to ensure maximum flow, this being achieved by manual expression at the end of the feed. The milk so obtained is fed to the baby by spoon or by bottle. If the milk supply is still inadequate a *complementary feed* of cow's milk should be given after each breast feed. This can be given by spoon rather than bottle if there is any evidence that the baby is starting to prefer the bottle to the breast. The quantity may be decided by a *test feed* or assessed in relation to the infant's likely needs. A test feed measures the amount of breast milk taken at one feed. The baby is weighed before and after the feed, no napkins being changed during the interval. In this way any stool or urine passed is still weighed with the baby, so that the difference in the two weights indicates the amount of milk taken. The weighing of the baby required in test feeding is likely to increase a mother's anxiety, thereby reducing her flow of milk. For this reason it is preferable to estimate the approximate amount of extra milk required for her baby. The complementary feed should not be sweetened lest the infant comes to prefer it to the breast.

There is no evidence that the drugs termed 'galactogogues' (e.g. iodine) increase the flow of milk and their use is not recommended. It has been shown that forcing mothers to drink beyond their natural desires has the effect of reducing the amount of milk produced, apart from the nuisance of causing frequency of micturition (Illingworth & Kilpatrick, 1953). Once complementary feeding has caused the baby to gain weight a mother's anxiety usually lessens and her flow of milk increases, so that the complement can be stopped. Mothers should be encouraged not to become over-concerned about their baby's weight gain. Provided a baby is thriving and sleeps between feeds, his rate of weight gain does not matter. In such cases regular weighing only serves to maintain an unnecessary state of maternal anxiety.

### 'Sleepy feeder'

A baby sometimes falls asleep at the breast. This is common in preterm babies but in others it is usually due to an inability to obtain milk, either because there is none or because an inverted nipple makes it impossible for the baby to grip the nipple. Sometimes a baby is forced to suck too long on the first breast when it has already been emptied; he is then left crying, finally going to sleep from exhaustion. All these possibilities must be investigated and if no obvious cause is found it may be helpful to increase the interval between feeds, thereby increasing the baby's hunger and making him more keen to suck.

### Engorgement

To some extent, engorgement always occurs at the onset of lactation, but painful breasts which may lead to reflex suppression of lactation must be prevented. This involves careful antenatal attention, a special watch after delivery being kept on mothers in whom engorgement is anticipated. A history of engorgement following previous births, small breasts with inelastic skin, and deformities of the nipple are all liable to lead to engorgement.

The engorged breasts become full and painful, the overlying skin being red and oedematous. At the first sign of engorgement the baby should be put to the breast in the hope that he can relieve the situation by drawing off some of the milk. This will be possible in early cases, but if engorgement is severe the infant will not be able to draw off milk and will only cause a cracked nipple. Such a situation must not be allowed to develop. Therefore the decision as to whether the baby is put to the engorged breast requires considerable judgment. If normal sucking is impossible, manual expression should be tried; the removal of a small quantity of milk may make it possible for the baby to feed from the breast. Manual expression is preferable to the use of a hand breast pump since this may damage the epithelium of the nipple and lead to a crack, but mechanical breast pumps are comfortable and efficient. In severe cases manual and mechanical expression will be impossible owing to pain. Such mothers should be given oral stilboestrol in doses of 5–15 mg in order to reduce lactation without complete suppression. The dose should be repeated, if necessary, at 4-hourly intervals but on each occasion the breasts must be examined to determine if engorgement is less, and the mother questioned about pain. It is usual for the pain to lessen before there is any visible evidence of reduction of the engorgement, but if either occurs the dose of stilboestrol should be withheld. Analgesics such as Tab. Codeine Co. should be given and considerable relief is obtained from the local application of warm cotton wool, the breasts being well supported. In the home the cotton wool can be warmed in an oven. Manual expression should be carried out as soon as the relief of pain permits.

### Cracked nipples

From what has been written already it will be appreciated that cracked nipples are preventable. The baby must never be permitted to suck at a breast from which no milk is flowing, a situation which arises if the milk has not yet come in, or if the breasts are much engorged, or if the infant has already emptied the breast. A crack may also result from the forceful removal of the baby at the end of a feed. During the feed a baby may produce a strong vacuum in the mouth and this should be released by placing a clean finger in the mouth before extracting the nipple.

Treatment of a cracked nipple requires the immediate temporary cessation of feeding from the breast. Early diagnosis is essential to prevent further damage and to reduce the risk of breast abscess; the nipples should therefore be inspected before and after each feed. If a mother complains of pain in the nipple but no crack is visible, treatment should still be the same. Feeding from the breast is stopped for 24 hours and 1 per cent aqueous gentian violet applied to the crack. During this period the milk should be expressed by hand and fed to the baby. Feeding from the breast is restarted after 24 hours if the crack has healed, but if this causes any pain in the nipple, feeding should be stopped for a further period.

### Breast abscess

This is usually due to a staphylococcal infection, commonly a sequel of a cracked nipple or of milk retention. The first sign is either flushing of the skin over one area of the breast or a hard painful lump, due at first to retention of milk but later becoming secondarily infected. At the first sign of infection, intramuscular penicillin should be given (unless a penicillin-resistant staphylococcus is known to be common in the unit, in which case the appropriate alternative antibiotic according to known sensitivities should be used). In early cases feeding from the affected breast should be continued, the breast being emptied of retained milk by manual expression. In late cases the affected breast should be firmly bandaged, feeding being permitted from the normal breast only. By this means lactation can be maintained in the normal breast but suppressed in the infected breast. Once the infection has subsided, and in some cases incision will be required, the baby can be put to the breast; full lactation will be resumed in a few days. If necessary, lactation can be completely suppressed by oestrogens but in countries where breast feeding is essential, everything possible should be done to maintain lactation.

### Contraindications to breast feeding

If the mother's health is liable to suffer from breast feeding, lactation should be suppressed. The decision must be taken in the light of the likely duration of the illness and the possible alternative arrangements for the baby. Open tuberculosis in the mother always used to be regarded as a definite contraindication to breast feeding. Modern management with isoniazid (INH) and INH resistant BCG (p. 528) has made this unnecessary, which is very fortunate since the condition particularly occurs in developing countries where the baby is likely to perish if not breast fed.

Severe inversion of the nipple may make breast feeding impossible, but the use of a nipple shield to which a teat is attached may make it possible to feed from the breast. Between feeds it may help if the nipple is pulled out at intervals. The use of breast shields in the postnatal period is not recommended since they are liable to cause oedema of the nipple which predisposes to the development of a crack.

If the mother is emotionally disturbed by breast feeding she should be allowed to stop, care being taken to ensure that she does not feel she has failed her baby. On the other hand, puerperal insanity is not necessarily a contraindication to breast feeding. In the newer mental units where babies are admitted with their mothers, it has been found that permitting the mother to breast feed has assisted her recovery.

The only condition in the baby which may prevent breast feeding is a deformity of such severity as to make feeding impossible; this occurs particularly with a severe cleft lip and palate. However, it is wise not to suppress lactation at once but to feed expressed breast milk for a few days in the hope that the baby, with increasing strength, will be able to feed from the breast.

### Suppression of lactation

The breasts should be well supported and, if painful, analgesics should be given but no expression of milk permitted. It is traditional to give oestrogens for the suppression of lactation but there is no need since breasts which are unstimulated by a sucking baby soon switch off completely. Many obstetric units no longer prescribe these drugs.

## ARTIFICIAL FEEDING

If breast milk is not available, cow's milk should be used. This can be given fresh, dried or condensed. Fresh milk is not recommended since in this form the protein is less digestible for the human baby. The choice between dried or condensed milk is largely a matter of individual preference. In the past, condensed milks have been used more widely in America than in Great Britain but their popularity over here is now increasing. It used to be thought that the risk of infection in the can was greater with condensed milks, but this is incorrect. If anything, the risk of infection is greater with dried milks since the unsterile hand is repeatedly introduced into the tin. The incidence of sore buttocks has been reported to be less with condensed milk feeding (Moss, 1957). Bulk preparation in maternity units is simplified by the use of condensed milk.

**Dried milks**

These are available as half-cream and full-cream. Half-cream milk should not be used for longer than the first month, in fact most babies can be fed on full-cream milk from the start. Half-cream milk is available because some very young babies, particularly preterm infants, develop loose fatty stools on a full-cream milk.

To calculate how to make up the feeds the following facts are used:

| | |
|---|---|
| Fluid requirements | 150 ml/kg. (2½ oz/lb) per 24 hours |
| Calorie requirements | 110 calories/kg. (50 calories/lb) per 24 hours |
| Full-cream milk | 20 calories per 30 ml (1 oz) |
| Half-cream milk | 16 calories per 30 ml |
| Sugar | 120 calories per 30 ml |

The total fluid required is calculated from the infant's *expected* weight, otherwise an underweight baby would be fed less than he required. This is divided by the number of feeds in the 24 hours to determine the amount to be given in each feed. On a normal 4-hourly régime there are five feeds and on a 3-hourly régime six feeds a day. Half-cream milk is reconstituted at full strength, that is, 4 grams of powder (a measure is provided) to 30 ml of boiled water. Full-cream milk is generally given at slightly less than full strength; instructions are given on the tin. Sugar should be added to both these mixtures in order to bring the calorie content up to 20 calories per 30 ml. For practical purposes one teaspoonful of sugar (providing 15 calories) for every 100–150 ml of feed is satisfactory. Most half-cream milks have added sugar and for these no more is required.

The change from half-cream to full-cream should be gradual. One measure of half-cream is replaced by full-cream each 24 hours until the change-over is complete.

**Unsweetened condensed milk (evaporated milk)**

This is milk from which a large amount of water has been evaporated, it is therefore reconstituted by adding boiled water calculated as follows:

| | |
|---|---|
| Undiluted evaporated milk | 50 calories per 30 ml |
| Daily requirement of undiluted milk | 60 ml/kg (1 oz/lb) |
| Standard dilution | 30 ml milk: 60 ml water |

This provides 17 calories per 30 ml.

This dilution is suitable for preterm as well as for mature babies. The calorie content is brought up by adding one teaspoonful of sugar for every 100–150 ml of diluted milk as with dried milk.

Sweetened condensed milk is not recommended since the sugar content is too high and the protein too low.

### Fresh cow's milk

This is less digestible than a dried or condensed milk. When given to newborn babies it should be diluted with an equal quantity of water, then boiled and sugar added.

### Preparation of feeds

Some mothers find it more convenient to make up the day's supply of feeds at one time, this method being satisfactory provided they can be stored in a refrigerator. Mothers must be instructed to use a level measure of powder and not a heaped one which produces too concentrated a feed, especially in its electrolyte content. To obtain a level measure the excess powder is removed with the flat of a knife.

Scrupulous attention should be paid to sterility, bottles and teats being boiled between each feed. Sodium hypochlorite (Milton) is a useful disinfectant in which to store bottles and teats between feeds, but it is essential that the bottles are filled with the solution and the teats immersed. Immersion of the teats is achieved by placing them under glass covers, or on the bottle which is laid on its side, in a bowl containing hypochlorite.

Most mothers like to give a warm feed, although babies will take a cold feed just as well. To ensure that the feed is not too hot it should be tested by shaking out a little on to the back of the hand. The teat itself should never be touched or it will be contaminated. The hole in the teat should be of such a size that when the bottle is inverted, milk comes out rapidly in drops but not in a stream. To enlarge the hole a red-hot needle should be used. If the hole is too large the baby will vomit from feeding too rapidly. If it is too small the baby is likely to swallow excessive air as a result of his vigorous sucking attempts to obtain enough milk. A hole which is too small is liable to become completely blocked with milk; blockage of the teat sometimes accounts for an infant falling asleep during a feed ('sleepy feeder').

The baby should be comfortable during the feed and this requires that the mother should be comfortable. A low chair with a seat which slopes backwards is preferable to an ordinary chair; alternatively, the use of a footstool may be satisfactory. The baby's head should be raised to prevent aspiration of regurgitated feeds or their passage into the Eustachian tube. Swallowed air can be brought up when the baby stops feeding—not at repeated intervals during the feed. The ideal approach is for a mother to cuddle her baby at the end of a feed and see whether he has any wind to bring up by himself. In teaching mothers how to bring up swallowed air great care must be taken to prevent them becoming obsessed with 'the wind'. This is essentially a 'Western' problem, some mothers spending an hour or more trying to bring up 'the wind'. The approach should be that if no air is brought up when the baby is held correctly then there is insufficient to bother about.

COMPLEMENTARY FEED
This feed of cow's milk is given after a breast feed when there is insufficient breast milk (p. 77).

SUPPLEMENTARY FEED
This indicates the replacement of a whole breast feed by cow's milk. It is unphysiological and should be used only in an emergency when the mother is unavoidably absent. If possible, the mother should express her breasts about the time the feed is due in order to maintain lactation.

## FEEDING DIFFICULTIES IN YOUNG INFANTS

**Mucus vomiting**

Vomiting in the first 2–3 days of life is frequently associated with mucus, aspiration of this vomit being one cause of cyanotic attacks. In many cases the vomiting results from swallowing maternal blood, so that altered blood in the vomit is usually maternal in origin. Incoordination of the pharyngeal muscles during the early days of life may not be uncommon and could account for some cases of early vomiting.

The frequency of vomiting in babies born by Caesarean section, whose stomachs contain more mucus, amniotic fluid and blood than babies delivered normally, is due to lack of the usual thoracic compression during delivery. This has led to the use of routine gastric aspiration at birth of all Caesarean babies (p. 99).

*Treatment.* A stomach tube (EG8; FG16) should be passed and the gastric contents aspirated. This is often all that is necessary and it also excludes oesophageal atresia (p. 151). If vomiting persists and no other cause is found, gastric lavage is performed. One per cent sodium bicarbonate is used for this in preference to saline since the mucus disappears more rapidly with its use. One gastric lavage may be sufficient but it can be repeated if necessary.

**Aerophagy**

Excessive air-swallowing can occur in greedy feeders who gulp air with their first mouthfuls of milk. This can be prevented by giving boiled water or milk by spoon before the start of the feed. Air-swallowing is difficult if the feed is given by spoon, and the baby's initial greed is thereby reduced. It may also result from faulty technique such as too small a hole in the teat, or permitting the baby to suck air from the bottle because it is empty or not held fully inverted. Excessive air-swallowing may also result from the hole in the teat being too large; this forces the baby to gulp in order to prevent drowning from the rapid flow of milk, but in so doing he takes in a lot of air. Excessive crying, due often to underfeeding, will also lead to air-swallowing.

Aerophagy may lead to vomiting and may cause intestinal hurry with consequent loose stools from excessive air in the intestine. In such cases the stool may be a normal yellow colour in one part and green in another.

## Vomiting

This is a very common symptom in the first few days of life, the most frequent cause being mucus vomiting (see p. 83). The possibility of intestinal obstruction must be considered in every case, particularly if the vomit is bile-stained (p. 161). It is also necessary to exclude infection although this does not usually occur so early.

In a breast-fed baby, vomiting is not due to the milk failing to suit the baby as mothers so often allege, and is rarely due to errors in technique leading to aerophagy (see above). In an artificially fed baby there is a greater possibility of technical errors and some of these cause vomiting from aerophagy. Vomiting may also be caused by an incorrect milk mixture. Vomiting from allergy to cow's milk is rare (see below).

## Evening colic

During the first 3 months of life it is common for babies to scream for long periods after the 6 p.m. feed. This is frequently ascribed to colic, a meaningless and unscientific label which in this situation is merely providing another name for screaming. It is usually related to the fact that this is the time when a mother's exhaustion is greatest and she is in a panic to try to get everything finished before her husband returns home. An explanation that a mother's haste and anxiety soon conveys itself to the baby may relieve the situation, particularly if she can delay the feed until after her husband's return. This should make it possible for the baby to be played with after the feed instead of being put straight back into his cot.

Those who believe in 'colic' as a cause of screaming give dicyclomine hydrochloride syrup ('merbentyl') in a dose of 5–10 mg ($\frac{1}{2}$–1 teaspoonful) 20 minutes before the feed. I find it more helpful to work out ways of reducing early evening family pressures.

## 2 a.m. crying

It is understandable that many young babies cry about 2 a.m. when they might be expected a feed. No harm comes from giving a feed at this time, but the possible habit of a nightly feed which may develop and tire the mother can often be prevented by delaying the 10 p.m. feed instead. It is common to have to wake the baby for this feed so it is delayed as long as possible. When he does wake in the night it will be later so that the feed he is then given takes the place of the 6 a.m. feed. Adjustment of feed times back to 10 p.m. and forward to 6 a.m. can be achieved later.

### Regurgitation and rumination

Many babies bring up partially digested milk and spill it out of their mouths. This is termed *regurgitation* and it may lead to *rumination*, the milk then being chewed over as a cow chews the cud. Rumination is a habit, the patients usually being bright babies who are bottle fed. It is sometimes a sequel of aerophagy, the baby having first developed a taste for the habit when milk came back with the wind. The infants derive obvious pleasure from the habit but their mothers become very distressed by it. They are worried by the 'vomiting' and by the continuous presence of partially digested milk on clothes and bedding which spoils them as well as making the baby smell. The mothers are often the type who keep dabbing at the baby's mouth thereby encouraging the habit. Sometimes the primary problem is maternal, the mother being anxious or depressed.

The diagnosis is made by watching the baby and by his very characteristic smell. It seldom causes harm so that, provided the baby is thriving, the emphasis should be removed from trying to stop the baby vomiting. Once the mother realizes it is only a habit and has been told to dress the baby (and herself if necessary) in suitable protective clothing, she is usually able to accept the situation with relief. Thickening the feeds with cereal and propping the baby up may reduce the symptom, but it often continues until the child is walking.

A small group of babies who ruminate, best described as 'malignant ruminators', will lose so much food as to kill themselves if something is not done rapidly to break the habit. For these a continuous intragastric drip of thickened feed is required, together with sedation.

### Milk allergy

Most infants fed on cow's milk develop antibodies to it (Gunther *et al.*, 1960, Coe & Peterson, 1963). The frequency with which these cause symptoms is much debated, but there is a growing feeling that symptoms from cow's milk allergy occur much more often than was formerly believed. It is possible that cow's milk feeding in the first 2 days increases the risk.

*Clinical features.* Three systems in the body are liable to be affected: the gastrointestinal—leading to diarrhoea, often with blood in the stools, vomiting and failure to thrive; the respiratory—leading to recurrent rhinorrhoea recurrent bronchitis (wheezy bronchitis, p. 351), asthma and possibly idiopathic pulmonary haemosiderosis (p. 364); the skin—leading to eczema.

Complete proof of the condition is not possible, but the diagnosis is likely if the symptoms disappear when milk is withheld and recur on at least 2 occasions when milk is reintroduced. Eosinophilia may be present but is not diagnostic. It has been suggested that a higher than usual level of milk antibodies may be present, but this also is not diagnostic. Other members of the family may share a dislike of milk, and there may be a family history of atopy.

Before diagnosing milk allergy as a cause of diarrhoea it is important to consider a secondary disaccharidase deficiency (p. 570) which can result from damage to the bowel wall caused by any severe intestinal disorder.

It has been suggested that sudden cot death in infancy can be due to an acute anaphylactic reaction in sensitive infants, following the inhalation of regurgitated cow's milk during sleep (Parish *et al.*, 1960). This is discussed on p. 368.

*Treatment.* If the diagnosis of cow's milk allergy seems likely, milk and meat from the cow are removed from the diet. Soybean milk can be given instead, though sometimes the children become sensitive to this. After about 1 year a gradual reintroduction of cow's milk is tried. Active desensitization is dangerous and should not be attempted.

## MIXED FEEDING

In planning the introduction of solid feeds, attention should be paid to a number of principles:

1. The earlier a new tasting food is introduced, the more likely is it to be accepted. Babies are conservative individuals who dislike change, but in the early months the sensation of taste is not fully developed so that less antagonism is encountered.

2. Only one new feed at a time should be introduced; if the baby is then upset if will be known which is the offending article of diet.

3. Small quantities only should be introduced at first. A baby who refuses a new food at the beginning of a feed when he is very hungry and wants only milk, may accept it without difficulty in the middle of the milk feed.

4. No new foods should be given when the baby is off colour or in very hot weather when he is more likely to be upset.

5. Cup and spoon feeding should be introduced early in order to make the change more easy and reduce the possibility of the baby refusing to give up the bottle.

Mothers should be encouraged to use their initiative and to develop an experimental approach, rather than feel they must rely on the nurse or doctor for every instruction. No single method will suit every baby; mothers should understand that there are many methods of equal merit and the dogmatic statements of friends and relatives should be assessed in that light. For this reason the instructions given here are intended only as a guide. There is no doubt that most babies could be started on solids when only a week or two old and this is practised in some centres. There is no particular advantage in this practice and it is not recommended since it may lead to obesity, especially if cereals are given early.

It is usual for cereal to be the first solid introduced but, if the baby is getting too fat, it is preferable to start with a protein-containing food such as meat. Cereal is introduced at about the age of 2–3 months. It is conveniently given before the 10 a.m. feed, being mixed with milk and given by spoon. After about 2 weeks, when the amount has been increased from one teaspoon to four, the cereal can also be given before the 6 p.m. feed. Egg yolk is started at about 4 months and may be given as a sponge or custard.

Between the ages of 4 and 6 months, bone broth with finely minced meat, liver or chicken may be given before the 2 p.m. feed and, if desired, the lightly cooked yolk of an egg can be mixed into it.

Once the baby starts to chew his fingers and even before he has any teeth he can be given fried bread or a hard rusk to chew on. At no time should the baby be left alone while feeding, for fear of choking. This is particularly vital when he is eating solid material such as a rusk, which might block the air passages. Every mother should be warned that if this does occur she should immediately hold the child upside down by the legs and smack his back until the piece is dislodged. Mothers must also be warned against the dangerous practice of leaving a baby feeding with the bottle propped up against the pillow. The risk of vomiting and consequent death from inhalation is very great.

Vegetable purée should be started by the age of 6 months when the iron stores in the liver are falling low. From the age of 6 months a baby can be given undiluted cow's milk, but, although pasteurized, it should be boiled until at least the age of 1 year in case infection has been introduced in the home.

Breast feeding can be gradually tailed off from the age of 4 months, stopping completely at 6 months. In countries where hygiene is poor and the risk of gastroenteritis great it is safer to encourage breast feeding alone up to the age of 12 months, only then introducing local foods. By this means, fewer babies will die of gastroenteritis although some will become anaemic, but this is the lesser of the two evils.

### Vitamin supplements

The supplements required by babies are principally vitamin C to prevent scurvy, and vitamin D to prevent rickets. The requirements for daily prophylaxis are vitamin C 30–50 mg; vitamin D 400 units. These may be given as orange juice and cod liver oil, or as proprietary preparations, usually in the form of drops.

One of the problems with cod liver oil which distresses mothers is when the child knocks the spoon with his hands and spills some oil on to his clothes, since the stain caused is likely to be permanent. This can be prevented by giving the oil during the daily bath. Mothers must be taught that the oil is given to prevent rickets. Many of them are unaware of its function or believe it is given to regulate the bowels; consequently they are liable to stop giving it for no good reason.

Vitamin C supplement is given as orange juice or rose-hip syrup concentrate. One teaspoon of the concentrate should be diluted with about 60 ml of boiled water and given by bottle at any suitable time during the day. Mothers should be specifically told not to boil the orange juice which would destroy the vitamin; a few will otherwise make this understandable mistake as they have been so repeatedly instructed to boil the milk feeds. For the same reason the boiled water should be cooled before mixing with the fruit juice.

## FEEDING DIFFICULTIES IN OLDER INFANTS AND CHILDREN

Today's parents have three major anxieties about their children's upbringing: feeding, sleeping and bowels. Of these, probably the greatest is their anxiety over the amount their children eat. To put it more accurately, the parents' worry is the amount of food their children do not eat.

The primary error is often the mother's belief that her child must eat a certain amount of food. The fear that her child may starve to death is very real, even if not expressed. Such fears and the resultant error of forcing the child to eat may be particularly strong if there are extra reasons for parental anxiety. The long awaited baby or the one who was born prematurely and required 'special care' are very likely candidates for undue parental anxiety. From the very earliest days of their child's life, preferably even before he is born, parents should be helped to adopt an attitude of unconcern over the amount eaten by their child. There is no fixed amount that a child should eat; mothers should allow their own common sense to tell them whether their child is well, not permitting the figure on a weight chart to dictate to them. Parents would be far happier if they could be weaned from weight charts and regular weighing sessions. There is no such thing as a 'normal' weight for a child; charts may show the average weight for a given age group but parents are liable to mistake the average weight for the 'normal' weight. This error in concept can be corrected only by parental instruction.

Parents must also be taught that the normal child gains weight erratically, in a step-ladder fashion, rather than as a simple steady gain. The child of small build is likely to put on weight at a slower rate than one who is of heavy build. Yet it is the mother whose child is of a light build who is likely to be the very one to become concerned by a slow weight gain and mistakenly to compare adversely his rate of weight gain with others of a larger build. Mothers should be told that a baby's rate of growth decreases during the first year (p. 242). Consequently, there is a reduction in the relative amount of food he requires.

The phrase 'a bonny baby' is mostly applied to those who are too fat. In prosperous countries today it is rare to find a healthy child whose weight is too low but it is common to find babies of excessive weight.

Weight is a very poor indication of health, whereas energy is an excellent guide. The child who is starved just sits about; nature knows that she must not waste any of the precious calories in needless activity. By contrast, the child who is energetic has a sufficient intake of calories even though his mother insists that he does not eat anything. Mothers must be helped to accept the fact that a child who is thriving is getting enough to eat, no matter how small his appetite.

It is about the middle of the child's first year of life that the majority of problems arise in relation to feeding. At this time a mother is starting her child on new foods which he may decide to refuse. Babies are very conservative individuals who dislike change; in such circumstances it is a mistake to force the child to take a food which he obviously dislikes. Mothers commonly force their children to eat vegetables, thereby putting the child off this particular food for many months. A child is much more likely to enjoy a certain food if, when young, he is not forced to eat it.

Children sometimes refuse food because they want to feed themselves, whereas the mother makes the mistake of insisting on feeding the child by spoon herself. Such mothers are commonly those who cannot bear their children to be messy; the tidy mother creates many extra problems for herself in the upbringing of her children. You cannot hope to have children and be tidy!

An additional factor behind a mother's concern that her child should eat is the fact that she has spent all morning cooking it for him. Some mothers are helped by being told not to prepare special dishes, but to purchase them ready-made beforehand.

It will be appreciated therefore that mothers must be prevented from coaxing their children to eat since this gives the child an opportunity to develop his natural negativistic tendencies. The bright child will be quick to exploit any gap in his parents' defences in this field. Dawdling over meals is one ruse used by the child whereas others who eat slowly do so because they enjoy playing with their food. Whatever the reason for dawdling, the mother must not make the mistake of having battles with her child to make him eat faster. Much better to give him less food in the first place and see how he reacts.

In addition to these methods of handling the child, the food should be made as appetizing as possible. Children, unlike adults, do not object to monotony; they enjoy having the same food day after day. Helpings should be small so that he can return for more, rather than large in the mistaken hope that he will at least eat some of it; children do not like plates piled high with food. Bright colours should be used whenever possible in cooking, more use being made of dyes such as cochineal to produce the coloured foods so much enjoyed by children.

Cheese, an excellent source of protein, is popular with children though, for no obvious reason, it is commonly regarded as an adult dish only. It may be grated on top of many dishes or given as processed cheeses which, in their attractive wrappings, are much appreciated. Raw carrots, a good source of vitamin A, are enjoyed by many children, providing an excellent mid-morning snack instead of biscuits.

Although babies are conservative in their habits they also have a great desire to experiment. Some of those who have turned away from being spoon-fed are delighted by an opportunity to feed themselves. In this connection it is relevant to point out that many babies from 6 to 18 months are too fat and that leaving them to feed themselves is a way of reducing their intake without causing tears.

Parents should view the problems of feeding through their child's eyes. They should picture how they would feel if, as soon as they sat down, a giant proceeded to nag them about their appetite and then spooned food into them. Looked at in this way a child's misery at mealtime or his refusal to feed becomes more understandable.

### The follow-up clinic

It is ideal that every newborn baby should be followed up in a special clinic for young babies, staffed by doctors and nurses with a wide experience of the problems involved. The title given to this clinic varies in different countries. In America the term 'well-baby clinic' is often used whereas in this country the clinic, run by the local authority, has been known as the Infant Welfare Clinic. This is a term which is likely to change in the future now that a wider concept of its work is accepted. The word 'welfare' is outmoded, suggesting something which the rich do for the poor. The emphasis should be on health but even the title 'Child Health Clinic' which has been proposed is too limiting. It has already been stressed (p. 5) that a child and his problems must be viewed in the context of his whole family; for this reason a more suitable term for the follow-up clinic would be 'Family Health Clinic'.

In the United Kingdom the doctor running such a clinic is increasingly likely to be a family doctor who is a member of a group practice and has received special postgraduate experience in paediatrics and child health.

Prior to the National Health Service it was necessary for the local authority to staff the infant welfare clinics because many families were without general practitioners. Today, such re-duplication of doctors is unnecessary. It is preferable that the doctor caring for the child when sick should be the same as the one looking after the child in health. He should be assisted by a Health Visitor who, as a highly trained nurse, is an essential member of the team. She is a member of the staff of the local Medical Officer of Health but should be seconded to work with one or more general practitioners.

The doctor will carry out the clinic in his own surgery or in Local Authority premises. If the surgery is used it is essential that a special session should be provided for the clinic rather than it being included as part of an ordinary surgery. The major function of the clinic lies in a positive approach to the provision of good health by means of health education and immunization procedures. Health education takes a great deal of time, more being achieved through group discussion than by didactic lectures. Mothers should not feel they are being hurried and should be encouraged to talk about their babies' ills and their own worries. A mother may need to be told that she is not abnormal if she does not feel maternal towards her baby as soon as he is born. It takes time to fall in love. She must be helped to learn to look for the need behind her child's behaviour so that she can interpret his needs.

The doctor must understand that if he treats feeding difficulties, crying or rashes as unimportant, because the baby's life is not in danger, he is ignoring the fact that these apparently minor problems cause mothers a great deal of anxiety and can affect the development of the normal mother-child relationship.

The frequency with which an individual attends such a clinic will vary according to the needs of the mother and the child. Attendances will be more frequent during the first year of life and with first children whose mothers are therefore less experienced. During the examination the child will be physically checked and will undergo developmental examinations and screening tests, such as those for vision and hearing, to determine that growth is proceeding normally. From these examinations the mother will learn something of the variation of normal.

Another essential function of the clinic is the early detection of handicaps. All children must be checked for these but to reduce the risk of delay in diagnosis those at special risk must be particularly watched. For this purpose it is usual for the Local Authority to keep a list of those infants 'at risk'. The 'at risk' register (Sheridan, 1962) comprises babies who have been subjected to any of a number of possible noxious influences such as:

*Family history*
Deafness, blindness, congenital dislocation of the hip. Family in a 'social problem' group including those born illegitimately and not adopted.

*Prenatal*

Rubella in early pregnancy. Bleeding in early months. Severe illness or major surgery in early months. Maternal diabetes.

*Perinatal*

Low birth weight. Post-maturity. Fetal distress. Asphyxia.

*Postnatal*

Prolonged poor sucking. Cyanotic attacks. Convulsions. Jaundice. Congenital abnormalities.

Children on the 'at risk' register will be seen more frequently than others and will usually attend a special follow-up clinic at a hospital run by a paediatrician. It has been suggested that the running of an 'at risk' register will cause undue parental anxiety. This can be avoided if the parents are handled wisely and are told that their babies are being carefully observed. The clinic is not of course termed an 'at risk' clinic but for those wishing a specific name it could be called an 'observation clinic'. The problem, however, revolves not round the name but how the parents are handled.

Once utopia has been achieved whereby the progress of every baby is checked by the family doctor and his health visitor in his own well-baby clinic, there should be no further need for an 'at risk' register which in any case is bound to miss a proportion of those who later turn out to be handicapped.

In developing countries it is unrealistic to separate the well and the ill children into different clinics. Such an arrangement could prevent a mother from bringing an obviously ill child if the clinic were held at a different time or place. Obviously this increases the risk of cross-infection, though this risk is less than appears at first sight since it is greatest in the early days of an illness, for example measles, and before such a mother appreciates that her child is ill. Separation of well and ill children into different clinics demands a sophisticated understanding by mothers; in most situations prevailing in a developing country it would lead to delay in diagnosis. For this reason it is preferable to organize an 'under-fives' clinic' (Morley, 1966). This should be staffed by as large a number of paramedical staff as possible, working under the supervision of a doctor. This method allows for further training of the staff as well as reducing the individual case load for the doctor.

## BIBLIOGRAPHY

AGATE F.J. & SILVERMAN W.A. (1963) The control of body temperature in the small newborn infant by low-energy infra-red radiation. *Pediatrics*, **31**, 725.

ANDREWS B.F. (1970) The small-for-date infant. *Ped. Clin. N.A.*, **17**, 1.

APGAR V. (1962) Further observations on the newborn scoring system. *Amer. J. Dis. Child.*, **104**, 419.

AVERY M.E. (1968) *The Lung and its Disorders in the Newborn Infant.* 2nd ed. Saunders, Philadelphia.

BAIN K. (1965) Personal communication.

BAIRD D. (1947) Social class and foetal mortality. *Lancet*, **2**, 531.

BAIRD D. (1952) Preventive medicine in obstetrics. *New Engl. J. Med.*, **246**, 561.

BAIRD D. (1964) The epidemiology of prematurity. *J. Pediat.*, **65**, 909.

BARTER R.H., HSU I., ERKENBECK R.V. & PUGSLEY L.Q. (1965) The prevention of pre-maturity in multiple pregnancy. *Amer. J. Obst. & Gynec.*, **91**, 787.

BOZIC C. (1963) Pulmonary hyaline membranes and vascular anomalies of the lung. Description of a case. *Pediatrics*, **32**, 1094.

BUETOW K.C. & KLEIN S.W. (1964) Effect of maintenance of 'normal' skin temperature on survival of infants of low birth weight. *Pediatrics*, **34**, 163.

BURNARD E.D. (1959) The cardiac murmur in relation to symptoms in the newborn. *Brit. med. J.*, **1**, 134.

BUTLER N.R. & BONHAM D.G. (1963) *Perinatal Mortality.* Livingstone, Edinburgh.

BUTLER N.R. & ALBERMAN E.D. (1969) *Perinatal Problems.* Livingstone, Edinburgh.

BUTTER N.R., GOLDSTEIN H. & ROSS E.M. (1972) Cigarette smoking in pregnancy: its influence on birth weight and perinatal mortality. *Brit. med. J.*, **1**, 127.

COE J.I. & PETERSON R.D.A. (1963) Sudden unexpected death in infancy and milk sensi-tivity. *J. Lab. clin. Med.* **62**, 477.

COOK R.C.M. & RICKHAM P.P. (1969) Neonatal intestinal obstruction due to milk curds. *J. Ped. Surg.*, **4**, 599.

DALY C., HEADY J.A. & MORRIS J.N. (1955) The effect of mother's age and parity on social class differences in infant mortality. *Lancet*, **1**, 445.

DAVIE R., BUTLER N. & GOLDSTEIN H. (1972) *From Birth to Seven.* Longman, London.

DAVIES P.A., ROBINSON R.J., SCOPES J.W., TIZARD J.P.M. & WIGGLESWORTH J.S. (1972) *Medical Care of Newborn Babies.* Heineman,n, London.

DAWES G.S. (1958) Changes in the circulation at birth and the effects of asphyxia. In *Recent Advances in Paediatrics* 2nd ed. Ed. Gairdner, D. Churchill, London.

DAY R.L., CALIGUIRI L., KAMENSKI C. & EHRLICH F. (1964) Body temperature and survival of premature infants. *Pediatrics*, **34**, 171.

DOUGLAS J.W.B. & BLOMFIELD J.M. (1958) *Children under Five.* Allen & Unwin, London.

DOUGLAS J.W.B. (1960) 'Premature' children at primary schools. *Brit. med. J.* **1**, 1008.

DRILLIEN C.M. (1972) Abnormal neurologic signs in the first year of life in low birth weight infants: possible prognostic significance. *Develop. Med. Child Neurol.*, **14**, 575.

DUBOWITZ V. (1968) Nerve conduction velocity—an index of neurological maturity of the newborn infant. *Develop. Med. Child Neurol.*, **10**, 741.

GLUCK L., KULOVICH M.V., BORER R.C., JR., BRENNER P.H., ANDERSON G.G. & SPELLACY W.N. (1971) Diagnosis of the respiratory distress syndrome by amniocentesis. *Amer. J. Obstet. & Gynec.*, **109**, 440.

GOLD E.M. (1970) Perinatal mortality. *Clin. Obstet. & Gynec.*, **13**.

GOMEZ P.C.W., NOAKES M. & BARRIE H. (1969) A prognostic score for use in the respira-tory-distress syndrome. *Lancet*, **1**, 808.

GRUENWALD P. (1963) Chronic fetal distress and placental insufficiency. *Biol. Neonat.*, **5**, 215.

GRUENWALD P. (1964) The course of the respiratory distress syndrome of newborn infants as indicated by poor stability of pulmonary expansion. *Acta Paediat.* (*Uppsala*), **53**, 470.

GUNTHER M., ASCHAFFENBURG R., PARISH W.E., BARRETT A.M. & COOMBS R.R.A. (1960) The level of antibodies to the proteins of cow's milk in the serum of normal human infants. *Immunology*, **3**, 296.

HARLEY J.D. & HERTZBERG R. (1965) Aetiology of cataracts in childhood. *Lancet*, **1**, 1084.

HARRISON V.C., HESSE H. DE V. & KLEIN M. (1968) The significance of grunting in hyaline membrane disease. *Pediatrics*, **41**, 549.

HEADY J.A., DALY C. & MORRIS J.N. (1955) Social and biological factors in infant mortality. Variation of mortality with mother's age and parity. *Lancet*, **1**, 395.

HEADY J.A., STEVENS C.F., DALY C. & MORRIS J.N. (1955) The independent effects of social class, region, the mother's age and her parity. *Lancet*, **1**, 499.

HEY, E.N. & KATZ G. (1970) The optimum thermal environment for naked babies. *Arch. Dis. Childh.*, **45**, 328.

HEY E.N. & O'CONNELL B. (1970) Oxygen consumption and heat balance in the cot-nursed baby. *Arch. Dis. Childh.*, **45**, 335.

HYTTEN F.E. (1954) Clinical and chemical studies in human lactation. *Brit. med. J.* **1**, pp. 175, 249.

HYTTEN F.E. & BAIRD D. (1958) The development of the nipple in pregnancy. *Lancet*, **1**, 1201.

ILLINGWORTH R.S. & KILPATRICK B. (1953) Lactation and fluid intake. *Lancet*, **2**, 1175.

JAMES L.S. (1965) Physiological adjustments at birth. *Anesthesiology*, **26**, 501.

JOLLY H., MOLYNEUX P. & NEWELL D.A. (1962) A controlled study of the effect of temperature of premature babies. *J. Pediat.* **60**, 889.

KEITEL H.G. & CHU E. (1965) Breast nodule in premature infant. *Amer. J. Dis. Child.* **109**, 121.

KINCARD-SMITH P. & BULLEN M. (1965) Bacteriuria in pregnancy. *Lancet*, **1**, 395.

LEBOYER F. (1975) Birth without violence. Knopf, New York.

LIGGINS G.C. & HOWIE R.N. (1972) A controlled trial of antepartum glucocorticoid treatment for prevention of the respiratory distress syndrome in premature infants. *Pediatrics*, **50**, 515.

LIND J. (1965) Physiological adaptation to the placental transfusion. *Canad. med. Ass. J.* **93**, 1091.

LIND T. & BILLEWICZ W.Z. (1971) A point-scoring system for estimating gestational age from examination of the amniotic fluid. *Brit. J. Hosp. Med.*, **5**, 681.

LOWE C.R. (1959) Effect of mothers' smoking habits on birth weight of their children. *Brit. med. J.* **2**, 673.

LUBCHENCO L.L. (1970) Assessment of gestational age and development at birth. *Ped. Clin. N.A.*, **17**, 125.

McCANCE R.A. & WIDDOWSON E.M. (1957) Physiology of the newborn animal. *Lancet*, **2**, 585.

McDONALD A.D. (1964) Intelligence in children of very low birth weight. *Brit. J. prev. soc. Med.* **18**, 59.

McKAY R.J. & LUCEY J.F. (1964) Medical progress—Neonatology. *New Engl. J. Med.*, **270**, 1231, 1292.

MORLEY D. (1966) In *Medical care in developing countries*. Ed. King M. Oxford University Press, Nairobi.

MORRIS J.N. & HEADY J.A. (1955) Social and biological factors in infant mortality. Objects and methods. *Lancet*, **1**, 343.

MORRIS J.N. & HEADY J.A. (1955) Mortality in relation to the father's occupation. *Lancet*, **1**, 554.

Moss P.D. (1957) Evaporated milk in infant feeding. *Brit. med. J.* **1**, 1453.

Neligan G.A., Parkin J.M. & Paul C. (1964) The use of an elastic band to prevent haemorrhage from the umbilical cord. *Arch. Dis. Childh.*, **39**, 630.

Office of Population Censuses and Surveys (1970) Classification of Occupations (1970) HMSO, London.

Parish W.E., Barrett A.M., Coombs R.R.A., Gunther M. & Camps F.E. (1960) Hypersensitivity to milk and sudden death in infancy. *Lancet*, **2**, 1106.

Prechtl H. & Beintema D. (1964) The neurological examination of the full-term newborn infant. *Clinics in Developmental Medicine*, No. 12. Spastics Society/Heinemann Medical, London.

Rawlings G., Reynolds E.O.R., Stewart A. & Strang L. (1971) Changing prognosis for infants of very low birth weight. *Lancet*, **1**, 516.

Robinson R.J. (1966) Assessment of gestational age by neurological examination. *Arch. Dis. Childh.*, **41**, 437.

Schulte F.J., Michaelis R., Linke I. & Nolte R. (1968) Motor nerve conduction velocity in term, preterm & small-for-dates newborn infants. *Pediatrics*, **42**, 17.

Scott K.E. & Usher R. (1966) Fetal malnutrition: its incidence, causes and effects. *Amer. J. Obstet. Gynec.* **94**, 951.

Sheridan M.D. (1962) Infants at risk of handicapping conditions. *Mth. Bull. Minist. Hlth Lab. Serv.* **21**, 238.

Silverman W.A., Fertig J.W. & Berger A.P. (1958) The influence of the thermal environment upon the survival of newly born premature infants. *Pediatrics*, **22**, 876.

Silverman W.A., Agate F.J. & Fertig J.W. (1963) A sequential trial of the non-thermal effect of atmospheric humidity on survival of newborn infants of low birth weight. *Pediatrics*, **31**, 719.

Sjöstedt S., Engleson G. & Rooth G. (1958) Dysmaturity. *Arch. Dis. Childh.*, **33**, 123.

Smallpeice V. & Davies P.A. (1964) Immediate feeding of premature infants with undiluted breast-milk. *Lancet*, **2**, 1349.

Swyer P.R. & Levison H. (1965) The current status of the respiratory distress syndrome of the newly born. *Canad. med. Ass. J.*, **93**, 335.

Usher R. (1963) Reduction of mortality from respiratory distress syndrome of prematurity with early administration of intravenous glucose and bicarbonate. *Pediatrics*, **32**, 966.

Usher R., McLean F. & Maughan G.B. (1964) Respiratory distress syndrome in infants delivered by Cesarean section. *Amer. J. Obst. Gynec.*, **88**, 806.

Usher R., McLean F. & Scott K.E. (1966) Judgement of fetal age. *Pediat. Clin. N. Amer.*, **13**, 835.

Waller H. (1946) The early failure of breast feeding. A clinical study of its causes and their prevention. *Arch. Dis. Childh.*, **21**, 1.

Wharton B.A. & Bower B.D. (1965) Immediate or later feeding for premature babies? *Lancet*, **2**, 969.

Wiener G. (1962) Psychologic correlates of premature birth: a review. *J. nerv. ment. Dis.*, **134**, 129.

Wigglesworth J.S. (1966) Foetal growth and retardation. *Brit. med. Bull.*, **22**, 13.

Wilson M.J. & Mikity V.G. (1960) A new form of respiratory disease in premature infants. *Amer. J. Dis. Child.*, **99**, 489.

Yerushalmy J. (1970) Relation of birth weight, gestational age and the rate of intrauterine growth to perinatal mortality. *Clin. Obstet. & Gynec.*, **13**, 107.

Zinkham W.H. (1963) Peripheral blood and bilirubin values in normal full-term primaquine-sensitive negro infants: effect of vitamin K. *Pediatrics*, **31**, 1963.

# CHAPTER 5

# NEONATAL DISORDERS

## BIRTH INJURIES

### INTRACRANIAL INJURY

This is the most serious of all birth injuries since it is very liable to be fatal. Even if not fatal it may leave the child with mental retardation, cerebral palsy or epilepsy, either alone or in combination. Damage to the brain may result from direct injury or anoxia and very often these two cannot be differentiated. Direct injury to the vital centres of the brain leads to impairment of respiration and therefore anoxia, while anoxia causes increased venous pressure leading to intracranial haemorrhage. In the mature baby intracranial haemorrhage is more often subdural, due to trauma, frequently in association with a torn falx. In the low birth weight baby it is usually due to anoxia and is either intraventricular, intracerebral or subarachnoid. In addition, the respiratory centre is depressed by a lack of oxygen so that anoxia from any cause initiates a vicious circle which must be broken by an immediate supply of oxygen into the lungs.

### Direct injury

This may produce obvious damage such as cerebral haemorrhage or dural tears, but in many instances no alteration in brain structure can be found. The role of anoxia in such cases is difficult to assess and must be decided by the evidence of asphyxia in other organs, such as Tardieu's spots which are petechial haemorrhages on the surface of the lungs and heart. Petechial haemorrhages in the brain result from asphyxia and not direct trauma.

The stresses which cause brain damage are especially those due to shearing forces associated with an abrupt change in head shape. Such changes occur when an unmoulded head is delivered precipitately, as in low birth weight babies, breech delivery or high forceps. The result may be a tear of the falx or more often of the tentorium cerebelli, which may then lead to haemorrhage.

### Anoxia (asphyxia)

*Aetiology.* Of all the causes of anoxia the most important is blockage of the respiratory passages by mucus, blood and amniotic debris. The role of intra-cranial injury has been discussed above. Sedatives and general anaesthetics given to the mother act directly on the respiratory centre of the baby. For this reason pudental block for forceps delivery is preferable to general anaesthesia, causing a significant reduction in the incidence of asphyxia in such babies. Placental function is impaired by premature separation, due in some instances to accidental haemorrhage or placenta praevia. The placenta may be abnor-mally compressed as a result of malpresentation or excessively strong and rapid uterine contractions. Kinking of the cord may result from malpresen-tation and be associated with prolapse of the cord. Anoxia may also result from diminished space for pulmonary expansion, as occurs with a diaphrag-matic hernia. These factors may exert their effect during intrauterine life or immediately after birth.

Failure to breathe at birth may result from a congenital defect of the brain. In such cases, subsequent brain injury may be incorrectly attributed to the asphyxia instead of to the underlying defect.

## CLINICAL FEATURES OF INTRACRANIAL BIRTH INJURY

In its most severe form the infant is stillborn. The next most severe is white asphyxia, the features being those of shock. Less serious is blue asphyxia.

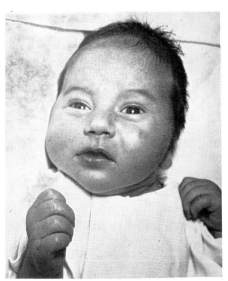

Fig. 17. Cerebral irritation. The eyes are widely open and staring. The fists are clenched and drawn up towards the face.

The infant with white asphyxia lies quite still, failing to respond to any stimulation. The baby is ashen-grey, hypotonic and often cold. The pulse rate is slow, thready and possibly irregular so that the situation may show itself before birth from examination of the fetal heart. The fetal heart should be assessed between uterine contractions because the normal heart may be slowed during these contractions. Slowing of the heart rate in the fetus or newborn baby is possibly the greatest indication of hypoxia. Additional ante-partum evidence of anoxia is the passage of meconium, since anoxia increases peristalsis and relaxes the anal sphincter. In such cases there may be meconium staining of the skin and umbilical cord. This sign is only of value in vertex presentation, since relaxation of the anal sphincter is common in breech delivery and has no significance. Intrauterine anoxia may cause excessive fetal movements for a short time.

Respirations are shallow, slow and irregular and life may gradually fade out despite all attempts at resuscitation. If the condition improves, the picture usually changes to one of cerebral irritation. However, this may be the state from the outset rather than a preliminary period of shock. In this stage the infant is hyperactive, the Moro reflex being heightened. Spontaneous twitching movements may occur which, in the severest cases, become generalized convulsions. Respirations are irregular and periods of apnoea may alternate with rapid respirations so that the baby is intermittently cyanosed. The facial appearance is very characteristic, the baby lying anxious and alert with wide open eyes as though awaiting an impending fit; the fists are usually tightly clenched with the hands drawn up to the face (Fig. 17). Raised intracranial pressure causes the fontanelle tension to be increased and a high-pitched 'cerebral' cry. Head retraction and nystagmus may occur, feeds being taken badly and often vomited. Some babies with asphyxia develop ileus, leading to green vomit and abdominal distension.

In the state of blue asphyxia the tone is relatively good and the pulse full and regular. In contrast to the baby with white asphyxia who makes no response to the stimulus of a pharyngeal or nasal catheter, the one with blue asphyxia grimaces or coughs when such a catheter is passed. The onset of respirations may be delayed, but these babies usually recover completely and only occasionally do they pass through a stage of cerebral irritation.

Most infants with intracranial injury show clinical signs from birth but, occasionally, these may be delayed for 2–3 days and such cases are usually severe. Similar symptoms may result from hypoglycaemia; differentiation is essential and is made by estimating the blood sugar level (see p. 641).

TREATMENT OF ANOXIA (ASPHYXIA)

The causes of anoxia are discussed on p. 96. The fundamental management of the condition lies in their prevention by good obstetric care. In treatment, the first requirement is a clear airway; this is followed by artificial respiration if the infant is not breathing, oxygen and, finally, drugs.

*Suction.* As soon as the infant is born he should be held upside down and pharyngeal suction applied using a rubber-ended mucus catheter. The tip should be moved gently in the mouth as it is very easy to damage the fragile buccal mucous membrane. Moreover, pharyngeal suction can cause slowing of the heart rate from vagal stimulation. Gastric aspiration should be routine in all asphyxiated infants since any material in the stomach is liable to be vomited and aspirated. It should also be routine for all infants born by Caesarean section, because the absence of the thoracic and abdominal compression of normal delivery leaves mucus, blood and amniotic debris in the stomach Gastric aspiration of infants born by Caesarean section reduces the incidence of respiratory and feeding difficulties.

*Artificial respiration.* If the infant is not breathing there must be no delay in providing artificial respiration since each minute lost increases the chance of permanent cerebral damage. In hospital practice this can be given by means of an endotracheal tube, but there must be safeguards to ensure that the pressure of oxygen does not exceed 30 cm of water otherwise the lungs can be overdistended and a pneumothorax result. Suction through the endotracheal tube must be obtained via a separate catheter inserted into the the tube and not by attaching the suction directly to the tube, since this may completely deflate the lung.

In home practice, mouth to mouth respiration after the insertion of a plastic oropharyngeal airway is the best alternative if the operator is not skilled in the technique of endotracheal intubation. The possible risk of infection is far outweighed by the fact that this is the most efficient simple method of artificial respiration for home use; prophylactic antibiotics can be given. Care must be taken to prevent overdistension of the lungs; the operator should be conscious of using his diaphragm rather than his cheeks, thereby keeping the pressure within safe limits. He must also remember to remove his mouth between breaths to allow the baby to exhale.

*Oxygen.* When oxygen is being given the baby must be breathing, either naturally or artifically. So often, oxygen is given to a baby who is not breathing. For emergency use a mask is used, but if required for long a tent or incubator is the most satisfactory. The only value of nasal catheters as a means of oxygen administration is that they are a powerful sensory stimulant, often causing a gasp to be taken when they are passed. Gastric oxygen should not be used as it is ineffective.

During the process of resuscitation the baby must not be allowed to get cold; this not only reduces the chance of survival but increases the oxygen requirements by raising the metabolic rate. If there is insufficient oxygen this metabolic response to cold fails, causing a drop in temperature. Hypoxia, therefore, can cause the body temperature to fall and for this reason a low or falling body temperature in an ill newborn infant is an indication for increasing the rate of oxygen flow to the infant, even though the baby is not cyanosed. In such cases the arterial $pO_2$ should be monitored in order to avoid excessive oxygen tension which in a preterm baby might lead to retrolental fibroplasia (p. 63).

It is of interest that newborn babies exposed to low temperatures do not respond by shivering. The subsequent rise in metabolic rate is possibly due to heat produced in the baby's brown fat. Brown fat is believed to be an important site of heat production in the human baby as in other newborn mammals (Hull, 1966).

*Drugs.* Immediate endotracheal intubation and artificial respiration have superseded the use of respiratory stimulants in babies with respiratory failure at birth.

Nalorphine (Lethidrone) is a specific antidote to morphine and pethidine, though of no effect against the barbiturates. Ideally, it should be given to the mother before delivery if birth is likely to occur soon after she has received one of these drugs. For the baby, 0·25 to 1 mg may be given into the umbilical vein for rapid action, but if the urgency is less the dose can be given intramuscularly.

If the infant is severely depressed and fails to respond to the combination of these measures he is probably acidotic and hypoglycaemic. Therefore, in addition to continuing lung inflation by artificial respiration through an endotracheal tube, the baby should be given 5 mEq of sodium bicarbonate and 5 g of glucose intravenously. In such babies external cardiac massage should also be performed if the apex beat is inaudible. For this the baby must be lying on a hard flat surface; rapid rhythmic depression of the lower left sternal border is then performed using two fingers.

TREATMENT OF INTRACRANIAL INJURY

The first essential is to deal with asphyxia as already described. The next is to prevent a convulsion since the risk of permanent brain damage is increased if a convulsion occurs. If the baby shows signs of cerebral irritation he must receive adequate sedation which in severe cases should first be given by intramuscular injection. Phenobarbitone is probably the best drug in these severe cases, given in a dose of 2–3 mg/kg every 6–8 hours. Therapy should be continued for at least 3 days in severe cases, though individual doses should be omitted if too heavy a sedation has been achieved. Babies with cerebral irritation who are being transferred to hospital must receive a dose of sedative before being moved so as to reduce the risk of a convulsion during the extra movement of the journey.

Nursing should be carried out with the head raised in order to reduce the increased intracranial pressure. The introduction of feeds should be delayed until the baby is well sedated, otherwise there is a risk of vomiting and aspiration of the feed. Tube feeding should be used if the infant does not suck and swallow satisfactorily.

Dexamethasone and mannitol can be given to reduce cerebral oedema. Vitamin K is often recommended for babies with intracranial injury to lessen the amount of bleeding but there is little evidence that hypoprothrombinaemia plays any part in the condition. If there is a deficiency of fibrinogen, fresh frozen plasma should be given intravenously.

PROGNOSIS IN INTRACRANIAL INJURY

It is very difficult to forecast the future mental and motor progress of these babies but the occurrence of fits gravely reduces the chance that they will be normal. All babies who have suffered intracranial birth injury should be kept under close observation for at least a year in order to detect cerebral palsy, mental retardation and deafness at the earliest opportunity.

The EEG is of considerable prognostic value in these children. In a study of 135 neonates with convulsions or suspected convulsions of multiple aetiology, 70 per cent of those with a normal EEG developed normally, whereas 64 per cent of those with an abnormal EEG died or were left with neurological damage (Tibbles & Prichard, 1965).

## SOFT TISSUE INJURIES

### Bruises and abrasions

These are often due to forceps or the ventouse extractor, but may be due to the attendant's nails which must always be kept short. Babies may also scratch their own face if nails are not cut. Mothers of first babies need to be shown how to cut the nails as it is not easy. Doing it when the baby is asleep makes it easier.

### Cephalhaematoma (Fig. 18)

This is a collection of blood lying between the pericranium (periosteum) and the underlying skull bone. Since the pericranium passes through the sutures, the haematoma is confined to the area of one bone, usually a parietal, and never crosses the midline. It should not therefore be confused with the caput succedaneum which is due to oedema of the presenting part and occurs anywhere on the head.

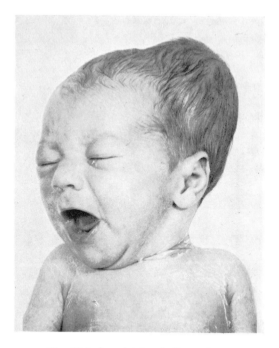

FIG. 18 Left parietal cephalhaematoma.

Cephalhaematomata, which may be bilateral, should be left strictly alone; they always subside although this may take a few weeks, and aspiration only runs the risk of introducing infection. Calcification may occur in the blood clot while ossification sometimes occurs at the edge of the haematoma where the periosteum is lifted (Fig. 19). This causes an irregularity of the skull surface which usually disappears in time.

### Traumatic cyanosis

This condition results from pressure on the neck veins and from temporary obstruction of the airway by a tight cord round the neck or by compression of the shoulders into the neck. Mucus in the air passages could also be a cause by producing temporary obstruction. The infant is cyanosed above the point of pressure and a normal colour below. The colour is due to the fact that venous congestion has been so intense that blood cells have extravasated into the tissues; these cells take several days to disappear and may cause jaundice.

Within a few hours of delivery petechiae appear on the forehead; after about 2 days a crescentic haemorrhage is seen over the sclera on one or both

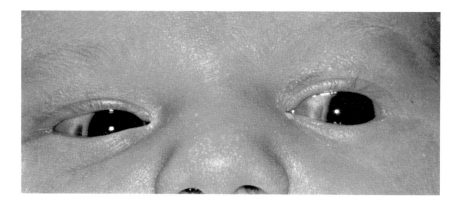

FIG. 20. Crescentic conjunctival haemorrhages in a child who had shown traumatic cyanosis. These are visible on the inner side of both eyes.

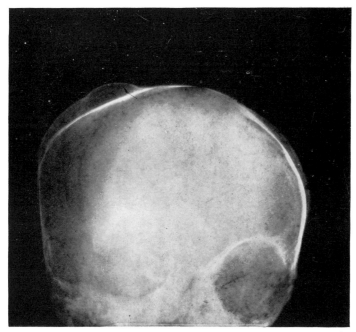

Fig. 19. Ossification of cephalhaematoma overlying the right parietal bone.

sides of the pupil (Fig. 20). The haemorrhage is sometimes most alarming to the mother who should be reassured that it will disappear within a few days and her child will be normal, unless there are any other complications. The condition is very common, though often missed unless a routine search is made for the haemorrhages. Retinal haemorrhages occur in about 35 per cent of newborn babies if examined in the first 6 hours.

### Sternomastoid tumour (Fig. 21)

This lump results from a tear of some of the fibres of the sternomastoid muscle, or damage to their blood supply during delivery. It particularly occurs following breech delivery when the muscle is more likely to be excessively stretched. The lump does not usually appear until the baby is about 2 weeks old; it is therefore unlikely to be only a haematoma as has been suggested in the past. Glairy material, resulting from muscle necrosis, has been found in addition to blood: the lump is probably composed of this material, of blood and of fibrous tissue formed during healing. The lump always diappears within a few weeks but, during healing, steps must be taken to prevent muscle shortening with its consequent torticollis. This is achieved by muscle stretching exercises. The mother is also instructed how to carry the baby and how to place him in the cot in such a way as to produce maximum stretching of the affected muscle.

## Subcutaneous fat necrosis

This condition consists of a subcutaneous indurated mass to which the overlying skin is adherent. It is due to necrosis of subcutaneous fat from compres-

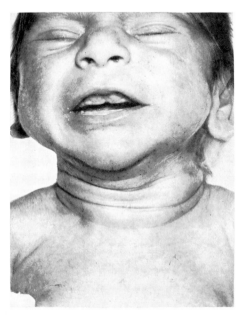

FIG. 21. Left sternomastoid tumour. A lump is visible on the left side of the neck.

sion during delivery and therefore occurs over bony prominences against which the fat has been compressed. The overlying skin is sometimes mauve. The most common sites are the cheeks and over the scapulae. There is no treatment, the lesion resolving in a few weeks.

## NERVE INJURIES

### Facial nerve

This is the most common nerve to be damaged at birth, the site of injury being the point at which the nerve crosses the ramus of the mandible. It usually results from the blade of a forceps, but may occur in a normal delivery from compression of the nerve against the sacral promontory.

The lesion is of the lower motor neurone type so that all facial movements are affected. At rest the affected side of the face appears smoother than the normal and the eye more widely open. The abnormality is more obvious on crying when the mouth is drawn to the normal side (Fig. 22). No blinking occurs so that the eye must be protected by nursing the child with the affected eye upwards and by inserting castor oil or liquid paraffin drops at frequent

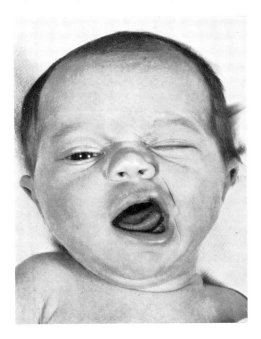

FIG. 22. Paralysis of the right facial nerve due to injury at birth. The right eye cannot be closed and the mouth is drawn to the left side.

intervals to keep it moist. Recovery is usually rapid and there is seldom any difficulty in sucking. Failure of recovery indicates that the lesion is due to agenesis of the nerve nucleus and not trauma. Such cases may be unilateral or bilateral and may be associated with other congenital anomalies (Möbius's syndrome).

### Erb's paralysis

This is due to a lesion of the brachial plexus affecting the fifth and sixth cervical nerves or their roots. It is caused by excessive stretching of the neck, particularly occurring in breech deliveries. The arm lies limply beside the trunk with the elbow extended, the forearm pronated and the fingers flexed in the 'porter's tip' position (Fig. 23). There is voluntary movement of the fingers but none of the arm.

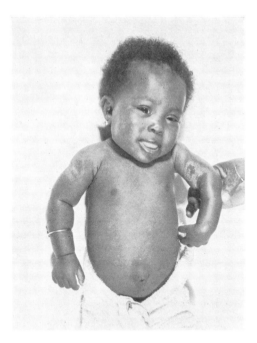

FIG. 23. Left Erb's paralysis. The forearm is pronated and the wrist flexed. In addition to the brachial plexus lesion the cervical sympathetic nerve supply has been damaged, producing a Horner's syndrome on the same side, indicated by ptosis and enophthalmos.

*Treatment.* The arm should be rested for the first week to allow haemorrhage and oedema in the nerves to subside, and any associated shoulder damage to heal. Splinting in abduction is no longer recommended since this may cause ultimate restriction of movement. Passive movements should be started at the end of the first week, the mother being taught how to put the shoulder, elbow and wrist through a full range of movement before or after each feed. Recovery may take several months and is not always complete.

### Klumpke's paralysis

This lesion is less common than Erb's and is due to involvement of the seventh and eighth cervical and first thoracic nerves. The result is a flaccid paralysis of the hand.

*Treatment.* The hand should be splinted in the neutral position. The prognosis is less good than for an Erb's palsy, especially if there is an associated Horner's syndrome due to sympathetic nerve damage.

## BONE INJURIES

The most common bones to be affected are the skull, clavicle and long bones.

### Skull

Considering the strains to which the head is subjected at birth, fractures of the skull are not so frequent as might be expected owing to its capacity for being moulded. Fractures may be linear or depressed, thereby causing a spoon-shaped depression. Such fractures occur more often during spontaneous delivery than forceps delivery and result from pressure of the skull on the sacral promontory or on the pubic ramus. It is not usually necessary to elevate a depressed fracture since elevation occurs spontaneously over the next few weeks.

The outlook depends on the associated brain damage; if there is none, the fracture need cause no anxiety.

### Clavicle

Unless a snap is heard during delivery, this fracture is not usually diagnosed until a lump of callus is felt during the second or third week. No treatment is required and recovery is perfect.

### Long bones

The humerus and femur are most commonly involved, the usual occasion being when a limb is brought down during delivery. Fortunately, healing takes place readily and no deformity results even if alignment is not perfect. For this reason, only minimal splinting is required, it usually being sufficient to bandage the arm to the side or the leg to its fellow.

## INJURIES TO ORGANS

Breech delivery frequently causes bruising of the external genitalia. If a baby is resuscitated with oxygen at too high a pressure the lungs can burst, causing an artificial pneumothorax. Lungs can also be damaged by manual artificial respiration, but with the availability of endotracheal intubation this method should now never be used.

The liver and spleen can be damaged by the operator's hand during breech delivery. The liver is particularly vulnerable since, in the newborn infant, it extends 2 cm below the right costal margin. Rupture of the liver or spleen causes sudden collapse associated with pallor and a thready pulse. The only hope is an immediate blood transfusion through the umbilical vein, followed by laparotomy. Evidence of rupture may be delayed a few hours after birth if a haematoma is held up under the capsule and later ruptures through it.

Massive haemorrhage may occur into the adrenals during birth. These glands are, usually congested at this time and a combination of asphyxia and trauma during breech delivery may cause bleeding. If the infant survives, subsequent calcification may occur in the adrenal haematoma.

## NEONATAL INFECTION

The newborn infant has incomplete immunity so that infections are more serious and may be fatal within a few hours. The most common organism is the staphylococcus but *E. coli*, acquired from the mother's intestinal tract during delivery, is a particular hazard at this age. Other organisms include *Haemophilus influenzae*, *Streptococcus faecalis* and *Klebsiella*. Thrush is a common infection, being discussed separately on p. 115.

The frequency of infection with gram-negative organisms in the newborn is correlated with a lack of immunoglobulin M (IgM). Most of the antibacterial activity against gram-negative organisms is carried in this fraction which is too large to pass across the placenta from the maternal serum. Synthesis of this fraction by the baby usually commences during the first week, so that a transient deficiency exists for the first two weeks of postnatal life which is partly made good by colostrum (p. 76). The only class of immunoglobulin of sufficiently small molecular size to cross the placenta is the IgG fraction which thereby comprises the bulk of the healthy infant's immunoglobulins at birth.

### CLINICAL FEATURES

These are separated into the general signs common to all forms of infection and local signs depending on the site. The risk of septicaemia is high so that a blood culture should be taken in all cases of suspected neonatal infection.

### GENERAL SIGNS

The most important symptom of neonatal sepsis is loss of appetitite. If a baby has been feeding well and then goes off his feeds, infection should be regarded as the cause until this is disproved. If feeds are then forced, vomiting occurs which is often associated with diarrhoea, causing the baby to become dehydrated. Dehydration is evident from the fontanelle and eyes which become sunken, from dryness of the mouth and from loss of elasticity of the skin. In the early stages the dehydrated infant is restless for fluid but he then falls into an apathy which may lead rapidly to death. Convulsions may occur in the terminal stage.

Fever is not always present with infection in the neonatal period and a fall in temperature associated with collapse is as common as a rise. Pyrexia is not therefore required for the diagnosis of infection in the newborn. Moreover, babies may develop fever from lack of fluid only, a situation particularly found in large babies who have been given insufficient fluid for their size during the first 2–3 days of life. The condition is sometimes called *dehydration fever*.

Three other signs are important, the presence of any one indicating a serious infection. These are oedema, haemorrhage and jaundice, and although there are commoner causes for each one, infection must be considered whenever these signs appear in the newborn period.

GENERAL TREATMENT

In view of the potential severity of any infection in the newborn period, prevention is the first line of treatment. This is effected by the avoidance of birth trauma and good nursing hygiene, particularly an efficient barrier technique. The risk of pseudomonas infection from equipment and from stagnant water used for humidification in incubators is great. For this reason equipment must never be washed in basins used for washing hands. The chance of cross-infection is much greater in hospital than in the home. Staphylococci in the intestines of healthy newborn infants are an important reservoir of infection in the nursery so that overcrowded nurseries are a particular danger. It is always safer for the baby to be nursed with his mother, especially if they can be together in a single room. Hexachlorophene powder used as described on p. 41 is both safe and effective in reducing staphylococcal infection. Scrupulous attention must be paid to the washing of hands after each baby is handled since this is the chief route by which infection is transferred from one patient to another. Mask and gown techniques must be faultless. If masks are touched the dangers are greater than if no mask is worn. Staff with colds, boils or diarrhoea should be excluded from dealing with babies.

PROPHYLACTIC ANTIBIOTICS

The administration of antibiotics prophylactically to healthy infants believed to be at greater than average risk of infection is debated, though opinion is hardening against this practice (Davies *et al.*, 1972). It used to be routine in most centres to give prophylactic antibiotics to all babies born following prolonged rupture of the membranes, but this is no longer common practice.

ANTIBIOTIC TREATMENT IN THE NEWBORN

Present policy is to give antibiotics at the earliest sign of infection without waiting for the results of bacterial investigations, although these must be initiated before starting treatment. In the absence of exact knowledge of the infecting organism a combination of antibiotics should be used to be effective against both gram-positive and gram-negative organisms. This combination will vary according to local information of likely bacterial sensitivity. Useful combinations are cephaloridine and gentamicin or ampicillin and cloxicillin.

A course of treatment should last at least 5 days and for severe infections treatment should be continued until there is clear evidence from the clinical picture and negative bacterial results that the infection has been eradicated. During the first week, the intramuscular route is usually safest because of uncertain absorption from the intestine.

Tetracycline should not be given since it stains the teeth yellow. It may also suppress growth, and for this reason should not be prescribed for pregnant women. Sulphonamides should be avoided since they increase the risk of kernicterus in the newborn period (p. 118).

Chloramphenicol must be used with great caution in young infants since in doses suitable for older children it can be toxic, leading to the 'grey baby syndrome'. Chloramphenicol, like bilirubin, is detoxicated by combining with glucuronic acid to form a glucuronide. In young babies there may be a deficiency of glucuronyl transferase, the enzyme responsible for this reaction. In this syndrome the baby goes grey, vomits and develops abdominal distension. Respiratory distress may occur; the baby then collapses and may die.

An infected baby must be strictly isolated. Parenteral fluids should be supplied if oral feeds are not retained.

### Gram-negative bacteraemia

This very serious condition presents with the acute onset of extreme shock, the infant being pale, cold and with a blotchy cyanosis. It may be associated with pyelonephritis, meningitis or pneumonia, but there may be no local signs of infection. The common organisms are *E. coli*, *Klebsiella* and *Proteus*. The most effective antibiotic is gentamicin given intramuscularly. Hydrocortisone and plasma should also be given.

LOCAL SIGNS AND TREATMENT

The local signs of infection may be much less obvious in the newborn than in later life and a fulminating infection with septicaemia may show only general signs. Only special points of difference relating to the newborn period are discussed here as infections are described in full under each system. The commonest sites for infection are the eyes, skin and umbilicus.

### Eyes (Ophthalmia neonatorum)

A 'sticky eye' is common, producing a purulent conjunctival exudate. The eyeball is not usually inflamed, though in severe cases there may be considerable oedema and inflammation of the eyelids.

A swab should be sent for culture, though this will be sterile in the majority of cases appearing in the first 2 days of life. The inflammation in such babies is due to irritation from amniotic fluid, meconium and blood; it can be largely prevented by the use of moist cotton wool swabs to clean the eyes immediately after birth.

The infant should be nursed on the side, with the affected eye against the mattress. This prevents the downward spread of material to the good eye which would occur if the affected eye was uppermost. Since cases occurring in the first 2 days are usually sterile, it is sufficient to treat these with mechanical methods aimed at clearing the exudate from the eyes. This can best be achieved by irrigation of the eye with saline using an intravenous giving set. This is more efficient than the old method of using an undine or swabs. By the time the result of the swab is received the eye is usually clear, but if not, and if any growth is reported, a local antibiotic to which the organism is sensitive can be applied.

Cases occurring after the first 2 days of life should always be treated with a local antibiotic in addition to saline irrigation, without awaiting the bacterial results. The commonest organism is the staphylococcus for which the most suitable local antibiotic is chloramphenicol. This is better applied as an ointment than as drops, which are rapidly washed away. If the infection recurs or proves resistant to treatment, blockage of the nasolacrimal duct (p. 225) should be suspected. In the treatment of gonorrhoeal ophthalmia, penicillin is much more effective than chloramphenicol. It is given as eye drops, starting with one drop per minute for the first 30 minutes.

In previous times, when ophthalmia neonatorum was commonly due to gonococcal infection, it was routine to apply 1 per cent silver nitrate drops into the eyes of all newborn infants. The rarity of gonococcal infection and the effectiveness of penicillin against it had mainly stopped this procedure, which often caused chemical conjunctivitis. However, the recent increased incidence of venereal disease has caused some centres to re-introduce this prophylactic measure, particularly since the early discharge ('48 hour') of mothers and babies from maternity units could lead to delayed diagnosis.

## Skin

Staphylococcal skin sepsis is unfortunately common in maternity nurseries; the same organism may cause ophthalmia and umbilical sepsis in the babies, and mastitis in the mothers. The lesions, which are not usually seen until the end of the first week, consist of isolated pustules. Staphylococcal paronychia is also common. The best local treatment is to apply 0·5 per cent aqueous gentian violet to the lesions. The colour of the paint is a disadvantage but the mother will usually accept this if it is explained to her beforehand that this method is more satisfactory than ointment. In all but the mildest cases systemic antibiotics should also be given.

In some instances large bullae appear, to which the name pemphigus is often applied incorrectly; this condition should be called *bullous impetigo* (p. 664). These lesions must be differentiated from *urticaria neonatorum* which occurs earlier in life, produces weals as well as lesions like pustules, and disappears spontaneously within 2–3 days (see. p. 673).

### Ritter's disease

This is severe generalized exfoliative dermatitis of the newborn due to a staphylococcal infection. It is one variety of toxic epidermal necrolysis. The outer layer of the skin in undenuded areas can be easily rubbed off by gentle pressure (Nikolsky's sign) so that large red exposed areas result. The condition was often fatal before the advent of antibiotics.

### Umbilicus

A 'sticky umbilicus' is common, usually being due to the staphylococcus. The frequent application of 70 per cent industrial methylated spirits is the best local treatment. Powders such as penicillin are unsatisfactory since they cake, causing local irritation.

### Urinary infection

There are usually no local symptoms so that in every case of suspected infection the urine must be examined microscopically for pus cells and cultured. The frequency of urinary infections in the newborn baby is hotly debated at the present time because of the difficulties in making a definite diagnosis in young infants. This aspect is discussed on p. 388.

### Meningitis

The incidence of meningitis is greater in newborn infants than in older children and its mortality higher. The commonest contributory factors are obstetric complications, particularly birth trauma, low birth weight, prolonged rupture of the membranes and concurrent maternal infection. Unfortunately, prophylactic antibiotics are not really effective so that such babies must be very closely watched for evidence of meningitis. To add to the difficulties, meningitis in the newborn produces a different clinical picture from that in older children, the signs being much less definite. Neck stiffness and head retraction, which are useful signs in the older patient, occur only as late signs in the newborn. The baby becomes drowsy and irritable. The most useful sign is the increased tension of the anterior fontanelle which may even produce a visible bump on the head and be the chief reason for the mother calling the doctor. There is an absence of the normal pulsation of the anterior fontanelle.

Owing to the absence of the classic signs of meningitis, a lumbar puncture should be performed on all babies in whom the site of the infection is undetermined. *E. coli* is more often the cause of meningitis at this age than at any other period of life. It has a very high mortality and those who survive are liable to be mentally impaired.

### Gastroenteritis

Diarrhoea is a common symptom of infection anywhere in the body; it is then termed *parenteral gastroenteritis*. *True gastroenteritis* is commonly due to one of the specific types of *E. coli* or to one of the enteroviruses, but may be staphylococcal and follow broad spectrum antibiotic therapy. Parenteral fluids are indicated if dehydration is present. The subject is fully discussed on p. 299.

### Nose

Nasal infection such as acute coryza, occurring in young babies, causes a mechanical problem in addition to the infection. Normal infants have great difficulty in breathing through the mouth so that nasal obstruction causes considerable feeding difficulties. The use of nasal drops containing $\frac{1}{2}$ per cent ephedrine in normal saline is often helpful; 1–2 drops should be inserted into each nostril before feeds.

'Snuffles' are very common in young infants and are more often due to a congenitally low nasal bridge and small nasal passages than to infection. This accounts for the frequency of the symptom in mongols. Syphilis as a cause is no longer seen in Great Britain. Apart from the noise there are usually no symptoms. If there is any difficulty in breathing, ephedrine nasal drops should be tried. The symptom disappears as the nose enlarges with age and has usually gone by the first birthday.

### Ears

Otitis media (p. 337) is not common in the neonatal period but the ears should be checked if infection is suspected.

### Mouth

Infection of the throat is more often due to pharyngitis than tonsillitis which is a disease of older children (p. 333). The most common oral infection in the newborn is thrush (p. 115).

## Lungs

### PNEUMONIA

*Congenital.* Infection acquired *in utero*, possibly ascending via the genital tract, can cause pneumonia within the first 48 hours of life. Histological examination of the placenta in such cases shows inflammatory changes. The commonest causal organisms are *E. coli* and *Streptococcus faecalis.* The autopsy findings differ from those in pneumonia acquired postnatally in that the bronchi are clear but the alveoli are filled with cellular exudate.

*Acquired.* This type of pneumonia may develop within a few days of birth, the predominant organism being *E. Coli* and *Staphylococcus aureus* (see p. 347). This may follow staphylococcal skin sepsis and lead to epidemics of staphylococcal pneumonia in maternity nurseries. The autopsy findings differ from the congenital type in that the emphasis is on acute inflammatory changes in the bronchioles. Abscess formation and empyema are frequent in staphylococcal pneumonia.

*Clinical features.* Whether congenital or acquired the predominating clinical picture is that of cerebral irritation resulting from anoxia. Respiratory symptoms are not only minimal but are commonly absent in babies dying from pneumonia in the first 48 hours of life. Since pneumonia is the most frequent severe infection in the newborn, all babies ill from infection on the first day must be regarded as having pneumonia until this is disproved. The chest X-ray may show few changes but if the lung pattern is altered there will be coarse irregular opacities.

*Treatment.* The general management of pneumonia is discussed on p. 346 and of staphylococcal pneumonia on p. 348. All cases of pneumonia in the newborn must be treated immediately and vigorously. Until bacterial studies are completed the best combination of drugs is cephaloridine and gentamicin.

*Prevention.* The prevention and immediate treatment of asphyxia go far to reduce the incidence of pneumonia in the newborn.

### MECONIUM ASPIRATION

This may cause severe asphyxia and shock at birth, with irregular gasping respirations and bradycardia. Once breathing is established, severe respiratory difficulty resembling RDS (p. 64) is obvious. These two disorders are differentiated radiologically since meconium aspiration causes mottled densities from lobular collapse.

Immediate assisted respiration is essential since death can occur within a few minutes. Recovery is likely if the infant survives 24 hours although this may take up to one week to be complete.

The stomach should be aspirated in any baby born with meconium stained liquor in order to reduce the risk of further aspiration.

ATELECTASIS

This term indicates failure of lung expansion after birth. Its role cannot be separated from pneumonia in the neonatal period since the two are often associated. Complete aeration of the lungs does not take place with the first breath, but over a matter of hours or even days. Failure of expansion renders the atelectatic portion more liable to infection while respiratory infection makes full expansion less likely.

**Thrush**

This fungal infection is caused by *Candida albicans* and its occurrence often indicates faulty technique. In hospital it is particularly liable to appear in nurseries which are overcrowded and understaffed. Special care baby units run a special risk because the increased heat and humidity favour the organism. In the home it results from lack of hygiene in feed preparation. Vaginal thrush in the mother may be transmitted to her baby, sometimes from contamination of the skin of the breast. Broad spectrum antibiotics cause a more rapid spread of thrush though they do not increase its incidence. The fungus exists as filaments and spores; the latter, being resistant to drying, remain in nurseries for long periods.

The lesions occur chiefly on the buccal mucous membrane but also on the tongue and palate. They consist of white patches which differ from milk-curds in being attached so firmly to the mucous membrane that they can be scraped off only with difficulty, leaving a bleeding granular surface. Thrush on the tongue causes a fur which is thicker and whiter than ordinary fur. These lesions cause discomfort so that the baby goes off his feeds and often vomits. In hospital it should be a routine for the nurse to check the mouth for thrush before every feed.

Lesions may occur in the oesophagus and, since the fungus is excreted in the stool, it may also cause a buttock rash consisting of an erythematous maculopapular eruption with a perianal distribution.

*Treatment.* Either nystatin, an antibiotic, or gentian violet is used. Nystatin has the advantage that it is colourless and less messy than gentian violet, although for home use the colour of the gentian violet makes it possible to check that the mouth has been painted. It has the disadvantage that it is much more expensive. Gentian violet occasionally causes ulcers in the mouth, especially in low birth weight babies for whom it should not, therefore, be prescribed.

Nystatin is used in a strength of 100,000 units per ml, and is inserted into the mouth with a dropper. Gentian violet is used in an aqueous solution of

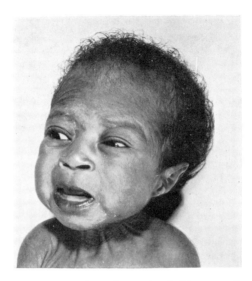

FIG. 24. Neonatal tetanus. Trismus is associated with contraction of the facial muscles, especially the mouth, and the neck muscles.

0·5 per cent. Both methods of treatment should be continued for 1 week after the disappearance of the last visible lesion in order to reduce the risk of recurrence from fungi still present in the mouth.

Buttock lesions are treated by the local application of gentian violet.

**Tetanus**

Neonatal tetanus is now confined to areas where there is ignorance of the normal methods of infant hygiene. The organism usually enters the body through the umbilicus, either because the cord has been cut with a dirty instrument, or because dirty dressings have been applied. The onset of symptoms is usually in the second week; the earlier the onset the worse the prognosis. The infant becomes rigid and is unable to feed because of intense trismus (Fig. 24). There are repeated spasms of the whole body and the more frequently these occur the worse the outlook.

For mild cases the best treatment is sedation using chlorpromazine and diazepam, keeping paraldehyde in reserve should spasms occur. For severe cases the ideal treatment, carried out in a special unit, is a combination of intermittent positive pressure respiration with the administration of curare. Penicillin and antitetanic serum (ATS) should always be given. The lowest dose of ATS for full therapeutic effect has not yet been determined but 10,000 units is as effective as larger doses (McCracken et al., 1971). If available, human tetanus immune globulin (TIG) should be given in preference to ATS.

This disease will die out completely once proper methods of hygiene are understood, but meanwhile *it can be completely prevented if full immunization against tetanus is given to the mother during pregnancy.*

**Cytomegalic inclusion disease**

This virus disease is widely disseminated in the animal kingdom but only occasionally causes disease in humans. However, although rare, it is becoming increasingly recognized in the neonatal period; it is therefore considered in this chapter although its manifestations are not confined to this period. A group of viruses, rather than a single one, is responsible and infection takes place *in utero* in most instances, producing the generalized form of the disease. A focal form, which is confined to the salivary glands, is probably the result of infection acquired after birth.

The brunt of the infection falls on the brain and liver. Until recently every congenital injection was considered serious, but a survey in 1970 (*Arch. Dis. Childh.*, 1970) showed that the majority of congenital infections do not produce obvious clinical signs. Only in the minority was there serious brain involvement causing microcephaly and severe mental retardation. Such patients may also have cerebral palsy, convulsions, choroidoretinitis, optic atrophy and cerebral calcification. Another group develop hepato-spleno-megaly and may show jaundice, thrombocytopenia, purpura and petechiae. In the survey the majority in this group improved, only a few progressing to mental retardation.

The clinical features have much in common with congenital toxoplasmosis (p. 541) from which it must be differentiated. The disease can be recognized in life by examination of the sediment from freshly passed urine when the characteristic 'owl's eye' intranuclear inclusions may be found. The virus has been cultured from liver biopsy material and the urinary sediment; serological tests are also available.

Improvement has occurred in some cases following the administration of idoxuridine.

## NEONATAL JAUNDICE

PHYSIOLOGY

A knowledge of bilirubin metabolism is essential for the understanding of neonatal jaundice. Phagocytosis of red cells in the reticulo-endothelial system releases haemoglobin which is broken down to bilirubin. Under normal circumstances it is only the ageing red cells which have completed their life span of about 120 days that are destroyed, but in pathological conditions causing haemolysis this process is accelerated.

The bilirubin so formed is released into the plasma and is known as indirect bilirubin because it gives an indirect Van den Bergh reaction. Indirect bilirubin is insoluble in water, cannot be excreted by the kidneys and is toxic to the brain. It is transported in the serum attached to serum albumin with which it forms a complex. When attached to albumin, indirect bilirubin loses its toxicity; but not all of it is bound, the remainder, being unbound or 'free', is toxic.

In the liver, indirect bilirubin is conjugated with glucuronic acid by the action of the enzyme glucuronyl transferase to form bilirubin glucuronide which gives a direct Van den Bergh reaction. This direct or conjugated bilirubin is water soluble and can be excreted by the kidneys; it is not toxic to the brain.

During intrauterine life, excess bilirubin in the fetus passes across the placenta to be metabolized by the maternal liver and possibly within the placenta as well. Consequently, accumulation of bilirubin does not occur during intrauterine life but after birth several factors may cause this to occur. The two principal reasons for an accumulation of unconjugated bilirubin are a defective enzyme system and excessive haemolysis. Accumulation of conjugated bilirubin results from obstruction to the flow of bile.

Conjugated bilirubin is not reabsorbed from the intestine, but unconjugated bilirubin can be absorbed into the blood and pass back to the liver via the enterohepatic circulation. In the adult, conjugated bilirubin is largely reduced to urobilin by the action of intestinal bacteria and there is minimal enterohepatic circulation of bilirubin. However, in the newborn, bacteria for this action are absent. Moreover, there is significant beta-glucuronidase activity in the gut which causes deconjugation of the bilirubin. The enterohepatic circulation of this unconjugated bilirubin increases the load on the neonatal liver. It is possible that increased enterohepatic circulation accounts for the hyperbilirubinaemia commonly found in neonates with small bowel obstruction.

An excess of unconjugated bilirubin can lead to kernicterus (p. 129), that is—biliary staining of the basal ganglia. The risk increases as the level of bilirubin rises, especially when over 20 mg per cent. This risk is greatest with preterm babies, partly because of the immaturity of their livers and partly because the low serum albumin level of the newborn is still greater if the infant is preterm. Asphyxia, by causing acidosis, also increases the risk, since the lower the pH the less the albumin binding capacity.

A number of drugs compete with bilirubin for albumin binding and can displace bilirubin from its attachment to albumin, thereby increasing the risk of kernicterus. These drugs include sulphonamides, salicylates and intramuscular diazepam which should not, therefore, be given to mothers in labour nor to newborn babies.

Delayed introduction of feeds to preterm babies is a factor causing hyperbilirubinaemia (Smallpeice & Davies, 1964; Wharton & Bower, 1965).

This is partly due to relative dehydration, but it is also possible that early feeding stimulates peristalsis, thereby diminishing the enterohepatic circulation of bilirubin. It may also introduce bacteria which aid the reduction of bilirubin to urobilin.

A further factor predisposing to hyperbilirubinaemia is delayed clamping of the cord (Saigal *et al.*, 1972). This is not a problem in the full-term baby but could be significant in the preterm infant.

Jaundice in the newborn commonly results from a combination of these mechanisms, though one is likely to be dominant. Thus there are three main types:

1. Defective conjugation.
2. Excessive haemolysis.
3. Obstruction.

## DEFECTIVE CONJUGATION

### 'Physiological jaundice'

It is common for normal newborn babies to develop jaundice about the second or third day of life as a result of defective conjugation with glucuronic acid. This is due to an immaturity of the enzyme system involving glucuronyl transferase and therefore occurs more often in preterm than in full-term babies. It is believed that this immaturity of the enzyme system in the preterm baby involves an actual deficiency of glucuronyl transferase during the first days of life.

The role of haemolysis as a factor in physiological jaundice is small. It has commonly been stated that the fall in haemoglobin occurring after birth is due to excessive haemolysis but, for the reasons discussed on p. 583, this is not a significant factor. However, in preterm babies an increased rate of haemolysis does occur and this plays a part in the development of physiological jaundice in such infants.

The accumulation of unconjugated bilirubin in cases of physiological jaundice may be sufficient to cause kernicterus. This risk is greater in preterm infants because such babies have a lower level of serum albumin. Consequently, unconjugated bilirubin is free to enter the central nervous system at lower levels of indirect bilirubin. This mechanism explains why full-term babies can tolerate higher levels of indirect bilirubin than preterm babies.

Babies with physiological jaundice become drowsy as do any jaundiced babies. They do not become anaemic or look ill as do babies with haemolytic disease of the newborn. The jaundice lasts only a few days so that jaundice persisting into the second week should never be regarded as truly physiological, even if no other cause for it can be found.

## Cretinism

Prolonged jaundice is common in cretins. The action of thyroid on bilirubin metabolism is obscure, but it possibly stimulates maturation of the conjugating system.

## Novobiocin

This drug causes hyperbilirubinaemia in the neonatal period because it competes with bilirubin for the very limited amount of glucuronyl transferase in the liver at this age. It should not therefore be given to babies. It does not have this effect in adults since they have an excess of glucuronyl transferase.

## Breast milk jaundice

A number of cases have now been reported (Gartner & Arias, 1966; Arthur et al., 1966) in which persistent jaundice occurred in breast-fed infants from inhibition of glucuronyl transferase activity. The inhibiting substance in the milk of such mothers was originally thought to be 3-alpha, 20-beta pregnanediol, but this is incorrect. It has now been shown that the inhibitory factor is in the lipid fraction of breast milk and that milk with a high content of free fatty acids is highly inhibitory (Bevan & Holton, 1972; Hargreaves, 1973).

Jaundice is slight in the first few days of life presumably because colostrum contains much less fat than ordinary breast milk. It becomes severe by the seventh to tenth day. Kernicterus has not been reported. The jaundice disappears when breast feeding is stopped.

## EXCESSIVE HAEMOLYSIS

### Haemolytic disease of the newborn (Erythroblastosis fetalis)

There are two main varieties of this disease, Rhesus (Rh) incompatibility and ABO incompatibility.

### RHESUS INCOMPATIBILITY

For this to occur the mother must be Rh-negative but the father Rh-positive so that the infant can be Rh-positive. Approximately 17 per cent of Caucasian (white) mothers are Rh-negative, whereas only 1 per cent of Negro mothers are Rh-negative. This difference accounts for the greatly reduced incidence of rhesus incompatibility among the Negro population. The escape of the infant's Rh-positive cells into the mother's circulation causes her to become sensitized and to form Rh antibodies which being IgG antibodies can pass back across the placenta to haemolyse some of the infant's cells. The effect on these cells depends on the quantity of the antibodies and the duration of their contact with the cells. As with all forms of antigen-antibody reaction, the more frequent the stimulus the greater the amount of antibody reaction. First babies may be affected but their risk is less than that in succeeding pregnancies. Sufficient transplacental haemorrhage to sensitize the mother can occur with a pregnancy ending in abortion. A transfusion or intramuscular injection of Rh-positive blood to a Rh-negative mother at any time in her life acts as the same immunizing stimulus as a Rh-positive baby.

The passage of fetal cells into the maternal circulation occurs usually at the time of delivery and is often associated with placental circulation. This is the reason why first babies are seldom affected. This transplacental haemorrhage is increased by manoeuvres such as caesarean section, manual removal of the placenta, amniocentesis, forceps delivery and external cephalic version, and by an accidental haemorrhage. Red cells also reach the mother's circulation via blood leakage into the peritoneum as occurs in a ruptured ectopic pregnancy. It is important, therefore, that blood should not be spilled into the peritoneal cavity during caesarean section.

Other factors must also be involved since only one in twenty Rh-negative mothers with a Rh-positive baby develop antibodies, so that a mother may have several unaffected Rh-positive babies and then start to produce affected infants. This is probably due to factors preventing the passage of fetal cells across the placental barrier or causing the immediate destruction of the cells in the maternal circulation. For example, ABO incompatibility protects the infant from Rh incompatibility since, if the fetus is ABO incompatible with the mother, the fetal cells which have entered the maternal circulation are rapidly eliminated by maternal anti-A or anti-B haemolysins.

Rh-negative babies born to a Rh-negative mother are not affected; the prognosis with regard to future babies born to a Rh-negative mother with a Rh-positive husband will therefore depend on whether he is homozygous or heterozygous positive. If he is homozygous all his babies will be Rh-positive but if heterozygous, only half will be positive.

Haemolytic disease of the newborn causes three clinical conditions depending on the severity of the haemolytic process: congenital haemolytic anaemia, icterus gravis, and hydrops fetalis. In its mildest form there is anaemia only—congenital haemolytic anaemia. If the rate of haemolysis is greater than the body's capacity to eliminate the bilirubin there is jaundice as well as anaemia—icterus gravis. If haemolysis is very severe, the anaemia can cause heart failure leading to oedema—hydrops fetalis.

*Hydrops fetalis.* These babies show gross generalized oedema with pleural effusions and ascites. Many are born dead or take only a few breaths and it is rare for one to survive, even with full treatment. The infant may be so large that delivery is possible only after puncture of the fetus to drain off some of the fluid. The clinical features are those of cardiac failure. Jaundice is not a feature since the maternal liver has metabolized the infant's excess bilirubin. However, the liver and spleen are much enlarged from additional haemopoietic tissue formed in an attempt to compensate for the excessive destruction of red cells. The placenta is grossly enlarged and oedematous.

*Icterus gravis.* These infants are either born jaundiced or become so within the first 24 hours. The degree of anaemia is variable but it is not so severe as in those with hydrops. The liver and spleen are enlarged from an abnormal degree of haemopoiesis. Jaundice increases for the first 2–3 days and may become intense. During this time the infant is obviously unwell (cf. physiological jaundice, p. 119), feeds are taken poorly and lethargy is present. If the jaundice reaches a dangerous level, kernicterus (p. 129) may develop.

*Congenital haemolytic anaemia.* These babies are the least severely affected. They show evidence of anaemia only and this is not usually severe.

MANAGEMENT OF RHESUS INCOMPATIBILITY

When a pregnant woman is found to be Rh-negative steps must be taken to determine whether the fetus is affected and, if so, how severely. Three methods are available: the previous obstetric history, the maternal antibody titre and the presence of bilirubin in the liquor.

The previous obstetric history is of considerable value in forecasting the likelihood of an affected baby since the worse the history of rhesus disease in previous pregnancies, the greater the risk of early intrauterine death of the fetus.

Maternal antibodies should be tested at the twenty-eighth and thirty-fourth week of pregnancy. Opinions differ on the predictive value of the level but a rising titre is most significant, indicating that antibodies are being formed in the current pregnancy rather than carried over from a previous pregnancy. The test should be carried out in every pregnancy, no matter how many unaffected Rh-positive babies the mother has had.

The major value of antibody titres is in selecting patients for amniocentesis since this procedure is potentially dangerous and cannot therefore be used as a routine. A sample of liquor is obtained by amniocentesis and examined for the presence of bilirubin. The higher the level of bilirubin the worse the prognosis for the baby. Amniocentesis can cause premature onset of labour; it can also damage the placenta leading to an escape of fetal cells into the maternal circulation with consequent increase in antibody production.

If these investigations show the baby to be affected, the question of premature induction of labour must be considered since the longer the fetus remains *in utero*, the greater the destruction of its red cells. On the other hand, prematurity brings its own problems which must be set against the advantages of early delivery. No baby should be allowed to go beyond term and there are grounds for induction at the thirty-eighth to thirty-ninth week in all cases, with earlier induction in special cases where the baby is thought to be severely affected.

Intrauterine transfusion of severely affected babies is now being carried out, the blood being infused into the baby's peritoneal cavity under X-ray control. By this means some babies have been kept alive *in utero* and thereby enabled to grow. Most of the babies still need an exchange transfusion after birth.

At birth the infant is examined clinically and haematologically for evidence of Rh incompatibility. A specimen of cord blood is taken for haemoglobin, bilirubin and direct Coombs' test. A positive Coombs' test indicates that the baby's cells are coated with antibody and therefore that the baby is affected.

If the baby is Coombs' positive the haemoglobin and bilirubin levels determine whether an immediate exchange transfusion is required to correct the anaemia or prevent kernicterus. Each case must be treated on its own merits but, in general, if the haemoglobin is less than 80 per cent (11·9 g per cent) or the bilirubin more than 5 mg per cent, an exchange transfusion with fresh blood should be carried out within the first 10 hours of life, or immediately if anaemia is severe. For less severely affected infants it is an advantage to wait a few hours to give the baby time to get over the trauma associated with birth so that he withstands the operation better. But in doing this the unconjugated bilirubin must not be allowed to rise to a level at which there would be a danger of kernicterus. Moreover, if the bilirubin is allowed to reach too high a level, an exchange transfusion is less effective in bringing it down.

More than one exchange transfusion may be required if the bilirubin rises again after the first transfusion. This secondary rise results either from continued haemolysis or because bilirubin is leaving the tissues and entering the blood. Only about one-quarter of the total bilirubin is in the circulation and therefore removed by the exchange transfusion, meanwhile continuous equilibration is taking place between the vascular and extravascular bilirubin. The maximal level of jaundice is usually reached by the fourth day. Repeat exchange transfusions, like the initial one, are carried out through the umbilical vein and/or artery; this route usually remains available for the first week of life.

During the exchange transfusion the heart should be continuously monitored, using an electrocardiogram with an oscilloscope. Particular attention should be paid to acid–base control during the transfusion in order to prevent changes in the pH of the infant's blood.

Because of its binding properties with bilirubin, albumin has been used to increase the amount of bilirubin removed during an exchange transfusion. More bilirubin is removed during the exchange if the blood has been fortified with added albumin or the infant given intravenous albumin beforehand.

An exchange transfusion is only one method of lowering the bilirubin level, and all the other methods for treating neonatal jaundice described on p. 126 are also used. It is more likely to be required in hyperbilirubinaemia due to rhesus incompatibility because of the additional need to correct the anaemia and remove antibodies.

Rhesus affected babies are very liable to develop anaemia during the first 6 weeks of life owing to marrow hypofunction and persistence of Rh antibody. For this reason all such babies, whether or not they have received an exchange transfusion, should have weekly haemoglobin estimations. This anaemia is not influenced by the administration of iron and if the haemoglobin falls below 50 per cent (7·5 g per 100 ml) a simple blood transfusion should be given.

PREVENTION OF RHESUS IMMUNIZATION

Because it is mainly during labour that the infant's red cells cross the placenta into the maternal circulation it is possible to prevent most cases of Rhesus immunization. One injection of anti-D gammaglobulin (obtained from male volunteers) is given to all Rhesus-negative mothers of Rhesus-positive babies immediately after birth.

This antibody destroys any of the infant's red cells which have reached the mother, thereby preventing them from stimulating her antibody forming mechanism. The injected antibody lasts only a few weeks and will have disappeared long before the next pregnancy.

It is essential that Rh-negative women undergoing an abortion—whether planned or spontaneous—should also be protected in this way as they are at as great a risk of immunization as the mothers of live babies.

ABO INCOMPATIBILITY

In almost all instances of this form of incompatibility the mother is Group O and the baby A or B. The reason for this limitation lies in the size of the antibodies and thereby whether or not they can cross the placenta. In O sera the anti-A and anti-B activity lies in the IgG fraction which can cross the placenta. The anti-A and anti-B antibodies have distinct serological properties in addition to molecular size—they are termed 'immune' antibodies. On the other hand, the anti-A antibody in B sera and the anti-B antibody in A sera is in the IgM fraction and therefore too large to cross the placenta—these are termed 'natural' antibodies.

The presence of immune antibodies in the mother's serum does not require previous stimulation by the passage of fetal cells, therefore ABO incompatibility occurs equally in first and in subsequent pregnancies and cannot be predicted.

Among white races this form of incompatibility is less common than the

Rh variety but in negro races, where the frequency of Rh-negative individuals is less, ABO incompatibility is more common.

The clinical effect is less severe than in Rh incompatibility and jaundice is not present at birth. It may not develop until the third day, then easily being confused with physiological jaundice. The Coombs' test is negative or only weakly positive. Anaemia is absent or mild, though spherocytosis may be present as a result of haemolysis; being changed to a spherocyte is the first stage in the action of haemolysis on a red cell.

The diagnosis is made largely by excluding other causes of jaundice in a newborn baby of A or B blood group whose mother is group O. Treatment (p. 126) is the same as for other causes of neonatal jaundice and an exchange transfusion is rarely required.

GLUCOSE-6-PHOSPHATE DEHYDROGENASE DEFICIENCY

This enzyme is contained in the red cells and is necessary for their stability. Deficiency of the enzyme impairs glutathione metabolism which is essential for the maintenance of normal red cell structure. Consequently, deficiency of the enzyme increases the liability to haemolysis. Deficiency of the enzyme is widely distributed throughout the world. It is uncommon among Caucasians, except for the Mediterranean races with whom it is extremely common. It is also very frequent in Negroes so that in some parts of Africa almost 25 per cent of the population may be deficient. It is common in Singapore owing to a high incidence among Malaysians and Chinese.

These races are affected by different types of the deficiency with differing clinical severity. The condition is discussed on p. 610.

VITAMIN K

An excess of vitamin K causes hyperbilirubinaemia. It seems probable that this is due to haemolysis rather than to interference with the activity of glucuronyl transferase. This action may occur in any baby but particularly in a preterm infant. For this reason the prophylactic dose of vitamin K to prevent haemorrhagic disease of the newborn should not exceed 1 mg per day.

Vitamin $K_1$ is the natural occurring vitamin and is fat soluble. It is less liable to produce hyperbilirubinaemia than the water soluble, synthetic analogues of vitamin K. Its action is also more powerful, more prolonged and more rapid in onset so that it should be used for preference.

The administration of vitamin K is particularly liable to cause haemolysis in individuals with glucose-6-phosphate dehydrogenase deficiency since it is one of the challenging drugs to which such patients react (see above). However, it has been shown that a dose of 1 mg is not dangerous to such individuals (Capps *et al.*, 1963).

EXTRAVASATION OF BLOOD

A number of babies have been reported (Rausen & Diamond, 1961; Nelson, 1965; Davis & Schiff, 1966) in whom hyperbilirubinaemia developed in association with a large extravasation of blood. Such bleeding has occurred into the tissues, into the intestine or as a cephalhaematoma. The result of the haemorrhage is for the immature liver to be presented with a large quantity of bilirubin to be metabolized. In these cases the liver has been unable to deal with the extra load so that jaundice has resulted.

HEREDITARY SPHEROCYTOSIS (p. 602)

In this condition the red cells are spherical and therefore more liable to haemolysis. Some of the affected babies may have such severe haemolysis as to cause jaundice. If the condition is so severe there is almost always a family history of the disorder.

TREATMENT OF NEONATAL JAUNDICE

Whatever the cause of the hyperbilirubinaemia it is essential that the bilirubin level is kept low enough to prevent kernicterus (p. 129). The danger level of unconjugated bilirubin is usually taken as 20 mg per cent, but there is no single figure below which kernicterus will not occur and above which it always will. One reason for this is that the serum bilirubin is not a complete estimation of the total bilirubin in the body since excess pigment diffuses into the extravascular space and possibly into the brain. Moreover, the serum level does not indicate whether the bilirubin is bound to albumin or not, and yet it is the concentration of unbound bilirubin only which determines how much bilirubin enters the brain. Because of its lower serum albumin the preterm baby may develop kernicterus at a lower level of bilirubin than a full-term baby.

However, it is certain that the risk of kernicterus below 20 mg per cent is small and that there is an increasing risk as the level rises. The faster the rate of rise the greater the danger, so that more than one daily estimation of bilirubin may be needed. The earlier the jaundice develops the more likely is it to reach dangerous levels.

METHODS

*Exchange transfusion*

An exchange transfusion immediately after birth may be required for Rhesus incompatibility for the reasons given on p. 123, but this is not required so urgently for the other causes of neonatal jaundice. Other methods, used early, may well remove the need for an exchange transfusion in the milder cases of Rhesus incompatibility; they may also prevent the need for a second transfusion in Rhesus babies.

*Fluids.* All jaundiced babies must receive adequate fluids to ensure there is no unnecessary concentration of bilirubin in the body fluids. Such fluid must be given by tube if the baby is not taking sufficient by mouth.

*Phototherapy.* Light decomposes bilirubin and phototherapy was first used as a method of treatment by Cremer *et al.*, in 1958. It did not immediately catch on since it was feared that the products of decomposition might be harmful to the baby. It is now known that there is no such risk and in fact photodecomposition is a normal alternative route of excretion of bilirubin from the body.

Phototherapy should not be used to prevent the occurrence of jaundice but only to help in preventing it from reaching a dangerous level. It is usually started when the bilirubin reaches about 10 mg per cent. Special units for the source of light are used and since this is a cold light an incubator may be required for the naked baby unless the ward or nursery is sufficiently hot.

Phototherapy can damage the retina, therefore the eyes must be bandaged while the baby is under the lamp. The baby can be removed from the lamp while feeding and during this time the bandages can be removed. Many mothers are distressed by being unable to handle their babies as often as they would like, and it is essential to pay particular attention to giving them the opportunities to feed their babies with the bandages off. Some babies develop diarrhoea and rashes but these are seldom severe.

The effect of light therapy is not influenced by skin pigmentation so that the response is the same in white and non-white babies.

*Phenobarbitone.* This drug enhances the activity of liver enzymes, thereby increasing the rate of bilirubin conjugation. It can be given to mothers for 7–10 days before birth or to the newborn baby—it is more effective when given prophylactically to the mother (Trolle, 1968). The dose of phenobarbitone for a newborn baby is 8 mg per kg per day, usually given for 3 days.

## OBSTRUCTIVE JAUNDICE

This cause of neonatal jaundice differs from the other two (defective conjugation and excessive haemolysis) in that the bilirubin is conjugated. It is not therefore a cause of kernicterus. The urine contains excessive bile while the stools are pale due to lack of bile.

Congenital obliteration of the bile ducts is described on p. 172. Jaundice from this cause does not appear until the second or third week of life and should not therefore be confused with the other causes already described. Neonatal hepatitis (see below) is a frequent cause of obstructive jaundice.

GALACTOSAEMIA (p. 572)

Jaundice occurs in these babies from the accumulation of galactose-1-phosphate which causes hepatocellular damage and impairment of the excretion of bilirubin. Consequently, there is a rise in indirect and direct bilirubin. In order to exclude galactosaemia, all jaundiced babies must have their urine tested for reducing substances.

## MISCELLANEOUS CAUSES OF NEONATAL JAUNDICE

### NEONATAL SEPSIS

Babies with any form of neonatal infection may become jaundiced (p. 109). Such infants are usually very ill but an *E. coli* urinary infection may cause jaundice without the child being seriously ill.

Although it could be expected that such severe disease would depress the conjugating mechanism, Zuelzer & Brown (1961) have found the mechanism of jaundice to be excretory failure from damage to the liver cells.

### NEONATAL HEPATITIS

Very occasionally jaundice in the neonatal period results from hepatitis. Such infants differ from those with physiological jaundice in being obviously very ill as well as jaundiced, their death rate being high. The clinical and biochemical picture may suggest obstruction so that differentiation from congenital obliteration of the bile ducts may be possible only by liver biopsy.

A number of viruses can cause the condition, particularly serum hepatitis (p. 319) which may merely be carried by the pregnant mother but cause severe infection in the fetus while *in utero*. On the other hand, the virus of infective hepatitis is seldom the cause, even if the mother is attacked by this virus during pregnancy. Gammaglobulin may protect the fetus and should always be given to pregnant mothers who develop infective jaundice.

Other viruses which can cause hepatitis in the neonatal period are Coxsackie, herpes simplex and the virus of cytomegalic inclusion disease. Hepatitis may also be due to congenital syphilis, although this is now uncommon, and to toxoplasmosis.

Neonatal hepatitis may lead to cirrhosis of the liver and is possibly the cause of some of the unexplained cases of cirrhosis in childhood.

## Kernicterus

This condition is due to a toxic effect of unconjugated bilirubin on the basal ganglia; these take up the bile pigment and show as yellow areas on the cut surface of the brain at autopsy. It results from an excessive accumulation of unconjugated bilirubin in the tissues from any cause, and it is to prevent the bilirubin in the body from reaching a dangerous level that an exchange transfusion is performed. Conjugated bilirubin differs from the unconjugated form in being water soluble and therefore not damaging to the brain.

The risk of kernicterus is increased by a level of serum bilirubin over 20 mg per cent (p. 118), by a birth weight less than 1500 g because of liver immaturity and low serum albumin concentration (p. 118), and by asphyxia because it causes acidosis, thereby lowering the albumin binding capacity.

In the majority of cases of hyperbilirubinaemia occurring during the first week the bilirubin is almost entirely unconjugated and there is seldom more than 1 mg per cent of conjugated bilirubin. Occasionally, the conjugated bilirubin also rises, due to an obstructive element within the liver. This produces a greenish-yellow colour as opposed to the orange colour resulting from a high level of unconjugated bilirubin.

Kernicterus causes cerebral irritation; it is diagnosed by refusal of feeds and vomiting, head retraction and arching of the back, a full fontanelle, high-pitched cry and involuntary 'windmill-like' movements of the arms. Death is likely, but even if the child survives he will suffer from mental retardation, deafness or athetosis.

It is possible that a partial hearing loss may occur in infants whose bilirubin had not risen sufficiently high to cause athetosis. It is essential, therefore, that all jaundiced infants should be followed up for evidence of hearing loss.

## MISCELLANEOUS DISORDERS

### Haemorrhagic disease of the newborn

During the first few days of life there is usually a fall in the prothrombin level but only occasionally is this severe enough to cause bleeding. If the degree of hypoprothrombinaemia is sufficient to cause bleeding the disorder is called haemorrhagic disease of the newborn. This condition occurs almost exclusively among breast-fed infants since cow's milk contains approximately four times the amount of vitamin K present in human milk.

Vitamin K is a fat soluble vitamin occurring in plants and egg yolk and synthesized in the human intestine by the action of bacteria. It is, therefore, so readily available to the adult that even experimental deficiencies are difficult to induce. In the newborn infant, however, deficiencies may occur from lack of intake and from the fact that the organisms which synthesize it in the gut have not yet fully colonized the intestine.

Vitamin K is essential for the synthesis in the liver of prothrombin and probably also of factor 7. Both of these are proteins which are required for clotting to occur. Immaturity of the liver enzyme system in the newborn may, therefore, result in an inadequacy of prothrombin and factor 7, thereby accounting for the greater frequency of haemorrhagic disease in preterm infants.

Clinically, bleeding may take place into the alimentary canal causing haematemesis or melaena, into the skin causing purpura, or from the umbilical cord. Pulmonary haemorrhage (see below) and cerebral haemorrhage are seldom due to this disorder.

Confusion sometimes arises when maternal blood, which has been swallowed by the fetus during delivery, is later vomited. However, if there is any possibility of haemorrhagic disease, the baby should be given treatment. The source of the vomited blood can be determined by testing it for fetal and adult haemoglobin (see p. 585).

*Treatment.* 2 mg vitamin $K_1$ (phytomenadione) intramuscularly is sufficient for most patients and is given once daily. In severe cases a blood transfusion is necessary and this can be given most rapidly through the umbilical vein.

Prophylactic vitamin K has, in the past, been widely given to newborn babies in order to prevent the disease, but its use must now be restricted in the light of present knowledge regarding its effect on hyperbilirubinaemia (p. 125) and not more than 1 mg given.

SECONDARY HAEMORRHAGIC DISEASE OF THE NEWBORN

This name has been applied to those causes of neonatal bleeding which are not due to a lack of vitamin K. In most instances this bleeding tendency is due to *disseminated intravascular coagulation* (see p. 601). This state results from a heavy consumption of platelets and labile coagulation factors. It is not a primary disease but is precipitated by a number of events, particularly anoxia, infection, hypoglycaemia and hypothemia. Babies who are small for dates are therefore particularly at risk.

Clinically, the baby is shocked and pale. Petechiae are visible and there is likely to be oozing from puncture sites. Other features depend on the site of bleeding. Haemorrhage into the lungs (see below) and brain occurs more often in this condition than in vitamin K deficiency. Bleeding may also occur into the intestine and the adrenals.

**Massive pulmonary haemorrhage**

Massive haemorrhage into the lungs is a relatively common finding in autopsies on newborn infants. Bleeding takes place into the alveolar spaces and into the interstitial tissue. The condition occurs particularly in babies who have suffered intrauterine malnutrition and are small for dates at birth.

Pulmonary haemorrhage is especially caused by disseminated intra-vascular coagulation (see above) and is therefore associated with anoxia, infection, hypoglycaemia and hypothermia. It is also found in babies with kernicterus.

Clinically, the condition usually develops within 24 hours of birth. There is increasing respiratory distress and irritability which may be severe enough to cause convulsions, thereby causing a mistaken diagnosis of a cerebral disorder to be made sometimes. Bleeding from the respiratory tract so that blood wells up into the throat occurs in many of the infants, making an immediate correct diagnosis possible. The chest X-ray shows granular opacities similar to hyaline membrane disease. Death occurs in most cases.

The disorder bears many similarities to hyaline membrane disease with which it may be associated; it has been suggested that abnormal surface forces in the lung may, at times, produce pulmonary haemorrhage (Rowe & Avery, 1966).

### Fetal haemorrhage into the maternal circulation

It is now appreciated that severe blood loss from the fetus via the placenta may occur about the time of delivery; the anaemia so caused may be sufficient to kill the infant. This blood loss can occur in a number of ways:

1. Rupture of one or more placental vessels as the result of an anomaly such as vasa praevia, a velamentous insertion or a succenturiate lobe of the placenta.

2. Damage to an anterior placenta during Caesarean section. On no account should the placenta be entered in order to reach the baby. A technique must be used which circumvents the placenta, the cord being clamped as soon as the baby's face is delivered.

3. Damage to the placenta during artificial rupture of the membranes, particularly if a high rupture is performed, or amniocentesis. This may cause external bleeding or fetal blood loss into the maternal circulation.

4. Damage to the placenta during amniocentesis.

5. In twin pregnancy associated with a single placenta, bleeding can take place from one twin into the other (see twin-transfusion syndrome p. 135).

6. In some cases fetal haemorrhage has occurred into the maternal circu-lation for which no cause can be found. That this should take place is under-standable when it is remembered that within the placenta the infant's capillary loops lie inside the maternal sinusoids. The pressure is higher on the fetal side so that any break permitting a leak results in the passage of fetal cells into the maternal circulation.

Fetal cells can be detected in the maternal circulation by special staining methods. These should be applied within 12 hours of a suspected feto-maternal transfusion in case destruction of the fetal cells occurs from their incompatibility with the mother's serum. Where vaginal bleeding is suspected to be fetal in origin, a test for fetal haemoglobin should be made on the blood lost. Such a test should be performed routinely if bleeding occurs when artificial rupture of the membranes is performed.

## Neonatal cold injury

Babies who are accidentally exposed to cold during the neonatal period develop a remarkably uniform syndrome; this is more liable to occur in low birth weight babies but may occur in any baby. The infant becomes sluggish with his feeds, develops puffiness of the eyes, hands and feet and often a runny nose. The face, hands and feet become pink from vasodilatation giving a false impression of good health. The baby feels cold, but it is re-markable how many mothers and even doctors and nurses fail to take note of this sign. In severe cases *sclerema* develops. This is a state of diffuse harden-ing of the subcutaneous tissues which causes the affected area of the body to feel solid. The skin can no longer be picked up separately from the muscle and an absence of pitting on pressure is characteristic. It usually starts in the thighs and buttocks but, if the child fails to improve, spreads to involve the whole body. The rectal temperature is usually below 32·0° C (89·6° F) and may be below 26·5° C (79·7° F). Pulmonary haemorrhage from disseminated intra-vascular coagulation is liable to occur.

In some instances cerebral birth injury or sepsis are additional factors causing the condition.

*Treatment.* This should aim at preventing the condition by ensuring warm surroundings for all newborn babies. A wall thermometer should always be placed above the cot in home deliveries. Provided the attendants are aware of the syndrome the condition seldom occurs. A low-reading thermometer which records down to 25° C should be used for babies; an ordinary clinical thermometer only records to 35° C and so may give a falsely high reading of the baby's temperature.

In many tropical countries there is a marked drop in temperature during the night. In these circumstances mothers should be encouraged to have their babies with them in bed in order to maintain the babies' body heat.

Patients should be slowly warmed by hot-water bottles or in an incubator. Adequate oxygen must be given since, when the environmental temperature falls, oxygen consumption in the newborn infant increases in association with the rise in basal metabolic rate (BMR) resulting from the baby's attempt to keep himself warm (see p. 99). Additional glucose should be given in the feeds since glycogen reserves are depleted by the increased BMR. Antibiotic cover should be given, owing to the increased risk of infection.

### Infants of diabetic mothers

These babies are larger than normal and it is likely that this is due to the maternal hyperglycaemia causing fetal hyperglycaemia. This stimulates the fetal pancreatic beta-cells, hyperplasia of which accounts for the unusual size of the pancreatic islets in these babies. Consequent increased insulin production in the presence of copious glucose, promotes fetal obesity and may cause hypoglycaemia. Since increased growth hormone results from hypoglycaemia, this may be an additional reason for the large size of these babies.

The skin is bright red so that the babies have been described as looking like over-ripe tomatoes. Much less commonly they present the appearance of being small for dates (p. 54) owing to maternal arterial disease. They are often born prematurely and are particularly liable to the respiratory distress syndrome (p. 64). Care must be taken not to overlook the fact that the baby has been born before term since they are seldom of low birth weight.

In some of the babies, a form of neonatal tetany may be seen in which there are periods of sudden generalized wild hyperactivity, followed by complete lack of movement. Chvostek's and Trousseau's signs, carpopedal spasm and laryngeal stridor are rarely seen in this type of tetany, although hypocalcaemia has been found and may be the cause.

During pregnancy, women who are diabetic should be strictly controlled, it being best to change to soluble insulin so that this is achieved. A history of progressive increase in birth weight with each succeeding baby may indicate the pre-diabetic state in the mother. Such women show a diabetic type of glucose tolerance curve and their babies may be as severely affected as those of mothers with overt diabetes.

The survival of the babies is dependent on meticulous attention to medical and nursing care and all should be managed as though preterm, regardless of their birth weight. They should be nursed in an incubator with high humidity, a careful watch being kept for the development of the respiratory distress syndrome. The blood sugar levels of these babies are so variable that there is no indication for the routine use of oral glucose, but a close watch should be kept for symptoms of hypoglycaemia, treatment being given immediately if they appear (see p. 641). Feeding should be started early in all cases to reduce the risk of hypoglycaemia and hyperbilirubinaemia. If tetany occurs, calcium should be given (see below).

There is an increased risk of venous thrombosis, especially renal, in the babies of diabetic mothers. The umbilical vein should, therefore, be avoided for the rehydration of these babies for fear of portal vein thrombosis.

### Neonatal tetany

In the first 2–3 days after birth, tetany may be due to cerebral damage or because the mother is diabetic (see above). From the end of the first week and for several weeks after, the condition is almost confined to infants fed on cow's milk, owing to its high phosphate content. During fetal life, normal levels of calcium and phosphorus are maintained by maternal factors, the infant at birth being in a state of functional hypoparathyroidism. Adaptation to the high phosphate content of cow's milk does not always occur rapidly and, in such cases, a low level of serum calcium may develop, with consequent tetany. Such infants may also develop transitory convulsions.

Some of these babies have a low serum magnesium as well as a low serum calcium. In this situation, treatment with intravenous calcium may be ineffective until the associated hypomagnesaemia is corrected. As a different problem, isolated hypomagnesaemia is a rare cause of neonatal convulsions.

Babies who develop neonatal hypocalcaemia are more liable to later hypoplasia of the dental enamel.

*Treatment.* Immediate therapy requires the intravenous administration of 0·2 ml/kg of 10 per cent calcium gluconate which must be given very slowly owing to the risk of cardiac arrest. If hypomagnesaemia is present or is suspected, 0·1 ml/kg of 50 per cent magnesium sulphate should be given by slow intravenous injection.

For the next 2 days the infant should be given 2 g calcium gluconate daily as a 2 per cent solution (contains 20 mg per ml) with the feeds. Calcium chloride is more irritating than calcium gluconate and therefore less suitable.

In addition, it is essential to change to a low phosphate-containing milk such as breast milk or SMA.

## PROBLEMS IN TWINS

Twins present special difficulties in pregnancy and labour which cause their prognosis to be less good than that of singletons. The perinatal mortality of twins is four times that of all babies and their average intelligence is lower than the normal.

The second twin is the more likely of the two to suffer since it is usually the smaller, has a longer labour and is more likely to require obstetric manipulation. The smaller of the two is particularly liable to neonatal hypoglycaemia.

The death rate among monochorionic twins is three times greater than that of dichorionic twins, one reason for this being the twin transfusion syndrome.

## Twin transfusion syndrome

When twins possess a single placenta there is always a connection between their vessels in the placenta. The site of this connection will determine whether bleeding occurs from one twin into the other. When this takes place one twin is plethoric at birth, the other being anaemic. The plethoric twin is the larger of the two and the increased circulatory volume may cause cardiac failure. Hydramnios occurs in the amniotic sac of the plethoric twin and it is this which can lead to an antenatal diagnosis of the condition.

Twin transfusion accounts for the marked disparity in size between twins which sometimes occurs (Rausen *et al.*, 1965).

**Neonatal hypoglycaemia** (see p. 641)

## BIBLIOGRAPHY

ARTHUR L.J.H., BEVAN B.R. & HOLTON J.B. (1966) Neonatal hyperbilirubinaemia and breast feeding. *Develop. Med. Child. Neurol.*, **8**, 279.

BERMAN P.H. & BANKER B.Q. (1966) Neonatal meningitis: a clinical and pathological study of 29 cases. *Pediatrics*, **38**, 6.

BEVAN B.R. & HOLTON J.B. (1972) Inhibition of bilirubin conjugation in rat liver slices by free fatty acids, with relevance to the problem of breast milk jaundice. *Clinica Chimica Acta*, **14**, 101.

CAPPS F.P.A., GILLES H.M., JOLLY H. & WORLLEDGE S.M. (1963) Glucose-6-phosphate dehydrogenase deficiency and neonatal jaundice in Nigeria. Their relation to the use of prophylactic vitamin K. *Lancet*, **2**, 379.

COLLABORATIVE STUDY (1970) Cytomegalovirus infection in the north west of England: a report on a two-year study. *Arch. Dis. Childh.*, **45**, 513.

CREMER R.J., PERRYMAN P.W. & RICHARDS D.H. (1958) Influence of light on the hyperbilirubinaemia of infants. *Lancet*, **1**, 1094.

DAVIES P.A. (1971) Bacterial infections in the fetus and newborn. *Arch. Dis. Childh.*, **46**, 1.

DAVIES P.A., ROBINSON R.J., SCOPES J.W., TIZARD J.P.M. & WIGGLESWORTH J.S. (1972) *Medical care of Newborn Babies.* Heinemann, London.

DAVIS J.A. & SCHIFF D. (1966) Bruising as a cause of neonatal jaundice. *Lancet*, **1**, 636.

ESTERLEY J.R. & OPPENHEIMER E.H. (1966) Massive pulmonary hemorrhage in the newborn. I. Pathologic considerations. *J. Pediat.*, **69**, 3.

GARTNER L.M. & ARIAS I.M. (1966) Studies of prolonged neonatal jaundice in the breast fed infant. *J. Pediat.* **68**, 54.

HARGREAVES T. (1973) Effect of fatty acids on bilirubin conjugation. *Arch. Dis. Childh.*, **48**, 446.

HULL D. (1966) The structure and function of brown adipose tissue. *Brit. med. Bull.*, **22**, 92.

MAISELS M.J. (1972) Bilirubin. On understanding and influencing its metabolism in the newborn infant. *Ped. Clin. N.A.*, **19**, 447.

MANN T.P. & ELLIOTT R.I.K. (1957) Neonatal cold injury due to accidental exposure to cold. *Lancet*, **1**, 229.

McCRACKEN G.H., DOWELL D.L. & MARSHALL F.N. (1971) Double blind trial of equine antitoxin and human immune globulin in tetanus neonatorum. *Lancet*, **1**, 1146.

NELSON T.C. (1965) The relationship between melaena and hyperbilirubinaemia in mature neonates. *Biol. Neonat.*, **8**, 267.

RAUSEN A.R. & DIAMOND L.K. (1961) Enclosed hemorrhage and neonatal jaundice. *Amer. J. Dis. Child.*, **101,** 164.

RAUSEN A.R., SEKI M. & STRAUSS L. (1965) Twin transfusion syndrome. *J. Pediat.*, **66,** 613.

ROWE S. & AVERY M.E. (1966) Massive pulmonary hemorrhage in the newborn. II. Clinical considerations. *J. Pediat.*, **69,** 12.

SAIGAL S., O'NEILL A., SURAINDER Y., CHUA L. & USHER R. (1972) Placental transfusion and hyperbilirubinaemia in the premature. *Pediatrics*, **49,** 406.

SCOPES J.W. (1965) Metabolic rate and temperature control in the human baby. *Brit. med. Bull.*, **22,** 88.

SMALLPEICE V. & DAVIES P.A. (1964) Immediate feeding of premature infants with undiluted breast milk. *Lancet*, **2,** 1349.

TIBBLES J.A.R. & PRICHARD J.S. (1965) The prognostic value of the electroencephalogram in neonatal convulsions. *Pediatrics*, **35,** 778.

TROLLE D. (1968) Decrease of total serum-bilirubin concentration in newborn infants after phenobarbitone treatment. *Lancet*, **2,** 705.

WHARTON, B.A. & BOWER, B.D. (1965) Immediate or later feeding for premature babies. *Lancet* **2,** 969.

ZUELZER W.W. & BROWN A.K. (1961) Neonatal jaundice. *Amer. J. Dis. Child.*, **101,** 87.

# CHAPTER 6

# CONGENITAL MALFORMATIONS

Any anatomical defect present at birth is classified as a congenital malformation. This term has no aetiological implication and must not be misused as a synonym for hereditary disorders.

Considering the complexity of human embryology it is not surprising if malformations of development occur with greater frequency in man than in the lower orders of plant and animal life. Now that the perinatal loss of life from obstetric causes and infection has been reduced, we are coming up against the hard core of death and impaired function resulting from congenital malformations. Approximately one baby in fifty is born with a severe malformation, this accounting for about one in five stillbirths and one in ten infant deaths. Some years ago it would have been considered impossible that these could be prevented, but there are now many hopeful lines of research; though while research is proceeding and some malformations are being prevented, fresh malformations are being produced by new drugs given early in pregnancy. Malformations are more common in babies born prematurely and possibly in those born to mothers with diabetes. Pedersen *et al.* (1964) found a significant increased incidence of malformations in newborn infants of diabetic mothers, particularly those with late diabetic vascular complications. On the other hand, Farquhar (1965) regards the argument concerning the possible increased incidence in babies of diabetic mothers as not yet settled.

Twenty to thirty per cent of aborted fetuses have a chromosomal abnormality and over half show abnormal development.

## AETIOLOGICAL FACTORS

There are many different aetiological factors, fresh ones being discovered every year. Each tends to have a specific effect, though this may be shared by other factors.

### Maternal age and birth order

There is a clear association between increasing maternal age and mongolism. It has been suggested that all congenital malformations are commoner in

older mothers, but statistical analysis does not support this, except in hydrocephalus, where there is a weak association.

Birth order does not affect the overall incidence of congenital malformations, despite earlier suggestions that all were more common in first-born
children. It is natural that malformations should be seen more often in first-
born children since about 40 per cent of the population are first-born. Consequently, the incidence of a malformation among first-born infants must
exceed this figure to be significant. Only in the case of congenital dislocation
of the hip, spina bifida, hydrocephalus and anencephaly is there such an
increase in first-borns. Pyloric stenosis is often described as occurring particularly in first-born children, but the increased incidence is not great and
probably of little significance.

### Paternal age
This does not affect the development of congenital malformations except in
the case of achondroplasia when advancing paternal age is a factor.

### Genetic determination
Genetic factors play a part in the production of a number of congenital
malformations, but a clear-cut dominant or recessive mode of inheritance can
be found only in a few diseases. Achondroplasia is due to a dominant gene
and cystic fibrosis to a recessive gene. A dominant gene affects development
in heterozygotes, that is, the abnormal gene is present on one member only
of the chromosome pair. Therefore, one parent only is affected and this one
shows the disorder. A recessive gene affects development only in homo-
zygotes so the abnormal gene must be present on both members of the
chromosome pair to produce its effect. Both parents are carriers but neither
shows the disorder. The chance that both parents will carry the same recessive gene is increased if they are related, hence the dangers of consanguineous marriages.

An alternative way of describing these differences is that a condition
inherited as a dominant one occurs with a single dose of the abnormal
gene, whereas a recessive condition occurs only with a double dose.

In an autosomal dominant disorder the abnormal gene probably acts by
producing a defect of body protein. Consequently the situation is comparable
to a house with half its bricks defective. There is therefore trouble from the
start so that a single dose produces a visible effect. The abnormal gene in an
autosomal recessive disorder causes an enzyme deficiency, but since enzyme
levels are higher than needed a 50 per cent defect causes no problem. Consequently, a double dose is required to produce the effect.

The chance of inheritance of a disease due to a dominant gene is one in two;

on the other hand, if one member of a sibship is suffering from a recessively inherited condition the risk to future siblings is one in four. In the case of a disease inherited as a dominant, one of the parents is not always affected since it is often due to a fresh mutation, particularly where the malformation reduces the chance of propagation. There is no increased risk for subsequent children born to parents following a fresh mutation. Fresh mutations seldom occur with recessive diseases.

Although the carriers of recessively inherited conditions are usually normal, it is now becoming possible to determine the carrier state in the heterozygous individuals of some disorders. For example, an enzyme assay is used in galactosaemia (p. 573). Deficiency of hexosaminidase-A can be detected in the serum of carriers of Tay–Sachs's disease (p. 579). Approximately 70 per cent of the women carrying pseudohypertropic muscular dystrophy have a raised serum creatine phosphokinase. In some conditions, if the carriers are subjected to sufficient stress a mild degree of the disorder becomes apparent. Thus, the sickle cell trait may become apparent if the patients are subjected to a low oxygen tension (p. 608). The female carriers of nephrogenic diabetes insipidus may develop polydypsia and polyuria during pregnancy (p. 622).

*Sex-linked genes.* These are mostly recessive and, since they are carried on the X chromosome, would be better called X linked. Examples are pseudo-hypertrophic muscular dystrophy and haemophilia. A female carrying such a gene is clinically normal since she is protected by a normal second X chromosome. A male bearing the gene exhibits the disease. When a female carrier is married to a normal male, half the sons are affected and half the daughters are carriers. An affected man cannot transmit the disease to his sons, since these inherit a Y chromosome and not an X chromosome from their father, but all his daughters will be carriers.

Some congenital malformations while not involving sex linked genes still show a differing incidence according to sex. Conditions which are commoner among females are anencephaly, spina bifida, patent ductus arteriosus, con-genital dislocation of the hip and cleft plate. Cleft lip on the other hand occurs more often in males.

There are a number of common malformations where genetic factors are probably involved: cleft palate, cleft lip, pyloric stenosis, mongolism, Hirschsprung's disease, anencephaly, hydrocephaly, spina bifida, talipes equinovarus and congenital dislocation of the hip are some of the disorders which occur in two or more members of a family more often than would be expected by chance. But, in none of these conditions does the distribution within the affected families follow the pattern of single factor inheritance and it is probable that environmental factors are also involved. This is suggested by studies of pyloric stenosis in identical twins, where as many as 50 per cent of their co-twins have been found to be unaffected. It is likely that most congenital malformations are multifactorial, resulting from a mixture of genetic and environmental factors.

Mongolism is due to a detectable chromosomal abnormality (see p. 218) and research is bringing to light other syndromes associated with abnormal chromosomes (p. 222).

Genetic counselling now occupies an important place in the handling of parents whose child has been born with a congenital malformation. In certain instances amniocentesis will be offered for the next pregnancy.

**Amniocentesis**

Antenatal diagnosis of chromosome disorders, especially mongolism, is now possible by growing fetal cells which have been shed into the amniotic fluid. This is now a service available for mothers of advanced age. The method also determines the sex of the fetus and is therefore of value to mothers who are carriers of sex-linked disorders such as pseudohypertrophic muscular dystrophy.

Anencephaly and severe spina bifida can be detected by assay of alpha-fetoprotein. It is believed that the rise in level occurring in such cases is due to the amount of choroid plexus exposed. A direct diagnosis of certain disorders, such as gargoylism (p. 575), can be made from examination of the fluid.

**Infection**

Rubella in early pregnancy is the greatest infection risk to the fetus by producing congenital malformations. Rubella causes malformations only if the virus strikes the fetus within the first 3 months of pregnancy, before organ differentiation is complete. The risk to the fetus is by far the greatest in the first month of pregnancy when about 50 per cent of infants are affected. In the second month the risk is about 25 per cent and in the third month about 5 per cent.

Rubella virus causes fetal growth retardation as well as specific organ malformations. The consequence of rubella in pregnancy ranges from death of the fetus *in utero* to birth of a normal but infected child. Virus may continue to be excreted by an individual for years after the original infection, especially in severe cases of the rubella syndrome. This persistence of the virus accounts for the appearance of malformations due to rubella in babies born to mothers who had an attack of rubella shortly before conception.

The developing organs principally affected by the rubella virus are the eye, ear, heart and brain. Cataract, nerve deafness and congenital heart lesions, especially patent ductus arteriosus, are the most common lesions but mental handicap may occur. More recently, evidence of systemic infection has been found in addition to the better known features of the rubella syndrome already mentioned (see p. 491).

Prevention of the rubella syndrome lies in the protection of all girls by vaccination before they reach child-bearing age. In the U.K. this vaccination is offered to girls from 11–13 years of age.

If the unvaccinated pregnant woman catches rubella in early pregnancy or if she has been in contact with someone with the illness, she is likely to seek advice regarding termination. About 90 per cent of adult women in the U.K. have rubella antibodies, leaving 10 per cent at risk when pregnant. A rising antibody titre, shown by two tests at an interval of 10 days, should determine whether a recent infection has occurred. If the titre does not rise significantly or if a decision regarding termination has to be made on a single serum sample, it is helpful to determine the presence of rubella-specific IgM. This is only present for 3–4 weeks after the onset of the infection (Banatvala *et al.*, 1970). In the case of contacts, serological tests of the patient can sometimes disprove the original clinical diagnosis of rubella.

It is no longer believed that gammaglobulin given to pregnant women who have been exposed to rubella provides any protection.

Evidence that other virus infections in the mother will produce malformations in the offspring is less definite, though it is suggestive in respect of influenza. Other viruses which may damage the developing fetus are infective hepatitis, mumps, Coxsackie B and vaccinia.

Increasing attention is being paid to the frequency of maternal toxoplasmosis as a cause of congenital malformations, especially hydrocephaly, microcephaly and abnormalities of the eye (p. 541). These malformations are due to a persistent infection of the fetus with the protozoon and are comparable to congenital syphilis. The abnormalities may not appear until a few weeks after birth and it is probable that the fetus is affected only if the maternal infection occurs during the second half of pregnancy, as in the case of syphilis. The virus of cytomegalic inclusion disease (p. 117) has a similar effect on the developing fetus.

### Nutritional deficiency

Animal experiments have shown that a deficiency of certain vitamins during pregnancy can cause the birth of young with multiple malformations. This effect can be most readily produced with deficiencies of some of the B group, but also with A, D, E and folic acid. Vitamin A given in excess also has this effect. These associations are unlikely in man but a well-balanced diet must be provided during pregnancy.

## Mechanical

Mechanical factors influence the position of the fetus *in utero*; a baby tends to adopt the intrauterine position for the first few days of life. Consequently, the newborn baby usually remains flexed, since this is the normal intrauterine position. A newborn baby who was delivered as a breech with extended legs will be found to bring the feet up to the head when the blankets are taken off the cot. These intrauterine moulding forces, by causing malposition, may cause dislocation of the hip or prevent the normal development of the limbs. This is often seen with talipes equinovarus, where the manner in which the abnormally placed feet must have interlocked *in utero* can be easily demonstrated. The malplaced limb may cause pressure on the head or trunk, leading to distortion of growth at the point of contact. Animal experiments have shown that limb abnormalities can be produced if normal intrauterine movement is prevented.

One cause for such immobility in man is oligohydramnios; in this case the mother may have noticed that fetal movements were less than normal, or that the head remained in one place, causing discomfort. Dimples or thinning of the skin may indicate sites of persistent local pressure.

## Irradiation

Exposure of the fetus to irradiation during the early weeks of development may lead to malformation; routine chest films of the mother should, therefore, be left till after the first 3 months of pregnancy. If carcinoma of the cervix is diagnosed in pregnancy, evacuation of the uterus is an essential preliminary to radiotherapy. A long-term problem is the possibility that irradiation of the gonads of either parent may cause gene mutation with consequent malformation of future offspring.

## Drugs

The risk that drugs given to the pregnant woman will affect the fetus is so great, that this is now the most important preventable cause of congenital malformations. Drugs, like viral infections, can alter the development of the fetus only if given during the first 3 months of pregnancy. The dosage and duration of treatment is important but, unfortunately, individual variation is such that malformations have been reported where only a single dose of a known teratogenic drug has been given. Presumably this results from an abnormal sensitivity of the affected fetus, but it indicates that there is no safe dose of such drugs.

Drugs may have two different effects on the developing fetus: one group, which includes the hormones, has the effect that might be expected from the known activity of the drug; the other group, a miscellaneous collection, has a totally unexpected action.

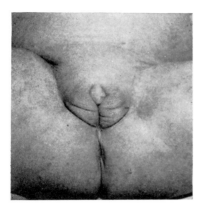

FIG. 25. Hypertrophy of the clitoris in a baby aged 10 weeks, which had been present from birth. During pregnancy, her mother had been treated with ethisterone for a threatened miscarriage.

In the first group are hormones given for threatened abortion. Drugs such as norethisterone and ethisterone which are powerful progesterone-like substances, also have strong androgenic activity which causes masculinization of the developing female fetus leading to female pseudohermaphroditism. A few cases have occurred following the administration of known androgenic compounds such as testosterone, for which the indications have been slender. The degree of masculinization of the female fetus shows the same variations as occur in congenital adrenal hyperplasia (see p. 195). If the drugs are given after normal differentiation has occurred, that is, after the first 3 months, only enlargement of the clitoris occurs (Fig. 25). Despite the anatomical similarity, there is no difficulty in differentiating the condition from congenital adrenal hyperplasia, since the androgenic excess does not persist after delivery and there is consequently no increase in the urinary excretion of 17 ketosteroids or pregnanetriol.

Cortisone is in this group and in experimental animals it has caused a cleft palate. This is presumably due to the action of steroids in suppressing growth, which in this case has prevented union of the two halves of the palate. There is some evidence that this has occurred in man.

Anticonvulsants, particularly phenytoin and phenobarbitone, given to pregnant women increase the incidence of congenital malformations in their infants (Lowe, 1973; Loughnan et al., 1973). This is presumably due to their action as folic acid antagonists. The risk may not be as great as was originally feared, but since the teratogenic effect is dose dependent it is essential to monitor the serum levels of anticonvulsants in pregnancy.

Hormones may also affect the fetus after development is complete. Antithyroid drugs such as thiouracil can cause goitre and hypothyroidism.

The second miscellaneous group of drugs is potentially more dangerous than the first, since the effect is less easily anticipated. The most disastrous drug in this group has been thalidomide which has caused phocomelia and other severe limb abnormalities.

### Socio-economic

The incidence of congenital malformations increases as social status falls. In the British Perinatal Survey (Butler & Bonham, 1963) the death rate from congenital malformations in social class 5 was six times higher than that of class 1. This increase particularly involves malformations of the central nervous system, especially anencephaly which is much commoner in the lower social groups.

### Geographical

There is an increased incidence of congenital malformations in the western half of England and Wales as compared with the eastern half. This unexplaned geographical factor is particularly well shown with anencephaly.

### Seasonal

Another unexplained factor is the seasonal variation in certain congenital malformations. Most of the disorders are not influenced by season but a winter excess has been found in anencephaly, spina bifida, cataract, oesophageal atresia and congenital dislocation of the hip. A summer excess has been found in pulmonary stenosis, some limb defects and some abnormalities of the lower alimentary tract (Slater et al., 1964). Conflicting reports have come from different regions in one country and from different countries, so that much more information is required.

## CLASSIFICATION

No satisfactory classification can cover all the varieties of malformations but Browne's is of value as a method of grouping the failures in development:

1. Failure of formation:
    (a) Complete absence e.g. absent limb, single kidney.
    (b) Small organ e.g. micrognathia.

2. Incorrect formation e.g. fused kidneys or fused radius and ulna.
3. Extra formation e.g. polydactyly.
4. Failure of fusion e.g. cleft lip, cleft palate, spina bifida.
5. Failure of atrophy e.g. syndactyly, imperforate anus due to persistent anal membrane, patent ductus arteriosius, branchial remnants, indirect inguinal hernia.
6. Failure of migration e.g. undescended testicle, malrotation of gut.
7. Failure of canalization e.g. hypospadias, congenital obliteration of the bile ducts.
8. Moulding deformities e.g. talipes.
9. New growth e.g. angiomata.

Congenital malformations are often multiple so that the presence of one should lead to a search for others. Hydramnios is commonly associated with congenital malformations, particularly tracheo-oesophageal fistula, and should always raise the suspicion that the child is abnormal. Multiple defects may be grouped as, for example, the occurrence of midline defects such as cerebral agenesis, cleft lip or palate, congenital heart disease, intestinal anomalies and pilonidal sinus.

An increased incidence of congenital malformations occurs in association with a single umbilical artery or a single palmar crease. The number of umbilical arteries and palmar creases should therefore be noted in every newborn baby.

## RESPIRATORY SYSTEM

In comparison with other systems the congenital malformations of this system are relatively rare.

### Posterior choanal atresia

This is due to a bony or membranous obstruction to the posterior nares; it is more often unilateral than bilateral. Unilateral obstruction causes little trouble and may not manifest itself until some time after birth. It produces a persistent white discharge which is so stringy that it can be wound round an orange stick. This characteristic of the discharge is of value in diagnosis. Bilateral obstruction causes severe respiratory obstruction from birth since the infant has great difficulty in breathing through the mouth. This difficulty in breathing occurs less when the infant is crying since this is associated with mouth breathing, whereas when quiet the baby attempts to breathe through his nose. Mouth feeding is impossible because the baby cannot breathe at the same time, food being blown out of the mouth. The nasal airway should be tested by observing the movement of a few threads of cotton wool placed in front of the nostrils.

*Treatment.* As an emergency measure a pharyngeal airway may make breathing easier. The obstruction is then pierced by blunt-ended forceps, a polythene tube being inserted to maintain the airway.

### Congenital laryngeal stridor

Although about half the cases are due to the 'infantile larynx' from which the child will almost always recover, congenital stridor should always be regarded as indicative of a potentially serious disorder. If the larynx is infantile the vocal cords are small so that the laryngeal aperture is narrow and the ary-epiglottic folds are lax; this causes the arytenoid cartilages to prolapse forward into the opening of the glottis with each inspiration. The edges of the epiglottis are folded back instead of flat, this being an exaggeration of the normal omega shape of the infantile epiglottis.

A less common cause of congenital laryngeal stridor is a vascular ring (p. 183) in which case associated dysphagia is common. Other rare causes are a laryngeal web, a laryngeal haemangioma, particularly subglottic, and a congenital mucous retention cyst. Few people now believe that enlargement of the thymus can cause laryngeal stridor.

The infantile larynx usually causes an inspiratory stridor only, whereas the other, more serious causes, often produce an expiratory as well as an inspiratory stridor. The association of hoarseness with stridor indicates a serious cause such as a laryngeal web or paralysis of the recurrent laryngeal nerve.

Laryngoscopy is urgent for all cases so that those conditions requiring surgery can be diagnosed and treated.

In most cases of infantile larynx the stridor is present at birth but occasionally it is not heard until the baby is a few weeks old. It usually disappears about the end of the first year when growth has sufficiently increased the size of the laryngeal aperture.

The great danger is laryngitis, causing sufficient laryngeal swelling to produce dangerous obstruction. Mothers should be warned to avoid the risk of infection, as far as possible, and to contact the doctor at its earliest sign.

### Lung anomalies

Anomalies of the lobes are common but seldom cause trouble. *Agenesis* of a lobe is usually associated with compensatory emphysema of the normal lobes. A diaphragmatic hernia is commonly associated with anomalies of the lung.

Congenital cystic disease is rare and many of the patients given this diagnosis in the past have had cystic fibrosis (p. 167).

*Intralobar sequestration of the lung* is a cystic malformation which most often occurs in the right lower lobe. The name implies that it is isolated from the rest of the lung but in fact there is frequently a bronchial communication so that the cysts contain air. The abnormality usually comes to light on account of infection and may therefore present as a lung abscess.

*Congenital lobar emphysema* causes overdistension of one or more lobes, usually the upper or right middle. It may present as acute respiratory distress immediately after birth but more often respiratory distress occurs after a few weeks, sometimes following a mild respiratory infection.

Lobar emphysema can be due to a number of different causes and should therefore be considered as a symptom-complex rather than as a single disease entity. It may result from a congenital deficiency of bronchial cartilage in one lobe, from partial obstruction of a bronchus with inflammatory exudate, aspirated mucus or foreign body, or from partial compression of a bronchus.

## ALIMENTARY SYSTEM

### Cleft lip (hare lip)

The cleft generally occurs to one side of the midline, may be single or bilateral and may exist by itself or in association with a cleft palate. A median cleft lip and palate is very rare; it is often associated with a cerebral malformation, particularly absence of the corpus callosum causing a single ventricle; these features may occur in trisomy 13–15 (p. 222).

The disorder may be familial and studies have shown that cleft lip, with or without cleft palate, is genetically distinct from median cleft palate alone. In its mildest form there is only a lip scar ('submucous cleft') indicating delayed intrauterine fusion of the maxillary process, but when severe the cleft extends into the nose.

*Treatment.* The cleft lip is usually repaired about the age of 3 months and surgeons commonly insist that the baby's weight has reached 5 kg. Some surgeons are prepared to carry out early repair provided the baby is referred to them within the first 2 days. There are advantages in this early closure, provided the operative risks are not increased, since feeding difficulties are avoided and breast feeding is more likely to be established.

### Cleft palate

In its mildest form this condition exists as a fish-tail notching of the uvula. From there, in order of severity, it proceeds to bifid uvula, cleft soft palate only and cleft soft and hard palate. Cleft palate may be lateral or median. A lateral cleft is often associated with a cleft lip and may be bilateral; a median cleft is very rarely associated with a cleft lip.

*Treatment.* Surgical repair of a cleft palate used to be left until the baby was about 12 months old, treatment being completed by the time speech had developed. However, a new approach, consisting of early orthodontic treatment (Burston, 1965) is producing much more satisfactory results. The basis of this treatment is the fitting, immediately after birth, of an oral appliance which is so placed as to stimulate the growth of the under-developed maxilla.

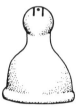

FIG. 26. Modified teat for use in babies with cleft lip or palate. Two parallel cuts have been made on either side of the normal hole.

By stimulating the growth of the palatal shelves the palatal cleft becomes smaller and the alignment of maxilla and mandible improved. This early orthodontic treatment helps the surgeon to achieve a good primary repair of the lip over a symmetrical and well-balanced facial skeleton. Timing of the lip repair depends on the progress of orthodontic treatment. Whatever method of treatment is used, early and prolonged speech therapy is necessary.

The immediate problem in cases of cleft lip or palate is difficulty in feeding, this usually being more severe with the palate defect. In all cases, breast feeding should be attempted since, despite the malformation, some babies feed well this way. If this is impossible, a bottle with an ordinary teat should be tried and this is usually satisfactory if treatment with the palatal prosthesis described above is being undertaken. For babies not being treated with a palatal prosthesis, a cleft palate teat can be used; this has a cowl on its upper surface so as to occlude the gap in the palate. Alternatively, two small parallel cuts can be made into an ordinary teat (Fig. 26). This is the only occasion when a teat may be cut. For normal enlargement of the teat hole a red hot needle should be used, since the hole made by scissors is always too large.

If these modifications to the teat prove unsatisfactory, the baby should be fed with a spoon whose edges have been turned over to make it funnel-shaped. It is then easier for the milk to be poured on to the back of the tongue, but great care must be exercised to avoid pouring it down the throat, with the risk of aspiration pneumonia. If all else fails the baby should be tube fed, but attempts at sucking should be made daily to keep him in practice. Manual expression of the breasts should be continued for as long as possible in the hope that feeding from the breast may be achieved after a few days, even though impossible at birth.

Close supervision should be maintained on all babies with cleft palate or cleft lip. It is a common finding that when these children are admitted from the waiting list for surgical repair, the operation has to be postponed owing to poor nutrition or anaemia. A particular watch must be kept for otitis media to which children with cleft palate are particularly liable (Paradise *et al*, 1969).

The immediate and intense distress felt at the time of birth by mothers of babies born with a cleft lip or palate can be greatly relieved by showing them photographs of similarly affected babies both before and after surgical repair. Such photographs should always be readily available since, to be really effective, they should be shown to the mother at the time of birth and not the next day.

### Epidermal inclusion cyst

Small white cysts are commonly seen on either side of the midline raphe of the palate (Bohn's nodules or Epstein's pearls) and occasionally on the inner surfaces of the gums. These are lined by stratified squamous epithelium and contain keratin. They are present at birth but disappear within a few weeks.

### Mandibulo-facial dysostosis (Treacher-Collins syndrome)

This syndrome results from disturbed development of the first branchial arch producing a very characteristic facial appearance (Fig. 27). The eyelids slope downwards and there may be a coloboma of the lower eyelids causing a notched defect. The malar bones are hypoplastic so that the cheeks are flat and the hypoplastic mandible causes a receding chin. The ears are deformed, the pinnae being low-set with deficient cartilage and the auditory meatus may be absent. The mouth is larger than normal (macrostomia), the palate is high and the teeth abnormally placed.

The condition is inherited as an autosomal dominant trait with variable manifestation.

### Micrognathia (Pierre Robin syndrome)

Severe under-development of the lower jaw is obvious and is often associated with a cleft palate (Fig. 28). Milder degrees are less obvious, but sometimes account for a baby's difficulty in sucking because he cannot get the lower lip sufficiently round the nipple or teat. The act of sucking in these cases helps to develop the lower jaw. The Pierre Robin syndrome is the one exception to the rule that the skeletal pattern of the jaws remains constant (see p. 353); the lower jaw in this condition can enlarge with age. This supports the suggestion that micrognathia can be due to intrauterine compression and that catch-up growth can occur after birth.

An infant with a poorly developed lower jaw is liable to excoriation of the chin from constant dribbling; this can be prevented by the regular application of a protective layer of vaseline. In severe cases the tongue falls back into the throat (glossoptosis) causing respiratory obstruction. Such babies should be nursed prone or on their side. They sometimes require an operation to fix the tongue to the floor of the mouth for the first few months of life.

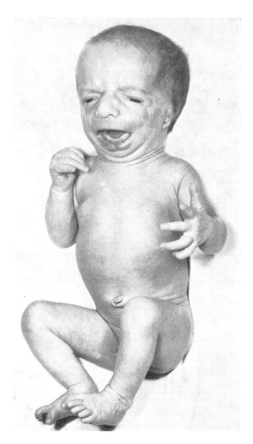

FIG. 27. Mandibulo-facial dysostosis (Treacher-Collins syndrome) illustrating the downward sloping eyes, large mouth and deformed ears.

## 'Tongue-tie'

Many babies are born with a short fraenum to the tongue so that its tip is tethered, but this is not a cause of feeding difficulties or delayed speech.

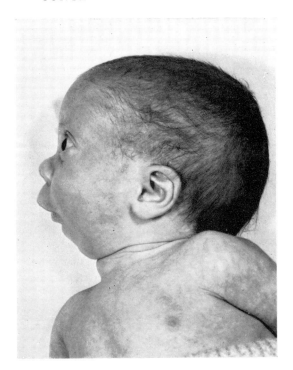

FIG. 28. Severe micrognathia (Pierre Robin syndrome). This baby also had a median cleft palate.

During the first year of life, the main growth of the tongue is in the tip so that the attachment of the fraenum comes to be sited farther back and the tongue can then be protruded. An explanation of these facts to an anxious mother is all that is required.

Very rarely the tongue remains tethered and this can cause interference with the pronunciation of some consonants and the playing of wind instruments. In such cases the operation of lingual fraenectomy may be necessary but never before the age of 4 years and only if the tongue is too weak to stretch the fraenum. The old operation of 'snipping' the fraenum may result in severe bleeding and should never be permitted.

### Oesophageal atresia and tracheo-oesophageal fistula

In 85 per cent of cases of oesophageal atresia, the upper oesophagus ends in a blind pouch and the lower oesophagus joins the respiratory tract by a fistula near the tracheal bifurcation (Fig. 29). A large proportion are associated with hydramnios, the most important clue to diagnosis.

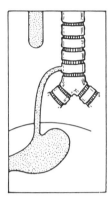

FIG. 29. The most frequent type of oesophageal atresia, which is associated with a tracheo-oesophageal fistula.

Hydramnios in these cases accounts for the high incidence of premature labour and is due to inability of the fetus to swallow. Under normal circumstances amniotic fluid is swallowed; evidence for this is the presence of dye in the fetal intestines after amniography. Further confirmation of i trauterine swallowing is the constant finding of lanugo and skin debris in the faeces of newborn infants. The bulk of this swallowed fluid is assimilated into the fetal tissues or removed through the placental circulation. A small quantity is returned to the amniotic fluid as urine. If the amniotic fluid is unable to reach the stomach, hydramnios is likely to occur (see also anencephaly and hydramnios, p. 217 and amnion nodosum, p. 199).

From birth, the infant pours liquid from the mouth due to an inability to swallow. This fluid, which is a mixture of saliva and mucus, often produces a fine foam round the mouth. As soon as the baby is fed he chokes, splutters and goes blue because the milk, having filled the oesophageal pouch, pours over into the respiratory tract.

Diagnosis rests on three facts; hydramnios in the mother, an excess of mucus from the mouth, and choking when fed. Confirmation can rapidly be made by the passage of a large tube (Jacques EG8; FG 16) which will not go down into the stomach. A large tube is essential since a small soft feeding tube may curl up in the blind pouch and mistakenly be thought to have entered the stomach. An ordinary rubber tube is sufficiently radiopaque to show on X-ray, a plain film being usually all that is required for confirmation. If necessary, a very little radiopaque material, such as aqueous propyliodone (Dionosil), can be injected down the tube in order to outline the pouch but this must be sucked out immediately after the film has been taken (Fig. 30). Barium should never be used as it is too thick to be sucked out properly and

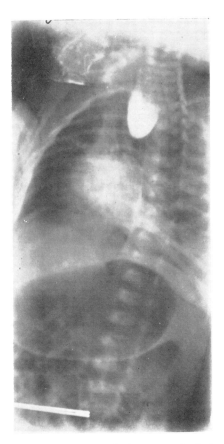

Fɪɢ. 30. Oesophageal atresia. The blind upper end of the oesophagus is
outlined by radiopaque dye.

would obstruct the respiratory passages if inhaled. Radiological evidence of
air in the stomach indicates the presence of a fistula.

It must be a routine to pass a stomach tube in all cases of hydramnios or
excess mucus, so that the diagnosis should be made before feeds have been
started. At the very worst, not more than the start of one feed should have
been given. Once the diagnosis is suspected no further feeds must be given
and, until the child is on the operating table, the pharynx must be constantly
sucked in order to keep the oesophageal pouch empty. The baby should be
nursed upright to prevent reflux of gastric contents through the fistula into
the lungs.

*Treatment.* With modern thoracic surgery a successful repair is possible in

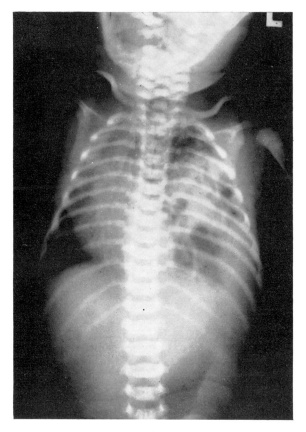

FIG. 31. Diaphragmatic hernia. The dark shadows in the left thorax are due to air in the intestine. The normal stomach bubble below the diaphragm is absent, since the stomach is in the chest.

95 per cent of patients where there is no other malformation, the situation in half the cases. In such patients the most important cause of death is pneumonia from inhalation of milk and saliva, and of regurgitated gastric contents if there is a tracheo-oesophageal fistula, these being even more irritating to the lungs than milk and saliva. This emphasizes the urgency of immediate diagnosis. Prematurity is another factor in mortality. If an additional malformation is present, survival may also be dependent on its severity.

### Diaphragmatic hernia

This most often occurs on the left side, permitting a variable amount of stomach, intestines and liver to pass up into the thoracic cavity. The left lung is collapsed and often malformed; pressure from the herniated organs pushes the mediastinum to the right.

The condition presents at birth, or shortly afterwards, with acute respiratory distress since increasing air in the stomach and intestines causes compression of the lungs. Chest expansion is poor and the air entry into the lungs diminished. The lack of viscera in the abdomen causes it to have a scaphoid appearance. Early diagnosis is essential, a plain X-ray film being sufficient for confirmation in most cases (Fig. 31). Difficulty in radiological diagnosis may sometimes arise from multiple lung cysts, but in the case of a hernia the deficiency of the bowel shadows in the abdomen will be apparent; it may also be possible to follow the line of the gas-filled bowel into the chest. If doubt still exists, a little radiopaque dye may be used but this should never be routine. Problems sometimes arise if the X-ray is taken very early in life before there is gas in the gut. A repeat X-ray a few hours later has given the diagnosis. A contralateral pneumothorax is common and seriously increases the mortality risk.

The disorder should be suspected in all newborn babies with respiratory distress.

*Treatment.* Immediate surgery offers the only hope for survival. If the child is *in extremis* an endotracheal tube should be passed immediately and the child ventilated by intermittent positive pressure. By this means the lungs can be efficiently inflated since the intestines are being compressed and the mediastinal displacement partially corrected. Oxygen must not be given by face mask as this inflates the stomach. If possible, a tube should be passed through the nose into the stomach to keep it empty of air.

### Hiatus hernia

In this condition, which is sometimes familial, a small knuckle of stomach passes upwards through an abnormally wide oesophageal opening in the diaphragm. As a result, the action of the cardiac sphincter is impaired and free reflux of stomach contents occurs, especially when the patient is lying down. An understanding of the physiology of the gastro-oesophageal junction is necessary for a better understanding of the problem (Chrispin & Friedland 1966; Chrispin et al., 1967). In the normal baby, reflux is prevented, not by the angle of entry of the cardia, but by the correct functioning of the vestibule; this is the bulbous lower end of the oesophagus lying partly in the thorax, partly in the hiatus and partly in the abdomen. Under normal circumstances the vestibule opens only during swallowing. Its muscosal folds produce a star-shaped tube, thereby increasing the resistance to flow through the tube. The 'mucosal choke' effect results in an all or none action so that when the vestibule opens it does so rapidly. The mucosal choke mechanism is assisted by the positive pressure on the intra-abdominal portion of the vestibule and the negative pressure on the intrathoracic portion.

When a hiatus hernia is present, no positive pressure is exerted on the lower part of the vestibule since this no longer lies in the abdomen. Consequently, crying alone or a dry swallow will cause the vestibule to open. This effect of dry swallowing probably accounts for the exacerbation of symptoms produced by upper respiratory infections, since these increase the amount of dry·swallowing.

Vomiting occurs from birth, particularly when the baby is laid down after a feed. It is common to find a little vomit and saliva on the pillow in the morning. The vomit contains mucus from oesophageal irritation (the oesophagus is particularly well supplied with mucous glands) and may contain flecks of

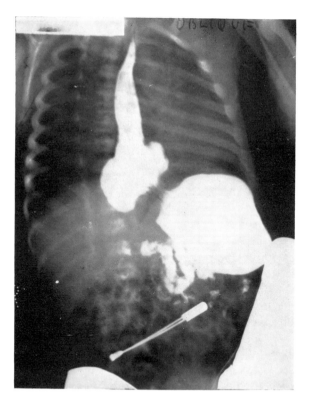

FIG. 32. Hiatus hernia. A barium swallow has been performed and the patient then placed in the head-down position. Free reflux from stomach to oesophagus resulted; a herniated portion of stomach can be seen immediately above the diaphragm.

altered blood. This blood results from oesophagitis due to gastric juice and passes down into the stomach before being vomited; it is therefore usually brown from partial digestion, rather than bright red. Pain may occur from oesophagitis and older children sometimes make peculiar writhing movements of the neck to facilitate swallowing. Oesophagitis is very liable to lead to stenosis and is the commonest cause of this condition in childhood; true congenital stenosis of the oesophagus is rare.

Diagnosis is made by barium swallow (Fig. 32). Free reflux is present when the patient is placed in the Trendelenburg position, but it may be more difficult to demonstrate the intrathoracic pouch of stomach. The so-called congenital short oesophagus results in most instances from a hiatus hernia. True short oesophagus is very rare, if it exists at all as a separate entity.

*Treatment.* This is either medical or surgical. Medical treatment involves keeping the baby propped up day and night in a special chair (Fig. 33). The feeds should be thickened by the addition of cereal or Nestargel to reduce their liability to reflux. Alkalis can be given to reduce the risk of oesophagitis.

The grave danger of this condition is oesophageal stenosis secondary to oesophagitis. So long as this does not exist medical treatment is satisfactory, a considerable proportion of cases spontaneously returning to normal within the first year. If stenosis is present, surgery should not be delayed.

## Congenital pyloric stenosis

Clinical evidence of pyloric stenosis seldom occurs in the first week of life and it is exceptional for a pyloric tumour to be found at birth. It seems that a short period of extrauterine life is required for the stenosis to develop sufficiently to cause symptoms. However, the liability to the condition is determined before birth and the increased familial incidence of the disease points to a genetic origin. There must also be some environmental factor to account for the observation that pyloric stenosis has quite often been found in only one of a pair of identical twins. Dodge (1973) believes that maternal stress in pregnancy is an aetiological factor and has experimental evidence in support.

The symptoms usually start in the second or third week of life, this holding constant for preterm as well as full-term babies, so that many preterm babies have been treated surgically before they were due to be born. It seems that the onset of feeding is one trigger mechanism which causes hypertrophy of the pylorus to develop in a susceptible individual. Clinical manifestations never develop after the end of the fourth month.

The condition is common and occurs in about three out of every 1000 live births. It is much commoner in boys than in girls, the ratio being four to one. About 50 per cent of affected children are first-born, but 40 per cent of children

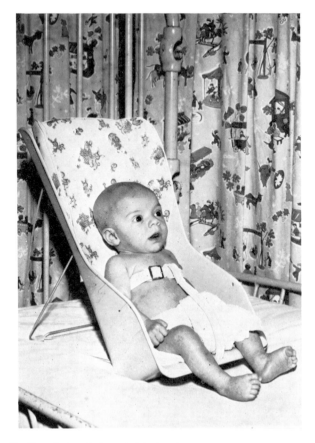

FIG. 33. Ekco baby chair, suitable for the continuous upright nursing of infants with hiatus hernia.

throughout the country are first-born. Therefore, there is only a slightly increased incidence among first-born children and probably little, if any, relationship between the two.

The presenting symptom is projectile vomiting. This may be so forceful that the baby vomits over the end of the bed, supporting the mother's common description that 'he pumps it up'. When the vomiting starts it may not be particularly forceful, only occurring with occasional feeds, but in a few days vomiting occurs during or after every feed. The vomit is characteristic since it contains curds of partially digested milk and is not bile-stained. Altered blood may be present if gastritis is severe, but this is more typical of a hiatus hernia.

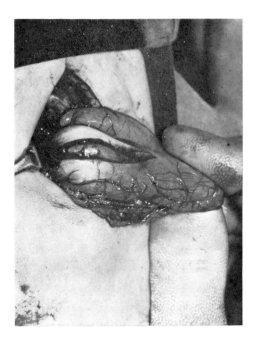

FIG. 34. Congenital pyloric stenosis. The glistening white pyloric tumour has been pulled out of the wound and the hypertrophied muscle incised down to the mucous membrane. This can be seen bulging up through the gap in the muscle. On the right of the photograph the incision is seen to extend as far as the stomach wall, where the hypertrophy ceases.

Constipation is usual since food is not getting through, but it is not invariable; some babies pass loose green motions which may mislead the doctor from the true diagnosis. The appetite remains good, in fact the baby is usually ravenously hungry unless he has become lethargic from dehydration and alkalosis. This good appetite is of diagnostic value when compared with the poor appetite of the baby whose vomiting is due to infection or to a simple feeding difficulty. Prior to the onset of symptoms the baby has been well and gained weight satisfactorily, but once vomiting commences there is an abrupt fall in weight. This rise and subsequent fall in weight is very different from the weight of a newborn baby with a feeding difficulty in whom no appreciable gain in weight occurs.

The babies have a very characteristic worried look, like the older dyspeptic patient; the experienced doctor or nurse may say that the baby 'looks like a pyloric'. Dehydration may develop and is diagnosed by the sunken fontanelle, dry mouth, inelastic skin and sunken eyes. Lethargy accompanies alkalosis, mothers sometimes remarking that their babies have become 'good' because they no longer cry so much. Shallow respirations are also a feature of alkalosis.

Gastric peristalsis, passing across the abdomen from left to right, will be observed in most cases, but is not diagnostic; it may be seen in babies who are wasted from other causes. The palpable pyloric tumour from hypertrophy of the muscle is diagnostic and has been aptly described as feeling like the tip of a nose. The abdomen should be palpated from the left side during a feed so that the abdomen is relaxed and the hypertrophied muscle contracted. The amount of insistence on the feeling of this tumour before making the diagnosis varies in different countries. In most centres in England the tumour will alway; be felt before the diagnosis is made, but this demands practice and patience. It is not always palpable first time and in such cases it is necessary to try to feel the tumour at subsequent feeds. It may be impossible to feel if the stomach is full of wind or feed and is most easily felt immediately after a vomit or a stomach washout. Barium radiography is sometimes used in the diagnosis by those who do not rely on palpation of the tumour.

*Treatment.* This may be either surgical by means of Ramstedt's operation, or medical with atropine methyl nitrate (Eumydrin) or methylscopolamine nitrate (Skopyl). The results of surgery are so excellent that medical treatment can be recommended only if no surgeon is available. The operation is not an emergency; the baby must first be rehydrated and any hypochloraemic alkalosis and hypokalaemia corrected. During this stage, gastric washouts using normal saline are carried out, up to three times a day if there is much residue. The operation may be performed under local or general anaesthesia; a longitudinal incision is made in the hypertrophied pyloric muscle down to the mucosa, special care being taken to avoid cutting the mucosa (Fig. 34). Feeds are commenced 2–4 hours later, and babies can usually return rapidly to full-strength feeds; the old slow schedules of diluted feeds for the first day or two need no longer be used. The most dangerous period for babies who have been in electrolyte imbalance is the 4 hours immediately after the operation, when they are liable to collapse. Warmth is essential in the operating theatre and when back in the ward. They should not be left alone during the danger period immediately after returning from the theatre. Mortality with Ramstedt's operation should be less than 1 per cent.

If the baby is treated medically a 0·6 per cent alcoholic solution of atropine methyl nitrate (Eumydrin) can be used, starting with one drop (0·2 mg) before each feed and working up to a dose of 4 drops before feeds, until vomiting ceases. It can then be reduced to 3 drops t.d.s. for 2 weeks and then stopped. Stomach washouts are required as in surgical treatment. The disadvantage of medical treatment is its uncertainty and its duration. It makes use of the fact that pyloric stenosis is a self-limiting disease and that if the patient can be tided over the first 2–3 months of life he will survive, although the hypertrophied muscle may be palpable for many months.

## Pylorospasm

This is an unsatisfactory diagnosis and not to be recommended. It can be confirmed only by radiology and yet it satisfies the conscience of those who prescribe Eumydrin without ever feeling a pyloric tumour.

## Congenital intestinal obstruction

There are many causes of congenital intestinal obstruction. The most common are intestinal atresia or stenosis, malrotation of the gut, Hirschsprung's disease and meconium ileus. Acquired intestinal obstruction due to milk curds (p. 314) may be mistaken for a congenital cause. Very often an exact diagnosis cannot be made until the abdomen is opened, but this does not matter. The essential is to make the diagnosis of obstruction as early as possible since successful treatment is dependent on early diagnosis. The classical triad for a diagnosis of intestinal obstruction is vomiting, constipation and abdominal distension, but in newborn infants the picture is not as simple as this suggests. Vomiting always occurs but not always as early as might be expected. Moreover, it is a very common symptom in newborn babies and could be of little significance. But if it is persistent and particularly if it is bile-stained, the chances that it is due to intestinal obstruction are great. Green vomit is always serious, though an obstruction above the ampulla of Vater would give rise to persistent vomiting of fluid which was not bile-stained.

The next difficulty with babies is that they may pass three to four meconium stools and yet have complete atresia of the bowel. The reason for this apparent anomaly is that meconium is formed *in situ* at all levels of the bowel during fetal life and any present below the level of obstruction will be excreted. Since in almost all cases the obstruction is below the entrance of the common bile duct, the meconium contains no bile and is of a lighter colour than normal. Moreover, the stools do not change to the normal yellow colour as occurs in the first few days if the bowel is patent. Nurses must therefore be trained to write down the colour of the stools of all newborn babies and specifically to record when the first 'changing' (i.e. yellow) stool is passed.

Abdominal distension is a relatively late sign; it is virtually absent in high intestinal obstruction. Occasionally, the distension of the stomach alone in duodenal obstruction may be sufficiently obvious for a clinical diagnosis to be made. It must be emphasized that the baby with intestinal obstruction does not look ill until the condition is dangerously far advanced, so the fact that the baby looks relatively well is no argument against the diagnosis.

One investigation only is of value and this is a plain antero-posterior film of the abdomen taken in the erect position. This will demonstrate fluid levels in the dilated loops of gut. Emphasis should be placed on the dilated bowels since fluid levels alone are not significant in the first year of life. An X-ray taken in the supine position is unnecessary and gives no additional information. The distribution of air within the intestines is also important, since normally this reaches the large gut within the first few hours of life. Absence of air below the obstruction may be obvious, particularly in small gut obstruction. In duodenal atresia the grossly dilated stomach and proximal duodenum, with absence of air elsewhere is very characteristic, causing the 'double-bubble'.

*Diagnosis.* This is usually obvious but the greatest diagnostic difficulty is ileus, secondary to sepsis. The infection may be within the bowel or separate, for example skin, umbilicus or septicaemia. Such children are extremely ill and there are no bowel sounds.

*Treatment.* Although surgical treatment for these babies is urgent it is important that any electrolyte disorder should first be corrected by intravenous therapy. During this period the stomach should be kept empty by repeated gastric aspiration.

### Intestinal atresia

Evidence suggests that this may be due to intrauterine interference with the blood supply to a segment of the developing bowel, thus explaining why the atretic segments are commonly multiple. This theory is supported by the observation that the anomaly is seldom associated with other malformations, except in the case of duodenal atresia which may be associated with mongolism; in this case it is probably due to failure of canalization of the duodenum.

### Imperforate anus

This ought to be diagnosed as soon as the baby is born since inspection of all orifices should be carried out at once. The routine taking of rectal temperatures of all newborn babies is a further safety precaution. The investigation required in this case is a lateral X-ray, taken with the child upside down and a small radiopaque marker on the site of the anus. A coin is too big and the variable amount of fat may cause it sometimes to lie far from the anus. Gas in the lower bowel indicates the gap between the end of the large bowel and the anus. The picture may be falsified by the presence of inspissated meconium in the lower bowel preventing the air from rising into the end of the blind pouch, or if the swallowed air has not yet reached the most distal portion of the bowel. A line drawn on the X-ray from the symphysis pubis to the coccyx gives the line of the levator ani. Provided the picture is not falsified, bowel ending above the line indicates an imperforate rectum, but if it comes below it is only an imperforate anus.

If there is any external evidence of the anus, such as a dimple, the rectum probably ends low down and surgery should be able to achieve continence. If the bowel ends above the levator ani, continence can seldom be established.

Congenital stenosis of the bowel occurs but may not cause symptoms for some time after birth. Anal stenosis causes the motions to be like ribbon, as though squeezed from a toothpaste container, and can be treated by dilatation from below.

### Malrotation and volvulus

If the gut fails to rotate normally during development, intestinal obstruction can occur in two ways. First, since the caecum remains on the left side, it carries peritoneal bands from its normal site which pass across the duodenum and may obstruct it. Secondly, the mesentery is attached by a short root, so that the chance of volvulus of the small intestine is much greater than with a normally attached mesentery.

### Meckel's diverticulum

This structure is a finger-like protrusion from the lower ileum and is due to persistence of a portion of the omphalo-mesenteric duct, which in the developing fetus runs from the mid-gut to the yolk sac. It may never cause symptoms but can give rise to a number of complications. It frequently contains aberrant gastric mucosa; this produces digestive enzymes which can cause peptic ulceration and haemorrhage from the mucosa of the diverticulum or adjoining ileum. It is therefore a possible cause of rectal bleeding.

Inflammation within the diverticulum leads to the same clinical picture as acute appendicitis and is very liable to cause perforation.

The omphalo-mesenteric duct may remain patent, causing a discharge from the umbilicus, or it may form a vestigial band and lead to intestinal obstruction. A Meckel's diverticulum may form the apex of an intussusception.

### Hirschsprung's disease

This condition, which is at least partly genetically determined, is due to congenital absence of the parasympathetic nerve supply affecting a variable length of the terminal bowel. In the majority of patients a short segment only of bowel is affected and in this group boys predominate. In those with a long segment, so that the small as well as the large intestine is involved, there is no difference in sex incidence. When two members of a family are affected the length of the segment is usually similar in both; the risk of recurrence in other members of the family is greatest in the long segment cases. No parasympathetic ganglion cells are to be found in the plexuses of Auerbach or Meissner in the affected portion of the bowel. This aganglionic segment of bowel always ends at the anocutaneous junction, but its starting point varies from case to case and may be anywhere from the splenic flexure downwards, or occasionally in the small intestine. Absence of the parasympathetic nerve supply prevents normal peristalsis, so that the affected portion becomes functionally like a piece of lead pipe through which the faeces must be forced from above. Consequently, the normal bowel immediately above the affected bowel hypertrophies in order to produce the increased power necessary for this action. The hypertrophied bowel dilates, while the aganglionic segment becomes narrow as a result of increased tone from the unopposed action of the sympathetic nervous system. The junction of the hypertrophied and narrow segments is characteristically funnel-shaped, a diagnostic feature in the barium enema (see Fig. 99, p. 307). Mongolism may be associated with Hirschsprung's disease.

An understanding of the pathology of the disease explains the clinical features. Constipation is the presenting symptom and dates from birth. There is delay in the passage of the first meconium stool which, in 90 per cent of normal babies, is passed within the first 24 hours. However, the age at which the child is brought to the doctor depends on the length of the narrow segment. A long narrow segment produces intestinal obstruction at birth, but a short narrow segment causes only intermittent constipation which may not be sufficiently severe to bring the child to the doctor for months, or even years. Very occasionally the condition presents as attacks of diarrhoea with distension in early infancy; this is due to enterocolitis and may easily be mistaken for gastroenteritis.

Examination of the abdomen shows the distension to be largely gaseous rather than faecal in origin. The rectum is found to be empty and the examining finger is gripped by the tight intestinal wall. Confirmation of the diagnosis is made by barium enema; the barium is seen to enter the narrow bowel and then to pass on to the dilated portion through the funnel-shaped connection. An additional diagnostic safeguard is a submucous rectal biopsy in order to demonstrate the absence of ganglion cells.

Intestinal obstruction from Hirschsprung's disease can usually be differentiated from other forms of obstruction in the newborn because flatus is often passed immediately after rectal examination. Children who have not presented at birth have a history of chronic constipation from birth, with acute episodes of severe abdominal distension, vomiting and complete constipation. These bouts build up for a few days and then, after the release of large amounts of flatus, the abdomen deflates, the child going back to his previous picture of chronic constipation and moderate abdominal distension. Such children are usually stunted in their growth. Unlike chronic constipation of functional

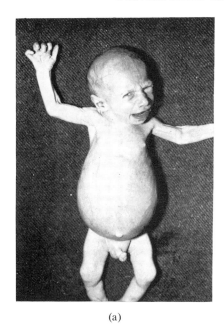 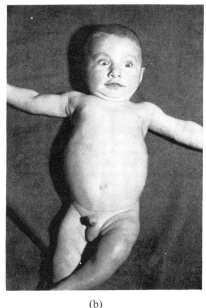

(a)                                    (b)

Fig. 35. Hirschsprung's disease.

(a) Aged 5 weeks—the infant is wasted and there is gross abdominal disten-
    sion.

(b) Aged 5 months—after preliminary treatment with bowel washouts only.
    Rectosigmoidectomy was successfully performed shortly afterwards.
    This child also has glandular hypospadias.

origin (see p. 304) pain is not a feature and there is no faecal incontinence; the
stools in the chronic stage are characteristically like pellets.

*Treatment.* The condition can be cured by surgical removal of the aganglionic segment of bowel. This should be preceded by a period of bowel washouts in order to deflate the bowel and remove the accumulated faecal material.
Saline rather than water should be used for the washouts since the absorption
of a large quantity of water could lead to water intoxication. If the aganglionic
segment is very long, the bowel washouts are unable to achieve their purpose
and a colostomy is required. Surgical removal of the bowel is not an urgent
matter and the child can be maintained on washouts until he is fit (Fig. 35).

## Meconium plug

Intestinal obstruction may result from a plug of tenacious, usually white
meconium in the ano-rectal region. It is not known whether this plug is the
sole cause of the obstruction, or whether its presence is the result of a delay in

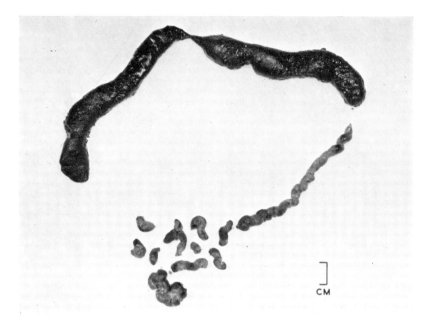

FIG. 36. Meconium ileus. Specimens of meconium removed at a successful operation. The upper and large portion came from the dilated proximal ileum and was extremely tenacious. The long, thin portion on the right was coiled within the undilated distal ileum. The hard pellets in the centre were removed piecemeal from the distal ileum.

the initiation of bowel evacuation in the newborn. The plug may be passed after rectal examination or require bowel washouts to achieve this. The baby is otherwise normal and the condition is not related to cystic fibrosis (see below). Some cases of supposed meconium plug obstruct for a second time and turn out to be Hirschsprung's disease.

### Meconium ileus

This cause of intestinal obstruction occurs as a manifestation of cystic fibrosis (see below). The meconium is extremely sticky owing to the absence of digestive enzymes. Consequently, the meconium cannot move down the intestine even though the gut is patent. The hold-up of meconium usually occurs in the lower ileum causing the large gut to be only of pencil size because its cavity has never been opened by the passage of meconium. It is understandable that before the condition was properly understood a diagnosis of stenosis of the large bowel was made.

The plain X-ray of the abdomen is characteristic because small quantities of air are mixed with the sticky meconium, giving a granular appearance.

Surgical removal of the sticky meconium is an extremely tedius and hazardous operation (Fig. 36) so that only a few children survive. Those that do are still left with the other problems of cystic fibrosis.

### Cystic fibrosis (fibrocystic disease of the pancreas)

This is an important and relatively common condition, its incidence lying between 1–2 per 2000 births. It is a frequent cause of ill health during childhood and an increasing number of patients are now surviving into adult life.

*Aetiology.* The cause is still obscure, this accounting for the different titles by which the disorder has been named. First recognized shortly before the Second World War, the pathology at that time was thought to be confined to the pancreas, hence 'fibrocystic disease of the pancreas'. At a later stage it was thought to be a generalized disease of mucous glands whose viscid mucus caused blockage and dilatation of the glands. It is now known that the mucus is not abnormally viscid. The only definite abnormality is the excessive quantity of mucus produced. The glands are histologically normal as is the chemical constitution of the mucus.

Even the concept of abnormal mucus proved too narrow when a disproportionately high number of these patients was found amongst those affected by heat stroke during a heat wave in New York. From this came the finding of an increased concentration of sodium and chloride in the sweat of those with cystic fibrosis.

The disorder is now regarded as a generalized disease affecting the exocrine glands. The basic abnormality is likely to be an enzyme defect, it being suggested that this inborn error of metabolism primarily involves the autonomic nervous system. It is inherited as an autosomal recessive, indicating a risk of one in four for future children born to families with one affected child. Early reports suggested the possibility of detecting the carrier state by a higher than average sodium and chloride level, but these reports have not been confirmed (McKendrick, 1962).

*Pathology.* Distension of the mucous glands leads to dilatation with consequent obstruction and fibrosis. The pancreas becomes progressively shrunken, being replaced by fibrous tissue. Obstruction of mucous glands in the lungs leads to bronchiectasis associated with alternating areas of emphysema and collapse. Secondary infection is almost inevitable, causing bronchopneumonia and lung abscesses.

At necropsy, cirrhosis of the liver is being increasingly found now that patients are surviving longer. The gall bladder is often small, thick walled and filled with a colourless mucoid fluid. The cause of the cirrhosis is not clear; in some it is associated with biliary obstruction from bile plugs but nutritional deficiency may be a factor.

*Clinical features.* About 10 per cent of the patients present with meconium ileus (see above) whereas the majority present as failure to thrive from birth, although this may not be obvious for the first few weeks. This failure to thrive is associated with steatorrhoea and recurrent respiratory infections due to the combination of intestinal and pulmonary pathology in varying degree.

Pancreatic failure causes steatorrhoea and gaseous distension, the distended abdomen contrasting sharply with the wasted body (Fig. 37). The stools are bulky, pale and so offensive that a diagnosis is usually possible on the mother's history alone. No other condition produces stools with such a revolting and clinging smell; a mother on returning home is likely to know whether her child indoors has passed a motion as soon as she opens the front door. One possible cause for error should be emphasized: while the child is on a pure milk diet the stools are less offensive than when on mixed feeding with a higher proportion of protein.

Unlike coeliac disease, the appetite remains good except during bouts of respiratory infection. The cheeks often have a characteristic mauve colour. The saliva is tenacious, thereby causing an additional problem for mouth hygiene.

The respiratory symptoms result from progressive bronchiectasis with pulmonary collapse and emphysema. This emphysema causes the chest to become increasingly barrel-shaped; at autopsy, the lungs remain inflated and may completely cover the anterior pericardium. Cough is particularly persistent and paroxysmal so that in young infants a mistaken diagnosis of pertussis may first be made, although no whoop develops. Clubbing of the fingers occurs early, becoming marked.

Secondary lung infection dominates the clinical picture, determining the length of survival. It also accounts for the retardation of growth which is so characteristic of the disease and may be associated with delayed puberty. *Staphylococcus aureus* and *Bacillus pyocyaneus* are the predominant secondary invaders; these are extremely difficult to eradicate as the anatomical changes in the lungs produce an environment in which they can flourish. Moreover, the high salt content of the bronchial mucus encourages the staphylococcus which, unlike most other pathogens, flourishes in a salt-rich medium. In long-standing cases the pulmonary changes lead to pulmonary hypertension and cor pulmonale. Death from right heart failure may then occur.

A few additional clinical features may be found. Rectal prolapse is fairly common, so that cystic fibrosis should always be considered as a possible cause in such cases (see p. 318). Sometimes, a mechanism similar to that causing meconium ileus leads to inspissation of faeces; this produces abdominal colic in association with a hard faecal mass found on palpation of the

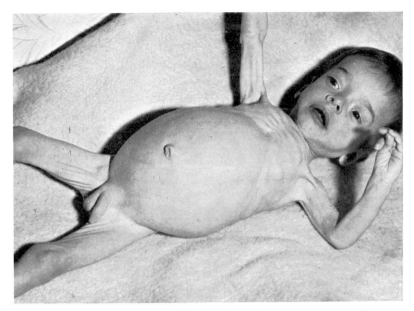

FIG. 37. Cystic fibrosis. The child is 9 months old but merely weighs 5·5 kg, a
gain of only 1·6 kg since birth. The limbs are wasted, the abdomen distended,
and the chest barrel-shaped from emphysema.

abdomen. The obstruction is usually transient so that laparotomy is seldom
required, but the faecal mass persists indefinitely. Occasionally an intussusception results.

Cirrhosis of the liver is a frequent necropsy finding but only in the long-
term survivors are there clinical signs of hepatic failure, portal hypertension
sometimes developing. Diabetes mellitus has also occurred in a few of the
oldest survivors. In a few cases a secondary deficiency of intestinal disaccharidases aggravates the diarrhoea (see p. 570).

Sinusitis is common. Nasal polypi frequently occur in the older patients,
leading to broadening of the nasal bridge, the facial appearance simulating
hypertelorism. A patient with nasal polypi should always be investigated to
exclude cystic fibrosis as a possible cause.

Sterility is almost universal in males with cystic fibrosis owing to anomalies
of the genital tract, particularly congenital absence of the vas deferens. There
is also a high incidence of inguinal hernia, hydrocele and undescended
testicles. No similar abnormalities exist in the adult females and these are
capable of bearing children.

*Investigations.* Many tests are available; more than one should be performed since the diagnosis cannot be made or excluded on the result of a

single test. The tests are based chiefly on the finding of an increased sodium and chloride content in the sweat or a reduction in the amount of trypsin in the stools or duodenal juice.

*Stools.* There is a raised albumin level in the meconium of babies suffering from cystic fibrosis. This has led to the development of a screening test which could be used routinely at birth. Microscopic examination of stools from patients on milk only shows an excess of fat, whereas those on a mixed diet show also an excess of starch granules and muscle fibres. Tryptic activity is determined by the ability to digest gelatin but, since bacterial action alone produces some tryptic activity, figures above one in fifty only should be regarded as normal. The presence of some tryptic activity does not therefore exclude the disease but very high activity is against it.

*Sweat.* Normal sweat contains not more than 64 mEq per litre of both sodium and chloride. Higher levels are found in patients with cystic fibrosis. Sweating is induced locally by the technique of pilocarpine iontophoresis. Since this electrolyte level rises with age the test is unsatisfactory in adults but of great value in infants.

*Duodenal enzymes.* This is a tedious examination because of the difficulty in obtaining the sample of duodenal juice. The determination of tryptic activity in the duodenal juice is more accurate than that in the stools but the test has to a large extent been superseded by examination of the sweat.

A duodenal tube is passed in the early morning when the stomach is empty. The child is left lying on the right side in the hope that peristaltic waves will carry the end of the tube through the pylorus into the duodenum. When difficulty is experienced in getting the tube through the pylorus, radiological screening can be used to guide it into place. Fluid is aspirated at short intervals to determine whether duodenal or gastric juice is being obtained. Duodenal juice is clear instead of turbid, yellow from bile instead of white, and alkaline to litmus paper rather than acid. Once duodenal juice is found, the sample is placed in a small bottle packed round with ice to reduce enzyme activity in transit to the laboratory. Serial dilutions are tested for their activity in digesting gelatin. Absence of tryptic activity in the duodenal juice is almost certain evidence of cystic fibrosis.

*X-rays.* An experienced radiologist will commonly be able to suggest the correct diagnosis in the light of the chest films. Apart from areas of collapse and emphysema it may be possible to make out the thickening of the bronchial walls. These thickened walls produce pairs of fine lines which branch and taper as they get farther from the hilum.

Other characteristic lesions are the small peripheral blob shadows which sometimes occur singly but more often in groups. These are first noticed during or after an acute respiratory infection and are due to small lung abscesses. Hilar gland enlargement occurs in the more advanced cases.

*Diagnosis.* Cystic fibrosis must be suspected in any patient with offensive motions. It must be differentiated from other causes of steatorrhoea, particularly coeliac disease (p. 308) and lambliasis (p. 328). It must also be suspected in children with recurrent respiratory infections and is an important cause of infants who fail to thrive.

*Treatment.* This is essentially palliative in that there is no cure for the condition, but where it is vigorously carried out survival rates have shown considerable improvement.

Control of infection is the key to survival. The aim must be to prevent the first respiratory infection from gaining a foothold, thereby leading to lung damage and chronic respiratory sepsis. Antibiotics must therefore be used with vigour and with strict bacteriological control so that a drug to which the bacteria are sensitive is employed. During the first year of life, antibiotics should be given prophylactically to all patients. Thereafter, prophylactic antibiotics should be given for 3 months after the successful treatment of each respiratory infection. Successful treatment demands the eradication of pathogenic bacteria and the return of the chest radiograph to normal. A wide spectrum antibiotic which is orally effective is chosen, this being combined with a suitable antibiotic administered by aerosol.

Adequate drainage of lung secretions is an essential part of treatment, being achieved by physiotherapy. Even young children can be taught simple breathing and postural exercises, these being combined with vigorous postural drainage and percussion. The mother should be taught these manoeuvres by the physiotherapist. Young children will be unlikely to cough out their sputum but will swallow it. This is reasonably satisfactory since drainage of the lungs is achieved, which is the aim of the procedure.

Optimum nutrition is maintained by careful attention to the diet. This should be high in calories and protein. The substitution of medium-chain triglycerides (MCT) for long-chain (LCT) facilitates fat absorption and reduces stool bulk. LCT require digestion by bile salts and pancreatic lipase in the intestinal lumen before they can enter the mucosal cell. Once inside the cell they have to be converted to chylomicrons by the addition of protein and phospholipid; this enables them to pass into the body via the lymphatics. On the other hand, MCT are absorbed directly into the mucosal cell without the need for bile salts and pancreatic lipase. Moreover they do not have to be converted into chylomicrons but pass directly into the portal blood stream instead of into the lymphatics. MCT is of value in children with severe steatorrhoea, especially if this is causing rectal prolapse.

Serial measurements of height and weight are plotted on a percentile chart so that a comparison with the normal can be made throughout. The diet is supplemented by a multi-vitamin preparation and pancreatin. The stated dose of pancreatin (B.P.) is 0·3–0·6 g, but this is insufficient. Pancrex V tablets and powder are satisfactory preparations, their strength being five times that of the B.P. preparation; the dose is 0·25–2·0 g given with each feed. It is wise to start with a low dose, gradually increasing it until there is no further reduction in the offensive nature of the stools. The stools should become considerably less offensive, but in childhood they seldom become completely normal though this may occur in older patients. The only complication from giving pancreatin is stomatitis and inflammation of the skin around the mouth and anus; this requires a temporary reduction in the dose. Care should be taken to avoid powder being left in contact with the skin round the mouth, and napkins should be changed as soon as a stool is passed.

Thoracic surgery has little part to play in the management of these patients since the bronchial dilatation is widespread. Occasionally, the area of bronchiectasis is localized; in such cases resection, combined with intensive antibiotic therapy to prevent infection in the remaining parts of the lungs, is of value.

All patients admitted to hospital must be nursed in isolation using the strictest of barrier techniques. Those living at home must, as far as practical, avoid unnecessary exposure to infection. They should not be taken to crowded places, and visitors with colds should be prevented from entering the home. Influenzal vaccine can be given every autumn and older patients should be strongly discouraged from smoking.

### Congenital obliteration of the bile ducts

This is the most common malformation of the hepatic system. It may involve the whole bile duct system, or only the extrahepatic ducts which may be totally absent or exist as fibrous cords. The child presents with jaundice but, contrary to expectation, this is not present at birth since the maternal liver has been able to function for the baby. Jaundice does not appear until the baby is 2–3 weeks old so that this cause does not enter into the differential diagnosis of the common problem of jaundice in the newborn infant. Somewhat surprisingly, the degree of jaundice may fluctuate from week to week, but after a few months the child will have become a deep olive green. Death does not usually take place until the baby is about a year old and can be prevented by surgery only if the extrahepatic system alone is involved; this is seldom the case.

Differentiation from neonatal hepatitis may only be possible by liver biopsy since this form of hepatitis can lead to biliary obstruction, the biochemical results therefore being similar in the two conditions. An exploratory laparotomy may therefore be required to make the diagnosis. It is now recommended that this is undertaken before the age of 3 months in order to prevent irreversible liver changes in those amenable to surgical treatment.

## HERNIAE

### Umbilical hernia

This is extremely common. In most white children the hernia comes through the centre of the umbilical ring so that the umbilicus itself is situated at the tip of the hernia. This is a true umbilical hernia and is due to delay in closure of the umbilical ring. In African children, the very common umbilical hernia is in fact supra-umbilical, so that it is shaped like an elephant's trunk with the umbilical scar on its inferior surface. There is an association between this type of hernia and the anomaly of 'cutis navel' which is more common in African children; in it the abdominal skin extends up the cord for a variable distance (Fig. 38).

*Treatment.* In both types of hernia, divarication of the recti occurs and both are likely to heal spontaneously, though the chances are greater in the true umbilical hernia. The herniae should be left alone in order to give the greatest

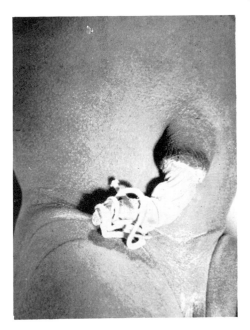

Fig. 38. Cutis navel. A common anomaly in African babies which is causally related to the later development of a supra-umbilical hernia.

chance of natural cure. Strapping may delay closure by preventing the normal movement of the recti and by encouraging umbilical sepsis (Woods, 1953). On no account should an umbilical hernia belt be used since the protruding knob on the inner surface keeps the gap open.

Since spontaneous closure of both types of hernia may occur up to the age of 5 years, parents and surgeons should be persuaded to leave them alone until then. Intestinal obstruction is exceptional in association with an umbilical hernia.

### Exomphalos (Fig. 39)

Between the sixth and twelfth week of fetal development, a portion of the intestine lies outside the abdominal cavity and within the umbilical cord. Normally it returns to the abdomen but occasionally, through an error of development, it remains outside, the child being born with exomphalos. The sac may contain other viscera, particularly the liver, in addition to the coils of intestine.

*Treatment.* The definitive treatment is immediate surgery; pre-operatively

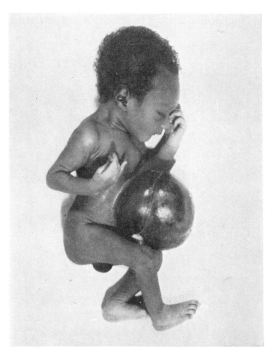

FIG. 39. Exomphalos. This was successfully treated by the daily application of 2 per cent mercurochrome.

the sac should be covered by a plastic bag to keep the exposed intestine warm and moist. Sometimes the peritoneum cannot be closed because it is overfilled by the new contents. In such cases it is sufficient to close the abdominal wall only, dealing with the peritoneum when the child is older. The development of new prosthetic materials to cover very large defects is a major advance. If expert surgery is not available, the old treatment of painting the sac every day with 2 per cent mercurochrome can be used because of the high operative mortality. This causes thickening of the wall of the sac and encourages its epithelialization; the large hernia is repaired at a later date. When using this treatment the possible danger of mercury poisoning must be watched.

### Inguinal hernia

In children this is an indirect hernia due to failure of closure of the processus vaginalis. It is much more common in boys and may be associated with an undescended testicle on the same side.

*Treatment.* Occasionally, the processus vaginalis may close after birth so that spontaneous disappearance of an inguinal hernia can occur in the early weeks of life. After allowing for this possibility, surgery is performed as early as practicable in infancy; trusses should not be used as they are very unsatisfactory. It is unnecessary to delay the operation on account of possible infection during the napkin stage, since this rarely occurs. Delay permits increasing separation of the walls of the sac and there is always the possibility of strangulation which is greatest during the first year of life. A further reason for advocating early surgery is the risk to the testicle if incarceration of the hernia occurs. The neck of the sac is tied off but no repair of the inguinal canal is required in young children. The condition is frequently bilateral, and some surgeons prefer to explore the other side at the same operation in order to reduce the chance of later herniation of intestinal contents through an existing sac. If an undescended testicle is associated with the inguinal hernia, orchidopexy should be carried out at the same time as herniotomy whatever the age of the child.

A direct inguinal hernia, which is the result of weakness of the inguinal muscles, is not seen in children and femoral herniae are rare.

## CARDIOVASCULAR SYSTEM

Congenital heart lesions are a relatively common malformation with an incidence of about 1 per cent. In post-mortems on infants dying within the first month of life about 10 per cent have been found to have this condition, so that congenital heart defects are a common cause of death at this age. Such a high frequency is not surprising when one considers the extremely complicated embryological development of the heart.

### Genetics

In a minority of cases the heart defect is part of a genetically determined syndrome such as Down's syndrome or other chromosomal abnormality. When these cases are excluded, congenital heart lesions are found to be the group of congenital malformations in which genetic predisposition appears least important, although it is not entirely absent. More impressive is the tendency for the same defect to be repeated in the family rather than any increased incidence of congenital heart defects among the relatives.

Although the overall sex incidence of these defects is equal in the two sexes, certain differences appear to be significant. Thus, aortic stenosis, coarctation of the aorta, transposition of the great vessels and Fallot's tetralogy are commoner in males whereas atrial septal defect and patent ductus arteriosus are commoner in females.

### Fetal circulation

Knowledge of the fetal circulation and the changes taking place at birth, are essential to a proper understanding of congenital heart defects. Much of the work on this subject has been carried out in Oxford by Dawes and his colleagues studying young lambs (see Avery for references).

The ductus arteriosus reduces the flow through the lungs by permitting blood in the pulmonary artery to pass direct to the aorta. In the fetal lamb about 55 per cent of the cardiac output perfuses the placenta, 18 per cent perfuses the hindquarters and only 12 per cent goes to the lungs. The liver is supplied by two systems: the left portion receives oxygenated blood from the umbilical vein, the right portion receives venous blood from the portal vein. It is this difference which probably accounts for the occasional finding of degenerative changes in the right portion.

Pulmonary vascular resistance is high in the fetus; the reasons for the reduced pulmonary vascular resistance in association with increased pulmonary blood flow at birth is not known. It is likely, however, that chemical factors associated with hypoxia are principally involved, hypoxia being associated with pulmonary vasoconstriction, while oxygenation leads to pulmonary dilatation. These appear to be more important factors than the mechanical effects of inflation of the lungs.

Occlusion of the umbilical cord after birth removes the placental vascular bed through which more than half the cardiac output has flowed. At the same time ventilation of the lungs introduces a vascular bed through which all the output from the heart must flow. This occlusion causes a greater rise in left compared with right atrial pressure, resulting in closure of the foramen ovale. This may not occur at once and in lambs some right to left flow through the foramen ovale has been shown for up to 48 hours after birth.

The main stimulus to closure of the ductus arteriosus is a high oxygen tension causing constriction of the vessel. However, although this constriction appears at birth, the ductus may remain anatomically patent for some days. During the first few hours of life the flow through the ductus may be in both directions when crying and other changes cause a rise in pressure on the pulmonary side. Hypoxia causes pulmonary vasoconstriction and the resultant rise in pulmonary vascular resistance, as occurs in the respiratory distress syndrome, causes the flow of blood to reverse, becoming right to left as in the fetus. A possible additional, though later-acting factor in closure is the action of stagnation of blood in a vessel causing fibrous and elastic proliferation of the intima.

These observations are confirmed by clinical findings. Careful auscultation of the newborn baby has shown the frequency of a systolic murmur in the first few hours of life which may indicate flow along the ductus, although it may be due to mitral regurgitation. The murmur is commoner in asphyxiated and premature babies, it being a frequent finding in babies with the respiratory distress syndrome (p. 64).

There is considerable variation in heart size in newborn babies. It is larger in expiration than inspiration but even allowing for this it is large for the first 1 to 3 days. Asphyxia causes an increase in cardiac size.

## Clinical picture

The condition may produce no symptoms and before the days of routine examinations some individuals with a congenital heart lesion lived to old age, entirely oblivious of their defect. This point is sometimes of value in helping the parents of a child in whom a murmur has been discovered, to get the problem into perspective.

### CYANOSIS

This is a serious symptom which usually implies a right to left shunt. Cyanosis may occur in attacks or be continuous; its presence serves to separate the different types of congenital heart lesions (see below). Clubbing develops when cyanosis is persistent, but is seldom seen before the age of 6 months.

### DYSPNOEA

This sign is of particular value in infancy where intercostal recession (Fig. 40) may be the first indication that the heart is abnormal. Recession is due to increased activity of the diaphragm which pulls on its attachment to the soft lower ribs. The exact reason for this extra diaphragmatic activity is debatable, but it appears that pulmonary congestion causes the lungs to be less elastic so that a greater pull is required by the diaphragm in order to achieve full expansion of the lungs.

FEEDING DIFFICULTY

Panting during feeds is characteristic. A congenital heart lesion should always be considered when a baby presents with difficulty in feeding, particularly if it tires him.

RETARDED GROWTH

This effect is mainly seen in cyanotic heart disease and results from the disturbance of nutrition to the growing tissues. The possibility of a congenital heart lesion must always be considered in infants who are brought for failure to thrive.

SQUATTING

Some cyanotic children adopt the trick of suddenly squatting on their heels during activity. This is seen particularly in Fallot's tetralogy; it seems that this increases the venous return. Pain and palpitations are uncommon in congenital heart disease, but screaming at the onset of a cyanotic attack is probably due to angina.

CARDIAC SIGNS

It is easy for examination of the pulse to be forgotten in infants, but the full bouncing pulse of the patent ductus is an important sign. Palpation of the femoral arteries is essential, since their absence is proof of coarctation of the aorta.

It should be possible by clinical examination to determine whether enlargement of the heart is due to hypertrophy of the left or right ventricle. Left ventricular hypertrophy produces a heaving apical impulse, so that when a hand is placed over the apex the whole hand is felt to move. Right ventricular hypertrophy produces a tapping beat which is best felt by a finger pushed upwards behind the sternum at the subcostal angle. Bulging of the sternum results from enlargement of the right ventricle and from altered lung compliance owing to vascular changes. (Fig. 40). Anatomically, it is easier to think of the right ventricle as being the anterior ventricle and the left as the posterior ventricle.

In a normal child the second sound in the pulmonary area is split on inspiration, though on expiration the splitting is slight or inaudible. The first element is due to closure of the aortic valve and the second to closure of the pulmonary valve. Only the aortic element is audible in the aortic area, therefore the normal aortic second sound is single. On the other hand, a single second sound in the pulmonary area is pathological in a child, occurring in conditions affecting valve closure, such as severe pulmonary stenosis or pulmonary atresia. Wide splitting which does not vary with respiration is a

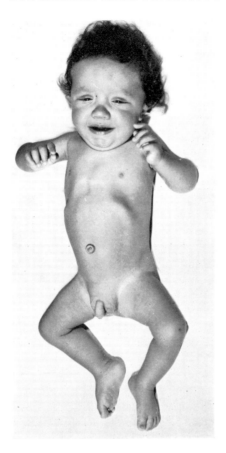

FIG. 40. Intercostal recession resulting from increased diaphragmatic activity in congenital heart disease. Forward protrusion of the sternum is visible, resulting from enlargement of the right ventricle.

feature of an atrial septal defect and is due to delay in the pulmonary element. In pulmonary hypertension there is accentuation of the second element of the split second sound.

A systolic murmur is audible in the majority of congenital heart lesions whereas a diastolic murmur is much less common. There is usually no murmur in uncomplicated dextrocardia or pulmonary atresia. In the early weeks of life the finding of a systolic murmur only, causes considerable diagnostic difficulty, since this may occur in a large number of babies with normal hearts, being probably due to blood flow through the ductus arteriosus which has not yet closed (see p. 177). This is also the likely cause of the murmur in babies with respiratory distress syndrome where there is increased pulmonary vascular resistance, with consequent shunting of blood through the ductus. Many children with a congenital heart lesion have no murmur for the first few weeks so that a systolic murmur heard in the neonatal period is often not due to congenital heart disease, whereas one heard later in the first year is very likely to be due to a heart lesion. A loud murmur, particularly if accompanied by a thrill, is almost certainly organic. The fact that a murmur in an infant is transient does not rule out organic disease. Therefore, all babies in whom a murmur has been heard, should be kept under observation for a long period before congenital heart disease can be excluded.

When taking the blood pressure of a child the cuff must cover two-thirds of the upper arm. A cuff which is smaller than this will give an abnormally high reading. Blood-pressure readings are difficult in babies but should always be attempted. In the absence of special apparatus the flush method is the most satisfactory, the systolic pressure being the point when an exsanguinated limb becomes pink as the cuff pressure is slowly lowered. A rise in blood pressure in the arms occurs in coarctation of the aorta.

X-rays should be taken from a distance of 2 metres if cardiac size is to be assessed. The heart of an infant is more horizontal than the adult, but the greatest diameter of the heart should not be more than half the width of the thoracic cage. The radiological size of the heart is extremely useful as an aid to diagnosis and, in general, a heart working against an obstruction, such as pulmonary or aortic stenosis, is still small when failure develops. On the other hand where there is an abnormal flow, such as occurs in a septal defect or valvular incompetence, the heart is always large by the time failure develops.

A valuable radiological sign is the degree of pulmonary vascularity. Overfilling of the lung fields (pulmonary plethora) is seen in atrial and ventricular septal defects, patent ductus and transposition of the great vessels. Pulmonary ischaemia is seen in pulmonary stenosis and Fallot's tetralogy.

The normal electrocardiogram of young children shows right ventricular preponderance.

**Diagnosis**

The principal diagnostic difficulty is to decide whether the murmur is innocent or organic. In a newborn child who is otherwise well it is likely that the murmur is innocent. A diastolic murmur is always organic though care must be taken to differentiate a venous hum (p. 186). At all ages the presence of other signs of a congenital heart defect will be helpful. Palpation of the femoral arteries is essential.

An innocent murmur is usually (but not always) softer than that caused by organic disease. It is heard to the left of the sternum, varies with posture and is not well conducted. The heart sounds are normal and, in young children, show normal splitting of the second sound in the pulmonary area. An innocent murmur is usually short and often has a muscial, sometimes 'gull-like' quality.

In a newborn baby with respiratory distress the diagnosis between cardiac failure, respiratory distress syndrome, meconium aspiration and pneumonia may be extremely difficult. Cyanosis, a systolic murmur and râles may be present in all three conditions. Babies with respiratory distress syndrome and meconium aspiration may show signs dating from birth, whereas it is unusual for babies with cardiac defects to develop failure as soon as they are born. Pneumonia seldom occurs on the first day. Hepatomegaly is an important sign of cardiac failure but secondary heart failure may occur both in the respiratory distress syndrome and in pneumonia.

An X-ray of the chest is essential in all cases of respiratory distress and may determine the diagnosis without difficulty (see p. 67). It will diagnose a diaphragmatic hernia or pneumothorax, important causes of respiratory distress in the newborn.

## TYPES OF CONGENITAL HEART DISEASE

Three types can be separated on the basis of cyanosis:

### 1. Acyanotic
Includes coarctation of the aorta, aortic stenosis and uncomplicated dextrocardia.

### 2. Potentially cyanotic
In this group the blood flow is usually from the left side, where the pressure is normally higher, to the right side. Reversal of blood flow through the shunt results from an increase in pressure in the lungs such as may temporarily occur during an attack of pneumonia, or permanently if pulmonary hypertension develops. Such a shunt can exist at one of three levels, ventricular septal defect, atrial septal defect and patent ductus arteriosus. In describing one of these conditions to parents it is sometimes helpful to ask them to imagine a four-roomed house with two chimneys. Communications normally exist between the upstairs and downstairs rooms on the same side, but there is no communication between the two rooms on the same level. A ventricular septal defect indicates an opening between the downstairs rooms, atrial septal defect an opening between the upstairs rooms and patent ductus an opening between the chimneys.

### 3. Cyanotic
Includes Fallot's tetralogy and transposition of the great vessels.

## ACYANOTIC GROUP

**Coarctation of the aorta**

This condition is more common in males and, although usually symptomless in children, may cause cardiac failure in infancy. It is diagnosed by finding a systolic murmur, often heard loudest at the back, absent femoral pulses and a rise in systolic blood pressure in the arms. The femoral pulses are not always easy to feel in fat babies so that repeated examinations may be required. Notching of the ribs on X-ray, due to the collateral circulation, will only be found in older children when sufficient time has elapsed for the notch to develop. Coarctation may be associated with aortic valve lesions or with a patent ductus arteriosus.

*Treatment.* Coarctation carries a high mortality from the age of 20 years onwards. Resection should be considered for all and is best carried out before

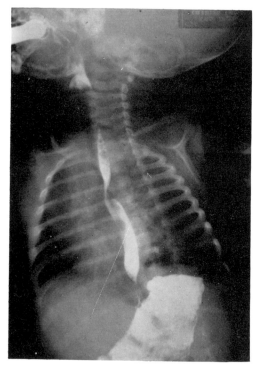

FIG. 41. Vascular ring. Left anterior oblique X-ray of barium swallow. The oesophagus is indented posteriorly by a ring formed by a double aortic arch. The tracheal shadow is visible anterior to the oesophagus.

the age of 5 years so that the child starts school without being regarded as a cardiac invalid. A child who shows any evidence of cardiac failure should have the defect repaired as soon as the diagnosis is made.

### Aortic stenosis

In childhood these patients are usually symptom free. The murmur is similar to that of pulmonary stenosis but heard on the right side of the sternum.

*Treatment.* Aortic valvotomy is indicated if there is a high pressure gradient across the valve.

### Dextrocardia

The heart is usually normal if associated with situs inversus but abnormal if it is the only organ affected. The electrocardiogram shows inverted p waves in lead 1 which resembles aVr. The tracings in leads 2 and 3 are interchanged.

### Congenital heart block

This is probably due to a malformation of the bundle of His and, although it may be associated with a septal defect, there may be no other detectable cardiac abnormality. The auricles and ventricles beat independently, the usual ventricular rate being about 60 per minute.

The child is usually without symptoms, the diagnosis being made on the chance finding of a slow pulse rate and the absence of any significant increase in rate on exertion. It is confirmed by the electrocardiogram which shows no relationship between the auricular and ventricular complexes. The prognosis is usually good, although syncopal attacks may occur.

### Vascular ring

An anomaly of the great vessels such as a double aortic arch produces a ring round the oesophagus and trachea. It is probable that the condition is often asymptomatic, but compression of these organs causes dysphagia, a harsh barking cough, and stridor. The baby tends to keep his head extended, thereby causing the trachea to be elongated and thrust forward. Presumably, the anterior portion of the trachea, being cartilaginous, can displace the compressing vessels whereas the posterior portion, being membranous, is more compliant. It is interesting that this is the position adopted by many infants with pneumonia (p. 344).

The diagnosis in cases with symptoms can usually be made by a barium swallow because of the indentation in the oesophageal shadow (Fig. 41). Such cases can be relieved by surgical division of the anomalous vessels.

## POTENTIALLY CYANOTIC GROUP

**Ventricular septal defect**

It is now realized that this defect may close spontaneously. Naturally, smaller defects can close more easily than large but the change is not confined to the small defects. Spontaneous closure has taken place in defects sufficiently large to have caused cardiac failure in infancy. The mechanism of closure is uncertain, but if it is going to take place it usually does so before the age of 5 years.

Large defects permit a torrential flow of blood into the pulmonary artery. This can cause pulmonary hypertension, being one variety of the Eisenmenger complex. It is reasonable therefore to regard the maladie de Roger type and the Eisenmenger complex as two extremes of a continuous series of cases of ventricular septal defect. The pulmonary hypertension may become so severe as to cause reversal of flow through the defect so that blood passes from the right to the left side.

In some patients with a large defect, acquired pulmonary stenosis develops. This mechanism protects the pulmonary circulation. The pulmonary stenosis may be 'real' or 'relative'. If 'real' there is a fixed rigid narrowing in the outflow tract of the right ventricle, or less often, in the pulmonary valve. In the other type the infundibulum and pulmonary valve are normal but the large left to right flow causes a relative stenosis.

Infundibular stenosis may develop to such a degree that there is reversal of the left to right shunt. This condition is indistinguishable from Fallot's tetralogy (p. 188) and represents an acquired form of that disorder.

CLINICAL FEATURES

*Small defect* (*Maladie de Roger*). There are usually no symptoms, the condition being discovered on a routine medical examination. A loud pan-systolic murmur is audible in the fourth left intercostal space, associated with a thrill.

*Large defect*. It is these children who present with clinical symptoms and sometimes with heart failure in the early months of life. The greatest risk of death from a ventricular septal defect is during the first 6 months of life. The systolic murmur is less loud than in those with a small defect and there is often an apical mid-diastolic murmur. The separated components of the second sound in the pulmonary area may come together to produce a single pulmonary second sound. Radiography shows enlargement of both ventricles and engorgement of the pulmonary vessels. The electrocardiogram shows right axis deviation.

TREATMENT

Children with symptomless small defects should be left untreated in the hope that spontaneous closure will occur. For those with large defects, especially where cardiac failure has resulted, the prognosis is bad. However, since there is a natural tendency for the child to improve if he can survive the first year of life, vigorous medical treatment should be applied. If this fails, surgery should be undertaken. The operation is a palliative one in which a band is tied round the pulmonary artery so as to equalize the pressure on the two sides of the defect. By this means the amount of flow through the defect is reduced, enabling the child to survive until old enough for direct repair; this is usually carried out between the ages of 5–7 years.

## Atrial septal defect

This is probably the most frequent single congenital malformation of the heart encountered in clinical practice; it is commoner in girls. The defect is of two types: *ostium primum* in which the defect is low down in the septum, the base being formed by the mitral and tricuspid valves which may also be malformed; and *ostium secundum*, in which the defect is higher so that only the septum is involved.

Patients with ostium secundum defects do not usually develop any symptoms until the second or third decade. The pulmonary second sound is widely split. In children the systolic murmur in the pulmonary area is not usually very loud. A diastolic murmur may be audible in the tricuspid area as a result of excessive flow through the tricuspid valve. X-rays show enlargement of the right ventricle; in fact the condition produces some of the largest hearts which are compatible with life. The pulmonary artery is dilated and there is pulmonary plethora. The aorta is usually small. The electrocardiogram shows right bundle branch block in almost all cases.

Ostium primum defects are less common, but are the more serious of the two, the patients presenting in childhood. The heart enlarges early and the prognosis is worse. There is a harsh long systolic murmur at the apex due to mitral regurgitation. The electrocardiogram shows left axis deviation, this being a characteristic sign. Although pulmonary hypertension is not common in association with atrial septal defects, it is more frequent in primum than secundum defects (see Eisenmenger complex, p. 186).

*Treatment.* An uncomplicated ostium secundum defect can be closed under hypothermia. The operative mortality is negligible and it should be carried out on all cases before the age of 20 years. An ostium primum defect requires a bypass and is a much more hazardous operation which should not be undertaken if pulmonary hypertension is present.

## Patent ductus arteriosus

This condition, which is twice as common in girls, is usually discovered by hearing the typical machinery murmur on routine examination. The murmur, which is accompanied by a thrill, is best heard in the pulmonary area and is continuous throughout systole and diastole, though louder in systole. There is no other murmur which sounds exactly the same, though a *venous hum* can cause difficulties. This is heard in normal individuals and results from the flow of blood in the great veins. It also is a continuous murmur and is audible just below the clavicles, especially on the right side. However, it is a softer murmur than the ductus murmur, is abolished by occlusion of the jugular vein in the neck and varies with extension and flexion of the head.

Diagnosis presents no difficulty if the typical murmur is heard and it should be possible to make a firm diagnosis on auscultation alone. The real problem arises in infants, since at that age patent ductus produces only a systolic murmur. Absence of the diastolic murmur is due to the pulmonary artery pressure in infancy being nearly equal to that in the aorta, thereby preventing flow through the ductus during diastole. The diastolic element of the murmur is usually present by the end of the first year when the aortic pressure has become higher than the pulmonary.

Infants form the age group when diagnosis is essential since if a patent ductus causes cardiac failure in childhood it does so during infancy. In such children the full or collapsing pulse, resulting from the high pulse pressure, is the most valuable clinical sign. X-rays show some left ventricular enlargement with pulmonary plethora and a varying degree of dilitation of the pulmonary artery. The electrocardiogram is normal, or shows left ventricular hypertrophy or a combined ventricular hypertrophy.

*Treatment.* A patent ductus should be tied or ligated in all cases to prevent later complications. If this is not carried out, adult life will almost certainly be shortened by the onset of cardiac failure and there is always the risk of bacterial endocarditis. The best time for the operation is 3–7 years of age.

### Eisenmenger complex

This term is applied to those cases of atrial or ventricular septal defect, or patent ductus arteriosus in which there is pulmonary hypertension. It occurs in a fair proportion of cases of ventricular septal defect and patent ductus, but is rare in atrial septal defect and is then mainly in ostium primum defects. The changes in the pulmonary vessels in many cases are present at birth and possibly result from a persistence of the fetal type of pulmonary circulation, the pulmonary arteries preserving their thick walls and narrow lumen after birth. Pulmonary hypertension results and in its turn causes more severe changes in the vessels. In other cases the changes in the pulmonary vessels are acquired; this is possibly more often the case in ventricular septal defect.

The pressure in the pulmonary artery is either equal to or, more commonly, greater than that in the aorta so that there is a reversal of the shunt through the defect. The patients are nearly always a little breathless and some are slightly cyanosed. Pulsation is visible in the pulmonary area. An ejection click is audible in systole, immediately after the first sound. The second heart sound in the pulmonary area is strongly accentuated and may be single. The systolic murmur is no longer harsh and no diastolic murmur is audible. The electrocardiogram shows right ventricular hypertrophy and right axis deviation, unless the underlying lesion is an ostium primum defect when left axis deviation is present.

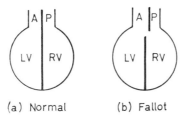

FIG. 42. Diagrammatic representation of Fallot's tetralogy.

(a) Normal. The truncus arteriosus is divided equally into the aorta (A) and pulmonary artery (P).
(b) Fallot. The dividing septum is off-centre causing the aorta to be larger than normal and over-ride the right ventricle (RV). The pulmonary artery is smaller than normal. Since the truncus septum is not central it fails to meet the intraventricular septum, thus leaving a ventricular septal defect.

The prognosis is poor and surgery is contraindicated. Closure of the ductus in such a case is likely to be fatal because of the need for a right to left shunt through the open duct. It should therefore never be undertaken if the patient is cyanosed or if the electrocardiogram shows right axis deviation.

**Pulmonary stenosis**

Although the majority of children with pulmonary stenosis are acyanotic this malformation is included in the potentially cyanotic group because about 10 per cent are cyanosed. This results from enlargement of the right auricle causing tricuspid atresia and regurgitation into the right auricle. The consequent rise of pressure in the right auricle above that in the left causes shunting of blood through the foramen ovale.

Simple pulmonary stenosis may be so mild as to be asymptomatic in childhood, or so severe as to cause serious cardiac embarrassment. In those who have no symptoms, some limitation of exercise tolerance is usually found, when this is specifically tested.

Giant *a* waves are visible in the jugular veins and the second sound in the pulmonary area is single if the stenosis is severe. A harsh systolic murmur is audible in the pulmonary area and is conducted into the neck.

Enlargement of the right auricle causes the cardiac shadow on X-ray to be oval in the horizontal axis, giving the appearance of an 'egg on a string'.

*Treatment.* Pulmonary valvotomy is available for suitable cases. If heart failure has occurred the prognosis is hopeless without surgery and death will occur within 4 years.

## CYANOTIC GROUP

### Fallot's tetralogy

This is a common form of congenital heart lesion and, if the mechanism of its production is understood, there is no need for the student to attempt to remember its four components as if they were isolated facts. Under normal circumstances the truncus arteriosus is divided equally into the aorta and pulmonary artery by a septum which grows down to meet the wall between the ventricles. In Fallot's tetralogy the septum is shifted to the pulmonary side, so that less of the truncus becomes pulmonary and more aorta, and it does not meet the interventricular wall. The result, as shown in Figure 42, is pulmonary stenosis, an over-riding aorta and a ventricular septal defect. The fourth component of the tetralogy is hypertrophy of the right ventricle due to the extra demands made on it.

Occasionally, the clinical state of Fallot's tetralogy is acquired in a child born with a ventricular septal defect (see p. 184).

Although this condition is considered in the cyanotic group, the babies are not usually cyanosed at birth. Cyanosis, which often becomes intense, usually develops about the first or second month. It has been suggested that the development of cyanosis is related to closure of the ductus but operative findings show that there is often no ductus present, and sometimes not even a fibrous cord to suggest one ever existed. Squatting is particularly associated with Fallot's tetralogy.

The enlargement of the right heart causes forward bowing of the sternum, the tapping beat of the large right ventricle being felt at the subcostal angle. The pulmonary second heart sound is invariably single. A loud systolic murmur is audible in the pulmonary area, being accompanied by a thrill in about half the cases. Radiological studies show the characteristic rounded apex, or 'boot-shaped' heart, due to right ventricular enlargement. The lung fields are clearer than normal because of diminished vascularity. The aortic arch is on the right side in about a quarter of the cases. The electrocardiogram shows right axis deviation and tall P waves.

The children are particularly liable to develop syncopal attacks associated with increased cyanosis. These are precipitated by excitement and exercise and result from spasm of the pulmonary artery due to the release of nor-adrenaline. This increased pulmonary obstruction causes more blood to be shunted from the right ventricle to the aorta. Propranolol, being an adrenergic blocking agent, can relieve this increased infundibular obstruction.

*Treatment.* The original surgical treatment (Blalock-Taussig operation) was to produce an artificial ductus by anastomosing the pulmonary artery to the subclavian artery. Nowadays, complete surgical correction is carried out, the best age for this operation being 7–8 years. If the child shows evidence of cardiac failure in early life, before full correction is possible, a preliminary palliative operation can be performed, such as pulmonary valvotomy or in-fundibular resection used separately or in combination, or the older type of shunt operation. By this means he is helped to survive until old enough for full correction.

### Transposition of the great arteries

In this condition the aorta arises from the right ventricle and the pulmonary artery from the left ventricle. This would produce two independent circuits and be incompatible with life, so that if the child survives there must also be either a septal defect or a patent ductus arteriosus.

Transposition is the most frequent cyanotic lesion causing congestive heart failure in infancy; without treatment few, if any, children survive the first year. Cyanosis occurs early and is present shortly after birth. The murmurs and thrills are of no diagnostic importance. The heart is always a normal size at birth but enlarges rapidly in the first 2 weeks. This produces a characteristic X-ray picture, since there is a narrow pedicle to the heart in the antero-posterior view because the aorta is superimposed on the pulmonary artery. By contrast, in the left oblique position, the pedicle is broad since the two vessels lie side by side. Both ventricles are enlarged and the lungs are over-filled, this being the only cyanotic lesion with pulmonary plethora. These findings differentiate transposition from Fallot's tetralogy, the other common cause of cyanotic congenital heart disease, in which the heart is relatively small and the lung fields clear.

*Treatment.* A valuable palliative procedure carried out in the early weeks of life is the creation of an atrial septal defect. Originally undertaken as an open heart operation, this can now be more safely carried out by the technique of balloon septostomy (Rashkind & Miller, 1966; Tynan, 1971). A catheter with a balloon at its tip is passed into the left atrium through the foramen ovale. The balloon is then inflated with contrast medium and pulled back so as to tear the septum. This is followed by a total corrective operation at about the age of 2 years using the Mustard technique (Mustard, 1964; Mustard *et al.*, 1964; Aberdeen *et al.*, 1965).

### Complications of congenital heart disease

The most frequent and grave complication is cardiac failure. All patients are more liable to suffer from recurrent respiratory infections which are often accompanied by bronchospasm. Bacterial endocarditis is always a possibility, although rare under the age of 5 years. Cerebral abscess is a particular risk in those with a right to left shunt, and cerebral thrombosis occasionally occurs.

### General management

One vital function of the doctor is to prevent the child from feeling that he is a cardiac invalid. The patient should rarely be sent to a special school and re-strictions on activity must be cut down to the minimum. The child will usually discover for himself the limits of his physical capacity, adjusting his activity accordingly. It is seldom necessary to stop him playing games if he wishes to take part. The only exception is in patients with aortic lesions in whom sudden death from cerebral or coronary insufficiency is liable to occur. These children should not take part in competitive games but otherwise their activity should not be limited.

The risks of infection are greater than with normal children so that steps must be taken to reduce the likelihood of contact. The young baby should not be taken to crowded places and visitors with colds should be kept away. Penicillin cover is required for all dental extractions and for any form of instrumentation or operation on the genito-urinary tract, as the disturbance may cause bacteria to be thrown into the blood stream. Regular dental care is needed to reduce the risk of dental sepsis.

Iron deficiency anaemia is common and must therefore be watched for and treated if present.

## CARDIAC FAILURE IN INFANCY

### Clinical picture

The majority of such infants will be under 6 months of age; the condition is frequently missed because the classical signs of heart failure, as seen in the adult, are not always present and the child is mistakenly thought to have pneumonia (see p. 345). Murmurs may be lost during an episode of heart failure and the most reliable sign is enlargement of the liver, particularly pro-gressive enlargement over a few hours. There is dyspnoea at rest with associa-ted difficulty in feeding and failure to thrive; restlessness is common and is largely due to anoxia. Oedema usually occurs in the face, as periorbital oedema, or on the dorsum of the feet. However, oedema is often not visible and cannot be relied on as a sign of cardiac failure. The heart rate is increased, averaging 140–180 per minute. Daily weighing may indicate the accumulation of fluid, a fall in weight being evidence of successful therapy. Cyanosis is useful in deciding the type of lesion but not the presence of failure; grey pallor is often a feature of cardiac failure. Pulmonary oedema causes a dry cough and ràles which are often associated with rhonchi from bronchospasm. The short neck of infants and the frequency of crying renders the jugular venous pressure of little value in this age group, though dilated veins on the scalp or back of the hands may be noticeable. These babies often sweat excessively, particularly about the head and neck.

Radiology may be helpful in determining the presence of a cardiac lesion but does not assist in the diagnosis of heart failure. Cardiac enlargement is not evidence of cardiac failure.

## Medical treatment

Babies should be nursed in an oxygen tent with high humidity to counteract the drying effect of the rapid respirations. Care should be taken to prevent overheating in the tent since this leads to peripheral vasodilatation and increased cardiac output. In view of the dangers of overheating, these babies should not routinely be transported to hospital in incubators.

Many restless babies will quieten with oxygen alone, because their restlessness is due to anoxia. They should be nursed in a high Fowler's position in order to assist respiratory movements by permitting free descent of the

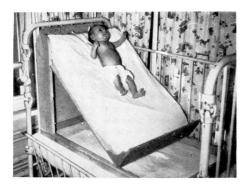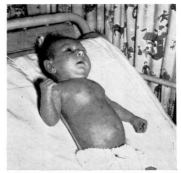

FIG. 43. Special bed for nursing infants with heart failure. The baby is suspended by tapes attached to two straps of adhesive plaster applied to the lateral aspect of the back; these are more easily visible in the photograph on the right. The skin is painted with Tinct. Benzoin Co. for protection, before applying the adhesive plaster.

diaphragm. This cannot be achieved by pillows, therefore a tilting board should be used to which the infant is strapped (Fig. 43).

Babies with heart failure are exhausted by feeding, a distended stomach adding to the respiratory difficulty. They should therefore be given small feeds by tube. If the infant will tolerate an indwelling tube, so that milk can be given by continuous gastric drip, the amount of disturbance is less than with intermittent tube feeds and the stomach is less distended. In severe cases, a low salt milk such as Edosol should be given, the serum electrolytes being checked regularly. Fluids should never be restricted and in cyanotic heart disease care must be taken to maintain sufficient intake in order to reduce the risk of venous thrombosis. Anaemia is common and must by treated at once by iron or, if necessary, by blood transfusion, since it may have precipitated the heart failure.

Rest is important and for the acutely ill infant morphine, up to 0·2 mg/kg (1/300 gr/kg) of body weight, is the drug of choice. For less ill babies and for maintenance therapy, phenobarbitone or chloral should be used. Digoxin should be given to all, the digitalizing dose being 0·08 mg/kg given in four equal doses in the first 24 hours. For maintenance therapy about a quarter of the digitalizing dose is required. The heart rate is used as a guide to decide the dose of digitalis, the drug being stopped if the heart rate falls below 100. Vomiting may be due to overdose but can also result from gastric irritation caused by cardiac failure; in such cases the digitalis should be given parenterally. When using diuretics, electrolyte balance should be watched carefully; hypokalaemia predisposes to digitalis intoxication.

If there is acute pulmonary oedema frusemide should be given intravenously or by mouth. Chlorothiazide may be used for maintenance therapy and for less acute cases, in a dose of 40 mg/kg. Antibiotic cover should be given to all cases, since an associated respiratory infection is common and may have precipitated the onset of cardiac failure. This should initially be given as ampicillin and later changed as necessary, in the light of bacterial investigations.

Bronchospasm is treated by oral salbutamol or aminophylline suppositories.

### Surgical treatment

In every infant with cardiac failure the doctor must decide whether a correctable abnormality is present. Nothing is more tragic than the finding of a patent ductus only in the autopsy of a baby who has died from heart failure. Cardiac catheterization is not easy in this age group so that a systolic murmur, with a collapsing pulse, may be sufficient indication for an exploratory thoracotomy lest a ductus is present. A few patients with coarctation of the aorta present with cardiac failure in infancy and, although many of these have additional cardiac anomalies, some can be successfully treated surgically. Many other conditions are amenable to surgery, though a preliminary period of medical treatment should always be given in order to offer surgery its best chance. The full effect of medical treatment will not become apparent for 2–3 days.

## GENITAL ABNORMALITIES

### Hydrocele

This is due to a collection of fluid within the tunica vaginalis. It is extremely common in babies and should be left alone since the fluid almost always disappears spontaneously. Only if the condition is still present at the age of 5 years should surgical treatment be carried out. A hydrocele of the cord does not disappear without surgical treatment.

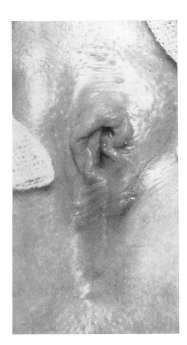 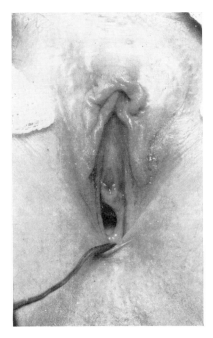

Fig. 44. Labial adhesions in a girl of 9 years.
*Left*  Before treatment.
*Right*  After separation with a probe.

**Labial adhesions** (Fig. 44)

This condition is quite common. The labia minora are fused along part, or the whole, of their adjacent edges, a thin line of cleavage being visible at the site of junction. The abnormalitity often passes unnoticed, the patient illustrated being 9 years old. Occasionally, the child may be referred because the sex is in doubt, but separation of the labia reveals the external genitalia to be quite normal.

These adhesions are not congenital as used to be thought since they have not been found in the newborn. They result from low-grade inflammation with the added factor of the low oestrogen status of a child. Evidence for the low oestrogen level being a factor is the absence of labial adhesions after puberty—presumably owing to spontaneous regression. Moreover, they can be made to disappear by the daily application of oestrogen ointment.

*Treatment.* Although oestrogen ointment locally causes the adhesions to disappear, it is laborious and takes time. Separation of the labia by a probe without anaesthesia is simpler and quicker. After separation, care is required to prevent the edges from re-uniting. The mother is shown how to separate and swab the labia daily and to apply vaseline, until epithelization of the edges is complete.


## INTERSEX STATES

Two major groups exist: in the first there is an abnormality of the chromosomes but the external genitalia appear normal in childhood; the second are the hermaphrodites.


**Chromosomal abnormalities**

The normal chromosomal pattern of a female is XX and of a male XY. During maturation of the ovum and sperm, reduction division occurs so that the two chromosomes separate. An ovum therefore always contains a single X chromosome, but a sperm may carry either a single X or a single Y. Fertilization of an ovum by an X sperm results in an XX zygote and a female is born, whereas a Y sperm produces an XY zygote and a male is born.

Occasionally, the two chromosomes fail to separate during reduction division (i.e. non-disjunction, see p. 218) so that one cell has both chromosomes and the other none. Numerous combinations result from the fertilization of these abnormal cells, the commonest being XXY and XO. XXY individuals have Klinefelter's syndrome (p. 643) and XO have ovarian dysgenesis (p. 646). YO individuals have not been found, presumably because the condition is incompatible with life.

## Hermaphroditism

There are two varieties: pseudohermaphroditism which is relatively common and true hermaphroditism which is very rare. In pseudohermaphroditism the gonads are normal but the external genitalia conform, in varying degrees, to those of the opposite sex. In female pseudohermaphroditism ovaries are present, but the external genitalia are masculinized; in male pseudohermaphroditism testes are present, but the external genitalia appear feminine. In true hermaphroditism both ovarian and testicular tissue are present, either in separate gonads or in one or two ovotestes.

### FEMALE PSEUDOHERMAPHRODITISM

There are three different varieties of this condition which are distinguished by their aetiology:

1. Female pseudohermaphroditism secondary to congenital adrenal hyperplasia. This accounts for the majority of cases.
2. Female pseudohermaphroditism secondary to androgens from external sources, particularly drugs.
3. Primary female pseudohermaphroditism. The cause is unknown.

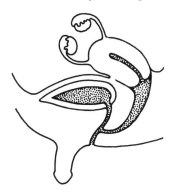

FIG. 45. The common type of female pseudohermaphrodite from congenital adrenal hyperplasia. The vagina and urethra join at the persistent urogenital sinus from which a single external orifice opens.

1. *Female pseudohermaphroditism with congenital adrenal hyperplasia.* Congenital hyperplasia of the adrenal cortex is due to a defect in the synthesis of hydrocortisone. The enzyme blocks responsible for this are discussed on pp. 629–631. The lack of hydrocortisone in the circulation causes the pituitary to secrete excessive adrenotrophic hormones in an attempt to correct the situation. This leads to hyperplasia of the adrenal cortex, causing an excessive production of androgens. Adrenal hyperplasia commences early in fetal life and, if the fetus is female, the excess of androgens prevents the normal separation of the genital from the urinary tract. The urogenital sinus persists and in most cases a single external orifice remains to serve both vagina and

urethra (Fig. 45). The clitoris is large at birth and, because the excess of androgenic hormones persists, as shown by the raised urinary 17-ketosteroids (17-oxosteroids), progressive virilization continues after birth. The child grows rapidly so that the bone age is advanced, she becomes very muscular, pubic hair develops early and the clitoris continues to enlarge (Fig. 46).

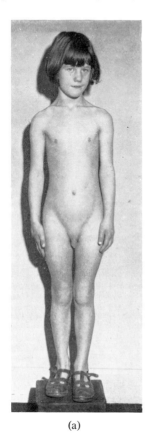

(a)

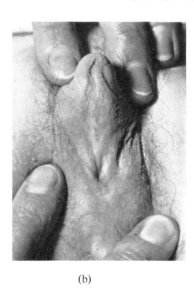

(b)

FIG. 46. (a) Female pseudohermaphroditism due to congenital adrenal hyperplasia in a girl aged 5 years who had received no cortisone therapy. She is tall and muscular, the clitoris is enlarged, and pubic hair is present, (b) Genitalia in the same patient. The enlarged clitoris is held up, revealing the single external orifice as illustrated in Fig. 45.

Severe salt loss may develop, causing vomiting and collapse. This may occur in either sex since affected males show no congenital malformation, the problem is discussed on p. 630.

*Diagnosis.* Confirmation of the diagnosis is dependent on finding an increased urinary excretion both of 17-ketosteroids and pregnanetriol. In small infants the rise in pregnanetriol is of more diagnostic value since the increase in 17-ketosteroids is relatively small. Nuclear sex chromatin is present indicating the normal female pattern (see p. 198).

Congenital adrenal hyperplasia is determined by an autosomal recessive gene. Affected males develop sexual precocity (see p. 285).

*Treatment*. This is discussed on p. 631.

2. *Female pseudohermaphroditism secondary to external sources of androgens.* The administration of androgenic hormones during pregnancy for the treatment of habitual abortion (see p. 143) has caused the same masculinization of the developing fetus as is seen in adrenal hyperplasia. The conditions differ in that drug-induced female pseudohermaphroditism does not cause progressive virilization after birth and there is no rise in 17-ketosteroids or pregnanetriol. Exactly the same mechanism has occurred in the rare cases where female pseudohermaphroditism has resulted from the presence, during pregnancy, of a maternal arrhenoblastoma, which secretes androgens.

3. *Primary female pseudohermaphroditism*. This is a very rare group of unknown cause. There is no androgenic stimulus.

## Male pseudohermaphroditism

No abnormality of hormone excretion is found in these patients, whose external genitalia vary from hypospadias with undescended testicles to a normal female appearance. Cases with normal female external genitalia are better termed the 'testicular feminization syndrome'.

### TESTICULAR FEMINIZATION SYNDROME

This is a rare herditary disorder in which the external genitalia are normal female but the gonads are testes and there is no uterus. The chromosome complement is XY. The testes are frequently ectopic, often being found in the inguinal canal in association with an inguinal hernia.

The condition is sometimes discovered in childhood because of lumps in the groins which prove histologically to be testes or because of inguinal herniae— a rare condition in girls. More often the child is thought to be a normal girl until puberty. At this time breast development occurs but there is primary amenorrhoea and sparse or absent pubic and axillary hair.

The patients should be brought up as girls but the gonads should be removed when fusion of the epiphyses indicates that growth is complete. This is necessary owing to their considerable risk of later malignant change. Cyclic hormonal replacement therapy should then be given. These patients, though sterile, can lead normal married lives. They should only be told that they were born without a womb; mention of the testes causes unnecessary psychological problems.

It has been suggested that the condition is due to a failure of end-organ response since even large doses of androgens have failed to produce virilization.

**Diagnosis of hermaphroditism**

In both varieties of pseudohermaphrodite the external genitalia may show every possible variation in male or female differentiation. Therefore, the diagnosis cannot be made from the external appearance. The first task is to differentiate congenital adrenal hyperplasia. This should not be difficult because of the evidence of excessive androgenic activity causing acceleration of growth and a rise in urinary 17-ketosteroids and pregnanetriol. In all other forms of hermaphroditism the rate of growth is normal, and there is no rise in 17-ketosteroids or pregnanetriol. Congenital adrenal hyperplasia may also be present in other members of the family.

*Nuclear chromatin.* The sexes of normal individuals can be differentiated histologically on the basis of nuclear chromatin which is present in females only. This 'sex chromatin' forms an intranuclear body lying against the inner aspect of the nuclear membrane and can be easily demonstrated in a buccal smear. Alternatively, polymorphonuclear leucocytes are examined in a blood smear. In these cells the sex chromatin body appears as a 'drumstick' projecting on a narrow stalk from one of the nuclear lobes. This is visible in about 2 per cent of female polymorphs and absent in male polymorphs.

Females are therefore 'chromatin positive' and males 'chromatin negative'. The explanation is that a single X chromosome is genetically active whereas additional X chromosomes are inactive; only inactive chromosomes are visible. This test is of the greatest value in the investigation of hermaphrodites. Female pseudohermaphrodites of all varieties are chromatin positive, whilst male cases are chromatin negative. Only with true hermaphrodites is a variable result obtained.

The possibility of female pseudohermaphroditism from adrenal hyperplasia must be considered in every case of apparent hypospadias if the gonads cannot be felt. This is almost certainly the diagnosis if such a patient collapses, this being due to adrenal failure. Vomiting from adrenal failure in such babies has been mistaken for pyloric stenosis.

A laparotomy is not required for the diagnosis of female pseudohermaphroditism due to adrenal hyperplasia and can be dangerous—adrenal failure may be precipitated. It should be carried out in other cases of hermaphroditism if the sex is in doubt, a biopsy being taken from each gonad.

## MALFORMATIONS OF THE URINARY TRACT

**Renal agenesis**

Unilateral absence is quite common, the ureter is also absent and there is asymmetry of the bladder trigone. The other kidney is usually hypertrophied and may therefore be palpable; it is often malformed.

Bilateral renal agenesis is incompatible with survival, although the patient may live for a few hours. A characteristic facies (Potter face) has been described so that diagnosis is possible before death. The space between the eyes in increased and a prominent epicanthic fold forms a wide semicircle on each side of the nose, which is flatter than usual. The chin recedes and the ears are low-set and large. Very little cartilage is present in the ears and the upper border of the pinna is flat. These characteristics may also be seen with other renal malformations, particularly in those with hypoplastic or polycystic kidneys. Renal agenesis occurs twice as often in boys and is often associated with pulmonary hypoplasia.

*Amnion nodosum* or vernix granulosum of the amnion occurs regularly in cases of renal agenesis and often in babies with severely hypoplastic or polycystic kidneys. It is associated with oligohydramnios, presumably due to lack of the urinary component of amniotic fluid (see p. 152).

### Renal hypoplasia

A single hypoplastic kidney is usually associated with other malformations of the renal tract. Bilateral renal hypoplasia usually presents with renal impairment and failure to thrive, and is the cause of one type of 'renal rickets' (p. 561).

### Polycystic kidneys

Cystic disease of the kidney exists in an infantile and an adult form. The majority of affected infants are stillborn or die within the first months of life. Both kidneys are involved, being grossly enlarged so that they are easily palpable; they may even be large enough to cause difficulty in labour. Those who survive longer than the first month show evidence of progressive renal failure with poor weight gain, anorexia and vomiting. Haematuria may occur and the intravenous pyelogram shows characteristic 'spider' calyces.

The infantile form may occur in more than one member of the family, but not in different generations, so that it is probably due to an autosomal recessive gene. However, the absence of a history of consanguineous marriages in recent large studies suggests that other factors may be involved. The adult form is also familial and does appear in succeeding generations; it is probably inherited as a dominant characteristic. Symptoms first appear in middle life.

### Hydronephrosis

This is usually unilateral although the other kidney may later become hydronephrotic. It is often due to ureteric obstruction by an aberrant renal vessel or adhesion, or from kinking or stenosis of the ureter. A ureterocele associated with an ectopic ureter ('ectopic ureterocele') is another important cause of ureteric obstruction.

The patient usually presents with recurrent attacks of severe loin pain, associated with vomiting and pallor. The condition must therefore be differentiated from intussusception and may sometimes simulate appendicitis, particularly if the affected kidney is ectopic and lying in the pelvis. This is one of the organic causes of recurrent vomiting which must be excluded before a diagnosis of 'periodic syndrome' is made (see p. 469).

There are usually no urinary symptoms, although the pain may be accompanied by oliguria and followed by diuresis. It is believed that this diuresis is reflex in origin, since the volume of urine passed is more than the amount which could have been held up in the dilated renal pelvis. The condition may present as a case of recurrent urinary infection, being discovered when routine urinary investigations are carried out.

*Treatment.* Surgical exploration should take place in all cases in the hope that the obstruction can be relieved.

### Ectopia vesicae (Ectopic bladder)

The bladder mucosa is exposed and acutely tender; the urine can be seen coming from the exposed ureteric openings. Epispadias is present and the child has a waddling gait due to the associated instability of the pelvis. Ureteric reflux of urine commonly occurs (p. 389).

*Treatment.* Reconstruction is extremely difficult and it is often necessary to transplant the ureters into the colon in order to obtain urinary control. The expectation of life is poor owing to the high incidence of secondary renal infection.

### Congenital urethral obstruction

BLADDER NECK OBSTRUCTION

Muscle hypertrophy in the region of the internal sphincter causes obstruction to the flow of urine from the bladder. Much confusion exists with regard to this condition, the main difficulty being that any obstruction in the urethra causes secondary hypertrophy of the bladder neck musculature, with consequent contracture of the vesical outlet. It is essential to determine the primary cause of the obstruction; bladder neck hypertrophy should only be regarded as the primary abnormality if the urethra is normal. In such cases, fibroelastosis has been found affecting the posterior urethra and this is probably the most common cause of primary bladder neck obstruction.

URETHRAL VALVES

These valves occur in boys and are found in the posterior urethra. When urine is passed they balloon out like a parachute so that great pressure is required to overcome the obstruction; even then only a few drops of urine escape at a time. The valves offer no obstruction to the passage of a catheter since it is pushed in the opposite direction to the urine flow; failure to appreciate this fact may prevent a correct diagnosis.

### URETHRAL DIAPHRAGM OR STRICTURE

The diaphragm is traversed by a central perforation. Congenital urethral stricture is only seen in males.

### Clinical features

The clinical picture from all these causes is the same. The majority of patients are male, the child being unable to pass a normal stream of urine. Dribbling of urine is a most serious occurrence and all mothers should be taught to recognize this symptom, just as they are able to recognize diarrhoea or vomiting. No newborn baby should be discharged from the care of the attending doctor or midwife until a normal stream has been witnessed (p. 43).

Unfortunately, the diagnosis is often not recognized until increasing urinary back pressure develops. There is then evidence of progressive renal impairment shown by failure to thrive, anorexia and vomiting. The bladder is palpable and the napkin always wet. Older children may be thought to have

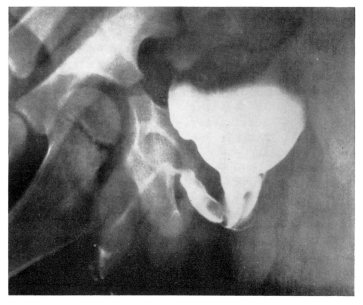

FIG. 47. Micturating cystogram in a child with congenital urethral valves. The dilated posterior urethra is visible below the bladder; it is divided into two portions by the outline of the valves.

enuresis but, when this is present by day as well as by night, an organic origin must be suspected.

Once the diagnosis is suspected, confirmation is a matter of radiology and endoscopy by the expert. Urethral valves are shown up by a micturating cystogram which also demonstrates the dilated posterior urethra immediately proximal to the obstruction (Fig. 47). Ureteric reflux of urine is also often seen (p. 389). Treatment by the endoscopic route is the method of choice, the final result depending on how much renal damage has occurred before a correct diagnosis has been made.

## Megaureter-megacystis syndrome

In thesé patients both ureters are grossly dilated and the ureteric orifices gape widely. The bladder is of large capacity but trabeculation is absent or slight. The aetiology is unknown, but it occurs equally in boys and girls and must be differentiated from a bladder neck obstruction. In that disorder the bladder is small and heavily trabeculated, while the ureteric orifices are normal.

Surgical treatment is not indicated, the children being taught the regime of triple micturition in order to empty the bladder completely.

## Absent abdominal muscles associated with malformations of the urinary tract

This syndrome, which occurs almost exclusively in boys, is not common. There is a deficiency of the abdominal muscles, the abdominal skin being wrinkled. It lies in redundant folds as though excessively stretched and bulges on standing. Bilateral cryptorchidism is constant and various associated malformations of the urinary tract have been found. The ureters are grossly dilated and tortuous and, although many hypotheses have been put forward

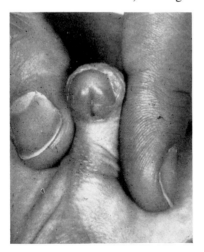

FIG. 48. Glandular hypospadias. The opening of the urethra can be seen below the blind pit at its normal site. The prepuce is 'hooded' instead of encircling the glans. A moderate degree of chordee is present.

to try to connect the two aspects of the syndrome on a causal basis, it is probable that they simply represent associated defects of development.

## Hypospadias

This is a common malformation in which the urethral opening is on the ventral surface of the glans or shaft of the penis. In glandular hypospadias the abnormal opening may be missed because it is small, and a pit, which proves to be blind, is present at the normal site. However, there should be no difficulty is diagnosing hypospadias of any variety because the prepuce is always abnormal and, instead of encircling the glans, is gathered as a hood on the dorsal surface (Fig. 48). Some degree of chordee is present causing the penis to be curved.

*Treatment.* Hypospadias should be repaired between the ages of 4 and 5 years. This allows the organ to be larger than at birth but ensures that the child, before starting school, no longer requires to sit down to pass urine. Circumcision must not be permitted as the prepuce is required for the repair. If the testicles cannot be felt, full investigation of the sex must be undertaken in case the child is a female pseudohermaphrodite.

## 'Congenital phimosis'

This is a misnomer since phimosis never occurs at birth. The error is made

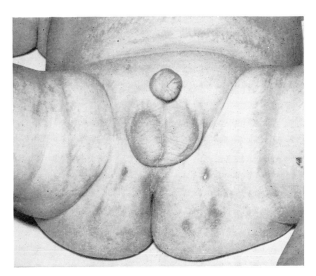

FIG. 49. Torsion of the penis. The penis is rotated anticlockwise; there is associated hypospadias.

from ignorance of the normal development of the foreskin. The penis, including the prepuce, develops *in utero* as a solid bud, the urethra being formed as an infolding of its under-surface. Not until late in fetal life does a line of cleavage appear, marking off the future prepuce from the future glans. At birth this plane is a visible division but not a free space. Separation of the glans from the foreskin is not complete until some time between 9 months and 3 years of age (Gairdner, 1949). Until this has occurred the foreskin can be retracted only with force which tears through the cellular link between them. Healing of this tear leads to fibrosis and an adherent foreskin.

Retraction of the foreskin should be carried out only when it is separate from the glans and should not be attempted before the third birthday. Forcible retraction, and the practice of inserting a probe and encircling the glans to 'break down the adhesions' are deplorable. Provided the child can pass a normal stream of urine no phimosis exists and examination of the urethral meatus is unnecessary. If phimosis is present it will have been acquired from forcible retraction or bad circumcision.

The function of the foreskin is to protect the delicate epithelial surface of the glans. Removal of the foreskin exposes the glans to continual contamination with urine if napkins are worn and often causes a meatal ulcer (see p. 394). Today, the arguments for ritual circumcision lie in the lessened incidence of penile and prostatic cancer among the circumcised and the lower incidence of cancer of the cervix in their partners (Abt, 1965). These are related to poor hygiene and the collection of smegma in those who have not been circumcised. However, the uncircumcised male, whose hygiene is good and who has not been subjected to early forcible retraction of the penis, does not carry an increased risk of cancer for himself or for his spouse. Moreover, detailed controlled studies by Terris *et al.* (1973) failed to support any association between circumcision status and carcinoma of the cervix.

For those newborn babies whose parents insist on circumcision the 'Plastibell' technique has simplified the procedure. This is a small plastic cup which fits over the glans and has a handle attached. The foreskin is drawn over the cup, ligatured into position and the foreskin severed. The handle is then broken off. No dressing is required and the ring with foreskin remnant drops off in about 4 days, leaving a clean healed line of excision.

**Torsion of the penis** (Fig. 49)

Occasionally the penis is partially rotated, an abnormality which may be associated with hypospadias. No treatment is required.

**Cryptorchidism**

This subject is discussed on p. 644.

# CONGENITAL MALFORMATIONS OF THE SKIN

## Haemangioma (vascular naevus)

This is by far the most common congenital malformation of the skin and is predominantly of two types: the capillary and the cavernous. The capillary haemangioma is pink or mauve and is superficial; the cavernous is red and extends more deeply. There are three common types of such haemangiomata which are best classified on a descriptive basis:

### 1. 'STORK'S BEAK MARK'

This consists of a pink capillary haemangioma found on the upper eyelids and over the occiput. The name indicates where the mythical stork might have marked the baby and is a reminder of the sites of this, the commonest of all congenital malformations. In some cases it is present in the middle of the forehead being shaped like a V whose junction lies just above the nasal bridge (*naevus flammeus*). No treatment is required, the lesion on the eyelid usually fading after a few months. The occipital lesion, though obscured by hair, often persists.

### 2. PORT WINE STAIN

This also is a capillary haemangioma, but with a very different outlook from the one described above; the colour is purple as opposed to the pink colour of the 'stork's beak mark'. It is superficial, often very extensive and disfiguring, and is particularly seen on the face, neck and limbs. Small raised areas like papillomata may be present in the main lesion.

A port wine stain on one side of the face, particularly if it involves the forehead, may be associated with an intracranial haemangioma on the same side (Sturge-Weber syndrome). The intracranial lesion may cause convulsions and mental retardation. A plain X-ray of the skull can confirm the diagnosis by showing calcification. Although there are parallel lines of calcification these are not in the walls of the haemangioma as often stated but in the substance of the cortex along the gyri. In most cases an arteriogram is necessary to determine the extent and operability of the haemangioma. If it lies behind the eye, glaucoma and buphthalmos may result.

*Treatment.* The condition is extremely resistant to treatment. No form of radiation should be used because of the serious risk of malignancy at a much later date, especially of the thyroid gland when the face and neck have been treated. Carbon dioxide snow may occasionally reduce the colour but in most cases it is better to accept the mark as untreatable, apart from diathermy for the papillomata, and learn how to camouflage it with modern methods of make-up. Many cosmetic firms now produce special types of powder base for these patients so that the lesion can be completely obscured.

3. STRAWBERRY HAEMANGIOMA (Fig. 50)

This is either a pure cavernous or a mixed capillary and cavernous haemangioma. It is soft, raised and red with a very distinct edge, which is usually
circular. Deeper cavernous elements of the naevus give a bluish colour. Unlike
the other two forms of haemangiomata this is seldom present at birth, but
appears during the early weeks, growing larger for the first few months. The
outlook is quite different from the port wine stain, since nearly every strawberry haemangioma will have disappeared by the age of 7 years and most of
them much earlier. This spontaneous disappearance first shows itself by the
appearance of small, sunken, pale areas in the centre; these gradually coalesce
leaving only a red rim which then vanishes. Neither size nor rapidity of growth
affect this natural regression. However, although spontaneous resolution is
the rule, this is sometimes incomplete, especially if mucous membranes are
involved. This may occur when the lips are affected, the lesion spreading on to
the buccal mucous membrane.

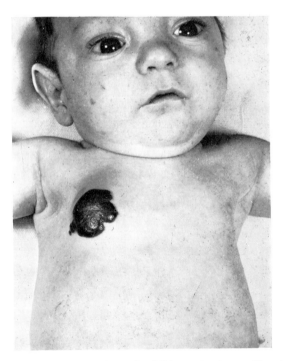

FIG. 50. Strawberry naevus. The easily visible portion is a capillary haemangioma; below this is a swelling due to a cavernous haemangioma. Sunken
pale areas are visible in the centre where spontaneous resolution has begun.

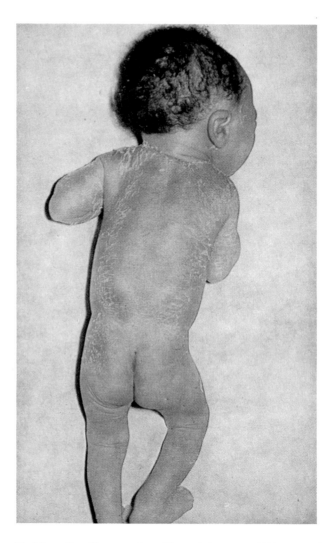

FIG. 51. Mongolian blue spot in a Negro infant. In addition to pigmentation at the typical site over the sacrum there are other blue areas on the back.

Sometimes, bleeding occurs from superficial ulceration. This is never dangerous since light pressure only is required to stop the ooze of blood. Unfortunately, ulceration leads to permanent scarring so that every effort should be made to prevent it.

In view of this natural history no treatment should be given before the age of 7 years, even for those which grow alarmingly in the first few months, apart from the exceptions mentioned below. Nothing is more tragic than to see the disfiguring scars left by surgical removal of these haemangiomata; scars which then grow with the child. There is usually no difficulty in persuading mothers not to have this naevus removed, but if there is, she should be shown serial photographs of a patient illustrating this spontaneous disappearance. If resolution is incomplete, later plastic surgery is safer and less extensive.

Oral prednisone can cause shrinkage of a strawberry haemangioma. This is not required for the vast majority which should be left to involute on their own. However, if the haemangioma threatens life, for example by involving the larynx or if a vital organ such as the eye is liable to be permanently damaged, steroid therapy should be used.

Prednisone should also be used for two rare types of haemangioma. In one there are multiple small haemangiomata which, though they usually disappear spontaneously, may be associated with intracranial haemangiomata; the other is a giant haemangioma associated with thrombocytopenia from destruction of platelets within the tumour.

### Spider naevi

These are common in children but usually insignificant. Their age incidence increases from 2 years until puberty when it levels off. There is a central red point, occasionally raised, from which a number of 'legs' radiate. The commonest sites are the dorsum of the hands and forearms. If the lesion is on the face and is unsightly, it can be removed by diathermy of the central area or by freezing with carbon dioxide snow.

### Pigmented naevus (mole)

This consists of a localized deposit of melanin which may be flat or papillomatous and may or may not be hairy. They are very common, the vast majority causing no trouble, except that they may be disfiguring so that removal by plastic surgery is required. Malignant change is exceptional; it is more liable to occur if the mole is subject to repeated trauma. In this case surgical removal is indicated.

### Cystic hygroma

This is a multilocular lymphangiomatous cyst most commonly found in the neck. The cyst is highly translucent and usually appears during the first year. It rarely regresses but tends to enlarge. For this reason surgical excision is the correct treatment.

## Ichthyosis
The children with this condition, often of familial origin, have a dry skin which comes off in flakes like 'fish-scales'. In older children, it is differentiated from the acquired dry skin of the child who has had severe eczema by the fact that it is generalized and no eczematous lesions are present. Treatment can be palliative only, the skin being kept well greased by means of frequent baths using aqueous cream, B.P. (ung. emulsificans aquosum) instead of soap. A trial of 10 per cent urea in emulsifying ointment (ung. emulsificans) is worthwhile since this application is sometimes dramatically effective in reducing the dryness of the skin.

## Supernumerary nipples
These are single or multiple occurring on either side of the trunk below and internal to the normal nipple. They are common, but their origin is often not realized until pigmentation occurs at puberty. In childhood they are pale brown and usually flat. Ectopic mammary tissue, usually in the axilla may or may not be associated with an extra nipple. This can cause problems from painful swelling during lactation.

## Mongolian blue spot (Fig. 51)
This is a racial characteristic and not strictly a congenital malformation. It is found in babies of negroid or oriental origin and in Eskimos. The lesions consist of dark blue areas of skin in the sacral region. The areas may be very extensive, involving all the back and there may be isolated blue spots on the limbs. The colour usually fades during the first year. The condition is often mistaken for a bruise if it has not been met before.

## Dermal sinus
These may be found anywhere in the midline of the scalp or spine. Their importance lies in the possibility that the sinus connects with the meninges, rendering the child liable to meningitis. A search of such a sinus should be part of the routine examination at birth and should also be made in all cases of meningitis, especially if recurrent. The opening of the sinus may be very small, though it may be associated with an abnormal growth of hair or telangiectasia of the surrounding skin.

## Congenital scalp defects

These are well circumscribed areas, usually found on the vertex which appear as punched out ulcers at birth. They are often familial and may be associated with an underlying defect of the skull.

Although much of the literature refers to the need for emergency plastic surgery this is unnecessary since spontaneous healing both of the skin and skull defect is usual. Epithelization of the skin occurs during the first few weeks of life leaving an atrophic hairless scar.

## Cutis hyperelastica (Ehlers-Danlos syndrome)

In this condition there is increased elasticity of the skin, hyperextensibility of the joints, and an increased fragility of the blood vessels due to poor connective tissue support of the cutaneous vessels. The skin bleeds very freely when injured, healing with fragile 'tissue-paper scars'. The disorder is inherited as an irregular autosomal dominant and 'formes frustes' occur.

*Diagnosis.* It is necessary to differentiate *cutis laxa* (*dermatomegaly*) in which there is looseness and hypertrophy of the skin, but no increase in elasticity, the skin hanging down in folds.

*Prognosis and treatment.* No specific treatment is available, but there is a tendency for improvement as the child grows older. The skin must be protected from injury as much as possible.

## Poikiloderma congenita

A rare disorder which particularly affects the face, limbs and buttocks. The condition is seldom present at birth, the first change being the development of pink, tense, inflammatory swellings in these sites during infancy; telangiectases then appear in the area, being followed by irregular pigmentation and fine atrophy. The affected skin is sensitive to sunlight and should be protected by an ultra-violet screening cream, such as Uvistat which contains mexenone(hydroxymethoxymethylbenzophenone). The development of cataracts is common.

## Ectodermal dysplasia

In this condition there is incomplete development of the epidermis and its appendages. It is divided into two groups according to the presence or absence of sweating:

### ANHIDROTIC TYPE

This is the more severe form of the disease which is associated with an absence of sweat glands and often of the sebaceous glands as well. The skin is dry and atrophic, the teeth are scanty and conical and the hair sparse and easily pulled out. The nails are brittle, the nipples poorly developed and the mammary glands may be absent. Atrophic rhinitis is common and there is depression of the nasal bridge. This feature, together with prominence of the supraorbital ridges, prominent ears and thick protruding lips, makes all the patients look alike, especially as they also have scanty hair and eyebrows.

The inability to sweat renders affected individuals very liable to heat stroke and they must adjust their activity accordingly.

Two forms of inheritance have been recognized—a sex-linked recessive type which occurs only in males but is transmitted by females, and an autosomal dominant type occurring in males, but possibly also in females.

### HIDROTIC TYPE

Except that they have sweat glands, these patients may have any or all of the other features of the anhidrotic type. It occurs in both sexes and is inherited as an autosomal dominant.

### CHONDRO-ECTODERMAL DYSPLASIA (ELLIS-VAN CREVELD SYNDROME)

A combination of ectodermal dysplasia with achondroplasia, polydactyly and congenital heart disease very occasionally occurs. It is inherited as an autosomal recessive.

## Epidermolysis bullosa

In this hereditary condition bullae appear on the skin as a result of minimal trauma. In severely affected patients similar lesions also develop on the mucous membranes.

### SIMPLE FORM

In this variety of the disease the lesions may not appear until the child begins to crawl and walk when they develop on sites of trauma. In some patients the lesions are limited to the hands and feet.

The disease is inherited as an autosomal dominant; it tends to improve after puberty and, apart from avoiding trauma and infection, no other treatment is required.

### DYSTROPHIC FORM

The lesions appear immediately after birth; they lie deeper in the skin than with the simple form of lesion so that scarring occurs and severe deformities of the hands and feet may result.

The mucous membranes are involved and the lesions in the mouth and pharynx may seriously interfere with feeding; stenosis of the pharynx or oesophagus can result from scarring. The conjuctivae can also be affected. Dystrophic changes occur in the nails and teeth and these structures may be lost.

This variety of the disease is inherited either as a dominant or as a recessive trait. The dominant form is the less serious so that the patients do not die in childhood but survive and reproduce. The recessive form is very serious, many of the patients dying within the first year of life. In those who survive the first year, there is a tendency for improvement with age.

*Treatment.* In this form of the disease steroids should be used and some of the patients respond well. The same care must be taken to avoid trauma and infection.

## Albinism

In *generalized albinism* there is an absence of pigment in the skin, hair and retina, though the iris usually possesses a little pigment; the pupils appear red with reflected light. Some of the patients are severely myopic. The disease is due to a failure of melanin production so that the skin burns easily when exposed to sunlight and carries an increased risk of developing epitheliomata. It is inherited as an autosomal recessive.

The condition is particularly striking among coloured races and is possibly more common amongst them. In addition to their colouring they have similar facial features. Those living in the tropics develop keratoses on the exposed areas, these being very liable to malignant change.

*Treatment.* Exposure to sunlight must be avoided. When this is impractical an ultra-violet screening cream should be used, such as mexenone (p. 209).

*Localized albinism* may affect one area of the skin (piebaldism) from a patchy lack of melanin or one area of hair, causing a white forelock. These forms of the disease are inherited by means of autosomal dominant genes. Localized albinism of the skin must be differentiated from *vitiligo*, an acquired depigmentation disorder, in which the white areas slowly increase in size and their borders are hyperpigmented.

*Waardenburg's syndrome* is an hereditary disorder, transmitted as an autosomal dominant and comprising congenital deafness, different coloured eyes and a white forelock.

## Urticaria pigmentosa (mastocytosis)

In a proportion of patients with this rare disease the condition is congenital. Brown macules appear during the early months which when rubbed produce weals; they may also become nodular. The trunk is the chief area to be affected but the mouth may be involved. The lesions may cause considerable irritation.

The histological picture is characteristic since accumulations of mast cells are visible in the upper parts of the dermis. Local applications to relieve itching, such as calamine lotion, should be used.

### Juvenile xanthoma

Small canary-yellow coloured papules are present at birth or develop shortly afterwards, particularly on the head and neck. The blood cholesterol is normal and the condition is unrelated to any metabolic or storage disorder.

The cause is unknown and the lesions usually disappear during childhood. Surgical excision is therefore seldom necessary.

### Naevo-xantho-endothelioma

This is a papule or flat raised lesion of reddish-yellow or brown colour. It may be single or multiple, particularly occurring on the face and scalp. Spontaneous disappearance usually takes place during the first 2 years of life.

## CONGENITAL MALFORMATIONS OF THE CENTRAL NERVOUS SYSTEM

Of all the different malformations which occur, those of the central nervous system are possibly the most devastating. The commonest of these are spina bifida with myelocele, hydrocephalus and anencephaly. A link exists between these three major central nervous system malformations since if one has occurred in a family, there is about a one in forty risk of a subsequent child being born with the same or one of the other two defects. Spina bifida and anencephaly are the only congenital malformations showing a significantly increased incidence among first-born children.

### Diastematomyelia

In this condition a bony, cartilaginous or fibrous spur traverses the spinal canal of a vertebra, splitting the spinal cord into two halves. A tuft of hair overlying the abnormality may be visible. As the child grows, the cord is split still further since it grows more slowly than the vertebral column. This causes increasing sphincter disturbances and neurological signs in the lower legs. These signs do not usually appear before the second year of life. The spur, if bony, will be visible radiographically. Surgical treatment is required.

The condition may be associated with spina bifida.

### Spina bifida

This condition varies from spina bifida occulta, which is of very little clinical significance, to rachischisis in which the neural tube is laid wide open. In spina bifida occulta the skin is intact, although the site of the underlying spina bifida may be marked by a dimple, haemangioma, lipoma, or tuft of hair. In the majority of patients with spina bifida occulta there are no symptoms and only very rarely is there paralysis. It is not a cause of enuresis unless neurological symptoms are present.

### Meningocele

A sac composed of the meninges protudes through the bifid vertebrae but the cord remains within the spinal canal. The overlying skin and spinal cord are usually normal. The lesion is most often found in the cervical and upper thoracic regions whereas a myelocele most often occurs in the lumbar region and sometimes in the occipital region. A meningocele is much less common than a myelocele, comprising only 5 per cent of the spina bifida cystica population. There are no motor or sensory defects, while hydrocephalus only occasionally develops.

### Myelocele (meningomyelocele) (Fig. 52)

This is a common malformation, about two to three thousand affected babies being born in Great Britain every year. The neural groove fails to close early in intrauterine life and the neural plate remains on the surface as a raw, reddish area surrounded by a blue, transparent membrane, which represents the meninges. The spinal cord is deformed and fibres run across the sac to the surface. The membrane remains transparent for the first few hours of life only, but during that time the nerve fibres can be seen through it. There is often a haemangioma at the junction with normal skin. The commonest site is the lumbar region and an *Arnold-Chiari malformation* is usually associated. This malformation is composed of a midline tongue of the vermis of the cerebellum, which extends for a variable distance down the spinal cord (Arnold malformation) and an elongated and abnormal medulla which passes through the foramen magnum (Chiari malformation). It is an important cause of hydrocephalus which occurs in about 85 per cent of cases, and can be demonstrated at birth by ventriculography, even before enlargement of the head is detected.

All cases of myelocele are associated with neurological signs from involvement of the spinal cord. The legs may be severely paralysed, causing talipes and congenital dislocation of the hip to be common. The paralysed legs are cold and, because of the neurological defect, do not sweat. Severe kyphosis may be present. The nerve supply to the sphincters is affected, resulting in dribbling incontinence of urine and a patulous anus with faecal incontinence.

*Treatment.* The management of the child with a myelocele has undergone enormous swings of opinion. In 1963 Sharrard *et al.* as the result of a controlled study advocated that the closure of the myelocele should be regarded as a surgical emergency to be undertaken immediately the child was born. This became standard practice in most centres. However, in the ensuing 10 years the enormous burden on the family of severely handicapped survivors became apparent and opinion changed towards selective surgery (Lorber, 1972; Stark & Drummond, 1973; Laurence, 1974).

It is now widely felt that only those babies with a favourable prognosis should have immediate surgery. Unfavourable signs which are used to exclude surgical treatment are severe paralysis or severe hydrocephalus at birth, gross spinal deformity such as kyphosis and severe associated malformations. Babies not treated surgically are given normal nursing care to ensure they do not suffer but are not nursed in incubators, not tube fed, not given antibiotics and not resuscitated.

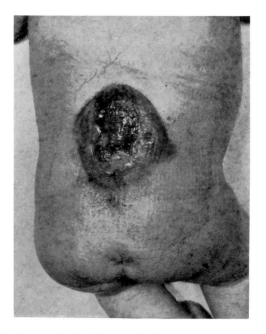

FIG. 52. Lumbar myelocele. The neural plate glistens in the centre of the defect, whereas the skin immediately surrounding it is dark from a capillary haemangioma. The anus is less taut than normal owing to involvement of the nerve supply to the sphincter.

Children surviving with faecal and urinary incontinence can be helped in a number of ways. Faecal incontinence can be prevented by once daily bowel washouts. Regular manual expression of the bladder using suprapubic pressure may be successful in keeping the child dry. Alternatively, the transplantation of the ureters into an isolated loop of ileum makes the fitting of an ileostomy bag for the collection of urine satisfactory. Urinary infection and consequent renal damage are the principal factors governing survival.

### Encephalocele

If a meningocele contains brain tissue it is called an encephalocele; this is most often found in the occipital region (Fig. 53). An occipital encephalocele is usually associated with severe mental defect, the children becoming microcephalic rather than hydrocephalic as might have been expected. To close the defect it may be necessary to remove a portion of the herniated brain.

### Hydrocephalus

This condition may occur alone or in association with spina bifida. The chances are particularly high if there is an Arnold-Chiari malformation (p. 213). The baby may be born with such a large head that decompression is required before delivery can be achieved, or the head may be normal at birth and enlarge progressively thereafter.

The disorder is due to an excess of cerebrospinal fluid under pressure. The majority of cases of congenital origin are due to a malformation of the brain causing blockage to the flow of fluid. Some are due to blockage from bleeding following intracranial birth injury. Occasionally, intrauterine toxoplasmosis or syphilis may cause the condition and every case should be investigated from this aspect.

Acquired hydrocephalus is less common; it results from blockage which in most cases is secondary to meningitis or intracranial tumour. Differentiation from congenital hydrocephalus is usually obvious from the history. In cases of doubt, the occurrence of convulsions or a raised protein in the cerebrospinal fluid favour an acquired hydrocephalus.

*Treatment.* Early treatment is essential if damage to the brain is to be stopped, therefore early diagnosis is vital. A special watch must be kept on those at risk, particularly low birth weight babies and those who have had birth trauma. The fontanelle becomes tense, remaining wider than normal for the age. The eyes are rotated downwards so that the sclera shows above the iris. Serial measurements of the head circumference indicate whether hydrocephalus is developing but diagnosis may be extremely difficult at first, especially in low birth weight babies, in whom normal growth is fast. Measurement of the head circumference at birth should be routine in all babies so that an abnormal rate of growth can be more easily detected. A difficult

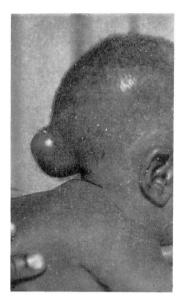

Fig. 53. Occipital encephalocele. This is the commonest site for the abnormality.

problem may be posed by those with a familial large head, but in these, the top of the head is flat in comparison with the globular head of the hydrocephalic.

Untreated hydrocephalus leads to mental impairment and sometimes optic atrophy. Spontaneous arrest may take place but brain damage is already likely to have occurred. It is of interest that papilloedema does not occur in the hydrocephalic infant since blockage of the cerebrospinal fluid prevents it from passing forwards into the orbital portion of the optic sheath. Consequently, no compression of the central vein of the retina occurs. Once a progressively fast rate of growth has been diagnosed, surgical treatment should be carried out. On the other hand, a period of observation is required if arrest appears to be taking place; this is reasonably certain if, after a gradual slowing of the rate of growth, the head circumference remains unaltered over a period of 3 months and the anterior fontanelle starts to close. Natural arrest occurs in up to 40 per cent of cases though the reason for this is unknown; it is possibly due to recanalization of the subarachnoid space. From a prognostic viewpoint, no correlation has been found in cases of arrested hydrocephalus between intelligence, head size, cortical thickness and duration of progressive disease.

Many methods of surgical treatment have been attempted, the most successful being techniques which drain the excess fluid directly into the heart.

This is achieved by means of a catheter passing from the lateral ventricle to the right atrium via the internal jugular vein. Inside the catheter is a valve, such as the Holter or the Pudenz-Heyer, which prevents blood flowing back into the catheter. The chance of success is greater in those developing after birth than if present at birth. A long-term complication of this operation is pulmonary hypertension and cor pulmonale.

### Anencephaly

In this condition there is almost complete absence of the cerebral hemispheres and the overlying skull. The patient is either stillborn or dies shortly after birth. About 90 per cent are female and the condition is commoner in first-borns. Interesting though unexplained facts are the higher incidence in the lower social classes, the peak incidence in mid-winter and the increased incidence in the western half of England and Wales. There is no seasonal variation in the incidence of hydrocephalus or spina bifida, but the risk of all three conditions appears to be higher in first pregnancies.

Anencephaly is usually associated with hydramnios due to an inability of the fetus to swallow (p. 152). This is due either to a neurological defect of the normal bulbar swallowing mechanism or to the position of the head in relation to the trunk.

### Hydranencephaly

In this condition resorption of damaged brain tissue occurs in fetal life. It is possible that this damage results from obstruction to the internal carotid arteries. The greater part of the cerebrum is destroyed, leaving only a thin membrane enclosing the ventricles.

The infants appear normal at birth, the head being of normal size. They feed normally so that the condition often goes unrecognized for the first 1–2 months. By this age the head has started to enlarge and it is obvious that development has failed to progress from the stage at birth. Diagnosis is made by transillumination of the head in a darkened room when the whole head lights up like a lantern (p. 14).

### Microcephaly

The size of the head is dependent on the growth of the brain, therefore, except for craniosynostosis (see below) all cases of microcephaly result from failure of brain growth. This may be affected by influences during pregnancy, during labour or in the first 2–3 years of life by which time brain growth is almost complete.

Microcephaly can result from a rare recessive gene causing cerebral agenesis. This can be difficult to differentiate clinically from microcephaly caused by intrauterine infection such as rubella (p. 491) cytomegalovirus (p. 117) or toxoplasmosis (p. 541) unless there are other signs of the infection. Antibody studies should confirm the diagnosis of these causes. The earlier the brain damage the greater its effect on head size.

Asphyxia at birth can cause such damage that the brain fails to grow normally thereafter. Such a child seen at the age of a few months would be difficult to differentiate from a child whose microcephaly had resulted from intrauterine causes unless the result of a clinical examination at birth, including head circumference, was available. Meningitis in the first 2–3 years of life could also cause acquired microcephaly.

All microcephalic children are severely mentally handicapped and they may have spastic cerebral palsy. The anterior fontanelle closes early and may even be closed at birth. The skull X-ray illustrates the brain growth failure since in addition to its small size there are none of the convolutional markings from pressure on the vault by the growing convolutions. In addition to this uniform density of the vault there is thickening of the tables. These features comprise the 'atrophic skull'.

Microcephaly due to brain growth failure must be differentiated from the much rarer condition of craniosynostosis (p. 237) in which failure of skull growth results from premature fusion of the cranial bones; consequent prevention of brain growth leads to mental impairment and blindness. In this condition there is evidence of raised intracranial pressure. The X-ray of the skull therefore shows increased convolutional markings as a result of this pressure and is totally different from the atrophic skull described above.

### Down's syndrome (mongolism)

This condition occurs about once in every 600 births but there is an increased chance if the mother is elderly. There are four types, all of which are due to a chromosomal abnormality. The commonest, forming about 90 per cent of the total is the 'regular' mongol. Such patients have an extra chromosome 21, instead of the usual pair, so that their chromosome complement is forty-seven instead of forty-six. They are termed 'primary' trisomics 21. This results from an error in germ cell formation termed 'non-disjunction'. Normally the chromosome pair divide equally, but when non-disjunction occurs the pair fail to separate so that one germ cell has both chromosomes while the other has none. Fertilization of a germ cell with two chromosomes results in a zygote with three. The other zygote only has one chromosome and as far as is known never develops into an embryo. The liability to non-disjunction increases with the age of the mother, accounting for the higher incidence of mongols born to older mothers. No chromosomal abnormalities can be detected in the parents of this type of mongol.

The second commonest group, comprising about 6 per cent of mongols, is the double trisomic. The chromosomal constitution in these is XXY plus trisomy 21 making forty-eight chromosomes in each cell.

The third group, comprising about 3·5 per cent of mongols are the inter-change or translocation trisomics. They have the normal complement of forty-six chromosomes but one is large and atypical. This abnormal chromosome results from a rearrangement whereby the extra chromosome 21 has become attached to a member of the D group (chromosomes 13–15). Sometimes the interchange takes place within the G group itself (chromosomes 21–22).

All these types of mongol look alike so that they can be differentiated only by chromosomal studies.

The fourth group, comprising about 1 per cent of mongols, are chromosome mosaics having some normal cells with forty-six chromosomes and other abnormal cells with forty-seven chromosomes. These patients may look like typical mongols but some of them have few features only of the condition. They are generally more intelligent than complete mongols and have different finger-print patterns. Obviously they are more difficult to recognize and therefore less often diagnosed at present.

Mongols are so named because their slanting eyes suggest an oriental appearance. Apart from mosaic mongolism they all look alike (Fig. 54) although not all the features are present in every case. The features may also be more obvious in some cases than in others. It is usually possible to make a clinical diagnosis at birth from the appearance and the striking hypotonia.

The eyes are small as well as slanting, the epicanthic folds prominent, the ears low set and the back of the occiput flat. Brushfield's spots are common, these being white or cream dots which are visible just inside the outer edge of the iris. The posterior fontanelle is usually open. There is often a high malar flush; a low nasal bridge accounts for the snuffles which are so common in these children. The mouth is small and the tongue may become fissured as the child grows older. The hands are short and broad, the little finger being especially short and in-curved due to an abnormal middle phalanx. A single transverse palmar crease is commonly present. There is often a wide gap between the great toe and its neighbour while a deep crease extends from the first digital crease towards the heel. Studies of palm and sole prints and of the dermal ridge patterns on the finger tips constitute dermatoglyphics. These studies show a specific pattern for mongolism so that the diagnosis can be made from the print.

All mongols are mentally handicapped, the IQ usually lying between 35 and 55. Very rarely the IQ may be as high as 70. Most mongols are friendly and they often show an unusual enjoyment of music. This friendly character-

istic probably reflects the fact that their parents, being aware of their intellectual limitations, did not subject them to pressure to do better. It is the
undiagnosed mentally handicapped child who is pressurized by parents
during the early years while trailing him from doctor to doctor seeking help.
Such pressure is likely to produce an aggressive reaction from the child, a
trait shown by a few mongols only.

Many have a congenital heart lesion and there is often an umbilical hernia.
There is a higher incidence of duodenal atresia and Hirschsprung's disease
among mongols.

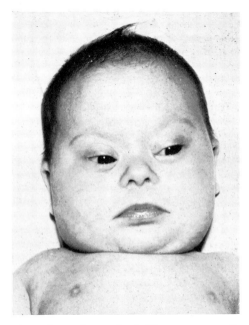

Fig. 54. Down's syndrome (mongolism). The eyes are small and slanting,
the epicanthic folds wide, and the ears low-set. There is a low bridge to the
nose.

Of great interest is the increased frequency of acute leukaemia among
mongols which is about three times the average incidence. The exact meaning
of this is not clear but it must be related to the finding of the Philadelphia (Ph)
chromosome in cases of chronic myeloid leukaemia. This is a small deleted
acrocentric chromosome which is assumed to have come from chromosome
21.

*Management.* Most mothers fail to notice the abnormality at birth but once the doctor is certain of the diagnosis he should tell the parents soon, rather than delay the information. Breaking the news should rarely be delayed beyond the second day and is probably best faced on the first day. This avoids the bitter reaction felt by parents who have already announced the arrival of a normal baby to their friends. In talking to the parents of mongols one rarely hears complaints that they were told too early but one often hears bitter resentment that they were not told early enough. I believe it to be wrong to tell only the father, asking him to keep it a secret from his wife since this creates an impossible relationship between them. On the other hand, it is often best to tell the husband alone and ask his advice as to how his wife should be told. Some husbands will prefer to break the news on their own, others will ask the doctor to talk to both parents together.

The approach to parents must emphasize that, as babies, mongol children differ very little from normal babies. In the past the parents were often frightened by the birth of a mongol as though it were a monster instead of a child with a handicap just like any other handicapped child. If the parents of a mongol child reject him at birth it usually means that they have been badly handled. The risk of rejection is always greater if the baby is separated from his mother, for example by being in a special care unit.

Although there is no cure for the condition, and this must be explained to parents, a great deal can be done to help the child and his family as with other mentally handicapped children (see p. 448). It sometimes helps parents to realize that their mongol child will be happier and have fewer worries than most people.

Although mongols are particularly liable to respiratory infections and may therefore die young, especially if they have a congenital heart lesion, they live to old age much more often than is realized.

Mongols are sometimes confused with cretins but this should never occur. Diagnosis between the two conditions is made, not by learning a list of different features, but by knowing that mongols are active even though backward, whereas cretins are sluggish and constipated. Mongols have a high colour while cretins are sallow.

*Genetic counselling.* Before discussing with the parents the possible risks for future children, the doctor must ensure that they understand something of the mechanisms involved so that guilt feelings are dispelled. If the mother is over 35 it is likely that the child is a regular mongol. However, chromosome studies are now routine in most centres in order to pick out the rare inherited forms of the disorder. If the child is a regular mongol the parents need not be studied. The risk for future children is about twice that for a mother of the same age. This risk is about one in 150 at 35 and one in forty or even higher at the age of 40 to 45.

If the chromosomes are irregular the parents should have chromosome studies. The mother is more likely to be abnormal than the father. By this means translocation parents can be discovered who must then be advised in a genetic centre of their greatly increased risks. Even higher is the risk if one parent is found to be a mongol mosaic.

## Other disorders due to chromosomal anomalies

Once the trisomic aetiology of mongolism had been established the search began for other disorders resulting from chromosomal abnormalities. Three of these have been established with certainty, it being possible to make a clinical diagnosis in each case. It is usual for all these babies to have a low birth weight despite a full gestation period. They are frail and puny, seldom living longer than a few weeks. All possess small ill-formed, low-set ears and are mentally retarded. It is likely that other trisomic states will come to light.

### TRISOMY 17–18 (E. TRISOMY, EDWARD'S SYNDROME)

Although less common than mongolism, this is not a very rare condition. The head has a prominent occiput, but receding chin. The sternum is usually short, resulting in a shield-shaped chest. One of the most constant features is the flexion deformity of the fingers which are rigidly fixed across the palm. The index finger deviates to the ulnar side, crossing behind the middle finger. Finger prints show the arches of the finger tips to be of a simple type.

The feet are characteristic since the prominent heel and convex sole simulate a rocking chair; hence the term 'rocker-bottom' feet.

### TRISOMY 13–15 (D. TRISOMY, PATAU'S SYNDROME)

This is a very rare disorder in a living child. There are gross deformities of the head and face. The head is small, nose deformed and jaw under-developed. Cleft lip and cleft palate are common. The eyes may be absent, small or of normal size but with coloboma or cataracts.

Capillary haemangiomata are common and may be diffuse. The fingers are often fixed in flexion and polydactyly is usual. The fingernails are hyper-convex and narrow. Characteristic palm, sole and finger prints are obtained. There is usually a congenital heart lesion.

At autopsy the frontal portion of the brain is particularly likely to be mal-developed. There are often no olfactory bulbs and tracts (arrhinencephaly). Agenesis of the corpus callosum may be found.

### 'CAT-CRY' SYNDROME ('CRI DU CHAT')

This is not a trisomic state but is due to the partial deletion of the short arm of one of the chromosome 5 pair. The presenting symptom is a weak but high-pitched cry which produces a characteristic, plaintive wail suggesting an animal in distress.

The babies also have a rounded face with hypertelorism, epicanthic folds and micrognathia. Some are microcephalic. The other systems are usually normal though there may be a congenital heart defect.

### Neurofibromatosis (von Recklinghausen's disease)

This disease, which is inherited as an autosomal dominant, comprises pigmented skin lesions, neurofibromata and other variable manifestations. The pigmented lesions on the skin are 'café au lait' spots which are irregular areas of light brown discoloration present at birth. The neurofibromata may be present at birth, but they especially appear and grow during later childhood. They are connective tissue tumours of the nerve fibre which particularly affect the peripheral nerves, but may also occur anywhere in the central nervous system. The peripheral neurofibromata may involve the skin; they are violet coloured at first, sometimes producing large, fleshy, pedunculated masses which are very unsightly. Neurofibromata involving the central nervous system produce symptoms from pressure and are likely to occur within the spine; of the cranial nerves the auditory is the most likely to be affected. The neurofibromata may undergo sarcomatous degeneration.

The patients may be mentally retarded and may have skeletal manifestations: these are cystic bone changes, scoliosis, local hypertrophy of a digit or limb, pseudoarthrosis and congenital bowing of the tibia.

## CONGENITAL MALFORMATIONS OF THE EYE AND EAR

### Strabismus

The natural position of the eyes at rest is to diverge; therefore, to have the eyes straight requires active muscle action. A squint is due to any disorder which disturbs the ability to use both eyes together. Binocular vision is not attained until the baby is about a month old so that up till that time a squint can be regarded as normal. Squints result from muscle imbalance, refractive errors and eye disease such as a retinoblastoma or toxoplasmosis.

A squint appearing at about the third month is usually due to muscle imbalance. This is sometimes associated with later clumsiness and poor speech in which case there may be a neurological basis (see Clumsy Child p. 434). The commonest variety of squint appears at about 3 years of age and is usually due to a refractive error, more often long sight, in a perfectly healthy child. This may have developed immediately after an illness such as measles which broke down the child's earlier ability to converge and so to overcome the refractive error.

All children with squints should be referred without delay for an ophthalmic opinion. Parents should be told that children do not 'grow out' of squints. The term 'lazy eye' is misleading and dangerous. Some squints can be fully corrected with glasses and without the need for surgery, others may continue to need glasses after surgery. Failure to treat a squint results in blindness of the affected eye from cortical suppression of the extra image ('amblyopia of disuse'). To avoid this calamity, routine visual tests, as described on p. 12, should be carried out on all children, the first being made before 6 months of age. Since there is a strong familial tendency to squints a special watch should be kept on those with a family history of the condition.

A unilateral squint is more likely to lead to amblyopia than an alternating squint in which either eye squints in turn or indiscriminately. However, there is always the possibility that an alternating squint will convert to a unilateral squint. The degree of squint is not related to the risk of amblyopia. It is also possible to develop amblyopia without a squint, as from a refractive error. Such a state of affairs would probably not show on a cover test but would on a visual acuity test; hence the importance of carrying out both tests (see p. 12).

Wide epicanthic folds may give a false impression of a squint. Pinching the nose of such a patient so as to reduce its width helps to determine whether or not a squint is present.

## Cataract

The principal factors leading to congenital cataract are nutritional and infective. Many of the children affected are of low birth weight though their maturity is greater than suggested by their weight (McDonald, 1964). These 'small for dates' babies have resulted from any of the causes of intrauterine malnutrition (p. 54), particularly maternal toxaemia, multiple pregnancy and poor diet in pregnancy (Harley & Hertzberg, 1965).

The principal infective agent is the rubella virus. Another cause is a chromosomal anomaly; there is an increased incidence of cataract in mongols (these patients may also develop degenerative opacities in later years) and in trisomy 13–15.

The effect of drugs given to mothers during pregnancy is suggestive but not proven.

In all cases of cataract, the child should immediately be referred to an ophthalmologist who will decide whether needling is required.

## Glaucoma (Buphthalmos)

This condition is not as rare as is sometimes believed since it accounts for 5 to 10 per cent of children admitted to schools for the blind. It is familial in 10 per cent due to a recessive gene. The disorder is due to a developmental anomaly

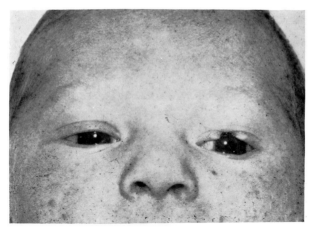

FIG. 55. Coloboma of the left upper eyelid.

of the filtration angle which impedes the flow of aqueous humour from the anterior chamber. Clinical features may be present at birth and 80 per cent develop during the first 3 months, the remainder during the rest of the first year. Photophobia from corneal oedema is the earliest symptom in those developing after birth, but will not be apparent in those present at birth. There is excessive watering from the eye, the cornea becomes hazy from oedema and the eye itself enlarges. Eighty per cent of cases are bilateral. If the condition is unilateral a difference in intraocular tension can be appreciated. Obvious pain is not a feature of the disease in infants.

*Treatment.* Surgery is essential since medical treatment is ineffective. Goniotomy is the operation of choice, an incision being made into the blocking tissue so as to open up a channel through which the aqueous fluid can drain. Provided it is carried out early, vision can be preserved in the majority of cases, though the prognosis is worse in familial cases.

### Coloboma

This is a notched defect which may involve the iris, choroid or eyelid (Fig. 55). The abnormality may occur as an isolated lesion or in association with other malformations, especially cleft lip or palate, mandibulo-facial dysostosis or arachnodactyly. If the defect in the eyelid leaves the cornea exposed when the eyes are closed, plastic repair should be undertaken at once.

### Obstruction of the nasolacrimal duct

This is due to failure of canalization of the duct. Wide epicanthic folds and a shallow nasal bridge are often associated. The disorder causes watering from the affected eye with an increased liability to infection. Secondary acute dacrocystitis may occur. The condition should be suspected in any baby with repeated infections in the same eye. In the majority of cases, spontaneous canalization of the duct occurs before the age of 6 months so that probing of the duct should be delayed until that age. Prior to this, pressure can be applied over the inner canthus in the hope of expressing fluid through the duct, so hastening its clearing. Management of the infection is discussed on p. 111.

### Accessory auricle and pre-auricular sinus

These conditions are commoner in Africans and both occur in front of the external auditory meatus. An accessory auricle can be removed without difficulty, but a pre-auricular sinus often contains rudimentary cartilage at its base which must be completely removed to prevent recurrence of the sinus.

### Congenital atresia of the auditory meatus

This condition may occur alone or in association with other anomalies such as the Treacher-Collins syndrome. It was an important associated anomaly in cases of phocomelia resulting from the administration of thalidomide to pregnant mothers.

During the first year of life an X-ray should be taken to determine whether ossicles are present. These are fully grown at birth whereas the pinna goes on growing until the age of 12 years. Consequently, the ossicles are less easily seen in older patients. If ossicles are found to be present, an operation to form an artificial meatus should be carried out. This permits the use of an air con-duction hearing aid which is more efficient than one designed for bone con-duction.

In babies with multiple problems such as the thalidomide children, atten-tion to the limb problem must not be allowed to overshadow the ear defect for which a hearing aid and surgical treatment must be provided at the earliest opportunity.

### Nerve deafness

Congenital nerve deafness is discussed with other causes of deafness on p. 339.

## CONGENITAL MALFORMATIONS OF BONES AND JOINTS

### Polydactyly

The possession of one or more extra digits often runs in families and is extremely common in Africans. Surgical removal is preferable to the old-fashioned method of tying a cotton thread round the base which may lead to oedema and infection in the gangrenous digit.

## Syndactyly

This term is applied to webbing of the fingers or toes. It is very common, usually bilateral and often familial. Partial webbing of the toes may be easily overlooked.

Repair of the fingers is best left until the age of 4–5 years. No treatment is required for webbing of the toes.

## Curly toes

Many deformities of the toes are encountered in childhood, these often being familial. This is the commonest congenital deformity of the lesser toes, affecting the fourth and fifth most frequently. As in every deformity affecting the toes the child must be examined when standing, since this is likely to increase the abnormality. The affected toe lies curled under its medial neighbour, it being the extent to which this occurs which determines whether surgery is required. In mild cases there is no disability but care must be taken over the fitting of socks and shoes.

Treatment by strapping to the neighbouring toes is often practised but is a waste of time since the condition relapses when strapping is discontinued. Surgery consists of transplantation of the long flexor tendon into the extensor tendon.

## Congenital flexed toe

This is less common and may affect a single toe or two adjacent toes. On walking, the affected toe takes the weight on the distal end instead of on the plantar surface. Surgical treatment is the same as for curly toes.

## Congenital dorsiflexion of the second toe

In this condition the affected toe tends to over-ride the third toe but surgery is seldom necessary.

## Congenital dorsal displacement of the fifth toe

The fifth toe lies on the upper and outer aspect of the fourth toe and is rotated laterally. Only surgery can correct the deformity, the most important element being correction of the skin by elongation of the web. This can be performed as an out-patient at any age after the first birthday.

## Hemihypertrophy

This condition ranges from enlargement of a single digit to enlargement of the entire half of the body. Some cases of limb hypertrophy are associated with a widespread haemangioma and it is probable that growth has been stimulated by the increased vascularity. Other instances of limb hypertrophy are

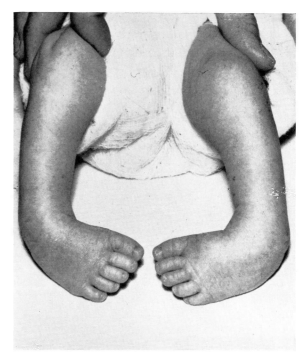

FIG. 56. Bilateral talipes equinovarus.

associated with an abnormality of lymphatics in the affected limb, such as lymphangioma. Haemangioma and lymphangioma may co-exist.

Increased incidence of malignancy involving the kidneys or adrenal glands has been noted in children with hemihypertrophy; careful watch should be kept for this possibility.

### Talipes (club foot)

The majority of these deformities are mechanical in origin, resulting from the abnormal position or restricted movement of the fetus *in utero*. In such cases it is possible to replace the child in the fetal position, thereby seeing how the deformities were caused. Hereditary factors also play a part, while a small number are associated with spina bifida and are paralytic in origin.

The varieties of talipes are named according to the position of the foot: equinus indicates plantar flexion and calceneus dorsiflexion; varus is inversion of the foot and valgus eversion.

TALIPES CALCANEOVALGUS ('TCV')

This is the commonest variety, though it is often missed. It is particularly seen

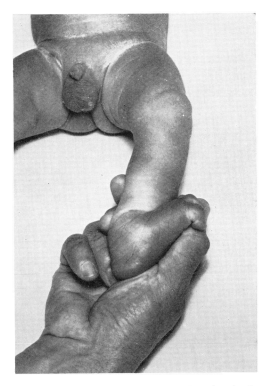

FIG. 57. The normal foot can be flexed and everted so that the dorsum can be made to touch the outer aspect of the lower leg. This is impossible if the child has talipes equinovarus.

in postmature infants whose feet are compressed in an exaggerated normal position from lack of amniotic fluid (p. 57). The foot is usually broad and flat. Orthopaedic surgeons are divided in their criteria for treatment, but there is a disability if the condition is left untreated, resulting from the long tendo Achillis. The foot is flat and unstable, girls finding themselves unable to wear high-heeled shoes.

### TALIPES EQUINOVARUS ('TEV')

This is the next most common variety and is often bilateral (Fig. 56). In bilateral cases there may be associated congenital dislocation of the hip. To test the foot it should be fully dorsiflexed and everted; in the normal the dorsum of the foot can be placed against the outer aspect of the lower leg (Fig. 57). Mild cases can be treated by manipulation and stretching exercises only. Serious cases require Denis Browne splints or repeated corrective plasters.

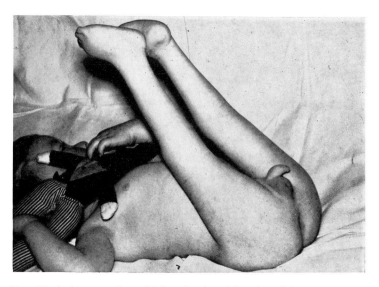

Fig. 58. Arthrogryposis multiplex showing deformity of legs and talipes equinovarus. Lack of muscle development in the buttocks is apparent.

### Metatarsus varus

A common malformation in which the forefoot is adducted on the rear part of the foot. No treatment is required if the deformity can be corrected passively, because it will therefore correct itself when the child begins to walk. Some of the remaining cases can be corrected by manipulation but repeated plasters may be necessary in severe cases. If the deformity is still present when the child starts to walk, the inner side of the sole should be raised.

### Arthrogryposis multiplex (Amyoplasia congenita)

A condition in which one or, more commonly, most of the limb joints are almost or completely fused as a result of replacement of muscle by fibrous tissue. The joints may be either extended or flexed, but more often the former, and a severe degree of talipes is present (Fig. 58). It is probable that in the majority of patients the malformation results from severe loss of mobility *in utero*, due to the effect of an extreme degree of moulding from increased intrauterine pressure. This occurs to a less extent in talipes alone. The condition may also result from muscle weakness and has occurred in patients with infantile muscular atrophy (Werdnig-Hoffmann disease) where the nerve disorder has commenced early in intrauterine life, and also in congenital muscular dystrophy.

The outlook is hopeless for those cases of primary neural or muscular

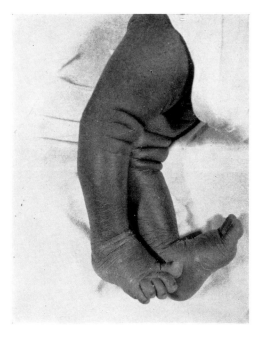

FIG. 59. Genu recurvatum associated with backward dislocation of the knees.

origin but, in those due to a moulding defect, the prognosis is much better than might be expected. There is a gradual loosening of the joints and development of joint movement. On no account should the limbs be splinted since, although this might hasten the improvement of position, function would be lost for ever. It is essential that the child should be left to move and kick freely, all unnecessary restriction by bed clothes being avoided. Associated congenital malformations are common.

**Genu recurvatum**

This is found in babies whose fetal position has been that of a breech with extended legs. The deformity at birth is most alarming and the knee may dislocate backwards with ease (Fig. 59). If left alone the leg returns to normal within a few weeks. The child should be nursed in a warm room so that the legs can be left uncovered, allowing them to flex without hindrance.

**Congenital dislocation of the hip**

This condition shows a female preponderance of about seven to one and has an incidence of four to five per 1000. Most dislocations occur in the last 4 weeks of pregnancy. The primary cause is simple laxity of the joint capsule.

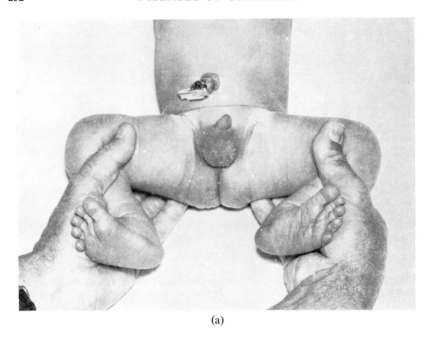

(a)

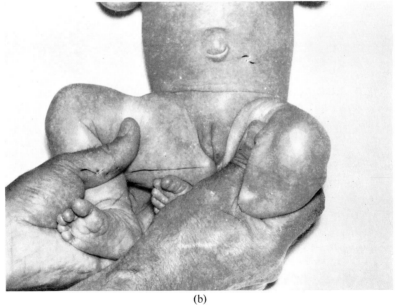

(b)

FIG. 60. (a) Normal hips permit full abduction.
(b) Congenital dislocation of the left hip. Abduction is restricted on the left side but full on the right.

There are two forms of generalized joint laxity which develop during prenatal life (Carter & Wilkinson, 1964). One is temporary, lasting only a few days after birth and is confined to girls; this is believed to be hormonal, resulting from the formation of relaxin in the uterus by the interaction of oestrogen and progesterone. The other is permanent, may occur in either sex and usually has a familial incidence.

The temporary joint laxity which is found in all girls accounts for their greater frequency of congenital dislocation of the hip. The permanent joint laxity is an important factor in the production of congenital dislocation of the hip in boys.

Breech position *in utero* is an additional factor since, in the presence of joint laxity, the flexed hips and extended knees favour the development of dislocation.

It used to be thought that a congenitally shallow acetabulum was the primary cause of congenital dislocation of the hip. In fact this is a rare condition causing fully established dislocation at birth associated with a false acetabulum. There is gross limitation of abduction and extension at birth so that the hips cannot be reduced by manipulation—quite a different condition from the usual type. In the common type the acetabulum is normal at birth, though untreated dislocation can lead to acquired shallowness of the acetabulum.

Congenital dislocation of the hip should be diagnosed at birth by two tests carried out during the routine examination of all newborn babies. First, the affected hip cannot be fully abducted (Fig. 60). Secondly, Barlow's modification of Ortolani's test is performed. With the child on his back the examiner grasps both thighs using his middle finger on the outer side and the thumb on the inner side as in Fig. 60 (b). Each hip is tested in turn with the hip half abducted. The leg is lifted upwards with the middle finger; if the hip is dislocated the head of the femur will be felt to slip over the posterior rim of the acetabulum into the socket. If the hip is dislocatable but not dislocated, in other words unstable, the head can be felt to slip over the posterior edge of the acetabulum and back again when the pressure is released. These movements of the femoral head may be associated with a 'clonk' or coarse click. A fine click can be produced by moving an undislocated head in its acetabulum, but in this case it is possible to feel that the head has not left its socket.

These movements of the femoral head are facilitated by the hypotonia which exists for the first few days of life. After 1–2 weeks the signs are much more difficult to obtain.

In any doubtful cases the hips should be X-rayed, although the absence of ossification of the femoral head at birth makes interpretation difficult in mild cases. In the early weeks of life preference should be given to clinical signs.

If by misfortune the condition is not diagnosed until later, it will be shown by asymmetry or shortening of the affected leg and a limp on walking. If treatment is delayed there is defective growth of the femoral head.

*Treatment.* A dislocated hip is rare whereas an unstable one is common and since this can change to complete dislocation it should be treated if the hip is still unstable when rechecked at one week of age. No manipulation is required for unstable or dislocated hips if the disorder is diagnosed shortly after birth. They should be splinted in a position of abduction at the hip for about 6 months and are then usually cured. Children in whom a fine click is detected should be checked again at 7–10 days, and provided the hip is stable and no click felt nothing further need be done.

It is interesting that congenital dislocation of the hip is rare in West Africa; this is possibly related to the fact that for the first 1–2 years babies are carried on their mothers' backs with the hips abducted so that cases could be cured. However, this cannot be the whole explanation and there must be a lessened genetic influence.

For late cases manipulative reduction is no longer favoured, unless the case is of very long standing. Slow reduction on a frame should be used. Once reduced, the legs are splinted in the medial position rather than the old fashioned 'frog' position of abduction, in which the hip is less stable.

### Funnel chest (Pectus excavatum) (Fig. 61)

This deformity is not due to rickets but to a congenitally short central tendon of the diaphragm. The patients are liable to suffer from repeated chest infections and in adult life cardiac embarrassment may occur. After the age of 6 months operative treatment should be advised in progressive cases, for cosmetic as well as for symptomatic indications (Chin & Adler, 1954).

### Pigeon chest (Pectus carinatum)

In this condition there is forward protrusion of the sternum. It may result from bronchial asthma or from right ventricular enlargement in congenital heart disease. It may also result from congenital overgrowth of the ribs; when this is bilateral the sternum protrudes and when unilateral there is unusual prominence of the costochondral junctions.

### Achondroplasia (Chondrodystrophia foetalis)

This condition, which in most instances is genetically determined by a dominant mode of inheritance, is due to an abnormality of cartilage development in the epiphysial plate. There is very little growth of the long bones so that the child is dwarfed, with strikingly short limbs but an almost normal trunk. The base of the skull is affected and remains small, but the cranium grows normally so that the appearance suggests hydrocephalus. Mental development is usually normal and these dwarfs often earn their living in the circus.

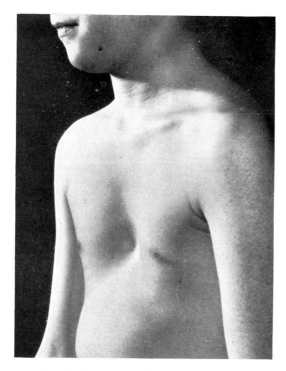

Fig. 61. Funnel chest in a boy aged 11 years.

Radiological diagnosis is best made from the appearance of the spine. In the lateral view the vertebral pedicles are short; in the antero-posterior view they are close together. The iliac bones are small and do not flare outwards as much as the normal.

### Marfan's syndrome (Arachnodactyly)

This is a widespread disorder of mesoderm determined by an autosomal dominant mutant gene with variable manifestation. There is overgrowth of the long bones (later named arachnodactyly) causing 'spider' fingers and toes with increased height. Although associated heart lesions may be congenital the majority are acquired, particularly aortic incompetence and dissecting aneurysm of the aorta. Dislocation of the lens is common. Excessive joint laxity may be present and can cause dislocation of joints.

This disorder must be differentiated from homocystinuria, an inborn error of methionine metabolism which is also associated with dislocation of the lens and arachnodactyly. These children are usually mentally handicapped and homocystine is present in the urine.

### Osteogenesis imperfecta (Fragilitas ossium)

Children with this condition have extremely fragile bones since very little bone is laid down owing to defective function of the osteoblasts, although the cartilage at the bone ends appears normal. The condition is determined by an autosomal dominant mutant gene with variable manifestation. Two forms occur: in the severest, the bones are thick and the infant is born with numerous fractures, seldom surviving long (Fig. 62); in the less severe form the bones are thin, the first fractures occur after birth and fewer bones are involved. Healing occurs readily since callus formation is abundant, but severe deformities result. The sclerotics are blue since they are thin, so allowing the choroidal pigment to show through. The skull is flattened and appears to bulge at the side giving the head a characteristic appearance. Deafness is common in later life.

### Hypertelorism

The eyes of these patients are set widely apart due to overgrowth of the lesser wing of the sphenoid. The patients are often mentally retarded.

### Cleido-cranial dysostosis

There is defective development or absence of the clavicles so that the shoulders can be brought abnormally close together. The membrane bones of the skull are also involved in the abnormal development, causing the fontanelle to be widely open and giving a globular shape to the head suggestive of hydrocephalus. Dentition is delayed and defective, and there is marked malocclusion. The condition is due to the inheritance of an autosomal dominant gene.

### Scoliosis

Congenital scoliosis is due to maldevelopment of one or more vertebrae; it is often associated with abnormalities of the ribs, such as aplasia or fusion. A common malformation is the hemivertebra. Very little treatment is possible, physiotherapy being of no value. However, if only one or two adjoining vertebrae are affected the ultimate prognosis may be better than seemed possible, owing to the development of compensatory curves above and below the abnormality.

### Klippel-Feil syndrome

The neck is short due to abnormalities of the cervical vertebrae which may be reduced in number, fused or abnormally shaped.

### Congenital elevation of the scapula (Sprengel's shoulder)

In this condition one or both scapulae are usually high and there is often a

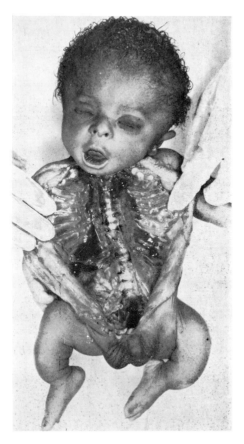

FIG. 62. Osteogenesis imperfecta in a baby dying shortly after birth. The skull bulges at the side from prominence of the soft parietal bones. The lower limbs are short and grossly deformed by multiple fractures. Numerous fractures of the ribs are present; on the inner aspect of the ribs glistening lumps of callus are visible through the parietal pleura.

bony or fibrous connection with the spine. The arm cannot be raised above a right angle. The disorder may be associated with the Klippel-Feil syndrome.

### Craniosynostosis

Premature fusion of the cranial sutures occurs in some infants, the resultant deformity depending on which sutures are affected. If the coronal suture is involved, the condition of *oxycephaly* (acrocephaly, turret skull) results (Fig. 63). The skull becomes turret-shaped due to the steep ascent of the parietal and frontal bones. In a number of patients there is also syndactyly, the

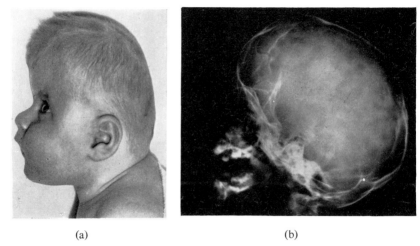

(a)                                    (b)

FIG. 63. (a) Oxycephaly, showing turret-shaped head.
(b) Skull in oxycephaly. Premature fusion of the coronal suture has
led to raised intracranial pressure, causing increased convolutional
markings ('beaten-silver appearance') on the vault.

term *acrocephalo-syndactyly* being applied. If the sagittal suture fuses early the
result is *scaphocephaly*; the skull becomes boat-shaped due to elongation of
the antero-posterior diameter.

Premature fusion of the skull bones may lead to raised intracranial pressure
which, if not relieved, can lead to blindness and mental retardation. Cerebral
function is more likely to be disturbed by coronal than by sagittal synostosis.
Retardation may sometimes be an associated condition rather than the result
of the early fusion. Some cases of craniosynostosis are associated with rickets.

Surgery is not required for every case but if there is evidence of raised
intracranial pressure this can be relieved by the operation of linear craniectomy. Refusion of the bones must be prevented by covering the cut edges with
polythene film or tantalum foil. The dura is left intact.

### Plagiocephaly (Fig. 64)

In this condition the head is asymmetrical. It is not a congenital malformation
nor is it the result of moulding during delivery since the abnormal shape is
not present at birth but develops during the first year, becoming most obvious
in its second half. The condition results from lack of synchronization of
fusion of the coronal suture on the two sides of the skull.

Parents should be assured that there is no abnormal pressure on the brain
and that the condition is harmless. As the child gets older the asymmetry
becomes less obvious as well as being obscured by the growth of hair.

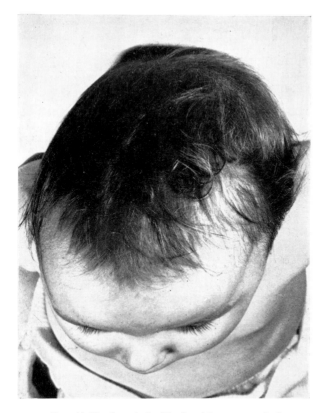

FIG. 64. Plagiocephaly. The head is asymmetrical.

**Osteopetrosis (Albers-Schönberg's disease, marble bone disease)**

This is a rare disorder in which there is defective ossification owing to lack of normal resorption of the cartilaginous ground substance. As a result, the bones are abnormally brittle and fracture easily. The disease is inherited both as an autosomal dominant and as an autosomal recessive trait; the sexes are equally affected.

The abnormal deposition of calcium is progressive, leading to gradual obliteration of the bone marrow and the development of leuco-erythroblastic anaemia (p. 592). Radiographically there is increased density of the bones with loss of the marrow cavity. The blood chemistry is normal. Optic atrophy may result from encroachment on the optic foramen and osteitis is a common complication.

No treatment is available, many of the patients dying in childhood.

However, the condition may progress sufficiently slowly for it first to be discovered in adult life.

## BIBLIOGRAPHY

ABERDEEN E., WATERSTON D.J., CARR I., GRAHAM G., BONHAM-CARTER R.E. & SUBRA-MANIAN S. (1965) Successful 'correction' of transposed great arteries by Mustard's operation. *Lancet*, **1**, 1233.

ABT A. (1965) Circumcision and prostatic cancer. *Acta med. scand.*, **178**, 493.

AVERY M.E. (1968) *The Lung and its Disorders in the Newborn Infant*. 2nd ed. Saunders, Philadelphia.

BAIKE A.G. (1965) Chromosomal Abnormalities. In *Recent Advances in Paediatrics*, 3rd ed Ed. Gairdner D. Churchill, London.

BANATVALA J.E., BEST J.M., BERTRAND J., BOWERN N.A. & HUDSON S.M. (1970) Serological assessment of rubella during pregnancy. *Brit. med. J.*, **3**, 247.

BARLOW T.G. (1962) Early diagnosis and treatment of congenital dislocation of the hip. *J. Bone Jt Surg.*, **44B**, 292.

BENNETT D.E. (1964) Problems in neonatal obstructive jaundice. *Pediatrics*, **33**, 735.

BETTMAN J.W. & CLEASBY G.W. (1963) Congenital glaucoma. *Pediatrics*, **32**, 420.

BURSTON W.R. (1965) The early orthodontic treatment of alveolar clefts. *Proc. roy. Soc. Med.*, **58**, 767.

BUTLER N.R. & BONHAM D.G. (1963) *Perinatal Mortality*. Livingstone, Edinburgh.

CARTER C.O. (1962) Human heredity. Penguin Books Ltd. London.

CARTER C.O. & WILKINSON J. (1964) Persistent joint laxity and congenital dislocation of the hip. *J. Bone Jt Surg.* **46B**, 40.

CHIN E.F. & ADLER R.H. (1954) The surgical treatment of pectus excavatum (funnel chest). *Brit. med. J.*, **1**, 1064.

CHRISPIN A.R. & FRIEDLAND G.W. (1966) A radiological study of the neural control of oesophageal vestibular function. *Thorax*, **21**, 422.

CHRISPIN A.R., FRIEDLAND G.W. & WRIGHT D.E. (1967) Some functional characteristics of the oesophageal vestibule in infants and children. *Thorax*, **22**, 188.

DAVIES P.A. & SMALLPEICE V. (1963) The single transverse palmar crease in infants and children. *Develop Med. Child. Neurol.*, **5**, 491.

DODGE J.A. (1973) Infantile pyloric stenosis. Inheritance, psyche and soma. *Irish J. Med. Sci.*, **142**, 6.

FARQUHAR J.W. (1965) The influence of maternal diabetes on foetus and child. In *Recent Advances in Paediatrics*, 3rd ed. Ed. Gairdner D. Churchill, London.

GAIRDNER D. (1949) The fate of the foreskin. *Brit. med. J.*, **2**, 1433.

HARE E.H., LAURENCE K.M., PAYNE H. & RAWNSLEY K. (1966) Spina bifida cystica and family stress. *Brit. med. J.*, **2**, 757.

HARLEY J.D. & HERTZBERG R. (1965) Aetiology of cataracts in childhood. *Lancet*, **1**, 1084.

KAPLAN S., DAOUD G.I., BENZING G., DEVINE F.J., GLASS I.H. & McGUIRE J. (1963) Natural history of ventricular septal defect. *Amer. J. Dis. Child.*, **105**, 581.

LAURENCE K.M. (1974) Effect of early surgery for spina bifida cystica on survival and quality of life. *Lancet*, **1**, 301.

LEAPE L.L. & LONGINO L.A. (1964) Infantile lobar emphysema. *Pediatrics*, **34**, 246.

LORBER J. (1965) The family history of spina bifida cystica. *Pediatrics*, **35**, 589.

LORBER J. (1972) Spina bifida cystica. Results of treatment of 270 consecutive cases with criteria for selection for the future. *Arch. Dis. Childh.*, **47**, 854.

LOUGHNAN P.M., GOLD H. & VANCE J.C. (1973) Phenytoin teratogenicity in man. *Lancet*, **1**, 70.

LOWE C.R. (1973) Congenital malformations among infants born to epileptic women. *Lancet*, **1**, 9.

MCDONALD A. (1964) Cataract in children of very low birth weight. *Guy's Hosp. Rep.*, **113**, 296.

MCKENDRICK T. (1962) Sweat sodium levels in normal subjects, in fibrocystic patients and their relatives, and in chronic bronchitis patients. *Lancet*, **1**, 183.

MUSTARD W.T. (1964) Successful two-stage correction of transposition of the great vessels. *Surgery*, **55**, 469.

MUSTARD W.T., KEITH J.D., TRUSLER G.A., FOWLER R. & KIDD L. (1964) The surgical management of transposition of the great vessels. *J. thorac. cardiovasc. Surg.*, **48**, 953.

NIXON H.H. (1964) Hirschsprung's disease. *Arch. Dis. Childh.*, **39**, 109.

NORMAN A.P. Ed. (1971) *Congenital Abnormalities in Infancy*. 2nd ed. Blackwell Scientific Publications, Oxford.

PARADISE J.L., BLUESTONE C.D. & FELDER H. (1969) The universality of otitis media in 50 infants with cleft palate. *Pediatrics*, **44**, 35.

PEDERSEN L.M., TYGSTRUP I. & PEDERSEN J. (1964) Congenital malformations in newborn infants of diabetic women: correlation with maternal diabetic vascular complications. *Lancet*, **1**, 1124.

PENROSE L.S. (1963) Finger-prints, palms and chromosomes. *Nature*, **197**, 933.

RASHKIND W.J. & MILLER W.W. (1966) Creation of an atrial septal defect without thoracotomy. A palliative approach to transposition of the great arteries. *J. Amer. Med. Ass.*, **196**, 991.

SHARRARD W.J.W., ZACHARY R.B., LORBER J. & BRUCE A.M. (1963). A controlled trial of immediate and delayed closure of spina bifida cystica. *Arch. Dis. Childh.*, **39**, 18.

SHARRARD W.J.W. (1963) The surgery of deformed toes in children. *Brit. J. clin. Pract.*, **17**, 263.

SLATER B.C.S., WATSON G.I. & MCDONALD J.C. (1964) Seasonal variation in congenital abnormalities. *Brit. J. prev. soc. Med.*, **18**, 1.

STARK G.D. & DRUMMOND M. (1973) Results of selective early operation in myelomeningocele. *Arch. Dis. Childh.*, **48**, 676.

TERRIS M., WILSON F. & NELSON J.H. (1973) Relation of circumcision to cancer of the cervix. *Am. J. Obstet. Gyncol.*, **117**, 1056.

TYNAN M. (1971) Survival of infants with transposition of great arteries after balloon atrial septostomy. *Lancet* **1**, 621.

VALENTINE G.H. (1966) *The Chromosome Disorders*. Heinemann Medical, London.

WOODS G.E. (1953) Some observations on umbilical hernia in infants. *Arch. Dis. Childh.*, **28**, 50.

# CHAPTER 7

# GROWTH AND DEVELOPMENT

## NORMAL GROWTH AND DEVELOPMENT

Growth and development are intimately related but are not identical. Growth is increase in size whereas development is increase in complexity. Growth can be accurately measured but the measurement of development is much more difficult.

The rate of growth in height is not constant throughout childhood. It is at its greatest when the child is born and, although the child is still growing very fast during his first two years, the rate is falling sharply all the time (Fig. 67). From the age of 3–10 years growth in height is comparatively slow and steady, often reaching its slowest period of all just before the onset of puberty. The adolescent growth spurt commences just before puberty, this being the only time in postnatal life when an acceleration of growth occurs. This rapid rate continues during puberty, followed by sharp deceleration falling to zero when adult status is reached.

The rate of growth influences the appetite so that it is natural for children to want more food during their first year and immediately before puberty. An explanation to parents of these basic facts will go far to allay one of their common anxieties. Growth in height is influenced by the seasons; it is faster in spring and slower in autumn. In view of this seasonal effect, the value of any drug given to promote growth must be assessed over periods of not less than 1 year.

Not all systems of the body grow at the same rate. This is illustrated by Fig. 65 in which the line marked *general* reflects the changes in the rate of growth in height described above. This is an indicator of bone growth, particularly the long bones and vertebral column. Individual bones grow at widely different rates, this being an important factor in the final body proportions. The pattern of muscle development is similar to that of bone but it is particularly laid down at puberty, especially in the male. Growth of the thoracic and abdominal organs also conform to this general growth pattern.

On the other hand, neural growth, representing particularly the brain, is entirely different. The human brain growth spurt begins in mid-pregnancy and is largely complete by the third year. This has a vital application to the man-

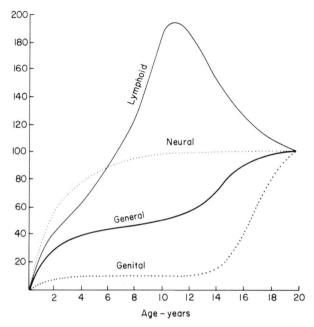

FIG. 65. Graph showing the major types of postnatal growth. The curves are drawn to a common scale by computing their value at successive ages in terms of their total postnatal increments. (After Scammon, R.E. (1930), 'The Measurement of Man'. Minnesota.)

agement of malnutrition in order to prevent it causing mental handicap. Priority feeding in famine areas must be given to pregnant women and children under the age of 4 years (see p. 444).

Lymphoid tissue shows another entirely different growth pattern. It grows progressively throughout childhood but ceases at the age of 10–12 years—before the puberty growth spurt. Moreover, this maximal growth is followed by regression so that the amount of lymphoid tissue in the body actually decreases. These changes can be watched in the tonsils which are barely visible at birth, become very obvious by the age of 4–5 years and get smaller in the early teens. If more parents were given this information, fewer tonsils would be removed because they were 'large'.

Fat increases rapidly during the first 12 months of life, being followed by a small steady loss until the age of 7 years; thereafter, the amount of fat remains constant until its pre-puberty spurt which occurs before that of bone and muscle. The increase in the amount of fat during the child's first year is of vital importance as to whether or not the individual becomes obese. It is only during fetal life and the first year that the number of fat cells increases as well as the total amount of fat (Brooke, 1972). Consequently, an overfed baby becomes provided with more than the required number of fat cells and these persist throughout life, demanding to be filled. Small wonder then that fat babies make fat adults and that their reduction in weight is so difficult. Mothers must be told these facts in order to prevent them from making their babies fat.

Genital growth is minimal during infancy and childhood but becomes very rapid with the onset of puberty.

The size of the newborn baby is only very slightly related to the size of the adult. The major factor deciding the size of a baby at birth is the environment during the last two months of pregnancy. The influence of these prenatal factors continues with diminishing strength during the first 2–3 years so that only after that period does the child get on to his own curve of growth; at this point his growth is said to be 'canalized'. This is regulated by his own hormonal system which during the first 2–3 years is only just beginning to take charge. This explains why growth hormone deficient children do not become apparent until the second or third year of life (p. 278). It also explains why future adult height is so difficult to predict from measurements taken during the first 2–3 years of life. Prediction is based on the correlation between bone age and the proportion of adult stature achieved (Bayley & Pinneau, 1952). Height prediction is particularly valuable for would-be ballet dancers whose ultimate height may eventually exclude them from dancing.

During a period of illness or starvation the rate of growth is slowed, but after the incident the child grows more rapidly than usual so that he catches up towards, or actually to, his original growth curve ('catch-up growth'). It is unknown how the body knows when to stop the catch-up phase of growth. The degree to which this catch-up is successful depends on the length of time growth has been slowed. If growth has been slowed for too long or into puberty, complete catch-up is not achieved (Prader *et al.*, 1963).

It is difficult to assess the influence of nutrition on growth since it is seldom the only factor involved. Retardation of growth occurs only if malnutrition is severe, and in such cases there is always the additional possibility of chronic infection such as malaria. If starvation has caused growth to be retarded, an adequate diet soon brings the child back to the normal height.

An interesting problem is posed by the fact that pure Japanese, born and reared in America, are taller than those living in Japan. However, the Japanese in Japan are now growing taller in common with all countries where nutrition has improved. Striking increases in height have occurred in Great Britain in the last 50 years. In fact, this increased height is possibly a better indication of improved social conditions than the infant mortality rate. It is believed to be due mainly to improved nutrition. The next question is when will this increased height in each generation cease. There is evidence from America (Bakwin & McLaughlin, 1964) that the end is in sight since the rate of increase for children from the higher income groups is now very slight.

The influence of food intake on height is also seen in the fat child who is taller than average; when weight is lost by diet the gain in height is less than anticipated from the previous pattern. This increased height is so constant that if a fat child is not taller than average, another cause, particularly hypo-thyroidism, should be suspected.

The hormonal control of growth during childhood is brought about by thyroxine and growth hormone working synergistically. Thyroxine is pre-dominantly required for skeletal maturation and growth hormone for linear growth. The adolescent growth spurt is largely brought about in boys by the rise in adrenal and testicular androgens and in girls by the rise in ovarian oestrogens together with adrenal androgens and oestrogens.

Growth hormone is derived from the anterior pituitary gland, exerting its influence through the metabolism of protein, fat and carbohydrate. Its action on protein metabolism is to simulate the transport of amino-acids across cell membranes and their incorporation into protein. Man responds optimally to human growth hormone only. This is a protein to which resistance may develop as a result of the development of antibodies. It accelerates bone age but only as much as it increases height. In comparison, anabolic steroids, androgens and oestrogens accelerate bone age more than height, thereby causing the ultimate height to be less than expected.

**Height**

When measuring the height of children it should be remembered that all individuals shrink a little during the day. The child must therefore be drawn out to the maximum by traction under the mastoids before making the measurement, checking that the heels are still on the ground. Similar pre-cautions must be taken with babies. They are measured lying down on a special table which has a fixed head-board and movable foot-board. Two people are required, one to keep the head against the head-board, the other to keep the knees firmly pressed down on the table and the feet flat against the foot-board.

To determine the rate of growth of an individual child, a number of meas-urements should be made at regular intervals, such as twice a year. These measurements give a growth curve which can be plotted in several ways: a *height distance curve* (Fig. 66) is obtained by plotting the height at each age and is the usual method; a *height velocity curve* (Fig. 67) is obtained by plot-ting the amount gained during each year and is a valuable addition; another method is to plot the annual growth against the bone age, thereby showing the height gained per bone age year. If these curves are plotted on a scale giving

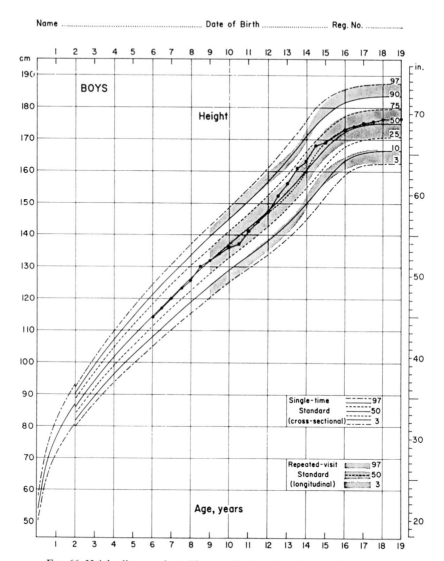

Fɪɢ. 66. Height distance chart. The growth of one boy is plotted between the ages of 6 and 19 years, showing his puberty growth spurt between the ages of 12 and 15 years.

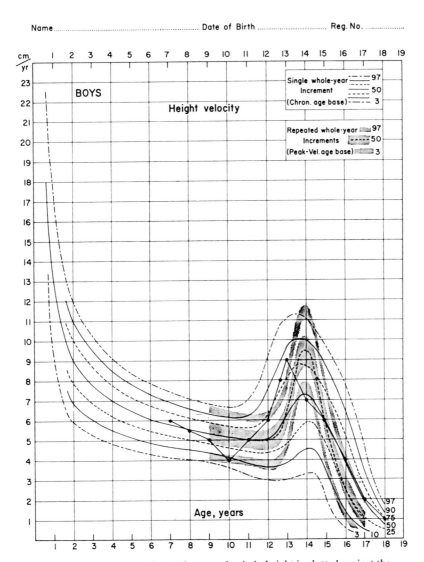

FIG. 67. Height velocity chart. The annual gain in height is plotted against the age. The curve shown is from the same boy as Fig. 66.

the average normals, a useful comparison can be made and it is here that percentiles are used. The fiftieth percentile is the median, so that 50 per cent of individuals are above and 50 per cent below. The limits of normality cannot be defined, but it is usually accepted that a healthy child should fall within the third and the ninety-seventh percentiles, indicating that only 3 per cent of a sample are above or below these limits. During the puberty growth spurt the normal child climbs up through the percentiles, dropping back to his own percentile once the spurt is over (Fig. 66). If he is a late developer, he drops down through the percentiles until the growth spurt occurs. The growth spurt starts earlier in girls, is less intense and stops earlier than in boys. Usually, boys have had an extra 2 years growth before their adolescent spurt. At all ages, adolescence included, the growth of girls is less affected than boys by stress such as illness or malnutrition.

In comparing the rate of growth of an individual with that of a standard, the standard used should have been made from a sample similar to himself as regards age, sex and race, since the variations with each of these is considerable. Many factors affect individual variation in body measurements but heredity probably accounts for 80 per cent of these, so that both parents should be seen when assessing individual growth problems.

From all this, the immense variation of normal can be appreciated, this being reflected in the tables for height, weight and head circumference on pp. 740–744. It is this normal variation which causes so much anxiety to parents who will over-emphasize the difference between one child and his siblings or worse still, the difference in size from the neighbour's children.

**Weight**

A child's weight is an indication of his growth and his deposition of fat. Growth is measured by height but insufficient attention is paid to the measurement of fat. Fat is measured by picking up the skin folds between special recording callipers; the folds over the triceps and subscapular muscles are the usual sites chosen. The measurement of skin folds gives a better indication of a child's progress than his weight.

During the first weeks of life the average baby gains 150–190 g (5–6 oz) a week, doubling his birth weight by about 4 months of age. However, many perfectly normal babies gain less than this and mothers should be reassured that provided the baby is contented, a slow weight gain is normal. At 1 year he will weigh about 10 kg, at 2 years 12 kg and at 3 years 15 kg. From the age of 3 to 7 years he gains an average of 2 kg a year and from 8 to 12 years about 3 kg a year. See Tables 12 and 13, pp. 742, 743.

**Head circumference**

The greatest increase in head circumference takes place during the first year of life, when it advances from 33 cm at birth to 46 cm at 12 months. At the age of 14 years it is 53 cm which represents an advance of only 7 cm in 11 years as compared with 13 cm in the first year. See Table 12, p. 744.

## Maturity

A child's maturity can be assessed in a number of different ways, such as skeletal, sexual, mental and dental.

### SKELETAL MATURITY

The skeletal maturity or bone age is determined by the appearance and state of fusion of the epiphyses. The wrist and hand are mainly used, with the addition of the elbow in older children. Comparisons are then made with a known standard.

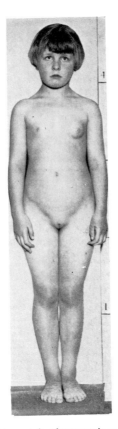

FIG. 68. Asymmetrical breast development in a normal girl at puberty.

SEXUAL MATURITY

This is determined from the age at which secondary sexual characteristics appear. In the male, these are facial, axillary and pubic hair, changes in the larynx causing alteration of the voice, and the size of the penis and testicles. In the female, they are axillary and pubic hair, development of the breast and external genitalia, and the onset of menstruation. The age at which the menarche occurs gives an exact date for girls so that comparisons are much easier than with boys. On an average, girls reach physical maturity about $2\frac{1}{2}$ years earlier than boys, their final height being about 15 cm (6 inches) less.

It is common for normal breast development to be asymmetrical, one breast sometimes showing considerable growth before there is any change in the other (Fig. 68). This is a normal variation of puberal development though the condition sometimes raises diagnostic difficulties if it has not been encountered previously. Occasionally the disastrous error has been made of amputating the breast in the mistaken belief that it was neoplastic.

In the majority of girls, the maximum growth spurt occurs before the onset of menstruation. This information will relieve mothers worried about tall daughters who have not menstruated, and who are under the misconception that there is much more growth still to come after the onset of menstruation. Children now mature earlier and are getting bigger for their age each year, so that in making comparisons recently collected standards must be used.

MENTAL MATURITY

The assessment of an infant's mental maturity is made from a study of his behaviour and his reactions to standard stimuli so that comparisons can be drawn. This comparative assessment can be made from the age of 1 month and gives the *development quotient*. Specific tests of intelligence can be carried out from the age of 2 years and give the *intelligence quotient*.

Development is a continuous process from conception to maturity but its rate varies greatly in different, though still normal, children. There is also a racial difference; the Negro baby at birth is more mature than the European (Geber & Dean, 1957), remaining ahead for the first year. This variation in Negro babies can also be detected in the electroencephalogram (EEG). The maturity of the baby is reflected in the amount of rhythmic movement in the EEG; there is a definite alpha rhythm in Negro babies by the age of 18–24 months, whereas in white babies this increase does not appear until about 24–28 months (Pampiglione, 1965). The sequence of development is the same for all children except that an unnecessary stage, such as crawling, may be left out. This particularly occurs in children given the walking frames now available; such children will learn to crawl only when it suits their purpose, this being likely to be some time after they learn to walk. In contra-distinction, children who learn to crawl may be late in walking since, having learnt to get about, they have a reduced stimulus to learn to walk.

Development is not a smooth continuous process but made up of lulls and spurts. Moreover, having achieved a skill, this may go into abeyance while another is being learned. Some skills develop separately, becoming co-ordinated later. The achievement of a new stage is dependent on the growing maturity of the nervous system so that development cannot be accelerated from outside sources. On the other hand, outside factors, particularly environment and to a less extent illness, can retard it.

Development is made up of many different fields: locomotion, manipulation, emotion, social relationships, understanding and memory, speech, visual and auditory behaviour, feeding behaviour, play behaviour and sphincter control. The rate of development in each field is likely to be very different so that one or more fields may be considerably retarded in comparison with the others. Uniform retardation usually denotes mental retardation, unless it is due to severe early emotional deprivation. But retardation in a single field such as walking or talking does not suggest mental retardation. It may just be the pattern for that particular child, or it may be due to insufficient stimulation in the particular fields. However, before accepting such causes it is essential to exclude organic disease, for example a motor defect in the case of delayed walking and deafness in the case of delayed speech.

The prediction of future intellectual performance on the basis of an infant's developmental assessment is impossible because intellect will be much influenced by future environmental factors.

During the examination for development it is essential to spend a long time watching the child. Four main areas of development are tested: Posture and gross movements; vision and fine movements; hearing and language; everyday skills and social behaviour. Particular attention should be paid as to how the child manipulates objects since this is much more important than gross motor development when assessing skills. In the consulting-room the spatula is a useful object for testing manipulation (see p. 11). It is also easy to remember the relative skills achieved at different ages if the same test object is used. Particularly important is social behaviour such as the age when smiling commenced, the amount of smiling, interest, alertness, concentration, vocalizations and speech.

The age at which most of the milestones (or 'stepping stones') are achieved varies considerably. Thus a normal child may sit without support at any age from 5–12 months. He may start walking alone at 8 months or not until the age of 2 years, or even later. To some extent the age at which a child learns to walk is determined by whether he has acquired other methods of propulsion. The expert crawler may dislike giving up this efficient way of getting about for the more hazardous method on two feet. Alternatively, a child may miss out the stage of crawling altogether, progressing straight from sitting to standing, to walking. Children who move about by bottom-shuffling, a habit which sometimes runs in families, are often late in walking.

On the other hand, certain milestones have only a narrow age range for normality, especially in the case of smiling. The normal baby smiles at about the age of 6 weeks. If a full-term baby whose mother had been making normal contact was not smiling by 8 weeks, I would begin to be concerned and I would be very worried if such a baby was not smiling by 10 weeks. By the age of 3 months the normally stimulated baby is vocalizing a great deal when talked to. Lack of vocalization at 4 months would begin to be a cause for concern, though in this instance it could be because his mother had not been talking to him.

At first the baby smiles at any warm human face but by 3–4 months his smile is particularly a reaction to recognizing his parents. At 6 months a baby can follow a rolling ball and since visual attention is related to IQ, this test gives information about intellect as well as actual vision.

The earliest sounds a baby makes result from vocal play. He discovers that by moving his lips and tongue he can vary the noises coming out of his mouth. His mother's subsequent reinforcement of relevant sounds such as 'da-da' causes him to copy such sounds while her obvious delight at his achievement causes him to experiment still more. A deaf child may produce sounds by vocal play but is unable to progress to the stage of copying his mother's sounds. Gesture is another important part of language development, the child excitedly pointing at objects; gesturing is seldom seen in the mentally handicapped.

Until the age of 6 months a baby will not follow a falling object, consequently a toy knocked off his cot appears to have disappeared completely from his world. By 6 months he is able to follow a falling object down to the ground. Also by this age he can pass a toy from one hand to the other but he cannot yet voluntarily let go an object; this skill is not achieved until the age of 9 months.

Different stages of normal development are best shown from photographs (Figs. 69–89).

### Critical periods of learning

It is now appreciated that there are 'critical' periods during the process of learning which are optimal for the development of various physiological and psychological functions. These periods are relatively short; in animal experiments, if the appropriate stimulation is not provided during the critical period for that aspect of learning, the animal ceases to progress in that respect.

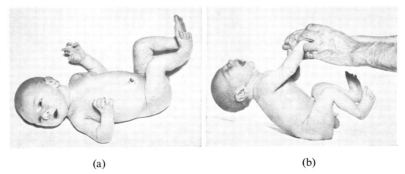

(a) (b)

(a) Supine. Head turns to one side, legs flexed, knees apart and soles turned inwards.

(b) Lifted from supine. Head falls loosely back.

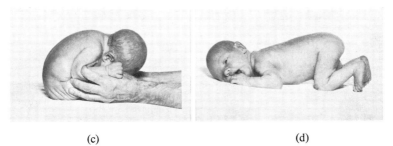

(c) (d)

(c) Held sitting. Head falls forward, the back making one complete curve.

(d) Lying prone. The head turns immediately to one side, limbs flexed under body and buttocks humped up.

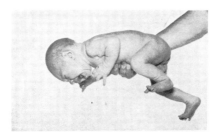

(e)

(e) Ventral suspension. The head is momentarily held in the horizontal position, the limbs are partially flexed.

FIG. 69. Newborn baby.

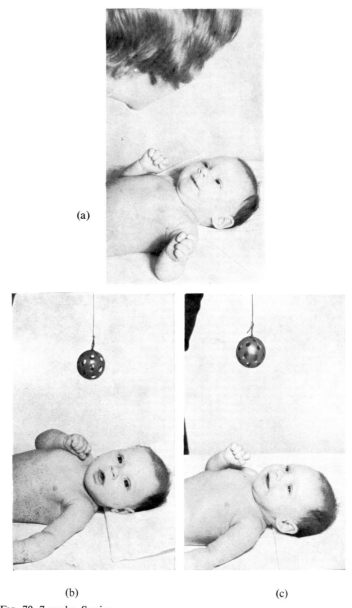

FIG. 70. 7 weeks. Supine

(a) Visually very alert; makes eye to eye contact and smiles.
(b) and (c) Follows a dangling toy held at 15–25 cm through a half circle from side to side.

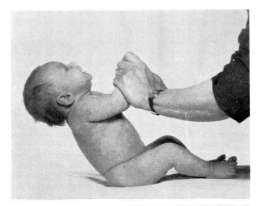

(a) While being pulled up the
    head lags.

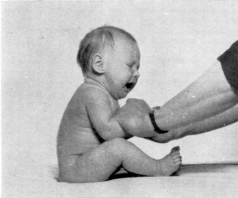

(b) When the vertical position
    is reached, the head is held
    erect for a moment.

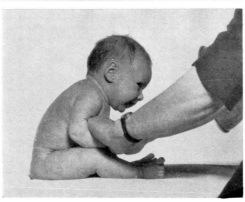

(c) Head then falls forwards.

FIG. 71. 7 weeks. Pulled to sitting.

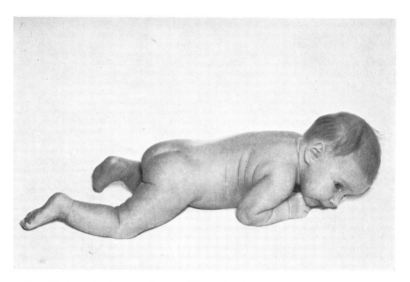

FIG. 72. 7 weeks. Prone. Elbows still remain close to the side with the hands near the sternum. Chin is lifted slightly from the couch. Buttocks flatter than in the neonate. Legs beginning to extend.

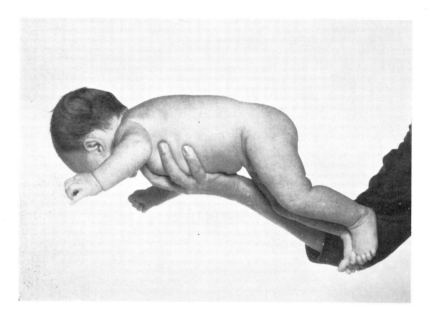

FIG. 73. 7 weeks. Ventral suspension. Head lifted slightly above the horizontal.

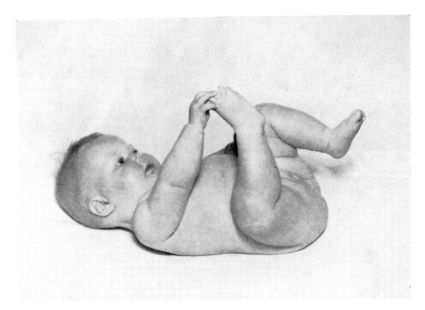

FIG. 74. 6 months. Supine. Plays with toes. Note intense visual concentration.

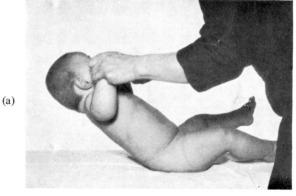

(a)

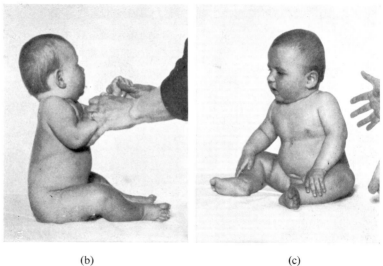

(b) (c)

FIG. 75. 6 months. Pull to sit.

(a) Braces shoulders and assists. No head lag.

(b) Back straight and head firmly erect at the end of the movement.

(c) Sits momentarily without support.

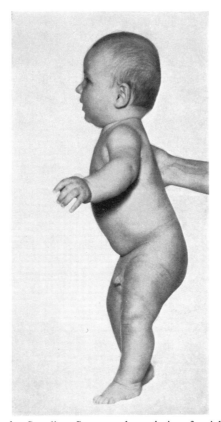

FIG. 76. 6 months. Standing. Supports the majority of weight on the feet.

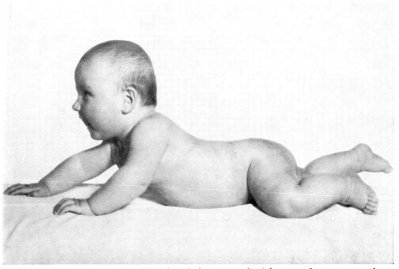

FIG. 77. 6 months. Prone. Head and chest are raised from surface supported on extended arms. Buttocks flat, thighs resting on couch.

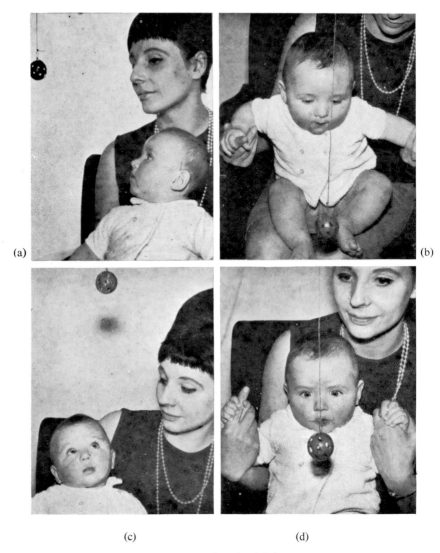

(a)

(b)

(c)

(d)

FIG. 78. 6 months. Visual following.
(a) Side to side.
(b) Downwards.
(c) Upwards.
(d) Convergence.

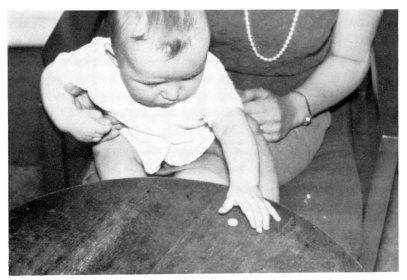

FIG. 79. 6 months. Hand and eye co-ordination shown in reaching for a sweet.

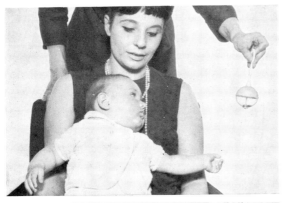

(a) On ear level.

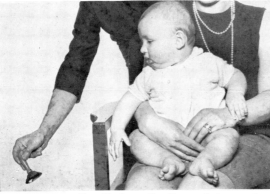

(b) Below ears.

FIG. 80. 6 months. Responds to sound.

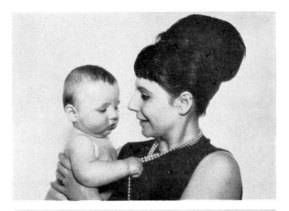

(a) Child is playing with mother's beads before sound is made.

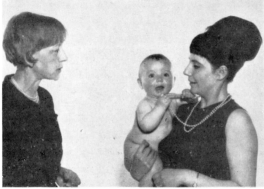

(b) Alerts to sound.

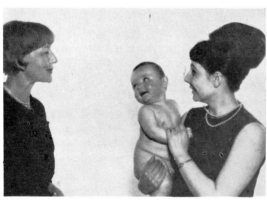

(c) Turns to source of sound.

FIG. 81. 6 months. Testing for hearing with whispered voice.

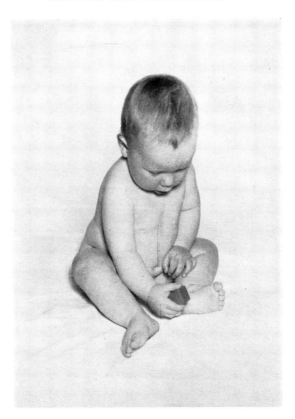

Fɪɢ. 82. 9 months. Grasping object between finger and thumb. Note intense concentration.

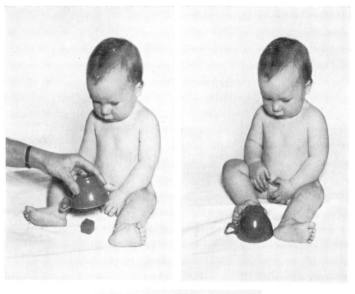

(a)

(b)

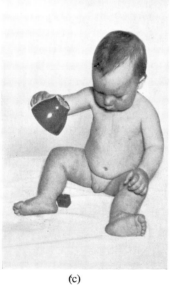

(c)

FIG. 83. 9 months. Demonstrating the developing awareness of the permanence of objects by finding the hidden brick.

(a) Brick is being covered by cup.
(b) Brick hidden by cup.
(c) Child finds brick by lifting cup.

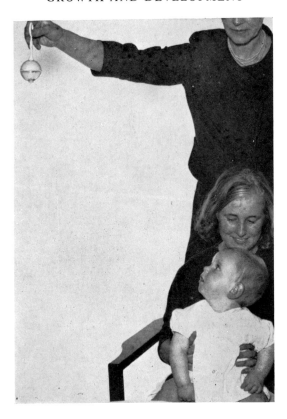

FIG. 84. 9 months. Demonstrating instantaneous localization of sound above ear level. In this hearing test the sound must not be made in the midline, directly above the child, since it is then heard equally in both ears and cannot be localized.

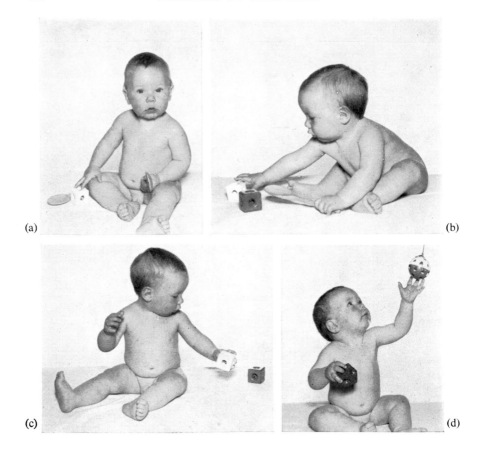

FIG. 85. 9 months.

(a) Sits completely on own.

(b) Reaching forward for object.

(c) Turning round for object behind.

(d) Reaching upwards for object.

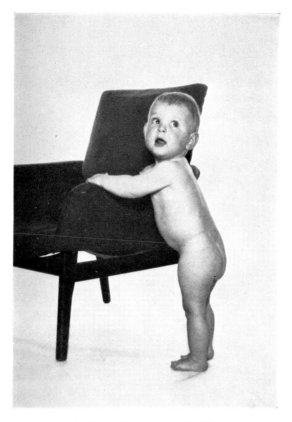

FIG. 86. 9 months. Can stand holding on.

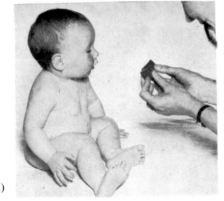
(a)

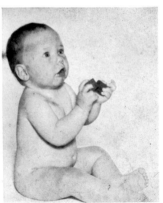
(b)

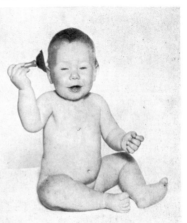
(c)

FIG. 87. 9 months. Imitation.

(a) Child shown the movement.
(b) Child imitates the movement.
(c) Child imitates ringing of bell.

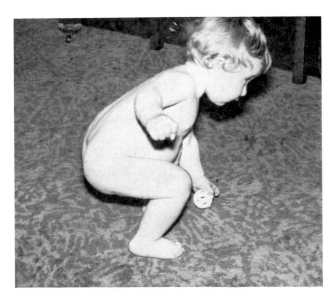

Fig. 88. 12 months. The child is now so stable on his feet that he can stoop down to pick up an object.

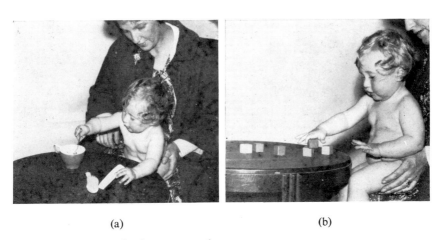

(a)                                            (b)

Fig. 89. 12 months. Spontaneous play.

(a) The child demonstrates her understanding of the use of a familiar object.
(b) Block building. The child is attempting to place one brick on top of another.

Alternatively, it seizes on whatever substitute stimulus is available, beginning to develop inferior or unsuitable patterns of behaviour. For a short time, while the central nervous system remains sufficiently plastic, the situation can be reversed but if left too long the immature or faulty habits of functioning become firmly established.

Learning takes place relatively slowly for the first 9 months but then becomes very fast. This is probably because the baby does not become fully

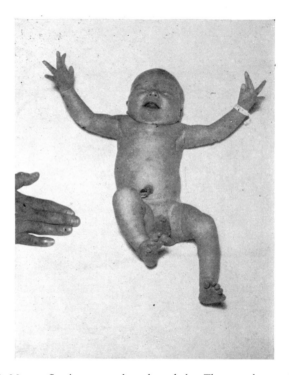

FIG. 90. Moro reflex in a normal newborn baby. The arms have extended, the legs are in the process of extending.

attached to his mother until about the age of 7 months. It is the child's movement out into space during the second half of the first year which increases the need for auditory as opposed to visual contact so that his mother must maintain contact through her speech. This aspect is of vital importance in the training of the deaf child (see p. 341). If the child fails to make this learning sprint he falls off in his learning ability about the end of the second year because of his inability to communicate. This inability to communicate can result in autistic reactions (p. 453).

*Influence of puberty.* Children who mature early do better at school than those who mature late. However, the early maturers are already doing better before the onset of puberty. It is not yet clear whether they still remain ahead after puberty.

NEUROLOGICAL MATURITY

During the first 6 months of life certain reflexes are present which later disappear. The age at which such reflexes disappear varies according to the reflex so that one way of assessing neurological maturity is to determine the presence of such reflexes and their subsequent disappearance within certain specified times. Persistence of the reflexes beyond the normal period indicates

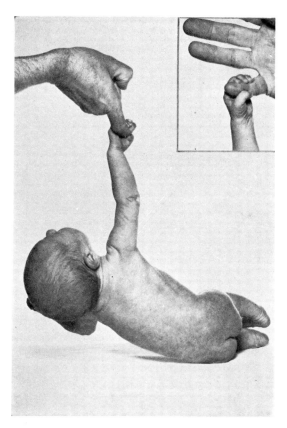

FIG. 91. Grasp reflex in a newborn full-term infant. The reflex is so strong that the infant is being lifted off the couch. Inset shows position of the infant's fingers during the reflex.

delayed cerebral development. While eliciting these reflexes careful watch should be kept for any difference between the two sides which might indicate a neurological defect on one side. It must be emphasized that although the normal baby in the early weeks may show asymmetrical patterns of movement—for example, the asymmetrical tonic neck reflex (p. 273)—by 4 months of age the baby becomes totally symmetrical in movement. Asymmetry after this age is usually due to cerebral palsy.

*Moro reflex.* This is dependent on the movement of the neck and can be elicited in two ways. The head can be supported in the palm 2 cm above the table and then suddenly released, or the baby can be pulled up by the hands for a short distance and again suddenly released. A sharp bang on the table will also induce the reflex but is a less satisfactory method.

The reflex consists of abduction and extension of the arms, the hands open but the fingers often remain curved (Fig. 90). This movement is followed by flexion of the arms ('embrace' movement) and extension of the legs; it is accompanied by crying. An asymmetrical response indicates a cerebral or brachial paralysis, or a fractured arm or clavicle. The reflex disappears by the age of 3–4 months.

The Moro reflex differs from the 'startle' reflex obtained by a sudden loud noise. In the startle reflex the elbow is flexed and the hand remains closed (Mitchell, 1960).

*Sucking and swallowing reflexes.* These are present in full-term babies and in all but the smallest preterm infants. Absence of these reflexes in a full-term baby suggests maldevelopment of the brain or brain injury.

*Rooting reflex.* It is this reflex which enables the baby to search and find the nipple when it is near. Contact between the baby's cheek and the mother's breast enables the infant to 'root' for the milk. The reflex can be elicited by touching the corner of the mouth, being best achieved shortly before a feed is due.

*Grasp reflex.* Any object placed in the infant's palm is grasped by the fingers (Fig. 91). This reflex should disappear by the fourth month but often does so earlier. Newborn babies commonly keep the thumb flexed across the palm during the first month, but persistence of this position after that period may indicate cerebral palsy.

*Placing reflex.* This is elicited by bringing the anterior aspect of the lower leg or forearm against the edge of a table. The leg is then lifted reflexly on to the table or the arm is raised so that the hand is placed on the table. This reflex is always present at birth in full-term infants.

*Stepping reflex.* This is elicited when the newborn baby is held vertical, with the feet touching the ground, and lightly propelled forward. Stepping movements of each leg alternate as the weight is brought to bear on the opposite foot (Fig. 92). This is termed the 'first walk' and lasts for about 2 months, but longer if the neck is extended. From the age of 2–6 months the reflex is lost, the feet merely dragging when the infant is propelled forwards. After the age of 6 months stepping again returns ('final walk'), the movement progressing so that the child walks alone by about the age of 15 months.

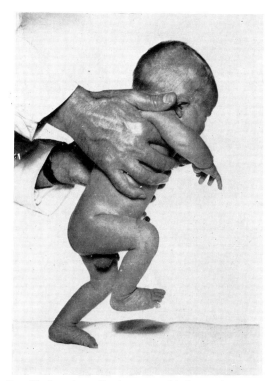

FIG. 92. Stepping reflex in a normal baby aged 2 days.

*Asymmetrical tonic neck reflex.* When the face is turned to one side the arm and leg on that side are extended and on the other side flexed. This reflex is well seen in preterm babies and in some full-term babies during the first week. It may persist weakly in normal babies up to the age of 4 months (Fig. 93), but a strong reflex after the first week, or persistence after the fourth month, probably indicates cerebral palsy.

All these primitive reflexes must be lost before voluntary movement is possible. By the age of 3 months most of the reflex actions have disappeared and there is a relative lull for a few weeks because voluntary action is not yet fully developed.

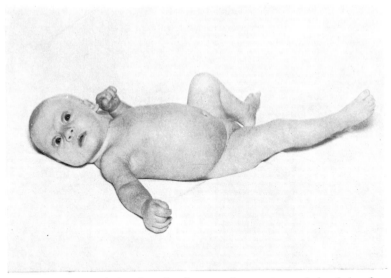

FIG. 93. Asymmetrical tonic neck reflex occurring spontaneously in a baby of
7 weeks. The head has turned to the right causing the right arm and leg to
extend, the left arm and leg to flex.

Although development from birth is a continuous process, it is not smooth
but comes in spurts and lulls. Moreover, although the sequence of development is the same for all children, its rate varies from child to child. Development is made up of many different fields, such as locomotion, manipulation
and understanding, and the rate varies for each field.

In addition to their value in the assessment of development these reflexes
are used in training methods. The reflex of defaecation ensures that the rectum
is emptied whenever it is full. By training, this reflex can be conditioned so
that the rectum is emptied whenever the buttocks come in contact with the
rim of the pot, though this is not without its disadvantages (see p. 305).

DENTAL MATURITY

Maturation of teeth can be affected by the same influences as those affecting
skeletal maturity, though variations in skeletal maturity are seldom accompanied by such marked changes in dental maturity. Moreover, illness does
not retard dental maturity as it does skeletal maturity. The first tooth to
appear is a central incisor, usually the lower, and the first dentition is completed with the eruption of the second molars by the end of the second year.
The first tooth of the permanent dentition is the first molar which appears at
the age of 6 years and is sometimes called the '6 year molar'.

The normal times of eruption are as follows:

| DECIDUOUS DENTITION | | PERMANENT DENTITION | |
|---|---|---|---|
| Incisors | 6–9 months | 1st molars | 6 years |
| 1st molars | 12–14 months | Incisors | 7–8 years |
| Canines | 18 months | Premolars | 10–11 years |
| 2nd molars | 2–2½ years | Canines | 9–12 years |
| | | 2nd molars | 10–13 years |
| | | 3rd molars | 12–25 years |

In developing countries where dates of birth are not kept, the number of teeth is useful for assessing a baby's age. To determine the age in months, 6 is added to the number of teeth present. This method holds good until 20 teeth are present.

### Cessation of growth

The absolute limit of growth is reached with fusion of the epithyses; this occurs later in boys than girls and accounts for their greater height. However, epithysial maturation is not the only factor in growth cessation since eunuchs of both sexes, although somewhat taller than average, stop growing even though their epiphyses have not fused. Growth probably ceases from lack of sufficient growth hormone. If the amount of available growth hormone in adults did not fall, normal adults ought, in theory, to become acromegalic.

### Sleep

Young babies spend much less time asleep than is usually believed. By the age of one month a baby sleeps for about 15 hours a day only. By 6 months he is asleep for about 13½ hours, this being the same length of time that an average baby of 12 months spends asleep.

Variation in sleep requirements of different children is enormous. Bright children seem to get bored by sleep and harass their anxious parents by not wanting to sleep (see p. 464).

### Tears

Crying is not associated with the production of tears at birth. Some babies do not produce tears until they are 2–3 months old, although the majority do so during their first week. Tears are produced later in preterm than in full-term babies (Penbharkkul & Karelitz, 1962).

### Eyes

All white children have blue eyes at birth, those eyes which are destined to be brown changing colour during the latter half of the first year.

These two terms are not synonymous. Puberty refers to the biological changes whereas adolescence refers to the new feelings caused by these changes and the individual's adjustment to them. Puberty and adolescence therefore interact but they can occur separately. For example, most young children with pre-cocious puberty do not experience adolescence at the same time.

Adolescence is caused largely by environment and the relationship between the individual and society. The more sophisticated the society the longer adolescence lasts, whereas a society with puberty rites creates such a sudden change in the individual's feelings that there is an absence of 'adolescence'.

# DISORDERS OF GROWTH AND DEVELOPMENT

Emphasis has already been placed on the normal variations in growth pattern; allowance must be made for the factors affecting normal growth, particularly heredity, before deciding that the growth of an individual is abnormal. 'Dwarfism' indicates small size; gigantism indicates excessive size. The term infantilism is used in several ways by different authors, but is best kept for those individuals who show sexual retardation as well as dwarfism; it is usually applied only when the individual has passed the expected age of puberty.

## SHORT STATURE (DWARFISM)

The term short stature is preferable since 'dwarf' suggests a mythical cause and is abhorrent both to the children and their parents. Moreover it is now clear that emotional factors can play a considerable part in the aetiology of small stature. Emotional deprivation alone is a major cause of small size in the U.K. today, and even in those with a physical cause such as congenital heart disease or asthma (without steroid therapy) it has become clear that emotional factors may also be playing a part. Physical and emotional factors are mutually reinforcing in children of small stature.

By definition a child is regarded as being abnormally short if his height falls below the 3rd percentile for his age. But the factors leading to this degree of small size may be operating in children whose height has not yet fallen to this level below normal. The factors involved are familial, nutritional, hormonal, emotional and physical. In most short children more than one factor will be operating. In listing the causes below, the disorders have been grouped according to the likely principal factor.

## Familial

### GENETIC SHORT STATURE

Allowance for parental height is essential in the assessment of short children. If a child's height is on the 10th percentile and that of his parents is similar then the child is probably normal. On the other hand, if they are on the 95th percentile then he is probably abnormal. Standards are now available which make allowances for parental height (Tanner *et al.*, 1970).

Apart from their small height these children are normal; they have a normal bone age and reach puberty at the usual time.

### GROWTH DELAY

These children have normal endocrine function but a delayed bone age. Their height remains proportional to their bone age throughout childhood. Puberty, although delayed, is eventually normal. Their final adult height is within normal limits, allowing for parental height.

In the past the term 'delayed puberty' has been used for this group of children, but this is unsatisfactory since the delay in growth antedates the delay in puberty. It is as though the whole tempo of growth is slower than normal and this slow tempo is seen often in other members of the family.

## Nutritional

Lack of food alone causes retardation of growth if it persists for sufficient length of time. There has been an increase of height of Japanese children since the end of the Second World War, this being due to improved nutrition. A similar increase has been observed in the new generation of pure Japanese who have emigrated to America.

Any chronic infection such as tuberculosis or malaria will cause delayed growth. An acute infection, if severe, can cause growth to cease during the illness. This temporary cessation of growth results in a line of increased density in the X-ray of the long bones which can be observed when normal growth is resumed (Harris's lines). It is likely that secondary hormonal factors are involved in this temporary cessation of growth and in the subsequent 'catch up' growth on recovery.

Chronic disorders of any major organ lead to stunting of growth. Thus:

*Intestine*—Malabsorption from intestinal disorders such as coeliac disease or cystic fibrosis. In the latter, pulmonary infection is an important associated factor.

*Heart*—congenital heart disease especially if cyanotic, less often rheumatic heart disease.

*Kidney*—congenital hypoplastic kidneys, chronic pyelonephritis and chronic nephritis.

*Liver*—congenital atresia of the bile ducts, glycogen storage disease and lipid storage diseases.

*Brain*—a disproportionately high number of mentally handicapped children are short. In part, this may relate directly to the disordered brain but other factors operate. Mongols are always shorter than average and this is probably a direct effect of the chromosomal abnormality which affects every cell in the body. Lack of food is a factor in many mentally handicapped children, but there are often associated disturbed family relationships leading to emotional problems comparable to those seen in the deprivation syndrome (see below).

SMALL FOR DATES (INTRAUTERINE GROWTH RETARDATION)

This condition results from lack of nutrition *in utero*, the causes of this being discussed on p. 54. Following a low birth weight the children are likely to grow up to be shorter than average; they also often possess characteristic physical features (Fig. 94). The face is elfin-like; there is a large forehead and well-developed nasal bridge but a small face which tapers down to a hypoplastic chin. These features sometimes lead to an initial impression of hydrocephalus, but there is no increase in the head circumference. The arms are short relative to the height, while growth on the two sides of the body may be asymmetrical. Intelligence may be retarded since intrauterine brain growth is affected.

It is probable that the 'Russell dwarf' and 'Silver's syndrome' are varieties of this condition.

## Hormonal

GROWTH HORMONE (GH) DEFICIENCY

This may exist as an isolated defect of pituitary secretion or as one element of panhypopituitarism in which case there is an associated lack of TSH and ACTH leading to clinical evidence of thyroid and adrenal failure also. Panhypopituitarism is most often seen following the removal of a craniopharyngioma. Fröhlich's syndrome should only be applied to those rare cases of a tumour involving the pituitary and the hypothalamus, leading to retardation of growth and obesity (see also p. 288).

Children with an isolated deficiency of GH are of normal weight and length at birth. Since GH is not essential to life it is growth only which is affected. This failure to grow becomes apparent during the second or third year and is then increasingly obvious as the gap widens between the 3rd percentile and the still lower height of the patient.

The children are plump and their bone age is retarded. This retarded bone age is commensurate with the retarded height age, whereas in hypothyroidism the bone age is even more retarded than the height age. There is a tendency to spontaneous hypoglycaemia despite a low serum insulin level because there is no GH to antagonize the insulin.

## HYPOTHYROIDISM

This condition is described on p. 623. There is early failure of growth associated with the other features of thyroid lack, particularly sluggish movements of the body and bowels (i.e. constipation).

## OVARIAN DYSGENESIS (p. 646)

## SEXUAL PRECOCITY (p. 282)

At first these children grow faster than normal and are therefore taller than average. However, because of premature fusion of the epiphyses they are ultimately shorter than normal.

## DRUGS

Long-continued steroid therapy retards growth. For this reason, in the case of children, such treatment should be avoided whenever possible. However, it may be required for those with asthma, nephrosis or rheumatoid arthritis. Since ACTH causes less growth retardation than steroids (Friedman & Strang, 1966) this is preferred except for the disadvantage that it must be given by injection.

Both androgens and oestrogens produce increased skeletal maturation, thereby inducing earlier epiphysial closure and a shorter ultimate height. These hormones are sometimes used in the treatment of constitutionally tall children to prevent excessive height (see p. 281).

There is some evidence (Cohlan et al., 1963) that tetracycline depresses normal growth, being deposited in the bones. Only long courses of tetracycline will have this effect and these should be avoided. It is also wise not to give the drug to pregnant mothers since fetal bones may be more readily affected.

### Emotional ('Deprivation dwarfism')

Children who are emotionally deprived fail to thrive and fail to grow. This is one end of the spectrum of child abuse, the other being the battered baby (p. 705). Such children have normal levels of growth hormone (Apley et al., 1971), and once admitted to hospital often develop a voracious appetite. It is difficult to determine whether their failure to grow results from a lack of calories only or whether emotional deprivation alone can also check physical growth; it seems likely that it can.

One child only in the family may be affected in this way as may occur in the battered baby syndrome. Failure of parenting has led to a failure of communication with the child who sits quietly and withdrawn.

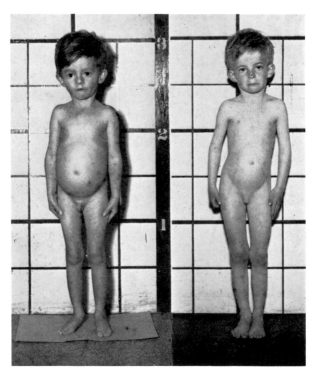

FIG. 94. Two examples of intrauterine growth retardation. Despite post-mature gestation in both, their birth weight was only 1·4 kg. At the age of approximately 5½ years their height is still ·089 m and weight 6·35 kg below the third percentile level. The head appears large in relation to the face, although the head circumference is normal; the nasal bridge is prominent. The characteristic circumflex-shaped mouth is obscured by the habit each has acquired of biting the lower lip in order to overcome the gap produced by the receding chin. Both show asymmetrical growth; the outer leg of both children is smaller.

Some children with growth failure of emotional origin have mothers who are obsessively concerned that their child should eat, resulting in severe negativism. The child refuses to eat what his mother provides and may develop bizarre eating habits.

## Physical

Children with skeletal disease may be of short stature. This may be congenital as in achondroplasia, osteogenesis imperfecta or Morquio's disease, or acquired as in rickets or spinal tuberculosis.

### MANAGEMENT OF A SHORT CHILD

In developed countries the majority of short children have nothing wrong with them, but treatable disorders must be excluded. Of these the most common is an emotional disorder, followed by hypothyroidism and coeliac disease. If the child is happy and energetic there is unlikely to be anything wrong, and this can be confirmed by showing that his height is not below the 3rd percentile after allowing for parental height and by finding a normal bone age.

In developing countries by far the commonest cause of short stature is malnutrition. In such children, chronic infection, especially malaria, is also likely to be a factor.

# GIGANTISM

## Constitutional gigantism

The commonest cause of excessive height is familial. This is not a problem for boys but can be for girls. If the prediction tables (p. 244) indicate a greatly excessive ultimate height, oestrogen therapy in order to cause premature fusion of the epiphyses can be given. The earlier this treatment is started the greater its success; it should preferably begin before signs of puberty present. Treatment is stopped when the bone age reaches 15 years. Menstruation may be irregular for a few months but regular periods are eventually achieved.

## Skeletal disease

Arachnodactyly (p. 235).

## Pituitary

An eosinophil adenoma of the anterior pituitary gland causes gigantism but is extremely rare in childhood. In the adult it causes acromegaly, since fusion of the epiphyses has occurred.

## Cerebral gigantism

A small group of children are large at birth and remain larger than average throughout childhood. The head is large, the forehead prominent and the ears very large so that there is a resemblance to acromegaly. The children are usually clumsy and somewhat mentally handicapped.

The cause is unknown, but a communicating hydrocephalus was demonstrated by Stephenson *et al.* (1968) in all the 6 cases they tested. It is suggested that the syndrome is due to dysfunction of the central nervous system leading to impaired intellect and altered hypothalamic control of anterior pituitary function.

### Thyroid

Thyrotoxic children grow faster than normal but the cause is not clear. There is no consistent tendency to faster skeletal maturation and the increased rate of growth occurs before they become thyrotoxic. Possibly both the faster growth and the thyrotoxicosis are due to a primary pituitary disorder. It is also necessary to take into account the increased amount of food eaten by these children.

### Sexual precocity

This disorder (see below) accounts both for cases of gigantism and dwarfism; during their period of growth the patients are taller than average but the end result is dwarfism from early fusion of the epiphyses.

### Obesity (p. 288)

Fat children are taller than the average (p. 245) and puberty is earlier than normal. It appears that the onset of puberty is more related to weight than to height.

### Local gigantism

Part or the whole of a limb may be much larger than its fellow, but otherwise normal. This may be developmental, but is sometimes associated with a haemangioma of the limb when the rapid rate of growth is due presumably to the increased blood supply (see also p. 227).

## SEXUAL PRECOCITY

This term is used to describe children who show normal sexual development before the usual age. It must not be confused with virilism which indicates the development of male characteristics in a female; in children this results from adrenal overactivity only (p. 629).

An age definition for sexual precocity is bound to be arbitrary in view of the wide variation of normal, but the tenth birthday makes a useful division between normal and precocious development. On this basis, a child showing any aspect of normal sexual development before the age of 10 years is regarded as sexually precocious.

'Precocious puberty' is a more restricted term indicating the early onset of puberty, that is, spermatogenesis in the male and ovulation in the female. It should be used only when gonadal maturation has taken place and can only

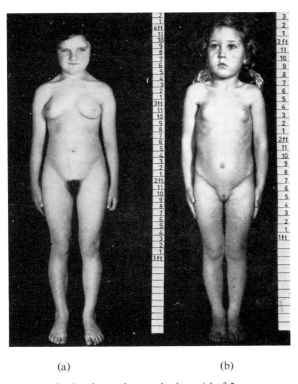

(a)                              (b)

FIG. 95. (a) Constitutional sexual precocity in a girl of 5 years.
(b) Premature development of breasts only in a girl of 4 years.
   The girl with constitutional sexual precocity is taller than normal, has adult curves and shows all the changes of normal puberty. The other girl is of normal height; she has retained her infantile shape and proportions.

occur in sexual precocity of constitutional or intracranial origin. Sexual precocity of adrenal or gonadal origin is never associated with gonadal maturation, although other signs of sexual precocity are present.

Sexual precocity is much more common in girls owing to the very large number of girls with constitutional precocity (Jolly, 1955).

## Constitutional

This indicates an early but otherwise normal puberty. It is much more frequent in girls (Fig. 95a) than boys (Fig. 96a) accounting for 90 per cent of all the girls with sexual precocity. A family history of the condition is common.

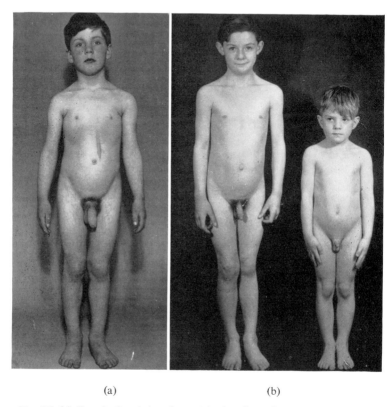

(a)                                    (b)

FIG. 96. (a) Constitutional sexual precocity in a boy of 5 years.
          (b) Adrenal hyperplasia in a boy of 5 years, with a control of the
          same age.
  The adult-sized testicles of the boy with constitutional precocity should be compared with the infantile testicles of the boy with adrenal hyperplasia whose testicles are of a similar size to those of the control.

Careful psychological handling is required since, being taller than average, they are taken for older than they are; thus more is expected from them than they are capable of giving. As they are sexually mature and can become pregnant, the same supervision is required as for any adolescent.

*Treatment*. Medroxyprogesterone acetate suppresses pituitary gonadotrophin excretion. It is valuable in girls, since it stops menstruation. This not only makes the girl's differences from normal less apparent but it also removes the parental fear of pregnancy. There is usually some regression of breast development, but the rapid growth in height is unaffected. The growth of pubic hair is also not altered.

### Intracranial

Intracranial lesions causing sexual precocity have helped in understanding the mechanism of normal puberty. These lesions have to involve the posterior hypothalamus but the anterior pituitary must be intact. In view of these facts, it is believed that the posterior hypothalamus normally exerts an inhibitory effect on the anterior pituitary during childhood. When this effect is removed, gonadotrophins are released which stimulate gonadal development. The commonest lesion is a tumour which is often pineal in origin because of the site of this organ. Although pineal tumours are much commoner in boys they do occur in girls, despite earlier writings to the contrary. The question as to whether the pineal gland has any endocrine function is still unsettled. Craniopharyngiomata and tuberculomata in this area may also cause the condition. Both these lesions may calcify.

### Gonadal

In boys, the lesion is an interstitial cell tumour of the testis; this causes enlargement of the affected testicle while the other remains infantile. In girls, it is due to a granulosa cell tumour of the ovary; this is exceedingly rare but fear of the condition has led to an unnecessary laparotomy in many girls with constitutional precocity. This error should never be made; a granulosa cell tumour in children is always palpable on abdominal or bimanual examination by the time it has produced evidence of sexual precocity.

### Adrenal

The cause is overactivity of the cortex, due usually to congenital hyperplasia and occasionally to a neoplasm. It causes sexual precocity only in boys (Fig. 96b); the result in girls is virilism (a feminizing adrenal tumour in girls is exceptional). Although the penis enlarges, the testicles remain infantile, a valuable differential sign since these mature to the adult size if the precocity is constitutional or intracranial in origin (Fig. 96).

### Premature development of breasts only ('premature thelarche')

In these children the breast development usually dates from birth, but there is no other sign of sexual development and their skeletal development is normal, thus distinguishing them from girls with constitutional sexual precocity (Fig. 95b). The nipple is not enlarged as in the adolescent breast and the body curves remain infantile. Puberty occurs at the normal age.

The condition is believed to be due to an abnormal sensitivity of the breast to the low level of oestrogens which exist throughout childhood, being referred to as a variety of 'end-organ' or 'target' sensitivity.

### Premature development of pubic hair only ('premature pubarche')

This condition is probably similar to the last and has been thought to be another variety of end-organ sensitivity. In this case the sexual hair follicles are unduly sensitive to circulating androgens.

## EUNUCHOIDISM

This results from failure of testicular endocrine function so that puberty does not occur. The failure may be either primarily testicular in origin or secondary to a pituitary disorder.

### Testicular

The testicles may be congenitally absent or have been removed or caused to atrophy as a result of surgery or an accident. Atrophy will also occur from infection, particularly mumps orchitis, irradiation or neoplastic disease. If eunuchoidism is the result of testicular failure, there is increased FSH after the age of 10 years because of the absence of the inhibitory action of testicular hormone.

### Pituitary

The failure may involve gonadotrophic function only, or there may be more widespread involvement of the pituitary so that the patient is stunted in growth and has evidence of thyrotrophic and adrenocorticotrophic deficiency. In cases of pituitary failure the output of FSH remains low throughout life.

The pituitary failure may be primary and of unknown cause, or secondary to damage from a local lesion such as a tumour of the gland itself, particularly a chromophobe adenoma, or of the region nearby, especially a craniopharyngioma.

*Clinical features.* Patients with eunuchoidism have very long arms and legs so that they are unusually tall; the span is greater than the height. There are no secondary sex characters; the face remains immature and has a yellowish tinge; the voice remains high-pitched.

*Diagnosis.* These patients must be differentiated from cases of delayed puberty due to slow maturation. Examination of the testicles is helpful, their absence suggesting eunuchoidism. If they are present but soft, the symptoms are testicular in origin, whereas in delayed puberty the testicles have the normal elastic feel of the infantile testicle. Failure of skeletal maturation in hypopituitary eunuchoidism causes considerable retardation of bone age, whereas this is only slight in simple delayed puberty. If the bone age is more than 4 years retarded, the cause is certainly pituitary in origin.

If hormonal therapy has been started, differentiation can be made only by seeing the effects of stopping the drug, since the signs of puberty will regress if they are due to its administration.

*Treatment.* Any lesion which can be corrected by surgery should be treated. Cases which are testicular in origin are given testosterone, those which are pituitary in origin being given chorionic gonadotrophin.

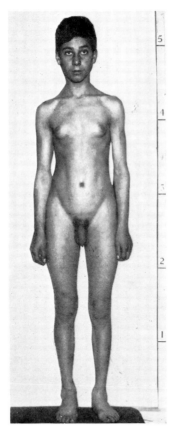

FIG. 97. Adolescent gynaecomastia. Transient enlargement of the breasts during puberty in the male is not uncommon.

## GYNAECOMASTIA

Transitory enlargement of the breasts occurs in about one-third of boys at puberty (Fig. 97). The usual explanation has been a presumed excess of oestrogens produced either by the adrenals or testes. Considering the intense hormonal activity occurring at puberty, a temporary imbalance of this nature would not be surprising. However, Jull & Dossett (1964) failed to find any rise in the excretion of oestrogens in boys with gynaecomastia. They suggest the condition is due to increased growth hormone at puberty which, in the presence of the small amounts of oestrogens already present, causes duct proliferation. The subsidence of gynaecomastia at the end of puberty coincides with a fall in growth hormone. Whatever the exact mechanism, no treatment is required for the condition.

Gynaecomastia is a feature of Klinefelter's syndrome (p. 643) and is also very rarely seen in association with an interstitial cell tumour of the testis, a feminizing adrenal tumour and hepatic disease. Its occurrence in liver disease results from disturbance of the normal androgen–oestrogen balance. Under normal circumstances, this is stabilized by enzyme activity in the liver which inactivates free oestrogen by conjugation and esterification. When the liver is damaged, free oestrogen circulates in the blood. Gynaecomastia may also occur as a result of accidental exposure to oestrogen preparations.

## OBESITY

Obesity in childhood is due to over-eating and is not an endocrine disease, with the exception of extremely rare conditions such as Cushing's disease (p. 632). Simple obesity, however, is accompanied by secondary hormonal changes. The fat child is taller than average; this is believed to result from secondary adrenocortical overactivity, shown by the increased production of cortisol and increased excretion of 17-ketogenic steroids. Whether secondary hyperpituitarism is a factor is uncertain.

The outstanding effect of the excessive intake of food is increased deposition of fat derived from fat in the diet and from the conversion of protein and carbohydrate into fat. Excessive protein increases anabolism and therefore accelerates growth; even when protein intake is not excessive, a high calorie intake will spare protein, thereby increasing anabolism. The seriousness of an excessive intake of fat during the first year of life has already been mentioned (p. 243); this leads to a permanent increase in the number of fat cells.

Much of the error in thought about fat children has arisen from Fröhlich's publication of a very rare fat boy whose illness was due to a tumour involving the pituitary gland. The child with simple obesity has not got a pituitary tumour and, moreover, Fröhlich's patient was stunted. It is therefore quite incorrect to refer to fat children as having 'Fröhlich's disease'.

Another misconception relates to 'puppy fat' which the child puts on shortly before the onset of puberty. It is commonly believed that this 'puppy fat' will be lost without difficulty and therefore no steps need be taken to correct the situation. It is true that a good deal of the fat will be lost during the next 2 years but it will return during the following 2–3 years unless the intake of food is restricted.

A further error regarding fat children is the idea that they are sexually retarded. In fact, both fat boys and girls start puberty about 1 year sooner than the average. The mistake made with boys is to believe that the genitalia are small, whereas they are merely lost in the rolls of fat.

*Aetiology.* The cause of excessive eating in any child is complex, probably comprising many factors. It is very likely that one or both parents are fat, but this does not indicate a genetic predisposition to obesity so much as a pattern in the house of having large meals. This pattern of overeating can be laid down early in life and accounts for why bottle-fed babies are commonly fatter than breast fed. It is likely that both breast- and bottle-fed babies stop feeding when they have had enough. Happily the mother who breast feeds does not know how much her baby has taken. Not so the mother who bottle feeds and who is often geared to feel that her baby must finish every bottle. Her pleasure when he achieves this leads her to reward him with praise, thereby encouraging still more a habit of overeating.

Many of the factors are psychogenic. A child who is insecure may eat for comfort because he lacks love. Some parents, mainly the mothers, overfeed their children as a method of demonstrating their love. Such mothers may have guilt feelings or feel unworthy, this leading them to try to tempt the child with sweetmeats in order to be sure of his love. An anxious mother who believes her child to be 'delicate' may overfeed him as one aspect of over-protection.

Fat children are inactive but in this case it is difficult to separate cause and effect. Inactivity certainly leads to fatness. Fat children are teased, thus causing them to withdraw from playing with others.

Mentally retarded children are often fat. This could in part be due to lack of activity, but there is the additional element that they are so unresponsive that the mother's only way of showing her affection is by giving food.

*Clinical features.* Overeating causes the child to show generalized obesity and to be taller than average. Secondary orthopaedic problems result, particularly genu valgum, and, to a lesser extent, flat feet. Backache may also occur.

Fat babies are more liable to attacks of acute bronchitis, often associated with wheezing (see p. 351).

*Prophylaxis.* The essential treatment lies in prevention by educational means. Propaganda aimed at parents must emphasize nutritional individuality, explaining that however little a fat child seems to be eating the intake is still excessive for his particular metabolic rate, since he is having to store excessive fat. Mothers (and doctors and nurses) must be got away from routine weighing of babies. For generations the weighing machine has been used to indicate whether a baby is healthy. Energy is the best indication of health, not a figure on a weighing machine. A fat baby is called 'bonny' whereas anyone who is thin is regarded as unhealthy. Mothers feel insulted if their baby is 'thin'. All this can be reversed once it is understood that fat babies make fat adults.

Doctors and nurses in well-baby clinics should lead the field of propaganda. The weighing machine should not be used routinely but should be kept in the doctor's room for his use when concerned about a particular baby. The clinic record card kept by the mother should indicate details of immunization but have no columns for weight measurements. Fathers are as bad as mothers in this respect, wishing to see the weight in the book when the child returns from the clinic. But all this can be corrected by an altered attitude on the part of the doctors and nurses.

*Treatment.* The only treatment for obesity is to reduce the intake of food. Fat babies should be dieted by reducing carbohydrate and increasing the amount of protein, vegetable and fruit. Cereal should be taken out of the diet and not more than one pint of milk per day permitted. Fat babies should be left to feed themselves rather than having everything spooned into them. In this way one hopes that more food will go into his hair and on to the floor but less into his mouth.

Older children will require a strict reducing diet. The problem with all reducing diets is one of monotony and hunger. However, the diet given below allows considerable variation and, provided green vegetables and salads are taken, the child should not feel hungry except when he first starts on the diet, before his body has become accustomed to a reduced intake. Meals should be taken at regular times, no eating being permitted between them.

Drugs which suppress the appetite are not recommended for children. They have side effects and the child is liable to believe the drug will cause him to lose weight, so that he fails to keep to his diet.

The greatest problem with regard to the success of the diet relates to the attitude of the parents. It will often be found that the child is keen to keep to the diet but his mother thinks he is being starved; strong pressure will need to be brought to convince her of the necessity for weight reduction. A successful discussion will often lead to her taking part in the diet as well. It is helpful to the child if he is given a target of weight to be lost by the next visit, instructing his parents to weigh him at home at least once a week. A loss of 1 kg a week should be achieved for the first few weeks of the diet and thereafter, a loss of 0·5 kg. Once the child begins to lose weight, his increased ability at sport and the fact that he is no longer teased for being fat, will encourage him to still greater efforts with his diet.

Owing to the tendency for childhood obesity to persist into adult life, long continued supervision is necessary. If the parents fail to keep the child to the diet they must be told the serious facts about fat children in a direct manner. Fat children become fat adults; the life expectancy of fat individuals is shorter than thin individuals and their incidence of illness greater. In some cases it may be necessary to take the child into hospital for the initial dietary treatment and to give less than 1000 calories per day.

## REDUCING DIET—1000 CALORIES

BREAKFAST
>90 *ml milk* ($\frac{1}{2}$ *teacupful*).
>30 *g bread* (1 *slice, size Hovis loaf,* $\frac{1}{2}$ *cm thick*).
>7 *g butter* (*size of half walnut*).
>1 *egg or* 1 *thin rasher of bacon, or piece of fish.*

MID-MORNING
>200 *ml milk* (*at school*).

DINNER
>30 *g lean meat, or* 60 *g fish* (*average helping*).
>60 *g potato* (1 *tablespoonful*).
>*Large helping of green leafy vegetable or salad.*
>90 *ml milk to drink* ($\frac{1}{2}$ *teacupful*).
>*or* 90 *ml milk sweetened with saccharine as a junket or jelly.*
>*Stewed fruit with saccharine or fresh fruit* (*average helping*).

TEA
>90 *ml milk* ($\frac{1}{2}$ *teacupful*).
>30 *g bread* (1 *slice as before*).
>7 *g butter* (*size of half walnut*).
>*With Marmite, fish or meat paste, salad or fresh fruit.*

SUPPER
>90 *ml milk* ($\frac{1}{2}$ *teacupful*).
>15 *g grated cheese* (1 *tablespoonful*) *or* 30 *g sardines* (3).
>30 *g bread* (1 *slice as before*).
>*Fresh fruit or salad.*

FOODS ALLOWED

*Green vegetables and salads can be used* ad. lib *to make up bulk. Raw fruit, or stewed fruits sweetened with saccharine. Meat, fish, cheese and eggs. Clear soups and meat extracts. Marmite. Milk not to exceed* 600 *ml daily. Butter not to exceed* 15 *g daily. Bread not to exceed three thin slices daily. Potatoes not to exceed one tablespoonful daily.*

FOODS NOT ALLOWED

*Fried foods—fish, chip potatoes, etc. Sugar, sweets, chocolate, jams, marmalade, syrup, honey, sweetened condensed milk. Biscuits, pastries, cakes, steamed and Yorkshire puddings, semolina, macaroni. Thick soups and gravies. Peas, beans and lentils. Oil and salad dressing. Fruit tinned in syrup. Bottled fruit drinks.*

## TEETHING

This is one of the commonest, though also one of the most trivial disorders of growth and development. The greatest danger is that symptoms are incorrectly ascribed to teething so that a serious underlying disease is overlooked. Convulsions should never be regarded as the result of teething and nothing is more dangerous than to consider teething as the cause of failure to thrive. The safest rule to apply is that a diagnosis of 'teething' is always retrospective and only made when a tooth has come through, the child having got better without any other diagnosis coming to light.

With these precautions in mind there are certain symptoms which can be ascribed to teething, though most children are never upset in any way and dentists now teach that the eruption of normal teeth is painless. A child may go off colour, become irritable, lose his appetite and develop a fever. The cheek on the same side as the erupting tooth may become pink and the gums red and swollen. Excessive salivation, leading to dribbling, may occur. Many mothers state that their children always cut their teeth with 'bronchitis', but in most instances they are only describing the cough and sounds in the throat which result from excessive salivation. Much less often does true bronchitis occur, presumably from lowering of the resistance to infection.

*Treatment.* This is seldom necessary, but occasionally a mild analgesic is required. Paracetamol is the safest analgesic for young children in a dose of 25 mg/kg.

## BIBLIOGRAPHY

APLEY J., DAVIES J., DAVIS D.R. & SILK B. (1971) Nonphysical causes of dwarfism. *Proc. roy. Soc. Med.,* **64,** 135.
BAKWIN H. & McLAUGHLIN S.M. (1964) Secular increase in height. Is the end in sight? *Lancet,* **2,** 1195.

BAYLEY N. & PINNEAU S.R. (1952) Tables for predicting adult height from skeletal age. *J. Pediat.*, **40**, 423.

BROOK C.G.D. (1972) Evidence for a sensitive period in adipose-cell replication in man. *Lancet*, **2**, 624.

COHLAN S.Q., BEVELANDER G. & TIAMSIC T. (1963) Growth inhibition of prematures receiving tetracycline. *Amer. J. Dis. Child.*, **105**, 453.

FALKNER F. (1962) The physical development of children. *Pediatrics*, **29**, 448.

FRIEDMAN M. & STRANG L.B. (1966) Effects of long-term corticosteroids and corticotrophin on the growth of children. *Lancet*, **2**, 568.

GEBER M. & DEAN R.F.A. (1957) The state of development of newborn African children. *Lancet*, **1**, 1216.

GELDEREN H.H. VAN (1963) Studies in oligophrenia. I. Growth in mentally deficient children. *Acta. Paediat.* (Uppsala), **51**, 643.

GRIFFITHS R. (1954) *The Ability of Babies.* University of London Press, London.

ILLINGWORTH R.S. (1962) An introduction to developmental assessment in the first year. *Clinics in Developmental Medicine.* No. 3. Spastics Society/Heinemann Medical, London.

JOLLY H. (1955) *Sexual Precocity.* Charles C. Thomas, Springfield, Illinois.

JULL J.W. & DOSSETT J.A. (1964) Hormone excretion studies of gynaecomastia of puberty. *Brit. med. J.*, **2**, 797.

MITCHELL R.G. (1960). The Moro reflex. *Cerebral palsy Bull.*, **2**, 135.

PAMPIGLIONE G. (1965) Brain development and the E.E.G. of normal children of various ethnical groups. *Brit. med. J.*, **2**, 573.

PENBHARKKUL S. & KARELITZ S. (1962) Lacrimation in the neonatal and early infancy period of premature and full-term infants. *J. Pediat.*, **61**, 859.

PRADER A., TANNER J.M. & VON HARNACK G.A. (1963) Catch-up growth following illness or starvation. *J. Pediat.*, **62**, 646.

RUSSELL A. (1954) A syndrome of 'intra-uterine' dwarfism recognizable at birth with cranio-facial dysostosis, disproportionately short arms and other anomalies. *Proc. roy. Soc. Med.*, **47**, 1040.

SHERIDAN M.D. (1960) The developmental progress of infants and young children. H.M. Stationery Office.

SILVER H.K., KIYASU W., GEORGE J. & DEAMER W.C. (1953) Syndrome of congenital hemihypertrophy, shortness of stature, and elevated urinary gonadotrophins. *Pediatrics*, **12**, 368.

STEPHENSON J.N., MELLINGER R.C. & MANSON G. (1968) Cerebral gigantism. *Pediatrics*, **41**, 130.

TANNER J.M., HEALY J.M.R., LOCKHART R.D., MACKENZIE J.D. & WHITEHOUSE R.H. (1956) Aberdeen growth study. The prediction of adult body measurements from measurements taken each year from birth to 5 years. *Arch. Dis. Childh.*, **31**, 372.

TANNER J.M., WHITEHOUSE R.H. & TAKAISHI M. (1966) Standards from birth to maturity for height, weight, height velocity and weight velocity: British children, 1965. *Arch. Dis. Childh.*, **41**, Part I 454, Part II 613.

TANNER J.M., GOLDSTEIN H. & WHITEHOUSE R.H. (1970) Standards for children's height at ages 2–9 years allowing for the height of parents. *Arch. Dis. Childh.*, **45**, 755.

# CHAPTER 8

# DISORDERS OF THE ALIMENTARY SYSTEM

## Stomatitis

The most common cause of inflammation of the mouth in the first year of life is thrush (p. 115). From the age of 1–3 years infection with herpes simplex virus is the most frequent.

### ACUTE HERPETIC GINGIVO-STOMATITIS (APHTHOUS OR ULCERATIVE STOMATITIS)

This is the most common manifestation of primary infection with herpes simplex. Children aged 1–3 years are those principally affected. The incubation period is 7 days and the onset is sudden, with fever and very painful lesions in the mouth which prevent feeding. The lesions may occur anywhere in the mouth but especially on the tongue, gums and buccal mucous membrane. They consist of small yellowish-white plaques (aphthae) which later erode to form ulcers. The disease is self-limiting, lasting about one week, for this reason idoxuridine, though possibly effective against herpes virus, is not recommended as a mouthwash since it is potentially mutant. Gentian violet is often prescribed, but in the mouth it is a messy preparation. The painting of glycerin is preferable, but since the mouth is kept moist by excess salivation resulting from the lesions and because these are very painful, it is probably kinder to the child not to do anything to the inside of the mouth.

This primary herpetic infection is followed by the development of antibodies but these are unable to prevent recurrent attacks of localized herpes, though they do prevent a generalized illness with viraemia. About half of those who have suffered a primary attack continue with 'cold sores' but some of the other half who do not get such attacks are symptomless carriers.

These recurrent bouts of 'cold sores' consist of vesicles which often become impetiginized, occurring in a group at the muco-cutaneous junction of the mouth or nose and never on the buccal mucous membrane. They principally occur when the resistance is temporarily lowered by an infection such as a cold or pneumonia. It is common to find a history of similar attacks in a close contact of the child from whom he has caught the primary infection.

The frequency of symptomless carriers is so high that the risk of a nurse or patient with cold sores on the ward probably does not increase the chance of cross-infection. However, it is always wise to keep such nurses away from children with eczema (see p. 683). Herpes of the eyes is so dangerous to eyesight that virologists consider parents should be warned never to kiss children's eyes.

### HERPANGINA

This condition is due to the Group A Coxsackie virus and occurs particularly in the summer. It is rare in England in comparison with North America. The lesion starts as a vesicle which becomes a greyish-white ulcer, differing from that due to herpes in that it is surrounded by a red areola. The site also differs since the lesions are principally on the fauces and soft palate. Pain is less severe than in herpes. The condition lasts 3–6 days.

### RECURRENT APHTHOUS ULCER

These are extremely common and are not due to the herpes virus since recurrent herpetic lesions are never intra-oral (see above). They may be secondary to dental sepsis, but often no cause is obvious. They are painful and difficult to treat but some relief may be obtained from sucking benzo-caine lozenges. Hydrocortisone ointment may help and even Vaseline gives relief by protecting the ulcer from rubbing on the gums or teeth. A light touch with a silver nitrate stick may shorten the course of the ulcer which untreated persists for about 10 days.

This condition is sometimes mistakenly called a 'gum-boil'. However, this term is correctly applied to a periapical abscess of a tooth which presents as a swelling on the gum margin, then discharging pus.

### VINCENT'S STOMATITIS

Vincent's infections is due to a combination of the anaerobic spirochaete *Treponema vincenti* and the fusiform bacillus, both of which are normal inhabitants of the mouth. They are commonly found in association with dental sepsis and as secondary invaders of herpetic lesions. The infection produces ulcers of the gums which are covered with a greyish slough, leading to a characteristic and unpleasant foetor. These ulcers occur particularly in debilitated and undernourished children and play an important part in the pathogenesis of cancrum oris (see below). Oral penicillin is usually effective. Alternatively, oral metronidazole (Flagyl) can be used (p. 735). Any dental sepsis present must be treated.

The term *Vincent's angina* is applied when the sloughing ulcers involve the tonsils; gum lesions may also be present.

CANCRUM ORIS (NOMA)

This condition is relatively common in developing countries. The majority of affected children are malnourished, the onset of the disease being precipitated by an acute infection. Tempest (1966) found that 70 per cent of cases followed an attack of measles. The disease is closely related to poor dental hygiene and ignorance. In the absence of a clean mouth, bacterial debris and tartar (dental calculus) build up on the teeth soon after eruption. Inflammation of the gum results, leading to facial gangrene by the direct spread of infection. Vincent's organisms are the most common bacteria to be cultured from the lesions, but clinical appearances and serological tests suggest that primary infection with herpes simplex virus is frequently the primary infection (Emslie, 1963).

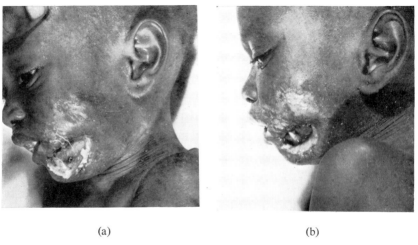

(a)                                                                 (b)

FIG. 98. Cancrum oris.
(a) The child presented with a visible sequestrum of the mandible.
(b) The sequestrum was removed without difficulty, in the out-patient department, revealing a large skin deficiency.

*Clinical features.* The first external sign of developing cancrum oris is an area of swelling and inflammation in the cheek. Examination of the mouth at this stage shows a sloughing ulcer of the buccal mucous membrane; this is in contact with an area of severe gingivitis and dental decay. The lesion proceeds so that the area in the cheek becomes black from necrosis and then sloughs away to leave a large defect which may include the lip or be quite separate from it. Involvement of the mandible or maxilla leads to osteitis and sequestrum formation (Fig. 98).

*Prophylaxis.* The build-up of dental calculus must be prevented by keeping the teeth clean. This is no problem in countries where mothers clean the teeth of their young children with a toothbrush or charcoal. However, in countries like Nigeria a chewing stick is used, but not until the child is about 8 years old. For these children good dental hygiene can best be achieved in young infants by the eating of fibrous cleansing foods such as oranges or sugar cane. The orange or the length of sugar cane is split into quarters and the flesh or pith bitten into and chewed thoroughly; by these means the teeth and gum margins are completely cleansed. For older children, like adults, the use of a chewing stick in place of a toothbrush is very effective.

*Treatment.* Oral hygiene and a course of intramuscular penicillin result in rapid cessation of further necrosis, with healing of the edges of the area. However, a large defect persists causing a hideous deformity which can be improved only by years of plastic surgical treatment. In many patients the jaws become completely fixed by fibrosis secondary to inflammation of the masseters. The first step in surgical treatment is a plastic operation to achieve some jaw movement. Such patients will have been existing on fluid feeds only.

**Recurrent parotitis**

This condition affects both children and adults and consists of a recurrent tender swelling of one or both parotid glands. During remissions the gland returns to normal, unless the recurrences are frequent; some enlargement may then persist between the exacerbations. The opening of Stensen's duct usually looks normal but turbid saliva can be expressed, this sometimes giving a 'snowstorm' appearance due to the suspension of small accretions of cells, mucus and the casts of ducts. Salivary calculi are not formed (in fact they seldom if ever occur in children).

The disorder is due to infection and dilatation of the ducts; sialectasis can be demonstrated by means of a sialogram. The organism is most often the *Streptococcus viridans*, but sometimes the pneumococcus. A source of infection in the teeth or tonsils is found in a proportion of cases. The pre-disposition of the parotid glands for this complication is due to the long narrow ducts which exist in this gland but not in the other salivary glands. The condition could result from congenital dilatation of the ducts, but there is no proof that this ever occurs.

*Diagnosis.* It is almost inevitable that the first attack will be regarded as mumps; differentiation on that occasion is difficult, but the mistake should not be made once a second attack has occurred. In mumps the opening of Stensen's duct in the mouth is usually inflamed and the saliva is not turbid.

*Treatment.* Antibiotic therapy is indicated, particular attention being paid to any source of infection in the mouth. The organisms are usually sensitive to penicillin which can also be injected direct into the duct. To improve drainage the mother should be shown how to massage the gland towards the duct entrance in order to prevent stagnation of saliva in the gland.

## Teeth

COLOUR

Tetracycline given to a pregnant mother may cause the deciduous teeth of her infant to be yellow when they erupt; a similar effect can follow the administration of tetracycline during early life. With age the yellow colour turns to brown. Severe neonatal jaundice may cause the deciduous teeth to be green when they erupt.

DENTAL CARIES

Once a cavity appears in a tooth it persists because the tooth, unlike all other parts of the body, has no method of reparation. The incidence of dental caries among school children is increasing; it is probably nutritional in origin and related to a high carbohydrate intake. The persistent sucking of a 'comforter' containing a solution of sugar is almost certain to lead to caries.

The quantity of sugar taken during meals is not serious but it is the length of time the sugar is in the mouth which is the chief factor in the production of caries. Sweets are particularly culpable in this respect. During sleep the flow of saliva is much reduced and swallowing almost stops, so that the contents of the mouth may remain there for hours. For this reason sweets and biscuits should never be given to children in bed at night.

Regular dental attention is essential for all children but particularly for those with heart lesions in whom the removal of a carious tooth increases the risk of bacterial endocarditis.

Conservative treatment of carious deciduous teeth should be carried out, if at all possible, in order to maintain adequate space in the jaws for the correct eruption of the permanent teeth.

Fluoride protects by hardening the surface of the teeth.

TEETHING
This subject is discussed on p. 292.

## Achalasia of the cardia (cardiospasm)

The oesophagus becomes enormously dilated and this is thought to be due to inco-ordination of the sphincter mechanism of the cardiac orifice of the stomach. It has been suggested that the aetiology might be similar to Hirschsprung's disease (p. 163), but, this is not the case, since the ganglion cells are normal. The condition is more common in children than is realized and many of those presenting in adult life have had symptoms dating back to childhood. Dysphagia and regurgitation of food are the major symptoms, but a history that mucus and saliva are found on the pillow in the morning is common. Some children present with recurrent pneumonia from spill-over of oesophageal contents.

The diagnosis is easily made by barium swallow when the dilated oesophagus is seen to end in the typical 'rat-tail' deformity. Occasionally a similar condition is produced by a congenital fibrous, or even cartilaginous, stricture of the lower oesophagus.

Treatment by Heller's operation has now largely superseded oesophageal dilatation. In this operation the oesophageal muscle is split for a length of at least 5 cm which must extend down to the junction of the oesophagus and stomach.

### 'Gastroenteritis'

This is a dangerous term since it is liable to be applied to any child with diarrhoea and vomiting, thereby giving the illusion that a diagnosis has been made and preventing further search for the cause of these serious symptoms. It should be a rule that the term 'diarrhoea and vomiting ? cause' be used until a specific intestinal infection has been proved.

Infection outside the intestine can cause diarrhoea and vomiting. This is common with respiratory infections, otitis media and urinary infections so that such disorders must be sought by intensive clinical and laboratory studies in all the patients. Serious disorders such as acute appendicitis or intussusception can also cause diarrhoea and vomiting and be labelled 'gastroenteritis'. Malaria is an important cause of diarrhoea.

True gastroenteritis may be due to one of the *Shigella* group of bacillary dysentery organisms (especially Sonne and less often Flexner or Shiga), or to one of the *Salmonella* organisms (especially in tropical countries) or a specific *E. coli*. Much attention is now being focused on the specific types of *E. coli* which may be carried harmlessly by some infants but cause severe gastroenteritis in others. It is for this reason that in hospital all babies under 6 months should be isolated; ideally, routine stool cultures should be taken on admission and once weekly. Occasionally an outbreak of diarrhoea in a newborn nursery may be due to staphylococcal gastroenteritis. In many cases no organism is isolated though the obvious infectivity of the condition is shown by spread to others. A considerable proportion of cases are due to viral infection or to simultaneous viral and bacterial infection. Rotaviruses are the most frequent cause of viral gastroenteritis.

In metropolitan countries, where standards of hygiene have improved, the severe outbreaks of gastroenteritis which used to occur in the summer are no longer seen. In developing countries, low standards of hygiene account for the appalling frequency of the disease. For this reason, breast feeding only must be the rule for all babies in these areas. Not even water should be given since this is likely to be contaminated. A mistaken belief in such areas is that the breast feed should be followed by a drink of water to cleanse the mouth.

*Clinical features.* In mild cases the stools are green, loose and offensive, but vomiting is not marked and the child continues to take an interest in his surroundings, even though the symptoms have been present for a few days. In severe cases the onset is usually sudden, the child refusing feeds and developing vomiting and diarrhoea. The stools may become so watery as to have little colour or consistency. A heavy cellular exudate in the stools on microscopy usually indicates one of the dysentery group, in which case the lesion is mainly in the large intestine and may produce blood in the stools and tenesmus.

Dehydration is the feature which marks out the severe case and is indicated by sunken eyes and fontanelle, loss of elasticity of the skin and dryness of the lips and tongue. When considering dehydration it is necessary to differentiate the hyponatraemic (salt deficit) and hypernatraemic (water deficit) forms. The clinical features of dehydration and other electrolyte disorders which accompany gastroenteritis are discussed on p. 722 (see also p. 70).

*Diagnosis.* Many mothers, especially those in developing countries, apply the word 'diarrhoea' to normal loose stools, especially in breast fed infants. It is therefore essential that a stool should be seen before treatment for 'diarrhoea' is commenced. If no stool is available for inspection a small glass tube should be inserted into the rectum to collect a specimen for observation and culture.

Stool cultures are necessary to determine whether the disease is bacterial in origin but throat specimens must also be examined for virus studies. The urine should always be examined to exclude a parenteral source of infection.

Amoebic dysentery (p. 302) is seldom acute; the stool contains mucus and red cells but few pus cells. Lamblia (p. 328) produces characteristic pale, bulky, frothy, offensive motions in which large numbers of the flagellar form of the parasite can be seen on microscopical examination of the wet stool.

The possibility of an acute intussusception must be considered in all cases of apparent gastroenteritis; its differentiation is discussed on p. 316.

*Prophylaxis.* Severe gastroenteritis is largely confined to artificially fed babies and is a disease associated with poor hygiene and dirty methods of feed preparation. Moreover, in a breast fed baby the colon is mainly populated by *Lactobacillus acidophilus* whereas in a baby fed on cow's milk it is mainly populated by *E. coli*, thereby increasing the chance of infection with a pathogenic *E. coli*. In poor and ill-educated communities every possible step should be taken to ensure breast feeding only, for 6–12 months. In hospital, infants under 6 months should be isolated, strict barrier nursing being carried out. Staff with infections, especially diarrhoea, should never handle babies.

In developing countries when breast feeding fails, the artificial feed should be given by spoon and not by bottle. A spoon can more easily be kept sterilized or at least kept clean, whereas a bottle is difficult to clean.

*Treatment.* Infants die from gastroenteritis, only if they become dehydrated; therefore, rehydration is the key to treatment. Breast milk is as bland a fluid as any electrolyte solution. For this reason, if the diarrhoea is unassociated with vomiting, a breast fed child should continue to be given breast milk only, the number of feeds being increased to increase the daily intake of fluid. In developing countries, the giving of water to such babies is a mistake since the risk that it is contaminated increases the chance of infection.

Artificial milk feeds should be stopped at once, since bacterial growth can flourish more easily in the medium provided by cow's milk; they are replaced by glucose saline.

If the child on either artificial feeds or breast milk is vomiting he can be tried on 5 per cent glucose and one-fifth normal saline by mouth. This solution is more likely to be retained than the boiled water commonly prescribed. The supply of breast milk is maintained by regular manual expression of the breasts until the baby is put back on them.

This strength of glucose saline can be made by the mother by adding 1 teaspoon of sugar and 1 saltspoon of salt to every 150 ml of boiled water. It is given for 24 hours, then a breast fed baby is put back on the breast; a baby on artificial feeding is given rapidly increasing strengths of milk.

An alternative method of giving the glucose-saline mixture with the advantage of wider electrolyte correction combined with simplicity is the use of glucose-electrolyte powder (Dobbs, 1974). These are particularly valuable in developing countries. The formula is:

|                          | Quantity (g) |
|--------------------------|--------------|
| Sodium chloride          | 10           |
| Sodium citrate           | 50           |
| Disodium phosphate       | 25           |
| Potassium chloride       | 25           |
| Magnesium hydroxide      | 10           |
| Glucose                  | 880          |
| Total hydration powder   | 1 kg.        |

15 g portions are placed in envelopes to be added to 250 ml (Coca-Cola

bottle) of boiled water. Alternatively, the contents of 2 envelopes are used with a one-pint beer bottle.

If the glucose saline is vomited, oral feeding is stopped for at least 24 hours and parenteral fluids given to correct the electrolyte imbalance (see p. 720). When the baby is fit to take oral fluids again he is given the glucose saline for 24 hours. A breast fed baby is then put back on the breast. An artificially fed baby is given increasing strengths of cow's milk. During this phase of recovery a quick return to full milk feeding should be made to prevent a marasmic state developing. Prolonged starvation because the stools are not perfect is a common mistake leading to marasmus.

Some babies who have made a good recovery while on glucose saline develop a recurrence of the diarrhoea when milk is reintroduced. This is usually due to a temporary deficiency of lactase as a result of damage to the intestinal mucosa. Such children should be given a low lactose milk for a period of days or weeks until it is found that they can tolerate normal milk.

The question of antibiotics is difficult. They play a minor part compared with rehydration, and there is a trend against them since they may prolong the carrier state. Their use should be dependent on the isolation of specific organisms and known sensitivities. Substances such as kaolin which may alter the consistency of the stool do not reduce the loss of fluid from the bowel; they are therefore not recommended.

If the baby is shocked he should be given oxygen and hydrocortisone. The ears should be examined every day as vomiting in babies predisposes to otitis media (see p. 337).

In assessing progress, attention is paid to the clinical appearance, cessation of vomiting, normal progressive daily weight gain and normal urinary output.

### Amoebic dysentery

This disease is due to infection with *Entamoeba histolytica*. The organism exists in a vegetative mobile form and a cystic form, both of which appear in the stool. The cysts may be carried by an individual without causing symptoms and they can survive in water for as long as 1 month. Infection is transmitted from a case or carrier through the cysts which are swallowed in contaminated water or food.

Although the disease is found particularly in the tropics its prevalence is related to bad sanitation rather than to climate. Infants and children are as susceptible to the disease as adults and where a lesser incidence exists in young children, it is due only to their reduced chance of contact with the infection.

*Clinical features.* The disease may present as an acute or a chronic illness.

*Acute type.* The onset is more often gradual than acute as in bacillary dysentery, though it is occasionally sudden with high fever. The stools are loose yellow and contain much mucus; blood may be present and in these cases tenesmus may be felt. The abdomen is tender and vomiting occurs in a considerable proportion of cases.

*Chronic and recurrent type.* Such children have recurrent bouts of bloody diarrhoea. They become irritable and wasted, growth being retarded.

*Diagnosis.* This is made by finding either form of the organism. The stool to be examined must have been freshly passed.

*Complications.* An amoebic abscess is very rare in childhood although amoebic hepatitis may occur.

*Treatment.* This must eradicate amoebae from the lumen of the gut, its wall and systemically—especially the liver. Prior to the introduction of metronidazole no single drug was effective at all three sites so that combinations of emetine preparations, chloroquine and tetracycline were used. Metronidazole being a direct-acting amoebecide which is effective against all forms of invasive amoebiasis is now the drug of choice.

### Trichobezoar

Occasionally, children develop the habit of chewing their hair which then forms a hair-ball in the stomach. Some of the patients are mentally handicapped; others are emotionally disturbed. The symptoms are indefinite but there may be a history of vomiting and abdominal discomfort. The mass may be palpable and the diagnosis may be obvious from the observed habit and lost hair.

The mass may take many years before symptoms are produced so that cases have occurred where the parents have entirely forgotten the child's earlier strange habits.

Diagnosis is made by barium meal which shows a filling defect in the stomach. The mass is removed surgically. If hair eating is still a habit, the cause should be investigated. Psychiatric treatment may be required (Friedlander & Kushlick, 1954).

### Intestinal polyps

These are of two varieties—the rectal polyp and multiple polyposis.

*Rectal polyp.* This is a benign hamartoma and is usually single. It causes rectal bleeding and can most often be felt by the examining finger. Treatment consists of ligation under anaesthesia through a proctoscope. Recurrence is rare and malignant change unknown.

*Multiple polyposis.* A rare familial adenomatous condition affecting the colon and carrying a grave risk of malignant change. Diagnosis is made by sigmoidoscopy and by double contrast barium enema, the colon being filled with air after injecting barium.

This condition comprises intestinal polyposis and oro-facial pigmentation. The polyps are adenomata which occur mainly in the small intestine. The pigmentation consists of melanin spots around the mouth which look like freckles, but the lips and buccal mucosa are also involved. The condition is inherited by means of an autosomal dominant gene.

## Chronic functional constipation

Mothers throughout the world are often more concerned by constipation, which seldom causes illness, than by diarrhoea which is often fatal. It is difficult to trace the origin of this fear though the association of constipation with some febrile states may be relevant since a return of normal bowel function accompanies recovery. The belief that a child will become seriously ill if he fails to have a daily bowel action is widespread; there are still many households where a weekly purge is the rule in order to cleanse the system. When a child is brought to a doctor for constipation it is common to find that at least one parent, usually his mother, is excessively bowel conscious. The imprint of the Friday night purge remains indelible and is very liable to be passed on from one generation to the next.

The word 'constipation' like 'diarrhoea' is frequently misunderstood, especially in developing countries where the words are often only an indication of the area of the child's body which the mother believes to be at fault and causing his illness. Constipation denotes hard stools as well as a long interval between motions. The breast-fed baby may have an interval of 1–2 weeks between bowel actions but the stool is always soft; consequently this is not constipation. These infrequent stools are a result of the minimum residue from breast milk. The anxiety of such mothers can be relieved by explaining that their breast milk is so ideally suited to the baby that little remains over to be excreted.

Babies fed on cow's milk pass firmer motions, more like those of an adult, and usually have a bowel action each day. Failure to do so is usually due to the excessive casein causing a hard alkaline motion. This can be easily corrected by increasing the sugar in the feed and, if necessary, by increasing the amount of water and fruit juice. Underfeeding produces 'hunger-stools' which are small, firm green pellets.

The frequency of bowel action in normal children varies as with any other physiological function. Some normal children, like some normal adults, have their bowels open only once every 2–3 days or longer. The child with true constipation passes hard stools infrequently and is likely to have faecal incontinence causing soiling. Abdominal palpation reveals faecal masses in the large intestine. Rectal examination shows a lax anus, often with perianal soiling, while the examining finger immediately comes on firm or very hard faecal masses (Fig. 99).

The basic cause of this problem is psychogenic. It has nothing to do with diet and 'roughage'. If mothers are concerned for a daily bowel action they are alarmed by its absence. These pressures and the indelible imprint of former generations lead many mothers to pot train at an early age. Any infant can be conditioned to defaecate reflexly when sat on a pot. This may save laundry, but unfortunately it is also associated in the minds of some mothers with the belief that their baby is now 'clean', the untrained babies still being 'dirty'. Having won this competition they run into trouble when the baby is about 1 year old. At this age, having developed his own willpower, he may refuse to sit on the pot. The correct action for a mother faced with this problem would be removal of the pot and a return to napkins. Sadly, many mothers regard such a child as wilful and force him to sit on the pot. This she can do but she cannot force him to have his bowels open, in fact he refuses to do so and becomes a stool withholder.

Whether or not he has been so trained the toddler, with his natural negativistic tendencies, will subconsciously fight any attempt of his mother to get him to have his bowels open. In the same way he will battle against her pressure in any other area of his developing skills, for example forcing him to eat or striving to make him talk (p. 476).

This negativistic reaction over bowel training may show itself in two different ways. The majority of such children concentrate so hard on fighting the pot that they hold on to their stools for as long as possible. After a period of days or weeks the call to evacuate becomes so great that the child starts to hold on to furniture with his legs stiff and held together. During this time his distress at the impending loss of stool causes him to be tearful and irritable, emotions which are usually wrongly interpreted by his mother as being due to pain on straining to pass the hard stool. She will commonly describe him during the few days before a bowel action as straining to evacuate instead of straining to hold on. Obviously if a child (or an adult) strains to pass a motion he does so in a squatting position not standing up with extended legs together which permit tight buttock contraction. Some children whose mothers have described them as straining to pass a motion actually push it back when it starts to come out—hardly the action of one who is straining to get rid of his stool.

Additional factors in school children, but much less important than the above, relate to the child who gets up late and dashes to school after a hurried breakfast without emptying his bowels. The reflex of defaecation is likely to come during class and to be suppressed.

Surprisingly, abdominal pain is not a feature of constipation. Some of the children have local pain from an anal fissure due to a tear while passing a hard stool, but the frequency of this has been exaggerated. If a rectal examination can be performed without pain and without finding anal spasm, a local cause for pain can be excluded. Far more important is the emotional pain felt by such children over the loss of what they are trying to hold on to.

The other but smaller group of children reacting negativistically to parental bowel concern do so by having their bowels open in inappropriate places such as the dining room. These children are not constipated, having found an alternative way out of the emotional pressures to which they are being subjected. The situation is comparable to the young child who refuses to use his pot but empties his bowels the moment his mother puts on his napkin.

It is interesting that constipation occurs about twice as often in boys as in girls. This could be that girls are less aggressive and defiant than boys.

Emphasis has been placed on the primary psychogenic cause of constipation but there is a secondary psychogenic element. Faecal incontinence, by causing the child to smell, leads him to be shunned and teased by his school fellows.

No mention has been made of a number of vague symptoms beloved of the laxative manufacturers. For example, sleeplessness, headache, bad breath and furred tongue. The evidence for such symptoms being caused by constipation is negligible.

*Diagnosis.* Differentiation from Hirschsprung's disease presents no problem, although chronic constipation of functional origin and Hirschsprung's disease are so often thought of together. The majority of children with Hirschsprung's disease present soon after birth with intestinal obstruction (see p. 164). The few who are less severe, presenting a picture of chronic constipation in childhood, have recurrent bouts of vomiting when abdominal distension builds up, until it is relieved by a large bowel action. Pain is not a feature, the abdominal distension being largely gaseous rather than due to faecal masses; faecal incontinence does not occur.

The differences to be found on rectal examination can be seen from Fig. 99. In Hirschsprung's disease the anus is clean and tight, the examining finger is gripped by the narrow segment, and no faeces are felt. In chronic functional constipation the anus is lax, there is faecal incontinence, the rectum is dilated, and the finger immediately comes on hard faecal masses. No barium enema is required for this diagnosis.

*Treatment.* In the light of the deep psychological causes of constipation it is obvious that an attack on the rectum is not the way to treat the problem. A 'bucket and spade' approach with washouts and laxatives will produce short-term success but long-term failure. The only hope is for the parents to understand the basic mechanisms of the problem. Once this is achieved their life will no longer be centred around their child's intestinal function as though he consists only of a bowel, requiring to be fed at one end and emptied at the other. Removal of parental pressure and helping the child to understand the problem allows him to relax and eventually to achieve normal control. But this takes a very long time since it involves a change in approach to bowel control which has been ingrained possibly for generations.

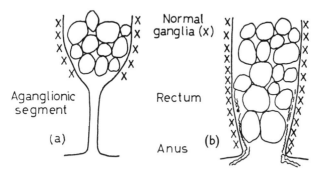

FIG. 99. Comparison between Hirschsprung's disease and chronic functional constipation
(a) Hirschsprung's disease. The narrow aganglionic segment immediately above the anus contains no faeces and there is no perianal faecal staining. Dilatation of the intestine and accumulation of faeces occurs in the area where there are normal ganglion cells.
(b) Chronic functional constipation. Intestinal dilation and faecal accumulation involve the rectum down to the anus which is lax, thus permitting the escape of semi-fluid faecal material leading to perianal staining.

Having practised both methods of treatment for a long time and having now not prescribed laxatives, washouts or enemata for many years, I am sure that psychotherapy is the answer. This can be at paediatric level in most cases though some families will require deeper psychiatric help. Stercoral ulceration is the fear of many doctors treating these children and is often given as the reason for washouts, but I have not met this oft repeated complication.

## Anal fissure

This results from a mucosal tear due to the passage of a hard stool and is commonly associated with a sentinel pile. It is the commonest cause of rectal bleeding. Healing is usually rapid once the constipation has been successfully treated. Digital dilatation of the anal sphincter reduces spasm and this can be combined with the local application of benzocaine ointment for the relief of pain.

### Recurrent abdominal pain

This is one of the most frequent complaints in childhood and is more often emotional than organic in origin. Cases of emotional origin present two different clinical patterns. In the first, there is an acute illness lasting 2–3 days in which the abdominal pain is associated with vomiting, and often with fever and headache. This is the 'periodic syndrome'.

In the second, the clinical picture is less dramatic though the abdominal pain recurs more frequently. Vomiting is unusual, but the child may also complain of recurrent headache or limb pains. The similar precipitating factors in those children with recurrent abdominal, limb or head pains and the fact that more than one of these frequently occur in the same patient, has caused them to be grouped together as the 'recurrent pains of childhood'.

When faced with a child with recurrent abdominal pain the doctor's first task is to exclude organic disease. The possible organic causes are manifold but diseases in the kidney, intestine or upper respiratory tract are the most frequent. Having excluded organic disease the doctor's next responsibility is to diagnose the emotional causes.

Since the symptom is more often due to emotional causes, the subject is discussed in Chapter 16, p. 469, together with the organic diseases from which it must be differentiated.

### Coeliac disease

During recent years a great deal has been discovered about the aetiology of this condition; it is now known to be due to intolerance to the protein gluten, present in wheat and rye flour. Further studies have shown the gliadin fraction of gluten to be the harmful substance and it is thought that there is an enzyme defect in the wall of the intestine which prevents the normal breakdown of gliadin. There is evidence to suggest that the toxic effect of the gliadin results from a harmful peptide produced in the intestine from incomplete digestion of gluten. Genetic factors are involved since there is an increased incidence of the disease among relatives of known cases.

*Clinical features* (Fig. 100). The symptoms do not develop until the child is given gluten, as in cereals, which usually occurs from the age of 3–6 months. Symptoms develop 1–4 months after first starting cereal foods. The infant loses his appetite, becoming miserable and irritable and developing loose, bulky, pale, offensive motions. Vomiting occurs at the onset and, as the stools may be very loose at this stage, a diagnosis of gastroenteritis is often made until the more typical fatty stools appear. Loss of weight is severe, the buttocks coming to hang in folds. The abdomen is distended, in marked contrast to the thin stick-like limbs. The liver is small and cannot be felt.

Malabsorption is widespread so that specific deficiencies occur; hypochromic anaemia from failure to absorb iron is almost constant and, in a few patients, the anaemia is megaloblastic from folic acid deficiency. Although megaloblastic anaemia is rare and a megaloblastic bone marrow alone only a little more common, a deficiency of folic acid, as shown by a lowered level of whole blood folate, is present in all coeliac children (McNeish & Willoughby,

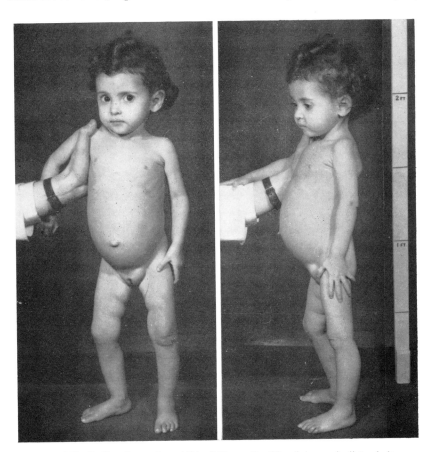

Fig. 100. Coeliac disease in a child of 18 months. The abdomen is distended; there is severe wasting of the limbs and buttocks.

1969). That megaloblastic anaemia is not more frequent, is possibly due to the absence of growth in these patients causing a diminished need for folic acid. Malabsorption of vitamin D may cause rickets and this is sometimes termed 'coeliac rickets', although this differs in no way from other forms of rickets due to lack of vitamin D. Malabsorption of calcium may lead to tetany and of protein to hypoproteinaemic oedema. Children with longstanding coeliac disease are dwarfed and their sexual maturity is delayed. Decreased activity of intestinal disaccharidases occurs in some patients as a secondary defect. This possibility influences the early treatment of patients with coeliac disease (see below).

There is an association between intestinal malabsorption and eczema so that some children with coeliac disease may be found with eczema. It is uncertain whether the primary defect lies in the bowel or in the skin but it is possible that chronic skin disease produces metabolic disturbances in the bowel mucosa.

*Investigations.* The glucose tolerance curve is a useful screening test since it is always flat, but it is not specific. The stools contain an excess of fat though splitting is normal; they should be estimated on a 4-day balance. The dextro-xylose test is more convenient than a fat balance and equally as accurate. 5 g xylose is given by mouth and its blood level after 1 hour measured. In normal children the blood level should be greater than 20 mg %. Clumping of barium is seen in the intestine after a barium meal, instead of the normal feathery pattern. Biopsy from the small intestine shows a typical flattened appearance of the villi and is the most reliable of the tests. There is little correlation between the severity of this lesion and the clinical symptoms. The villi can return to normal with treatment. Experimental work has shown that they can be induced to return to their former pathological state by the administration of gluten, this change occurring within a few hours.

*Diagnosis.* The disease can be excluded by the finding of a normal whole-blood folate. Coeliac disease must be differentiated from cystic fibrosis. Its onset is later, the stools are less offensive and the appetite poor in comparison with the good appetite in the patient with cystic fibrosis except in the presence of infection. There is normal tryptic activity and the sweat electrolytes are normal in coeliac disease. The dextro-xylose absorption test is abnormal in coeliac disease and normal in cystic fibrosis. This pentose sugar is not normally present in the diet. It requires active absorption from the intestine and therefore the test differentiates mucosal defects from other causes of malabsorption.

Infestation with *Giardia lamblia* produces similar stools, but the parasite is seen on microscopy of the stool or in fresh duodenal fluid, and there is an immediate response to mepacrine therapy.

*Treatment.* Gluten in all forms must be excluded from the diet by cutting out all foods made from wheat, rye or barley. Any food made from flour, such as biscuits, cake and bread, must be cooked with a gluten-free flour. In very severe cases a short period of high-protein skimmed milk, glucose and banana may be required before progressing to the full gluten-free diet. The frequency of a secondary disaccharidase deficiency, particularly lactase, warrants the exclusion of lactose from the diet during the first weeks of treatment in all cases. If the onset is so acute as to be life threatening, the child should also be given steroids until he is over the crisis.

Any associated specific deficiency such as iron, folic acid or vitamin D must be made good by supplements. If a megaloblastic anaemia is present, it is reasonable first to see the effect of the gluten-free diet alone before starting folic acid, since a normal blood picture may be induced as a result of improved absorption. It is interesting that some children with severe coeliac disease who are already on a gluten-free diet, suddenly thrive when given additional folic acid. A multivitamin preparation should be given to every patient and a particular watch kept to ensure that rickets does not develop during the period of rapid growth which follows the start of treatment.

The response to treatment is dramatic, there being an immediate gain in weight and height. The diet must be continued for life, therefore confirmation of the diagnosis by intestinal biopsy is always essential. The main reason for this is to remove the increased risk of intestinal cancer. However, the diet also ensures normal growth throughout childhood. It also prevents the risk of recurrence of symptoms during pregnancy and the vague abdominal discomfort which may be felt by the coeliac patient on a normal diet at any time, but especially after alcoholic indiscretion.

### Protein-losing enteropathy

This rare condition presents with oedema from hypoproteinaemia but the protein has been lost from leakage into the intestine. There is no proteinuria. The major cause in children is congenital lymphangiectasia of the small intestine. A barium meal shows thickening of the mucosal folds of the jejunum, the diagnosis being confirmed by jejunal biopsy. A number of other intestinal disorders in childhood can very rarely cause sufficient leakage of protein to have a similar effect; for example, ulcerative colitis, coeliac disease and Crohn's disease.

### Acute appendicitis

Though not an uncommon condition in childhood it does not occur as often as supposed. Diagnosis is made difficult by the fact that children often fail to conform to the picture of appendicitis as seen in the adult. The classical symptoms of the disease comprise the acute onset of central abdominal pain which after a few hours moves to the right iliac fossa and is associated with fever, vomiting and constipation. In children, although vomiting is almost constant, the abdominal pain often remains central. Constipation is by no means the rule and there may even be diarrhoea. Fever is not usually marked and may be absent. The condition is less common under the age of 2 years, but may occur at any age and it is in the very young patients that diagnosis is most difficult since they present with general symptoms such as irritability and refusal of feeds. However, even though they cannot complain of abdominal pain, their mothers usually soon realize from their behaviour that they have pain in the abdomen. Anorexia is a most important symptom. If a child is eating he is probably not suffering from an acute appendicitis.

The child's appearance may vary from seeming little different from normal to being desperately ill. The tongue is less often furred than in the adult and guarding in the right iliac fossa may not be obvious. The most useful physical sign is 'release tenderness'. This sign is elicited by gentle but deep palpation in the right iliac fossa, followed by sudden release. If localized peritonitis is present, the child jumps when the hand is released because of pain caused by the movement of the inflamed surfaces of peritoneum on each other.

The greatest problem with young children is the frequency with which the condition is complicated by local or generalized peritonitis. This is partly due to the time which lapses before operation because of diagnostic difficulties, and partly because the omentum at this age is small and immature, making it less effective in sealing off the infection. Consequently an inflammatory mass is common in young patients. The difficulty in diagnosis is increased by the child's resentment at being disturbed; great patience is therefore required to get the child to settle so that a full abdominal examination can be performed. If necessary, the child should be given a sedative, the doctor returning after an interval. This resentment of being either examined or made to sit up can be an indication of acute appendicitis, being due to pain on active contraction of the abdominal muscles; in this way they differ from children with gastroenteritis, tonsillitis or otitis media who are often restless and frequently change their position.

*Diagnosis.* The greatest difficulty arises in the differentiation from acute mesenteric adenitis. This condition is usually associated with an acute upper respiratory infection and the child complains of abdominal pain. The temperature is usually high, vomiting is less constant and there are no localizing signs in the abdomen. It must be suspected in any child complaining of abdominal pain who is found to have acute tonsillitis, but acute tonsillitis and appendicitis may coexist so that if there is any doubt a laparotomy should be performed. The white cell count should not be used in the diagnosis of acute appendicitis in children. The level is too variable to be of any value and if the surgeon has reached the position where a white cell count is going to make the difference between operation and not, then the abdomen should certainly be opened.

The possibility of gastroenteritis causes a very real diagnostic problem in young children with abdominal pain and diarrhoea. Diarrhoea often occurs in pelvic peritonitis from a pelvic appendix, and in the early stages no localizing signs are present. Repeated examinations at intervals to determine whether localizing signs are developing is the correct management, unless the child's condition will not warrant delay, in which case an exploratory laparotomy should be performed.

Urinary infection causes abdominal pain. Tenderness in the renal angle may be a useful diagnostic sign, but on the right side could be due to a paracolic appendicitis. Frequency of micturition may be secondary to pelvic peritonitis. In view of these difficulties, microscopic examination of the urine is essential in every case of suspected appendicitis. If this reveals no pus cells, or even just a few, then it is most unlikely that the child has a urinary infection since the urine of such patients is loaded with pus cells.

Pneumonia may cause difficulty since in children it often causes abdominal pain. Moreover, the pain of peritonitis may cause the reversed type of breathing with an expiratory grunt which is typical of pneumonia. The absence of any localizing signs in the abdomen and finally the chest X-ray should lead to the correct diagnosis. Diabetes, which in childhood is always acute, may present with abdominal pain; there will be thirst, polyuria and possibly drowsiness. The importance of the routine urine test for sugar in all children suspected of appendicitis is obvious.

There is usually little difficulty in differentiating recurrent abdominal pain of emotional origin from an attack of acute appendicitis. The history is typical and the child seldom looks ill. There are no localizing signs of inflammation.

A diagnosis of 'grumbling appendix' should never be made in children. This suggests chronic appendicitis which, apart from the exceptional causes of tuberculosis and actinomycosis, does not exist. If repeated attacks occur they are due to recurrent bouts of acute appendicitis and not chronic appendicitis.

### Peritonitis

In the majority of children, peritonitis is secondary to acute appendicitis. Primary peritonitis occasionally occurs but is much less common than it used to be. It is usually due to a streptococcal or pneumococcal infection; gonococcal peritonitis is not seen nowadays. Pneumococcal peritonitis has a tendency to occur as a complication of nephrosis. Very occasionally staphylococcal peritonitis occurs in the newborn, secondary to a staphylococcal lesion elsewhere.

Children with peritonitis are extremely ill and there is generalized abdominal tenderness associated with distension. Bowel sounds are absent, an important difference from acute intestinal obstruction in which they are loud. In most instances a laparotomy must be performed in case an acute appendicitis is present. The only exceptions could be a child with nephrosis, or one with septicaemia where the peritonitis was part of a generalized infection to be treated with antibiotics.

## Acute mesenteric lymphadenitis

This is usually secondary to an acute upper respiratory infection, particularly acute tonsillitis, and causes abdominal pain. There may be a history of a few days' malaise and sore throat associated with fever before the onset of the abdominal pain. The pain is usually colicky and is variable both in its site and intensity. Between the attacks of colic the child may appear completely well and be found sitting up playing with his toys. Vomiting may occur, but it is not constant and the fever is usually high. Constipation may be present whereas diarrhoea is unusual. Abdominal tenderness may be found but its site varies from hour to hour. The enlarged and inflamed mesenteric glands cannot be felt through the abdominal wall. Therefore the diagnosis can only be proven when a laparotomy has been performed for suspected appendicitis and enlarged glands are found, particularly in the ileocaecal region. They are bright pink, firm and discrete. In such cases the appendix should be removed so that the operation is not a wasted one. The symptoms usually disappear in 3–4 days. Treatment with chemotherapy or antibiotics is required for the upper respiratory infection.

## Neonatal intestinal obstruction from milk curds

This is a relatively new condition (Cook & Rickham, 1969) occurring in babies aged 1–2 weeks, which has only been found in those fed on cow's milk. It seems likely that it is due to the new vogue in some centres of early introduction of concentrated feeds, especially in low birth weight babies, in order to achieve a high calorie intake. It differs from congenital intestinal obstruction by presenting after the stools have changed from meconium to the usual brown colour.

It is possible that affected babies have a decreased absorptive capacity for protein.

## Acute intussusception

In this condition one portion of the intestine becomes invaginated into the next portion. It occurs particularly in babies between the ages of 3 and 12 months and usually affects healthy infants, but a recent history of a respiratory infection or gastrointestinal upset is common.

*Aetiology.* This is still uncertain but in a few instances a polyp or Meckel's diverticulum has been found to form the apex of the intussusception. This has supported the theory that enlargement of Peyer's patches of lymphoid tissue might act in the same manner. These patches are most numerous at the ileocaecal valve and in the terminal ileum, the commonest sites for the intussusception to start, and the usual age of the patient is such that dietary upsets, following the introduction of mixed feeding, might be expected to occur and to cause lymphoid hyperplasia. But an intussusception may originate in other parts of the bowel where lymphoid patches are much less numerous. Experience with polyps suggests that these must be much larger than a Peyer's patch could ever be if they are to start an intussusception. The theory of an enlarged Peyer's patch cannot therefore be the complete answer and abnormal or exaggerated peristalsis may well be a factor. This must sometimes take place as otherwise a retrograde intussusception, which is occasionally found, could never occur. Increasing attention is being paid to the frequency of a prodromal respiratory infection; an adenovirus has been found in a high proportion of these cases.

*Clinical features.* The children are almost always well nourished and the onset of symptoms is so sudden that the parents can usually give the exact time when the symptoms began. Vomiting is an early symptom and is associated with severe colicky abdominal pain. During the bout of pain the child draws up his legs and screams. The progression of the intussusception pulls on the mesentery and its nerve supply, this being so severe that during a bout of colic the child often becomes white and shocked; in a few minutes he returns to normal, falling into a peaceful sleep until the next bout. The stools may become loose and then cease altogether, but the passage of normal stools does not exclude the condition. Blood in the stool ('red-currant jelly') is often regarded as the feature of the condition, but it is a late sign unless the intussusception is low down in the bowel.

In early stages the child appears perfectly normal between bouts of colic and it is at this stage that the diagnosis should be made, not when there are grave signs of dehydration and intestinal obstruction. Palpation of the abdomen reveals a mass formed by the intussusception in a large proportion of cases, though diagnosis should not be delayed because this cannot be felt. In a restless child the doctor's hand should be left in contact with the abdomen under the bedclothes. When an intussusception is suspected, this part of the examination must be carried out first, since the chances of getting the child to settle after examining the throat or ears are slender. The tumour is sausage-shaped, lying anywhere along the line of the colon. It is tender and can be felt to harden during a bout of peristalsis. If the caecum has taken part in the intussusception, its absence from the right iliac fossa causes a feeling of emptiness in that area. Only rarely will the apex of the intussusception have moved far enough round to be felt on rectal examination but blood may be found on the examining finger. In difficult cases a barium enema may be required to confirm the diagnosis, though this is not usually necessary (Fig. 101).

*Diagnosis.* The greatest difficulty arises in cases of gastroenteritis and dysentery, particularly since an intussusception may be associated. It is the bouts of colic which are typical of an intussusception and if, as is so often the case, the child becomes pale during the bouts the diagnosis must be regarded

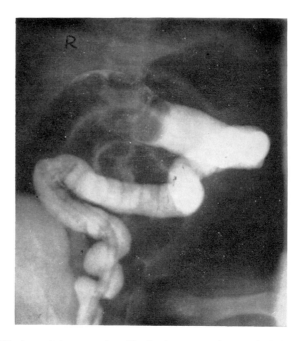

FIG. 101. Acute intussusception. The barium enema has reached the apex of the intussusception, revealing a characteristic concave filling defect.

as certain. A rise in temperature has sometimes been regarded as evidence in favour of gastroenteritis, but this is incorrect since a moderate fever occurs in most cases of intussusception. In gastroenteritis the stools have an offensive smell; this will be detectable on the finger after rectal examination even if no stool has been seen, whereas in intussusception no faecal odour will be smelt, even when the finger is smeared with mucus and blood.

Anaphylactoid purpura may be associated with considerable abdominal pain from purpura in the wall of the intestine; it is differentiated by its typical skin rash. Occasionally an intussusception occurs in association with anaphylactoid purpura.

Two other conditions produce screaming attacks in infants: acute otitis media and acute pyelitis, but these are not associated with pallor as in an intussusception.

*Treatment.* Once the condition is suspected a laparotomy should be performed, after preliminary resuscitation if necessary. It cannot be overstressed that the passage of blood is not required for the diagnosis; this is bound to be a late sign if the intussusception is high up in the intestine. In longstanding cases reduction may be impossible so that resection, which carries an increased mortality, is required.

The use of a barium enema for reduction is debatable. It is obviously an advantage to avoid an operation, but it is not always possible to be certain whether a small knuckle of bowel, not obstructing the lumen, has been left unreduced. Reduction by this method is impossible in late cases and should not be attempted, as valuable time may be lost. It can therefore be only an alternative to surgery in those cases where reduction is easy and surgical mortality nil.

There is always a chance that the intussusception may recur at a later date, but this seldom occurs owing to the adhesions and thickening of the intestinal wall caused by the first attack.

## Ulcerative colitis

This condition is one of relapsing diarrhoea associated with the passage of blood and mucus from ulcerative lesions in the colon. The cause is unknown, the disorder being more common in adults than in children. It must be considered whenever a child has a persistent bloody diarrhoea which is not due to bacillary or amoebic dysentery. The onset in children is less often fulminating than in adults and the first symptom is nearly always diarrhoea. Blood may be present in the stools from the start; occasionally there may be rectal bleeding only, or it may appear after a short interval. Tenesmus before defaecation, and abdominal pain are common. The children are always underweight and often anaemic. Many show evidence of emotional strain, and family tension is common. Psychological factors are important in the aetiology, probably accounting for the finding that other members of the family have sometimes been affected.

Diagnosis is confirmed by sigmoidoscopy when the typical ulcers in the colon are seen, but in some only a granular proctitis is present. Barium enema shows loss of haustration in the colon.

Perforation of the intestine may occur but arthritis is probably the most frequent complication. In longstanding cases malignant change may develop in the affected portion of the bowel.

*Treatment.* General measures are the first essential, the diet being high in protein and low in residue. Iron and blood transfusions may be required for anaemia. Steroid therapy has greatly improved the prognosis, being best given as a combination of oral prednisolone and local hydrocortisone hemisuccinate sodium, administered as a retention enema by drip. Sulphasalazine, which is an azo compound of salicyclic acid and sulphapyridine, is sometimes of value. It is less effective than the combination of oral and local prednisolone, bı . in mild cases it is reasonable to give the drug a trial in the hope of avoiding steroid therapy. Surgical treatment, consisting of ileostomy and possibly colectomy, is used in fulminating cases which fail to respond to adequate steroid therapy and in selected chronic cases.

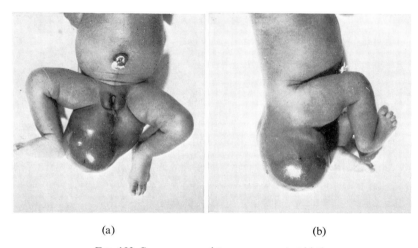

(a)                                                    (b)

FIG. 102. Sacro-coccygeal tumour present at birth.

## Rectal prolapse

This condition used mainly to occur in undernourished children but nowadays the patients are usually well-nourished toddlers of 1–2 years; only occasionally is it seen in wasting diseases such as cystic fibrosis. It is usually the result of straining, though by no means are all of them constipated. In some it is related to excessive pot-training and being left for too long on the pot.

*Treatment.* It is first of all necessary to reassure the mother that the condition is not as serious as the alarming appearance would make her think, and to explain that almost all children recover spontaneously in time. Visits to the lavatory should be short and one of the most effective treatments is to provide the child with a small seat for use on the adult lavatory. This reduces the amount of straining which occurs in the fully flexed position while sitting on a pot on the floor. If the child is constipated, the family should be managed as described on p. 306.

In most cases the rectum can be easily replaced digitally by the mother. Sometimes the prolapse immediately recurs in which case this can be prevented by strapping the buttocks between bowel actions. If there is difficulty in replacing the rectum it should be pushed back by placing a finger, previously covered in toilet paper, into the rectum. Withdrawal of the finger alone is then possible since the paper remains applied to the rectal mucosa and is passed with the next motion. Should the mother be unable to replace the rectum she should not panic but put the child to bed and encourage him to go to sleep, giving a sedative if necessary. The foot of the bed should be raised and a warm compress placed on the exposed rectum. Within a few hours the rectum will have gone back on its own or can easily be replaced by hand.

Surgical treatment is rarely required and then only if there has been no improvement after some months.

## Sacro-coccygeal tumour

This tumour is a teratoma and is usually present at birth. The large mass lies in the region of the coccyx displacing the rectum anteriorly (Fig. 102). It may sometimes be mistaken for a meningocele but is larger and continues to grow downwards and forwards so as to displace the rectum further, whereas any enlargement of a meningocele after birth is slight and occurs in a posterior direction. The sacro-coccygeal tumour, being a teratoma, feels solid and cystic since it contains many different forms of tissue, whereas the meningocele is purely cystic. About 25 per cent of these tumours are malignant and therefore surgical excision should be extensive and include the coccyx.

## Viral hepatitis

This condition is caused by two viruses which differ in their epidemiology but produce identical clinical pictures. Virus A causes *infective hepatitis* and is usually spread by faecal contamination of food and drinking water. The incubation period is about 1 month, the highest incidence being between 5 and 15 years.

Virus B causes *serum hepatitis*. It is associated with the finding of Australia antigen in the serum of infected persons. Whether this is the virus itself is uncertain but it is certainly a marker for the infective agent of serum hepatitis. Of those infected, many fail to develop a clinical attack of jaundice but all are liable to become carriers. Jaundice may then be transferred to another individual by the injection of serum products such as plasma or blood from a carrier. Transfer may also take place by the use of contaminated syringes and needles, therefore a freshly sterilized needle and syringe must be used for every form of injection; an obvious advantage is to have disposable need-les and syringes. A pregnant mother infected with either virus may transfer the infection to the fetus, though this is more likely to occur with virus B (see p. 128). The incubation period is much longer, being about 3 months, and the age incidence does not fall off in adult life. There is no cross-immunity between these two infections.

*Clinical features.* The patient is unwell for 4–5 days before the jaundice appears, anorexia being the outstanding early symptom. Fever, vomiting and general malaise occur and there may be upper abdominal pain. Signs suggest-ing an upper respiratory infection are sometimes present. The urine becomes dark from bile and the liver moderately enlarged and tender. Both these signs may be found before the jaundice is visible. When the jaundice appears the child usually feels much better; at this stage the stools become pale. In a considerable proportion of cases jaundice never appears.

*Diagnosis.* Once the child has become jaundiced the diagnosis is no prob-lem, but considerable difficulty arises in the premonitory stage and in those who never develop jaundice. The finding of an enlarged tender liver and the presence of an excess of urobilinogen in the urine are usually sufficient, but if necessary the abnormality of the liver function tests can also be demon-strated. In the early stages the child may present as a case of pyrexia of un-known origin and appendicitis may be considered, but the severe anorexia should point to the correct diagnosis. Early diagnosis is essential in order to limit the spread of the disease.

*Prognosis.* The majority of patients recover completely, but a very small number develop acute liver failure or progress to cirrhosis. In the early stages there is no means of picking out these serious cases, but among the most ominous signs is a persistent reversal of the albumin-globulin ratio. The disease is more serious in those with a deficiency of glucose-6-phosphate dehydrogenase.

*Treatment.* Because of the few cases which develop serious complications all must be kept under close supervision until they have returned to normal. They must be kept strictly in bed during the period of acute symptoms and encouraged to take frequent small feeds of a high-calorie diet rich in protein. Restriction of fat is unnecessary and patients can suit their own tastes as to the amount of fat they eat. Once the child feels well enough to get up it is probably safe to let him do so, even if still jaundiced, provided he rests for an hour after each meal. Full activity should not be permitted until there is no excess of urobilinogen in the urine.

Gammaglobulin reduces the severity of infective hepatitis but has no influence on serum hepatitis. Since infective hepatitis is usually mild in children and gammaglobulin is expensive it is seldom required. Gammaglobulin is effective prophylactically and should be given to close contacts of patients with infective hepatitis.

## Cirrhosis of the liver

This is a chronic diffuse hepatitis which is not a single disease, but the end-result of a number of damaging agents whose effects vary according to the part of the liver which they attack and the duration of their action. Damage to the parenchyma as in viral hepatitis can be followed by complete regeneration since the parenchymal cells can return to normal. But damage to the portal tracts leads to a disorderly regeneration only, with widespread fibrosis.

The noxious agent may be an infection such as viral hepatitis, syphilis, malaria or amoebic dysentery. Occasionally, pyogenic infection of the umbilical vein in the newborn may lead to cirrhosis and this may follow an exchange transfusion. Alternatively, the damage may be caused by obstruction of the bile ducts which, in children, is most often due to congenital atresia.

Cirrhosis may occur as a sequel of haemolytic disease of the newborn, though the mechanism of its production is uncertain. If there has been severe jaundice, obstruction in the bile ducts has possibly resulted from inspissated bile, this obstruction leading to cirrhosis. But the association has been found in infants without much jaundice and, to account for this, it has been suggested that the maternal antibodies may directly damage the liver cells.

Cirrhosis may develop in patients with cystic fibrosis. Its incidence in this disease increases with the advancing age of the patient, but its cause is uncertain (see p. 169).

The role of malnutrition in the production of cirrhosis is still not clear. Insufficient protein leads to fatty infiltration of the liver which predisposes to the later development of cirrhosis. But this is not the complete cause since cirrhosis is uncommon in African children and it is likely that other factors are also involved. For example, cirrhosis of the liver is common in Jamaica and results from drinking 'bush-teas' which are home-brewed infusions of herbs. The toxic factor is pyrrolizidine, the species of herbs particularly responsible being *Crotalaria* and *Senecio*. Since it commences as an obliterative process in the hepatic vein radicals it is termed '*veno-occlusive disease of the liver*'. The accumulation of chemical substances in the liver may lead to cirrhosis, such as copper in Wilson's disease or galactose in congenital galactosaemia.

### BILIARY CIRRHOSIS

Obstruction of the bile ducts leads to gross jaundice associated with an enlarged liver, bile in the urine but no bile in the stools. Evidence of portal obstruction is absent or occurs late only.

PORTAL CIRRHOSIS

In the early stages, general and gastrointestinal symptoms feature so that there is general malaise associated with anorexia, nausea and vomiting. Once portal obstruction has developed, ascites appears, a collateral circulation being formed which may lead to bleeding from an oesophageal varix. Jaundice is not a feature of this form of cirrhosis, but a haemorrhagic tendency results from the low level of prothrombin.

*Treatment.* This must be directed towards the causal agent and the surgical removal of any obstruction. The diet should be high in carbohydrate and protein, and supplements of vitamin B complex and vitamin K given. Portal hypertension may be relieved by shunt operations between the portal vein and inferior vena cava. The prognosis is better in those with swollen rather than shrunken livers. Some improvement has occurred in cases of active chronic hepatitis by the use of steroid therapy.

## Liver abscess

This is extremely rare in childhood. It may result from an ascending infection along the umbilical vein, or as part of a general pyaemia. A solitary abscess can occur in amoebic dysentery and occasionally results from a roundworm which has entered the bile duct.

## Leptospirosis

This condition is due to *Leptospira icterohaemorrhagiae* (Weil's disease) from rats, or *Leptospira canicola* (canicola fever) from dogs. The disease, which is not common in children, is caused either by a rat bite, or from contact with urine from an infected dog, or by swimming in infected water—the most common method of infection in children. The leptospirae enter the body either through a skin abrasion or through the mucosa of the mouth, nose or conjunctiva.

*Clinical features.* Weil's disease is more severe than canicola fever and more liable to be fatal, although fatal cases of canicola fever do occur. The incubation period is 1–2 weeks, the onset being sudden with high fever and headache. Jaundice occurs in about half the cases of Weil's disease but is less common in canicola fever; haemorrhages may occur into the skin. Pain in the muscles and conjunctival suffusion are characteristic. Meningeal involvement, producing the clinical features and cerebrospinal fluid changes of aseptic meningitis (p. 404) may be present; in some cases these features occur alone. A morbilliform rash may occur.

*Investigations.* Proteinuria from renal involvement is almost constant. Leptospirae may be isolated from the blood, urine or cerebrospinal fluid. Specific agglutination tests are available.

*Diagnosis.* The possibility of this condition must be considered in every case of apparent infective hepatitis. The greater severity of the illness and the presence of muscle tenderness and proteinuria are the distinguishing features. The disease must also be considered in all cases of the aseptic meningitis syndrome. In the absence of any other clinical features, diagnosis is dependent on isolation of the spirochaete and on agglutination tests.

*Treatment.* Penicillin is the drug of choice though not all cases respond; tetracycline is sometimes effective.

## BIBLIOGRAPHY

COOK R.C.M. & RICKHAM P.P. (1969) Neonatal intestinal obstruction due to milk curds. *J. Ped. Surg.*, **4**, 599.

DENNISON W.M. & SHAKER M. (1970) Intussusception in infancy and childhood. *Brit. J. Surg.*, **57**, 679.

DOBBS R.H. (1974) Glucose-electrolyte hydration powders for the management of gastro-enteritis. *Nigerian J. Paed.*, **1**, 71.

EMSLIE R.D. (1963) Cancrum oris. *Dent. Practitioner.*, **13**, 481.

FRIEDLANDER F.C. & KUSHLICK P. (1954) Trichobezoar. *Arch. Dis. Childh.*, **29**, 556.

JUEL-JENSEN B.E. (1969) Infections with the virus of herpes simplex (Herpesvirus hominis). *Brit. J. Hosp. Med.*, **2**, 1687.

MCNEISH A.S. & WILLOUGHBY M.L.N. (1969) Whole-blood folate as a screening test for coeliac disease in childhood. *Lancet*, **1**, 442.

PINKERTON P. (1958) Psychogenic megacolon in children: the implications of bowel negativism. *Arch. Dis. Childh.*, **33**, 371.

TEMPEST M.N. (1966) Cancrum oris. *Brit. J. Surg.*, **53**, 949.

# CHAPTER 9

# DISEASES DUE TO PARASITES

All forms of intestinal parasites are more common in the tropics where heavy infestation is one of the factors causing chronic ill health. In temperate climates they cause few symptoms, though the observation of live worms in the stools causes much emotional distress.

## Threadworms (pinworms, Oxyuris or Enterobius vermicularis)

These are the commonest worms of temperate climates, being most wide-spread where there is poor hygiene and overcrowding. The worms infest the large bowel, especially the caecum and appendix. The fertilized female emerges from the anus to lay her eggs on the perianal skin. This causes irritation and the consequent contamination of the hands from scratching results in reinfection of the host and transfer to others by direct contact or through food.

The symptoms are largely the result of perianal irritation and, since this is most marked at night, it can cause sleeplessness and sometimes enuresis. The worms may crawl into the vagina, producing vulvo-vaginitis. The association of abdominal pain with threadworms has been overemphasized, the majority of patients having no symptoms at all. Pain in some of the children is func-tional, being related to the attention paid to the bowels once worms have been seen, and to the disgust felt by the parents and the child on their discovery. The appendix is one of the main sites inhabited by threadworms and it is therefore understandable that worms are often found in those removed at operation. Their role in the aetiology of the inflammation of the appendix in such cases is less definite. It has been shown that the young larvae burrow into the upper layer of the mucosa of the appendix from where they emerge later as adults and migrate to the anus. Perforation of the intact mucous membrane renders it more liable to secondary infection so that the worms are sometimes the primary cause of appendicitis. In other cases they are only passengers in an appendix which has become inflamed from some other cause.

*Diagnosis.* Adult worms look like threads of cotton and are easily identified. Ova can be demonstrated by placing a short strip of scotch tape on the peri-anal skin in the morning before bathing or defaecation. The ova adhere to the scotch tape which is then mounted on a slide with decinormal sodium hydroxide solution and examined under the microscope.

*Treatment.* Piperazine is the most effective drug and acts by paralysing the worm. It can be given as a single-dose preparation (Pripsen, which comprises piperazine phosphate and senna). A second dose should be given 2 weeks later to deal with worms maturing from ova ingested after the time of the first dose. An alternative single dose oxyuricide is viprynium embonate (Vanquin), the dose being 5 mg per kg, repeated after two weeks. This drug stains the stools red. All members of the family should be treated since it is likely that more than one is infected, even if worms have not been seen. Possible transfer of eggs from anus to mouth is prevented by keeping the finger nails short and wearing gloves and pyjamas at night until cure has been achieved. An additional treatment is the local application of Ung. Hydrargyri Ammoniati Dil. (HAD) to the perianal skin at night. This deters the worms from coming out to lay their eggs and they are passed with the next motion instead. The life of a threadworm is only 5–6 weeks, so that prevention of auto-infection during that period is an additional safeguard to ensure the infestation dies out. These hygienic measures are essential for the certain eradication of the worms; a possible disadvantage of a single dose treatment is that the measures are less likely to be maintained for the required 6 weeks than if the patient is given a week's course of treatment.

Some authorities do not consider it worthwhile treating symptomless cases. However, the treatment available is now so simple and the disgust caused by the worm liable to be so great, that it would seem much wiser to treat all patients and their families.

### Roundworms (Ascaris lumbricoides)

These worms inhabit the small intestine and look similar to an earthworm, only white. The ova are passed in the stool and, where insanitary conditions exist, they can contaminate food and be swallowed. The eggs hatch in the small intestine and the larvae are carried in the blood stream to the lungs via the liver and right side of the heart. They then pass up the respiratory tract to the epiglottis and are swallowed. Finally, they become estabished in the small intestine where they mature.

The passing of an adult worm in the stools is usually the first sign of infestation, though colic may occur and heavy infestation can cause intestinal obstruction. Occasionally a worm is vomited. Sometimes the larvae, while in the lungs, cause transient pulmonary symptoms and X-ray evidence of infiltration; this is short lived. Eosinophilia may be marked.

*Treatment.* A single dose of piperazine as for threadworms is effective. Thiabendazole is an alternative single dose therapy.

### Hookworm (Ancylostoma duodenale and Necator americanus)

This is rare in Britain but a serious cause of anaemia and ill health in the tropics. The eggs are passed in the faeces, developing into larvae in the soil. These can penetrate the intact skin of bare feet coming in contact with contaminated soil. The larvae pass into the blood stream and reach the lungs from where they pass up to the epiglottis and are swallowed. On reaching the duodenum they attach themselves to the mucosa by means of hooks. They feed by sucking blood, growing into mature worms which are about 2 cm long.

Occasionally, the larvae penetrate to the deeper layers of the skin, where they are unable to enter the blood vessels. For months, therefore, they migrate through tunnels in the skin which are visible to the outside as inflamed raised channels (*larva migrans*).

A few worms in a healthy patient produce no symptoms, but a severe infestation causes increasing anaemia and oedema with eventual death from heart failure. The diagnosis is confirmed by a positive occult blood test and the finding of ova in the stools. The larvae may cause an itching papular eruption at the site of entry through the skin ('ground itch').

*Treatment.* Prevention lies in the proper disposal of faeces and the wearing of shoes. A single dose of bephenium hydroxynaphthoate is usually effective treatment, the dose being 5 g for patients over 2 years and 2·5 g for those under 2 years. Thiabendazole is also effective. An alternative drug is tetrachlorethylene, but this is much more toxic. The anaemia should be corrected by iron therapy or a blood transfusion.

### Trichuris trichiura (whipworm)

This parasite is about 5 cm long and is widely distributed in warm moist climates. The anterior portion of the worm is elongated into a thin whip-like filament with which it bores into the superficial mucosa of the caecum, lower ileum or ascending colon. The thicker posterior portion of the worm projects into the lumen of the bowel. The eggs are passed in the stools where they can be easily recognized microscopically. If deposited on moist soil the eggs hatch into larvae in two weeks. If ripe eggs are swallowed they hatch out in the duodenum, then becoming attached to the mucous membrane of the caecum or nearby bowel.

Infestation is frequently so mild that there are no symptoms. Heavy infestation causes abdominal pain which is usually right-sided, while massive infestation causes a severe and often bloody diarrhoea, sometimes associated with prolapse of the rectum.

The worm is difficult to eradicate. The most effective treatment is dithiazanine iodide but because of its side effects of nausea, diarrhoea and cramps it is wise to treat the child in hospital. The dose is calculated from the adult dose by the percentage method (p. 730). The basic adult dose is 100 mg t.d.s. for one day, then 200 mg t.d.s. for 5 days. If the patient is unable to tolerate this high dose then 100 mg t.d.s. is tried for 3–4 weeks. The tablets must be swallowed whole.

### Strongyloides stercoralis

In America this parasite is known as the threadworm. The parasite is only just visible to the naked eye as a delicate thread. It lives in the depth of the mucous membrane anywhere in the intestine, but mainly in the duodenum. The eggs hatch out in the intestinal canal to form larvae which undergo further development in warm soil. These larvae penetrate the skin, travelling through the lungs in the same way as the hookworm (p. 326) and may produce the same clinical effects. Chronic intestinal infestation causes epigastric pain and diarrhoea leading to emaciation.

Treatment is with dithiazanine iodide exactly as described for *Trichuris* (p. 326).

### Tapeworm

Infestation results from eating undercooked pork (*Taenia solium*) or beef (*Taenia saginata*) and the cysticercus stage is passed in these animals. Although gastrointestinal symptoms may occur, in most instances nothing abnormal is noted until the flat, moving, white segments of the worm are passed. Man is also liable to infection with the cysticercus stage of *Taenia solium* by swallowing eggs from his own or another individual's infection. These may lodge in the brain and cause epilepsy, or in the muscles where they cause pains.

*Treatment.* Mepacrine should be tried first. For a young child 4 tablets (100 mg each) are given and for an adult 8 tablets. One-quarter of the total tablets is given every quarter of an hour and a saline purge 2 hours later. The head of the worm stains yellow and should be looked for after filtering the stool through black gauze.

Dichlorophen is an alternative treatment, the dose being 60 mg/kg given as a single dose in the morning. No purgative is required as the drug has a laxative action. The worm is digested in the bowel after destruction by the drug so that no segments are passed.

### Trichiniasis

*Trichinella spiralis* is one of the smallest roundworms parasitic in man; it is acquired through eating inadequately cooked pork. The adult worms are 1–4 mm long and burrow into the mucosa of the small intestine. The larvae are not expelled with the faeces like other intestinal helminths, but pass into the blood stream and settle in skeletal muscle fibres where they form a fibrotic nodule.

Fever is usual and gastrointestinal symptoms may be marked during the acute stage, although they have been minimal in some outbreaks. There is stiffness and weakness of muscles and often there are signs that the central nervous system or the peripheral nerves have been affected. Two characteristic features are oedema of the eyelids and splinter haemorrhages under the nails. Eosinophilia is almost invariable.

*Treatment.* There is no specific treatment but steroid therapy should be given to reduce the acute symptoms.

## Lambliasis

*Giardia lamblia* is a protozoan with flagellae which also exists in a cystic form. It produces offensive fatty motions from secondary disaccharidase deficiency (p. 570) so that the patient is sometimes suspected of having coeliac disease. During the last war a high incidence of the condition occurred in day nurseries. The parasite is found in the stool, but since it lives in the duodenum and upper jejunum it may only be found in the duodenal juice.

The condition usually responds well to mepacrine, the dose being 50 mg t.d.s. for 5 days for children up to 4 years, 100 mg for children of 4–8 years and 200 mg for children over 8 years. Metronidazole is effective if mepacrine fails.

## Hydatid disease

This is produced by the larval stage of *Taenia echinococcus*, a minute worm which lives in the small bowel of the dog. The disease occurs mainly in sheep-rearing countries, since the animal is an alternative host, when sheep, dog and man are in close contact. Infection occurs from ova passed in the faeces of the dog, the larvae passing through the wall of the intestine to settle mainly in the liver, lung or brain. Here they become encysted and grow larger, producing symptoms as a space-occupying lesion.

The most sensitive indication of the disease is the complement fixation test (CFT) but there is also an intradermal test which should give a positive reaction. Eosinophilia is usual. Surgical removal is the only form of treatment and the CFT should become negative 9 months later unless more cysts are present, which is the case in about 60 per cent of patients.

## Schistosomiasis (bilharziasis)

This condition is caused by two intestinal blood flukes, *Schistosoma mansoni* and *S. japonicum*, and by one vesicle blood fluke, *S. haemotobium*. The eggs are passed in the stool or urine and hatch into ciliated larvae (miracidiae) which invade certain species of water snail. Here they mature into fork-tailed larvae (cercariae) which escape into the water and can penetrate human skin. They then make their way via the blood stream and the lungs to the liver, where they mature. After maturation, swimming against the portal blood stream, the female schistosomes deposit their ova in viscera: the intestinal varieties in the lower bowel and the vesical in the bladder.

The pathological effects are due less to the adult schistosomes than to their eggs. In all sites they produce inflammation and subsequent fibrosis. Hepatic cirrhosis and portal hypertension can be the end result of intestinal schistosomiasis while cardio-pulmonary involvement can complicate both forms.

A heavy primary infection can produce an acute febrile illness which lasts several weeks with remittent fever, headache, allergic skin reactions and marked eosinophilia. The chief effect is in the chronic stage and depends on the site where the eggs have been deposited. In the vesical form, haematuria is often the only symptom and typically it occurs at the end of micturition. In the intestinal form there are dysenteric symptoms.

*Treatment.* The essential is to prevent the disease by the proper disposal of faeces and the prohibition of bathing in infected water. Niridazole is most effective against *S. haematobium* but less effective and more toxic when used against *S. mansoni.* Trivalent antimony products are therefore still used against this variety and against *S. japonicum.*

## Malaria

This disease is distributed throughout tropical countries but its incidence is less in dry places and at high altitudes. Four types of parasite are known to exist in man—*Plasmodium malariae*, the cause of quartan fever, *P. vivax* and *P. ovale*, which cause benign tertian fever, and *P. falciparum*, which causes malignant malaria, the type responsible for all the more serious complications.

In the first stage of the life cycle in human beings the parasites develop in the liver. They then pass out into the blood stream for the asexual cycle within the red cells, destroying these cells in the process. The length of this cycle determines the interval between the bouts of fever in the classic form of the disease. After a time, certain of these ordinary parasites of the asexual cycle become sexually differentiated, developing into male and female gametocytes. When a patient is bitten by a mosquito these gametocytes enter its body and complete their development, later returning to infect another patient.

*Clinical features.* The classical disease with recurring bouts of high fever is seen only in the non-immune child. For the child living in an endemic area the illness is quite different, being dependent on his degree of immunity and therefore on his age. The newborn baby has a passive immunity acquired from his mother lasting a few months; congenital malaria is therefore extremely rare although the placenta is often infected, this being a major cause of low birth weight (Jelliffe, 1968). This is followed by a period of a few months when mild attacks occur as a result of waning immunity. Severe attacks develop between the ages of 9 months and 2 years; thereafter, increasing active immunity develops, so that despite the presence of parasites in the blood the feverish attacks become milder and less frequent. The child then lives in harmony with the parasite, a state reached by the third year, though immunity is never complete. The mechanism of immunity is not fully understood though there is a rise in gammaglobulin. Although it is exceptional for a baby in an endemic area to develop malaria before the age of 6 months this is now being seen occasionally. This could be due to maternal immunity being partial only, because she has taken some antimalarials which are now freely available in markets in developing countries.

During the period of severe attacks the child develops bouts of fever with anorexia, vomiting and particularly diarrhoea. Therefore, every young child with acute diarrhoea in a malarial area must be given routine antimalarial treatment in addition to other therapy. Convulsions are common and may result from the high fever only, but much more serious are the cases of convulsions from cerebral malaria which is due to *P. falciparum*. The capillaries in the brain become blocked with red blood cells, many of which contain the parasites. Such children are desperately ill with convulsions, shock and coma. The death rate is high and survival may be associated with mental retardation and paralysis.

Chronic malarial infection causes enlargement of the liver and spleen, anaemia and probably retardation of growth. This anaemia is sometimes megaloblastic because recurrent attacks of malaria in an individual whose folic acid intake is marginal may tip the balance into an actual deficiency of folic acid. When investigating such children for fever it is important to look for other causes, even though malarial parasites are seen in the blood. Prolonged fever in a child brought up in an endemic area is seldom due to malaria, though antimalarial therapy must be given as a routine.

*Prophylaxis.* General measures should be undertaken to eradicate the mosquito. For individual protection, mosquito nets should be used at night and prophylactic drugs taken, these being started 1 week before entering and continued for 4 weeks after leaving a malarial district. Pyrimethamine weekly (p. 737) or proguanil daily (p. 737) are now preferred to chloroquine or amodiaquine for prophylaxis.

The planning of large-scale programmes for the control of endemic malaria must take into account the cost of drugs, their means of distribution and a variety of sociological aspects such as whether the local population will accept the drugs even if they are given them. Prophylaxis during the early years of life is strongly recommended and will reduce the infant morbidity and mortality. However, it interferes with the development of natural immunity and, therefore, to be effective must be continued throughout the period of exposure. Sudden cessation of prophylactic drugs, as is likely to occur when infants stop attending infant health clinics, may lead to overwhelming malarial infection. In areas where malarial control is poor it is safer to provide treatment for acute attacks, hoping thereby to control morbidity without interfering with the development of immunity.

*Treatment.* Chloroquine and amodiaquine are the drugs of choice. For radical cure of vivax and tertian malaria a course of primaquine should follow this treatment in order to destroy the tissue forms of the parasite.

In severe cases of malignant malaria and in blackwater fever (see below) treatment is also required for shock using intravenous fluids and steroids if necessary.

*Blackwater fever* may occur in young children in endemic areas and is a manifestation of hypersensitivity in a patient saturated with malaria. The child becomes acutely ill with vomiting, haemoglobinuria and acute anaemia, and may die from anaemia, anuria and shock.

## BIBLIOGRAPHY

JELLIFFE E.F.P. (1968) Low birth-weight and malarial infection of the placenta. *Bull. Wld Hlth Org.*, **33,** 69.
MORLEY D. (1973) *Paediatric priorities in the developing world.* Butterworth, London.

# CHAPTER 10

# DISORDERS OF THE UPPER RESPIRATORY TRACT

## Epistaxis

Nose-bleeding is a common symptom in childhood. In most cases it is due to a local cause but it can result from generalized disease. The common local causes are trauma from contusion, nose-picking or the insertion of a foreign body, and acute coryza. The bleeding usually takes place from Little's area on the anterior portion of the nasal septum where there is a plentiful supply of blood vessels. In some cases of recurrent epistaxis the bleeding arises spontaneously from Little's area in which case a prominent vein is usually visible. Such cases are successfully treated by the application of cautery to the vein but before doing this it is worth trying the effect of twice daily applications of petroleum jelly to the nasal septum. This greasy application prevents the drying of the nasal mucosa which leads to desquamation of the epithelium over the superficial veins in Little's areas and subsequent bleeding. Nasal diphtheria is an important local cause of epistaxis which must not be forgotten even though it is now rare.

Epistaxis from generalized disease occurs at the onset of the specific fevers as part of the upper respiratory symptoms which accompany these infections. It may also occur in association with certain bleeding disorders such as purpura, leukaemia and haemophilia.

## Acute coryza (common cold)

The problem of colds in children is much the same as with adults, but children are especially susceptible when they start school and mix with large numbers of people in confined spaces. It is therefore common for a mother to bring her child to the doctor on account of frequent coughs and colds during his first winter at school. Most of these children improve once they develop resistance to the organisms which they are meeting for the first time.

A common cold in a baby is much more serious since the nasal obstruction causes severe respiratory and feeding difficulties. The newborn baby has the greatest difficulty in breathing through his mouth so that if, as an experiment, the nose of a normal baby is closed by pinching it will be found that the baby

332

becomes acutely distressed and cyanosed before taking a breath through the mouth. It is usually found that these symptoms cause the experimenter to be even more distressed than the baby! He therefore relaxes his hold of the nose without waiting for the baby to take the eventual breath through his mouth.

*Treatment*. Nasal obstruction from coryza in children of any age may be temporarily relieved by the instillation of nasal drops containing 0·5 per cent ephedrine in normal saline. Their chief use is for those babies who are unable to feed because of nasal obstruction; 2 drops are inserted into each nostril before feeds. Oily nasal drops should never be used in any patient in view of the risk of lipoid pneumonia. Antibiotics are not effective against the primary viral infection causing the cold but only against the secondary bacterial invaders. They are usually indicated for infants only in whom there is greater constitutional disturbance and an increased risk of spread of infection.

### Acute sinusitis

Nasal sinus infection in childhood is more often chronic and is discussed as sinobronchitis on p. 352. For practical purposes only the ethmoid sinuses are present at birth. The maxillary sinus is very small at birth, not reaching a significant size until about the age of 4 years. The frontal sinus appears about the age of 6 years, the sphenoidal sinus about 8 years.

Acute ethmoiditis may occur in infancy, although it is more common in older children; it is usually due to a streptococcal infection. The child rapidly becomes acutely ill with proptosis of the eye on the affected side associated with periorbital swelling and inflammation. An orbital abscess may develop. Acute osteomyelitis of the maxilla, which is confined to infancy, may affect the orbit similarly but there is also induration with swelling of the cheek and palate (p. 697).

## THE PHARYNX

### Acute tonsillitis

During the first year of life the tonsils are always small. Infection of the throat during this period affects the whole pharynx rather than the tonsils alone as in older children, so that it is more correct to refer to acute pharyngitis in babies.

In acute tonsillitis the tonsils become enlarged and inflamed, often with white exudate on the external surface of the gland when the term acute follicular tonsillitis is used. This white exudate must be differentiated from the creamy material which may be visible in the tonsillar crypts and does not necessarily indicate infection. The uvula and faucial pillars are usually involved at the same time, and the tonsillar glands at the angle of the jaw on each side become enlarged and tender. The commonest organism causing tonsillitis between the ages of 5 and 17 years is the haemolytic streptococcus. Under the age of 3 years pharyngitis is usually non-streptococcal, being caused by virus infections, especially adenoviruses, herpes simplex and Coxsackie viruses (Moffet *et al.*, 1968). They may be inflamed in association with many generalized infections, especially the infectious fevers of childhood.

In adults, acute tonsillitis is associated with considerable pain at the back of the throat. In children, the remarkable feature is that they may have severely inflamed tonsils but no pain in the throat. In such cases pain, if experienced, is usually felt in the abdomen. This accounts for the failure to diagnose such an obvious condition and emphasizes the need for the throat to be examined in every case.

Acute follicular tonsillitis must be differentiated from diphtheria. Diphtheria causes a single dirty-grey membrane which covers a large area of the tonsil and may spread to the fauces and palate, as opposed to the isolated white flecks on the tonsil in acute follicular tonsillitis. In diphtheria the faucial pillars and uvula are not red, the temperature is only slightly raised and the pulse rate may be disproportionately fast; in acute follicular tonsillitis there is a high fever. In diphtheria the child is usually more toxic and ill; there may be considerable swelling of the neck ('bull-neck') from periadenitis, in addition to inflammation of the lymph glands themselves.

*Treatment.* Although the majority of cases of acute tonsillitis will settle without any trouble, there is always the risk of a more generalized spread of infection and in children, especially, the complication of acute otitis media. There is also the special risk in children that an acute streptococcal tonsillitis may be followed by the development of rheumatic fever or acute nephritis. For these reasons acute tonsillitis should be treated seriously, antibiotics being administered.

Early treatment is not essential for the prevention of rheumatic fever, in fact a slight delay in initiating treatment possibly permits the development of some degree of immunity. The essential aspect of treatment is first to prove the presence of the beta haemolytic streptococcus and then to eradicate it by giving a full 10-day course of treatment. Although most cases will respond to sulphonamides these act more slowly and less effectively than penicillin which is therefore preferable. The penicillin can be given orally or intramuscularly. Paracetamol can also be given for the symptomatic treatment of pain and fever.

### Chronic tonsillitis

This condition results from repeated attacks of acute tonsillitis. Here the doctor should be far more influenced by the history of recurrent attacks than by the appearance of the tonsils. Enlargement of the tonsils is no indication that they are unhealthy. The tonsils, in common with lymphoid tissue elsewhere in the body grow throughout childhood (p. 243). The small tonsil is more likely to be the seat of chronic inflammation than the large one and there is a world of difference between the small fixed fibrotic tonsil which cannot enlarge and the large mobile pair of tonsils, sometimes so large that they meet in the mid-line, which if given time will revert to a normal size.

These large tonsils do not cause respiratory obstruction because they are in front of the airway through the nasopharynx. Only occasionally do they cause difficulty in swallowing; it is surprising how little the child is inconvenienced by a really large pair of tonsils.

In deciding whether the tonsils should be removed it is necessary to consider whether they are still functioning as the first line of defence. If they are removed when still able to function the child will be worse off, since he will then suffer from recurrent pharyngitis and more severe involvement of the tonsillar lymph glands. If the child is suffering from repeated attacks of tonsillitis and the tonsillar glands are enlarged, especially if the tonsils remain small and fibrotic, then their removal is indicated. Removal of the tonsils before the age of 4 years is rarely advocated.

If the child has once suffered from a peritonsillar abscess (quinsy) so much destruction of the tonsil will have taken place that they should always be removed. Tuberculous cervical adenitis is frequently associated with a primary tuberculous infection of the tonsil and sometimes of the adenoids also. In such cases the removal of tonsils and adenoids is a wise addition to chemotherapy, reducing the risk of later recurrence of the adenitis.

The removal of the tonsils in children who have had rheumatic fever or acute nephritis should be recommended only if the tonsils are the seat of repeated infection. The fact that a child has had one of these diseases does not alter the indications for the operation.

## The adenoids

The adenoids or nasopharyngeal tonsil are an aggregation of lymphoid tissue situated in the midline at the junction of the roof and posterior wall of the nasopharynx. They enlarge during childhood, reaching maximum development between the ages of 5–15; they may persist to adult life although they are seldom seen after the age of 20. During the first 4 years of life they cause much more trouble than the tonsils because hypertrophied adenoid tissue obstructs breathing and, by extending laterally, interferes with the musculature at the opening of the Eustachian tubes on the lateral wall of the nasopharynx. If there is gross enlargement the opening is blocked. If the opening of the Eustachian tube is not clear, free drainage from the middle ear cavity is prevented, thereby increasing the liability to otitis media.

The adenoids can be seen only by means of posterior rhinoscopy but a good idea of their size can be obtained from the appearance of the nasopharynx. A large pad of adenoids pushes the uvula forwards and upwards thereby increasing the depth of the pharynx.

Removal of the adenoids should be recommended if there is evidence that they are obstructing the nasal passages. The fact that a child keeps his mouth open is not in itself an indication for adenoidectomy (p. 353). Repeated attacks of otitis media are a clear indication for adenoidectomy in view of the risk that further attacks may cause impairment of hearing.

In general, the tonsils seldom require removal before the age of 4 years but the adenoids may. After the age of 4 years, if removal of the tonsils is necessary, the adenoids are usually removed at the same time since they also are likely to be the seat of chronic infection.

### Retropharyngeal abscess

This condition usually follows an acute upper respiratory infection, occurring when inflammation in one of the retropharyngeal glands proceeds to suppuration. It mainly affects infants, being most often due to the haemolytic streptococcus. There is an acute onset of dysphagia, the infant lying with his mouth open and head retracted. The accompanying toxaemia is usually severe.

The bulge in the pharynx can seldom be seen from the outside since it is too low down, but it can be felt with a finger inserted into the pharynx. A lateral X-ray of the neck for soft tissue shadows may show the pharynx to be pushed forwards.

*Diagnosis.* Tuberculosis of the cervical spine may produce a similarly placed abscess except that it lies deeper in the neck. The onset is less acute, there is more neck stiffness and an X-ray shows involvement of the cervical vertebrae.

*Treatment.* When opening a retropharyngeal abscess a guarded blade should be used so that there is no risk that this will be inserted too deeply. The guard is most simply made by winding a strip of adhesive tape round the blade at the required distance from its point. The infant's head must be well down and no anaesthetic given so that the cough reflex is retained and the risk of inhalation of pus reduced to a minimum. Suction should be used to remove the pus as soon as it emerges. Antibiotic therapy is always indicated.

### Acute epiglottitis

This condition affects young children. Its striking clinical effect is a profound toxaemia which develops rapidly and appears to be out of all proportion to the observed physical signs since the nasopharynx is seldom involved. Examination of the epiglottis, which can be achieved with a spatula by looking into the mouth from above and behind the patient as when using a laryngoscope, shows this to be bright red and oedematous. Death often occurs rapidly but if the child survives long enough, acute respiratory obstruction may develop. A tracheostomy should therefore be performed early if signs of obstruction develop.

The causal organism is usually *Haemophilus influenzae*. Ampicillin or chloramphenicol should be given. Autopsy examination shows a characteristic straight line of demarcation at the base of the epiglottis where its bright red swelling ends.

## THE EAR

### Otitis externa

This is not uncommon in children, usually resulting from swimming in baths; it is very liable to recur. The ear is extremely painful, this being exaggerated by movement of the pinna and by lying on the affected ear. The external auditory meatus is red, soggy and swollen and may be almost closed. Local furuncles or vesicles may be present, the discharge, which may be serous or purulent, usually being scanty. A painful enlarged lymph gland may be palpable in front of, below or behind the pinna. The insertion of a gauze wick which has previously been soaked in glycerine with 10 per cent ichthammol gives relief. Alternatively, hydrocortisone ointment or drops may be used. Penicillin should also be given since the infection is usually caused by the staphylococcus.

Swimming should be forbidden to children with any ear infection whether otitis media or externa.

### Acute otitis media

Infants and young children are particularly liable to this condition because at their age the Eustachian tube is short, wide and straight and they spend most of their time lying down. Consequently, bacterial spread from the nasopharynx into the middle ear takes place with ease, vomited feeds being also likely to pass along the same route. The pharyngeal opening of the Eustachian tube is easily blocked by enlarged adenoids, in which case the resulting stasis leads to infection of the middle ear.

The infant with otitis media is usually acutely ill with anorexia, fever and often vomiting and diarrhoea, but there may be nothing to point to the ear as the source of the infection. Routine examination of the ears is therefore essential. This should be repeated every day in children with an upper respiratory infection, or in those who are vomiting from any cause, or where a diagnosis has not yet been reached. Some infants will pull on the affected pinna and others will shriek from the pain caused by the infection. Examination of the ear drum reveals acute inflammation shown by loss of the light reflex, immobility, injection and perhaps bulging.

Facial nerve paralysis may occur as a complication of acute otitis media. The majority of cases occur early, no additional therapy being required and they usually recover rapidly. If the paralysis occurs later in the illness it may be due to acute mastoiditis for which surgery is required. Acute mastoiditis and lateral sinus thrombosis are now rare complications of otitis media.

The infection must be dealt with adequately from the start in order to reduce the chance that it will become chronic, leading to deafness. Ampicillin is the antibiotic of choice. Nasal drops containing ephedrine 0·5 per cent in saline can be prescribed with the aim of keeping the Eustachian tubes open. Treatment should be continued until the appearance and mobility of the ear drum returns to normal (mobility is tested by insufflation with the rubber bulb which can be attached to the auriscope).

Myringotomy is seldom required nowadays but should still be performed if a full drum fails to subside rapidly. Spontaneous perforation of the drum during treatment shows that myringotomy should have been performed.

*Serous otitis media (glue ear).* In this condition there is a sterile collection of glue-like fluid in the middle ear. It is now common in developed countries where it has largely replaced the discharging ear, but it is uncommon in developing countries. It seems likely that the difference relates to the greater use of antibiotics for respiratory infections in developed countries and associated incomplete treatment of many children with otitis media. Allergy has been suggested as a causal factor but without evidence.

The child may not complain of pain so that the condition presents as deafness. The principal finding is an immobile and often retracted tympanic membrane. Its light reflex is often lost.

Treatment with ephedrine 0·5 per cent in saline nasal drops is sometimes successful but the insertion of a grommet is often required after sucking out the fluid to ensure complete drainage.

Whatever the type of otitis media, it is essential for treatment to continue until normal mobility of the drum returns. Hearing should be checked before the child is discharged from care.

### Chronic otitis media

The ear drum is deformed, thickened and immobile. There is usually a purulent discharge and a visible perforation. Some impairment of hearing is present in the affected ear. This condition results from recurrent upper respiratory infections with consequent otitis media, indicating that therapy has been inadequate. It is to prevent this that adenoidectomy should always be considered if there have been more than two attacks of acute otitis media. The possibility of tuberculous otitis media or cholesteatoma should be considered in chronic otitis media.

### Acute mastoiditis

This condition is now very rare, its presence indicating inadequate or inappropriate antibiotic therapy. The mastoid process is tender and inflamed; the pinna may be pushed forwards. X-rays show clouding of the mastoid air cells. Most cases respond to correct antibiotic therapy, surgery rarely being required.

### Foreign body

Earache or deafness is occasionally caused by a foreign body which the child himself has inserted. It is obvious on examination though its removal may be difficult.

### Referred earache

Pain in the ear may be referred from a lesion in the throat and is one reason why considerable earache may be felt after tonsillectomy. Earache may also be felt by children while teething or in association with mumps. A local lesion in the ear must be excluded before accepting that earache is due to referred pain. Symptomatic relief for the pain can be obtained from a hot water bottle or a pad of warm cotton wool bandaged over the ear. In the home, cotton wool can be warmed in the oven.

## DEAFNESS

### Aetiology

From the practical point of view the causes of deafness should be subdivided into those which occur before the child has learnt to appreciate sound and those which develop afterwards. In the first group are the true congenital causes and those which affect the child during the neonatal period. In the second are those occurring after the neonatal period.

#### CONGENITAL AND NEONATAL DEAFNESS (EARLY DEAFNESS)

The cochlear nerve may be malformed at any point along the course from its nucleus to the end organs in the basilar membrane. Some varieties of congenital nerve deafness are inherited. The vestibular apparatus is usually intact. The middle or external ear may be similarly malformed and in some cases the middle ear is absent or the pinna grossly deformed and no external auditory meatus present (p. 226). Maternal rubella occurring during the first 3 months of pregnancy is very liable to cause damage to the cochlea with consequent deafness. The risk of deafness in such cases is about 30 per cent, being unilateral in about one-third of the cases. Kernicterus from hyper-bilirubinaemia is often associated with high-tone deafness (p. 129); in such cases pathological changes have been found in the cochlear nuclei. Intra-cranial birth injury and asphyxia may also result in deafness.

ACQUIRED DEAFNESS (LATE DEAFNESS)

The commonest cause of deafness occurring after the neonatal period is otitis media, the danger being greatest if the condition is allowed to smoulder on or become recurrent. Deafness may be a sequel of meningitis or encephalitis. It is a particularly important complication of mumps, usually developing during the first 2 weeks of the illness when it may be associated with mumps menin-gitis or due to isolated involvement of the eighth nerve. Traumatic or neo-plastic lesions may destroy some part of the auditory pathway. The toxic action of such drugs as streptomycin or neomycin is liable to cause nerve deafness. Deafness also results from such simple causes as blockage of the external auditory meatus by wax or a foreign body such as a bead. Congenital syphilis, toxoplasmosis and hypertension are rare causes.

**Management of the deaf child**

Early diagnosis is essential for successful treatment and the proper develop-ment of speech. All babies should therefore be given a screening test for hear-ing around the age of 6 months. Particular attention will be paid to those babies on the 'at risk' register (p. 91) but, since these account for only about 50 per cent of the deaf children, all babies must be tested. It is not necessary for the test to be carried out in a sound-proof room but the room should be sound-treated by means of acoustic tiling.

The testing materials should produce sounds the baby knows rather than sounds which are new to him. Simple materials only are required: a cup and spoon, high and low pitched rattles, and toilet paper for the noise made when it is crunched. The sounds should be made quietly at a distance of about 1 metre out of view of the child but not behind the ear. By 6 months of age a child is able to localize sound, therefore, to pass the test he must turn and look directly at the source of the sound (Fig. 81, p. 262).

Mothers are extremely competent at appreciating the inability of their young children to hear normally, being seldom wrong unless the child is mentally handicapped; their complaint must therefore be treated very seriously. They are less competent at appreciating acquired partial loss of hearing so that a careful follow-up of children who have had otitis media is needed.

In understanding the management of the deaf child it is vital to appreciate that the normal child has to learn to hear, the first year of life being the most crucial for this. The ability to learn auditory discrimination diminishes as the child grows older; thus adults can less easily learn a foreign language than a child and are always likely to have a foreign accent because they are no longer able to learn the difference between sounds as does a child. It is therefore obvious that the deaf child must be taught to hear as early as possible. Delays cause diminished capacity for hearing, the consequent impairment of speech being seen in its most severe form in the deaf-mute. Total deafness is exceptional and only 1–2 per cent of deaf children have no hearing at all. All children should therefore have a 2-year period of auditory training before being regarded as totally deaf.

Parent guidance starts from the day deafness is diagnosed, being undertaken by the audiologist and by the specialist teacher of the deaf. This teacher will visit the home in addition to her work at the auditory training centre. By visiting, she not only learns about the home circumstances but is able to relate her advice to the actual needs of a particular home and a particular mother. She will also train the other children so that they can help the deaf child.

For the first 1–2 years of life all the auditory training will be given by the mother who will be taught how to handle her child so as to bring sound to him. She must speak very close to her child's ear, repeating sounds again and again so that he can learn auditory discrimination.

A hearing aid should be fitted at the earliest age at which the child will accept it, this often being as young as 10 months. The aid should be a double one, since two ears are better than one, and must be worn continuously. It is particularly important that he should be wearing an aid when he starts to crawl since he will no longer be close enough to his mother for full instruction. Children of this young age enjoy their aids and do not pull them off. It is the child who has not been given an aid till later in life who refuses to wear it since sound means nothing to him, not having been taught how to hear. The function of a hearing aid is to make sounds louder. The child must still go through the lengthy process of learning to hear the sounds which now reach him. A child with normal hearing starts this learning at once but does not produce speech until he has been listening to it for a year. The deaf child must therefore be expected to take a year from the time he is given a hearing aid before he starts to talk.

The child should be kept in a normal environment so that he is able to listen to speech all day long; with auditory training it will be found that his capacity to hear, as measured by audiometry, improves. Lip-reading should also be taught in order to fill in any gaps in his hearing and this may be combined with sign language, the signs being made near the mouth so that mouth and hand movements lie within the same field of vision. A patient trained in sign language alone is only able to communicate with other deaf individuals who also know the language. This limits his contacts, also encouraging intermarriage with the possibility of propagating further deaf children if the parents have an inherited form of deafness.

A child should be taught in an ordinary school if possible. This can often be achieved by means of a hearing aid and sitting him in the optimal position in the classroom. If specialized training is required he may need to be sent to a school for deaf children but outside school hours he ought to be in contact with normal children as much as possible. A child who becomes deaf after speech has been acquired should never be educated in a school for deaf children since his problems are very different from those with congenital deafness.

There may be the greatest difficulty in differentiating the moderately mentally handicapped child from the deaf child; for this reason all children who are sent to a school for the educationally subnormal should have their hearing tested. It should also be remembered that some children react with behaviour problems because they cannot hear normally. To add to the difficulties of diagnosis some children with behaviour problems who have normal hearing may appear not to hear, this also occurring in the juvenile psychoses, especially autism (p. 453), where the children live in a world of their own.

## THE LARYNX

### Acute laryngitis

Acute laryngitis is seldom an isolated condition in children but occurs either in association with infection of the upper respiratory tract or as laryngo-tracheo-bronchitis (p. 351). It produces a barking cough. The particular danger in infancy is respiratory obstruction since the laryngeal aperture is so small that swelling of the cords from infection may be sufficient to obstruct the larynx. Antibiotics are required and in older children some relief may be obtained from inhalations containing Tinct. Benzoin. Co.

### Acute spasmodic laryngitis (croup, laryngitis stridulosa)

This name is given to those cases of acute laryngitis which are associated with stridor from laryngeal spasm. The degree of laryngeal spasm is often out of proportion to the severity of the inflammation. The spasm occurs particularly at night and can be most alarming. The child, who is usually aged between 2 and 4 years, wakes up struggling for breath and may be intensely cyanosed.

The spasm is more likely to be found in nervous children and may come on several times during the night. Attacks are self-limiting, although they tend to recur, possibly because they are due to a number of different viruses.

The condition must be differentiated from acute epiglottitis (p. 336) which is a fulminating bacterial infection but also causes laryngeal obstruction.

*Treatment.* The child's main need is for sedation; antibiotics are often unnecessary. Antispasmodics such as salbutamol should be tried and a cold air humidifier is of value.

In those subject to the attacks, sedatives should be given at bed-time at the earliest sign of respiratory infection. The frequency of attacks in these susceptible children is sometimes reduced by giving the last meal of the day earlier than usual.

## Laryngismus stridulus

This term is applied to a condition of spasm of the glottis which lasts a few seconds and ends in a long crowing inspiration. It is a manifestation of rickets and is now very rare. In children with rickets it may be associated with tetany and convulsions, this combination being called spasmophilia (p. 561).

## Papilloma of the larynx

This is the commonest new growth of the larynx in children and causes hoarseness. The tumours are often multiple and are liable to recur after removal.

## Congenital laryngeal stridor (see p. 146)

## BIBLIOGRAPHY

JONES R.S.(1972) The management of acute croup. *Arch. Dis. Childh.*, **47**, 661.
KEVY S.V. (1964) Croup. *New Engl. J. Med.*, **270**, 464.
MOFFET H.L., SIEGEL A.C. & DOYLE H.K. (1968) Nonstreptococcal pharyngitis. *J. Ped.* **73**, 51.
PRATT L.L. & WINCHESTER R.A. (1963) Etiology of auditory defects. *J. Pediat.*, **62**, 245.
WHETNALL E. (1965) Deafness. *Brit. med. J.*, **1**, 362.

# CHAPTER 11

# DISORDERS OF THE LOWER RESPIRATORY TRACT

## Pneumonia

The clinical picture of pneumonia has altered with the introduction of anti-biotics and there are now advantages in considering lobar and broncho-pneumonia together, although bronchopneumonia is by far the more serious. Lobar pneumonia tends to strike the healthy child, is more common in older children, and is most often due to the pneumoccocus. Bronchopneumonia has the unpleasant characteristic of striking the child who is debilitated or already down with some other disease such as gastroenteritis, occurring most often under the age of 5 years. It is commonly due to a mixed infection with the streptococcus, staphyloccocus, pneumococcus and Friedlander's bacillus. The respiratory syncitial (RS) virus can be isolated from a high proportion of infants with lower respiratory tract infections of varying severity. In a study in Newcastle, about 60 per cent of severe respiratory infections in childhood were found to be due to the RS virus (Gardner *et al.*, 1964). In such cases an association with *Haemophilus influenzae* is common. Bronchopneumonia may also be a complication of the acute specific fevers, especially whooping cough and measles. Parental smoking doubles the risk of pneumonia or bronchitis in the first year of life (Colley *et al.*, 1974).

*Clinical features.* Pneumonia can be diagnosed from the end of the bed by the child's appearance. There may be no physical signs in the chest, conse-quently the use of the stethoscope is a positive handicap if its owner believes he must hear something wrong before he can diagnose pneumonia. The child looks ill and anxious, the cheeks may be flushed and the skin hot and dry, but if the infection is severe he will be ashen and probably sweating. Respirations are rapid, the alae nasi are working and there is a reversal of rhythm so that expiration is forcible and the pause follows inspiration. This results in the expiratory grunt which is so characteristic of pneumonia in children. This grunt is probably a protective reflex brought on by anoxia, causing a rise in intra-alveolar pressure so that oxygen exchange is assisted. In the really severe cases there is restlessness, due particularly to anoxia, the head is thrown back to improve the airway (p. 183), and the eyes become more prominent, probably from raised venous pressure.

The onset of infection may be very rapid, with a high fever, particularly if it is of the lobar type. In bronchopneumonia the onset is more insiduous and in the very ill child the temperature, far from being raised, may be subnormal. It must be emphasized that the temperature is of no diagnostic value, but it is an important guide to the clinical state and to therapy, determining whether the child requires warming or cooling. Cough may be very troublesome but no sputum will be brought up as this is swallowed by children. Neck stiffness, due to meningismus (p. 400) may accompany the onset of pneumonia in childhood, particularly if the infection is in the apex of the lung; it must be differentiated from meningitis.

The child may become drowsy or delirious and convulsions may occur, especially if the temperature is high. Cyanosis is an indication of severity, usually indicating that both lungs are involved. Herpes of the lips may be present, though this is less common in children than in adults.

If there are signs in the chest they will be fine râles (crepitations) indicating an alveolar lesion. These are best heard at the end of deep inspiration but may be obscured by coarse râles from fluid in the bronchioles or bronchi. Bronchospasm, indicated by rhonchi, is not a feature of pneumonia but may be caused by irritation from fluid in the bronchi. If the infection is localized to one lung the fine râles may be similarly localized, but localization is difficult to determine in children and one is often confounded by an X-ray which shows the lesion to be on the opposite side from that suggested by the signs. This is probably due to the ease with which sounds are transmitted in the child's chest.

A change in the percussion note usually indicates extensive lung involvement at one site and is therefore more likely to be detected in lobar rather than bronchopneumonia. Direct percussion over the clavicle should not be forgotten as this is of value in the diagnosis of apical pneumonia. If there is marked impairment of the percussion note an empyema should be suspected. Bronchial breathing will be present only if the pneumonia is extensive; it is more usual to find diminution in the breath sounds. An X-ray gives the final proof of pneumonia, the opacity seen being due to collapse as well as consolidation. This collapse results from blockage of the bronchioles by mucus and infected material which occurs much more easily in children because of the small diameter of their respiratory passages. It is unnecessary for every child with suspected pneumonia to be X-rayed as the diagnosis should be made on clinical grounds, treatment being started without delay. On the other hand, there is much to be said for X-raying all cases on recovery, particularly if this is delayed, in order to ensure that there is no residual collapse which might lead to bronchiectasis.

*Diagnosis.* In infancy, the greatest diagnostic difficulty lies in differentiating cardiac failure from pneumonia, since rapid breathing, excessive activity of the alae nasi and restlessness occur in both. The presence of a cardiac murmur is strong evidence in favour of cardiac failure but is not always present; the most useful sign of cardiac failure is enlargement of the liver. Some children with pneumonia develop secondary cardiac failure; if in doubt appropriate treatment for both conditions should be given.

A common error in diagnosis is for bronchitis or asthma to be called pneumonia but these do not cause the typical respirations of pneumonia. Meningismus raises the question of meningitis and a lumbar puncture will often be required for certain differentiation. Peritonitis, most commonly from appendicitis, may be a real difficulty since distressed or even grunting respirations may occur, but it should always be possible to elicit guarding or tenderness in the abdomen. Acute pyelonephritis may produce the same high temperature, hot dry skin and meningismus as is seen in classical lobar pneumonia but renal tenderness and direct microscopy of a specimen of urine should remove any doubt. Acute otitis media may produce an ill, distressed child with high fever but not with the respiratory signs, although the two conditions may well exist together.

If the response to antibiotic therapy in a case of pneumonia is not immediate the possibility of underlying lung disease, particularly cystic fibrosis and less often nowadays tuberculosis, should be suspected.

*Treatment*. Pneumonia, and particularly bronchopneumonia, still calls for very great nursing skill, though with modern antibiotics it is unnecessary for all cases to be sent to hospital. Most children are more comfortable when propped up, but the position adopted should be the one which gives greatest relief, and some prefer to be flat. Small babies particularly, who are so distressed that they have adopted the head back position, are better if they are assisted in taking up this posture.

*Feeds*. The calorie intake must be kept up but the child is unlikely to want solids and should not be forced with these. High-calorie fluids containing sugar and vitamin supplements are best; small babies, if distressed by bottle feeding, should be fed by tube. It is bad therapy to tire a baby by making him take a bottle and he is more liable to vomit if feeds are forced in this way.

*Oxygen* should be given if the child is cyanosed or restless, cyanosis being an absolute indication for hospital treatment. Although older children may tolerate a mask, the majority will require an oxygen tent. Nasal catheters are irritating to the nasal mucosa and should not be used. Dry oxygen is irritating also; it should be moistened before entering the tent. Cooling the oxygen by ice is traditional and correct if the child's temperature is high, but often a collapsed baby with a subnormal temperature is given cooled oxygen routinely while other attempts are being made to raise his temperature. Restlessness, though possibly due to the illness itself, is more often due to anoxia. Oxygen should therefore be given in high concentration; it may be necessary to have two cylinders on full flow in order to achieve a sufficient concentration in the tent. Access to the infant must be only through the sleeves in the tent, thus avoiding unnecessary loss of oxygen. If a child is anaemic, cyanosis is less obvious, or absent; if in doubt oxygen should always be given.

*Sedation.* The child must be made to sleep, phenobarbitone or chloral being given in adequate dosage if he is restless. However, as so much of the restlessness is due to anoxia, the effects of full oxygen therapy should first be observed for a few minutes since many children go off to sleep once they have been given this urgent therapy.

*Clothing.* This must be light, the child being neither overclothed nor over-heated. Unfortunately, there is a tradition among mothers which dies hard, that children with fever require heating. Mothers must be impressed with the need for preventing high temperatures, being encouraged to open the windows to the fresh air. Temperatures above 39·5° C should be brought down by tepid sponging. Small infants are most easily nursed naked in an incubator. They can be more easily observed and if collapsed can be more satisfactorily warmed.

*Specific therapy.* In the long run the choice of antibiotic is dependent on isolation of the causal bacteria and sensitivity tests. For immediate use, while awaiting these results, a combination of intramuscular benzylpenicillin and gentamycin is likely to be the wisest choice.

*Suction* may be a life-saving measure in babies whose small bronchi and bronchioles have become blocked with infected material. This line of treatment is often forgotten; all general practitioners should carry a suitable mucus catheter in their bags. Postural drainage and percussion for a few seconds at a time, combined with suction, are remarkably effective, though to those who have not practised them they may sound drastic and even dangerous. Surprisingly, however, babies tolerate this treatment well, the improvement in their colour, once the obstructing material has been removed, being dramatic. If the child is collapsed, and this occurs particularly in small babies, immediate ventilation is required. Digitalis should be used if there is evidence of heart failure.

It is in small babies that pneumonia is most lethal. A previously healthy child may even be found dead in bed, the diagnosis being made only on full histological examination of the lung (see p. 367).

### Staphylococcal pneumonia

This is a severe form of pneumonia, occurring particularly in infants (see also

p. 114). Primary staphyloccocal pneumonia occurs only in the first year of life; in older children and adults it is usually secondary to measles or influenza. In some areas it has become the most important pathogen causing pneumonia in children because of the effective antibiotic control of other causes and the emergence of resistant strains of the staphylococcus aureus. In newborn babies it may follow staphylococcal skin sepsis and may cause epidemics of pneumonia in maternity nurseries. Staphylococcal pneumonia is the commonest cause of pneumonia in infancy.

The onset is acute, the picture being that of a toxic infant with grey cyanosis and respiratory distress.

The particular feature of infection by the staphylococcus is its ability to destroy tissue and form pus. Destruction of lung tissue leads to lung abscesses. If the lesions are near the periphery of the lung there is erosion of the pleura resulting in a tension pneumothorax, empyema or pyopneumothorax. The lung abscesses tend to cavitate to form air cysts (pneumatocoeles) which, if the child recovers, usually disappear spontaneously (Fig. 103).

*Treatment.* The general management is the same as discussed on p. 346. The best choice of antibiotics is a combination of ampicillin and cloxacillin, thereby covering the possibility of a penicillin resistant organism. Amoxycillin is better absorbed from the intestine than ampicillin but is more expnesive. Flucloxacillin is similarly better absorbed than cloxacillin.

### Congenital pneumonia

This condition is discussed on p. 114.

### Acute bronchiolitis

This is an extremely acute respiratory infection, usually due to the respiratory syncitial virus, in which bronchial obstruction predominates. The disease particularly affects infants in the first year of life. The obstructive picture is due to the very small calibre of the bronchioles so that the inflammation, which causes mucosal swelling and exudate, results in obstruction at a very early stage in the illness. The disease is most common in winter and early spring and may occur in epidemic form. It appears to spread to infants from older members of the family who are suffering from a mild upper respiratory infection.

*Clinical features.* The clinical picture is similar to an acute pneumonia but with the emphasis on bronchial obstruction; this shows on the X-ray as pulmonary overdistension without evidence of collapse or consolidation. Within a few hours of the onset the infant is fighting for his breath, cyanosed and very bubbly, with an extremely distressing paroxysmal cough; there is

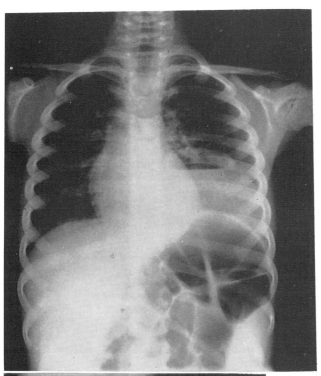
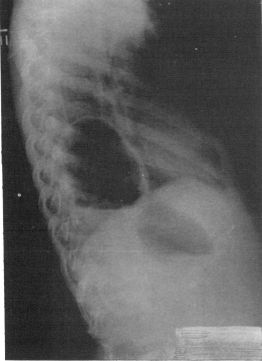

Fig. 103. PA and lateral films showing pneumatocoele in the left lower lobe. The fluid level results from pus within the air cyst.

seldom much fever. Differentiation from bronchopneumonia may not be easy and indeed the disease may proceed to that condition, but it forms a distinct clinical entity amongst the pneumonias of childhood.

*Treatment.* Although the response to antibiotics is poor, probably because the primary infection is a virus, these should always be given. A combination of benzylpenicillin and gentamycin given intramuscularly at first is a reasonable choice. Steroids are indicated if the baby is collapsed and there is some evidence that they may be of value in diminishing the inflammation in the bronchioles, thereby reducing the obstruction. Assisted ventilation may be needed. Digitalis is required for associated heart failure.

From the practical point of view it is essential to recognize and deal with the obstructive element by suction and by postural drainage with percussion, before commencing oxygen therapy. This should be repeated as often as necessary in order to achieve maximum patency of the bronchial tube.

Tracheostomy may be required in order to permit adequate bronchial suction. It is the baby with acute bronchiolitis whom the general practitioner is likely to find *in extremis* at home and tends immediately to put in his car and rush to hospital. But a few minutes spent first in suction at the home may make the difference between his bringing a live instead of a dead baby.

### Acute bronchitis

This is a diagnosis which should always be suspect until a full search has been carried out for underlying factors not at first obvious. Many children admitted with 'acute bronchitis' demonstrate after 1 or 2 days that this was part of the prodromal infection of one of the acute specific fevers, particularly whooping cough or measles. When a house physician has once incurred the wrath of his chief or ward sister for admitting such a child into the open ward he will remember in future that all cases exhibiting signs of acute bronchitis should be placed in a cubicle.

Acute bronchitis may occur whenever there is an underlying predisposing condition, the most important of which are congenital heart disease, bronchiectasis and cystic fibrosis. In previous times rickets was a common underlying cause but it is now rare, although the fat child previously subject to rickets, is still common and very likely to be 'chesty'.

The majority of parents of children with asthma give a history that when the attacks first occurred they were regarded as bronchitis. Bronchial asthma in the first year of life does not produce the typical attack of later years in which expiratory obstruction predominates.

A mother will often state that her baby 'cuts his teeth with bronchitis'. In many such cases, if a detailed history is taken, it will be found that the mother is describing not a child who is ill or off his food, but one with a wet type of cough from the excessive salivation accompanying the eruption of the teeth. A small number of babies do develop signs of bronchitis while cutting teeth and one can only assume that their resistance to infection is lowered at this time.

When all these underlying causes have been excluded, uncomplicated cases of acute bronchitis are found to be less frequent than is often realized. The illness may affect children of any age, being more common in those living in towns, especially slums, and in those who are habitually overclothed. Cough, fever and anorexia are the main symptoms but there is none of the constitutional disturbance of pneumonia, nor is there the severe obstructive element of acute bronchiolitis, although some degree of obstruction of the bronchi results from the accumulation of mucus and secondary bronchospasm. Infection and mucus in the bronchi are always likely to cause bronchospasm and this secondary spasm may dominate the clinical picture causing the distinct clinical entity of acute spasmodic bronchitis.

*Acute spasmodic bronchitis* ('Wheezy' bronchitis, asthmatic bronchitis). Wheezing is the chief feature but, unlike bronchial asthma, this is preceded for about two days by the cough and fever of acute bronchitis. The bronchospasm of bronchial asthma develops suddenly out of the blue. The term 'asthmatic bronchitis' for these patients is unsatisfactory and misleading. The condition has nothing to do with asthma and its prognosis is quite different; for this reason the term asthmatic bronchitis, which alarms parents, should be discarded.

Acute spasmodic bronchitis is more often found in fat children (Hutchinson-Smith, 1970). It tends to recur but the majority of children grow out of it by the time they are seven. The possibility that milk allergy is a factor should always be considered (p. 85).

*Treatment.* A wide spectrum antibiotic should be given and plenty of postural drainage combined with percussion and suction. Oxygen is needed if the child is cyanosed but this is not usually the case. Salbutamol is a satisfactory antispasmodic to relieve bronchospasm and has the advantage over ephedrine that it is less likely to produce tachycardia. A steam tent, with its risk of burns, should no longer be used. Mothers still like to rub camphorated oil into the chests of such children but this is liable to produce folliculitis of the skin and should be discouraged.

### Acute laryngo-tracheo-bronchitis

This condition mainly affects children under the age of 5 years, particularly those from 6 months to 2 years. Bacteriological studies have failed to show any uniform picture and the *Haemophilus influenzae*, haemolytic streptococci and staphylococci which have been isolated are probably secondary invaders.

The respiratory syncitial virus is probably the primary infection in a high proportion of cases.

The clinical picture is one of acute respiratory obstruction, although signs of a respiratory infection may have preceded this for 1–2 days. This obstruction results from a combination of viscid secretion and small air passages; death results from mechanical suffocation. If the child survives more than about 4 days bronchopneumonia usually develops.

*Treatment.* The urgent need for these infants is an adequate airway. Suction through the mouth is usually ineffectual, whereas tracheostomy is often life-saving, not only improving the airway but making adequate suction possible. Moist air in a tent is needed but not oxygen, since a lack of oxygen indicates the need for tracheostomy. A combination of intramuscular benzyl-penicillin and gentamycin should be given, pending bacterial results.

### Chronic bronchitis

The majority of children who are described as suffering from chronic bronchitis are in fact having recurrent attacks of acute bronchitis and in this respect there is a similarity with infection of the appendix. Any of the predisposing causes of acute bronchitis already described can produce these recurrent attacks but sinus infection and bronchiectasis are the particular offenders and may exist together.

### Sinobronchitis

So common is the association of sinus infection and recurrent bronchitis that the term sinobronchitis has been introduced. Sinobronchitis occurs most often in those living in towns, especially if there is overcrowding and poor ventilation. Malnutrition is not a factor, many of the patients being overweight. The symptoms occur mainly in the winter and consist of recurrent colds and coughs. The usual description given by the mother is that the child keeps catching colds and these always go down on to the chest.

Characteristically the cough is brought on by changes in posture and especially occurs on running, lying down in bed and getting up from the bed. This is due to mucus and pus trickling down the back of the throat where it causes irritation and consequent coughing bouts. This mucopus may be seen on the posterior wall of the nasopharynx during the examination of the throat, especially if the child is made to gag by touching the soft palate with the spatula; mucopus is then squeezed down into view. During the night this material may pass down the respiratory tract into the bronchioles, thereby leading to lobular collapse (Fig. 104) and the risk of bronchiectasis. The ease with which this journey is made can be well demonstrated by the insertion of lipiodol into a child's nose at night; in the morning it will be found in the bronchi.

Many of the children with sinobronchitis keep their mouths open, a condition often described as the 'adenoidal facies'. This is an inaccurate title since it suggests that the facial expression results from enlarged adenoids whereas the adenoidal hypertrophy is often secondary to the mouth being kept open. Skeletal pattern is constant, therefore large adenoids cannot affect the shape of the maxilla or cause 'adenoidal facies'. Many factors are involved in the

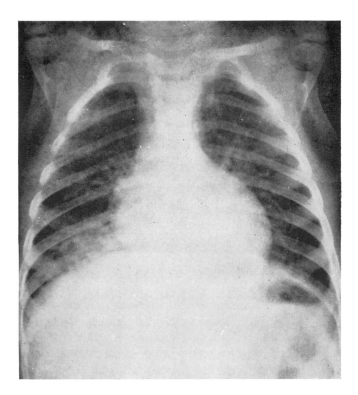

FIG. 104. Bilateral basal lobular collapse, mainly on the right, in a child with sinobronchitis.

production of this open-mouth habit. In infancy it is normal for the mouth to be kept slightly open, the infantile upper lip being bowed upwards in comparison with the straight upper lip of the older child (Fig. 105). It is this which accounts for the greater frequency of dribbling in infancy. Redness of the chin may result but this can be prevented by a barrier cream.

The change from the infantile pattern usually occurs during the second year. Persistence of this pattern may be genetically determined and the mother may be seen to have a similarly shaped mouth. Dental malocclusion may also be present and in order to achieve an adequate lip seal in swallowing, the tongue may be thrust between the teeth. This tongue-thrusting movement can cause progressive forward protrusion of the incisors. A stage may be reached in which incompetence of mouth closure is so great that during swallowing the lower lip has to be brought up to fill the gap between the teeth. Persistent thumb-sucking aggraves this deformity. During the years of facial development up to puberty there is also a tendency in the opposite direction to close the bite and improve the situation.

The adenoids may be enlarged but the whole mouth structure must be assessed to determine the part they are playing. It is incorrect to consider enlarged adenoids as the cause of the problem in every child who keeps his mouth open. The adenoids enlarge from repeated infection, but an abnormal mouth pattern and incorrect breathing habits may be the primary cause of such enlargement. Breathing tests with cotton wool should be made to decide whether the breathing is nasal, oral or a mixture of both. Only a minority of

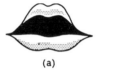 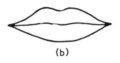

(a) (b)

FIG. 105. Normal lip pattern at different age periods.
(a) Infant. The mouth is open.
(b) Older child. The mouth is now closed.

those with an open-mouth habit are found to be mouth breathers, because a seal is formed between tongue and teeth instead of between the lips.

*Treatment.* A combined approach is required from the otologist, orthodontic surgeon, paediatrician, speech therapist and physiotherapist. Ideally, these specialists should work together in a combined clinic. If the adenoids are enlarged and obstruct the nasal passages they should be removed; this is only the beginning of the treatment programme, though it often constitutes the only treatment given so that the child is only temporarily improved. Once a satisfactory airway has been achieved the child should be taught by the physiotherapist to breathe correctly; if speech is affected the help of the speech therapist is required. If the adenoidal obstruction is incomplete, it is worth trying nasal drops of 0·5 per cent ephedrine in normal saline given three times a day for a few weeks in order to shrink the oedematous tissues sufficiently to permit correction of breathing habits, thus breaking the vicious circle. The drops must be correctly applied if they are to be effective. The head should be back and to one side, 3–4 drops being placed in the lower nostril. If the child is old enough he should be asked to sniff up while a finger lightly compresses the other nostril. This is repeated for the other side after the position of the head has been changed, and finally, with the head held far back in the median position, the child sniffs up for 2 minutes. Only by these means are the drops carried throughout the nasal passages. Maxillary antrum washouts are now seldom performed.

Many of these children have a poor posture with lordosis and rounded shoulders; this can be improved by postural exercises given in addition to the breathing exercises. Postural drainage and percussion are also required if pulmonary collapse has occurred following the aspiration of mucus from the nasopharynx, or if any moist sounds are heard in the bronchi.

The treatment of sinobronchitis is essentially mechanical; expectorant mixtures are useless. Antibiotics are indicated only if there is an acute episode of infection, being then an adjuvant to the basic mechanical methods.

**Bronchial asthma**

This condition occurs more often in boys than girls and its incidence is increasing. This increase is in part related to the faster pace of modern life with its accompanying stresses and strains which are conveyed from the parents to their children. The greater scholastic demand made on children today is also a factor. The basic feature of children with asthma is that they have inherited bronchi which are more labile than normal so that spasm of bronchial smooth muscle occurs more easily.

*Aetiology*. Three factors can act as triggers for the attacks: allergy, which is often inherited, emotion and infection. One factor only may be present in a single patient but more often it is a combination of factors, especially allergy and emotion.

Evidence for the allergic factor is the manifestation of some other allergic disorder by the patient, eczema being the most common, or by other members of the family. The common disorders present in the family are asthma itself, eczema and hay fever. It will often be found that the patient had eczema as a baby; residual eczematous lesions in the flexures of the knees and elbows may persist for many years. The natural history of eczema and asthma in the same patient is of interest; it is frequently found that they bear an inverse relationship to each other so that when one relapses the other improves. The frequency of hay fever in the patient or his family is not surprising since it indicates hypersensitivity of the upper respiratory tract whereas asthma indicates a similar sensitivity of the lower respiratory tract. In some children the attack of asthma may be preceded by allergic rhinitis which is the same as hay fever. Most important is sensitivity to the housedust mite. This microscopic animal lives on shed human skin and prefers humid, warm and dark living conditions. It is found in all houses except those previously unoccupied, thereby providing an explanation for the temporary reduction in attacks experienced by sensitive patients when moving to a newly-built house. Sensitivity is caused by dead mites as well as live and also by their droppings. The bedroom mattress and bedding produce ideal living conditions for the mite, hence sensitive patients commonly develop attacks at night. Sensitivity to pets may be due to the impregnation of their fur or feathers with house-mites. Sensitivity to the pet itself is due to allergy to its skin scales rather than to its hair. Short-haired animals are more liable to cause allergy than those with long hair.

In asthma the majority of allergic stimuli enter the body by inhalation rather than ingestion so that it is unusual for asthma to result from eating something to which the patient is sensitive. The reverse is true of urticaria. A seasonal history suggests the likelihood of pollen as the allergen, whereas the house-dust mite is the likely factor if attacks come on in bed.

The emotional factor is seen in the psychological make-up of these patients who are commonly nervous, disturbed children, often described by their parents as being unduly sensitive. They are often introspective, this state usually having been brought on by the parents, one or both of whom are likely to be over-anxious. It is because of this relationship that many children with asthma are free of their attacks when away from home and why many improve in boarding school. Their intelligence is above average (Mitchell & Dawson, 1973), this being understandable since such emotional interplay would be unlikely in the duller members of the community. The relative rarity of asthma in backward children emphasizes the importance of emotional factors in its aetiology.

If infection is a factor it is commonly viral.

*Clinical features.* The attack comes on suddenly, bronchospasm causing acute respiratory obstruction with greater difficulty in expiration than in-spiration. This difficulty has been graphically described by an asthmatic patient who remarked: 'If ever I get rid of this breath I shall never take an-other one!' The mothers of young children with asthma are seldom able to say whether inspiration or expiration is the more difficult, though clinical exami-nation demonstrates the difference. Bronchospasm results in an audible wheeze, prolongation of expiration and rhonchi which are audible in both phases of respiration, though more marked on expiration. In some children the onset of an attack is heralded by a running nose due to allergic rhinitis which the mother commonly describes as a 'cold'. This differs from the com-mon cold in that the nasal discharge is persistently clear and there is no history of coryza in other members of the family. In a severe attack the child becomes cyanosed and very frightened, thereby causing a vicious circle of increasing respiratory distress. Typically, exercise induces wheezing in children with asthma.

Bronchospasm usually stops as abruptly as it started, but the asthmatic attack itself tails off rather than having a sudden end. One reason for this is that secretions become retained in the narrowed bronchi and must be coughed away before the lungs are clear. These accumulated secretions cause an alteration in the adventitious sounds from the chest which commence with an audible wheeze and change to a rattle. It is this development of moist sounds which leads mothers to describe the attack of asthma as being followed by 'bronchitis', though in reality this is nothing more than the retention of mucus consequent upon bronchospasm.

In infancy, asthma is often not suspected at first, the attacks being thought to be recurrent attacks of bronchitis because the difficulty in breathing is less predominantly expiratory than in the older child. But because they are recurrent, short and not associated with any appreciable fever, unless they have lasted for a long time, asthma should be suspected.

*Investigations.* The history will point to the likelihood of a specific allergic cause and this can be checked by skin testing. Skin tests are not undertaken before the age of 4 years since antibodies have not become fixed in the tissues before then. A rise in IgE is found in those with an allergic cause.

Eosinophilia in the sputum or blood indicates allergy whereas polymorphs in the sputum are found in cases of infective origin. The severity of airways obstruction can be measured by respiratory function tests which are compared with the predicted normal values; these tests are also of help in assessing the effect of treatment.

*Treatment.* This comprises measures to prevent attacks and the treatment of the acute attack. The aim is to remove any increased airways resistance.

*General management.* Precipitating factors must be avoided or neutralized and perfect chest shape maintained. Particularly important are measures to reduce exposure to the housedust mite since this is the most common allergen. The child should be out of the room, and ideally out of the house, when the bed is made. The mattress should be vacuumed daily and turned weekly. Whenever possible the bedclothes should be shaken outside every day as well as being washed frequently. Feather pillows and eiderdowns should be removed, pillows of kapok or rubber being substituted. Damp dusting should be the rule. The bedroom should be kept dry but not with a paraffin heater since this gives off water. One reason for the common improvement of asthmatic patients on admission to hospital may be the reduced population of mites in wards from frequent changes of bedding and a relative absence of curtains and upholstered furniture.

The possibility of pets being an allergic factor should be tested by their temporary removal before any more drastic steps are taken.

The majority of children improve as they grow older, but it is essential to prevent the chest deformity which is liable to result from emphysema (Fig. 106). This causes a pigeon-shaped chest and poor respiratory excursion,

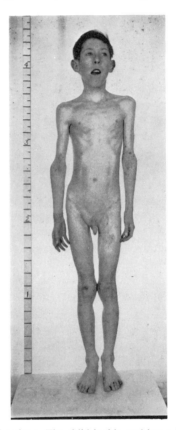

FIG. 106. Bronchial asthma. The child is thin and has a barrel-shaped chest from emphysema. Eczematous lesions are visible in the elbow flexures and groins. A right inguinal hernia is present.

breathing being largely diaphragmatic. If this occurs, the child will suffer from repeated chest infections throughout life even though asthma may have ceased. Physiotherapy is therefore a basic part of the treatment of all children with asthma. The children, with their mothers, are taught breathing and postural exercises, the mothers learning how to carry out postural drainage and percussion. These manœuvres should be carried out at least twice a day in the home, but when the mother is proficient, attendance at the physio-therapy clinic is required for occasional supervision only. Postural drainage and percussion are carried out during an attack in order to prevent the accum-ulation of secretions which otherwise occurs, provided the child is not dis-tressed by the treatment. By this means the attack can be cut short since there are no retained secretions to be coughed away when bronchospasm has ceased. Children should not be expected to cough up the sputum since they naturally swallow it, but this is almost as satisfactory since the bronchi are cleared.

An explanation should be given to patients that asthma is a liability with which you are either born or not, there being no 'cure'. Such instruction prevents parents from searching hopelessly for a cure and helps them to understand the methods of treatment which are aimed at keeping down the attacks. It gives them an added incentive for carrying out physiotherapy which should be continued for 1 year after the last attack. It is likely that there is a psychogenic element in the remarkable improvement brought about by physiotherapy, the parents having at last been given something positive which they can do to help their child. It should be emphasized that physiotherapy is not being tried out as one possible line of therapy but rather that the breathing methods taught should become a way of life for the child. He should be told to breathe as instructed whenever the opportunity arises, not only during the formal daily periods of exercises. In this way he may find he can cut short an attack when he feels it coming on.

It is important that the parents should not treat the child as an invalid nor overclothe him. Removal to a boarding school as practised in the past should seldom be necessary. If there are severe emotional factors, psychotherapy may be required.

Desensitization is available to many of the allergens including the housedust mite, but in all cases the effect of evasive measures should first be determined.

Disodium cromoglycate can prevent attacks of allergic asthma by inhibiting the release of histamine which follows the combination of antibody with allergen. It is of no value in the treatment of attacks. The drug is given as a powder which is inhaled through a spinhaler four times daily. This requires co-operation and is therefore not suited to very young children. By inhaling the drug half an hour before taking exercise a child can often take part in games which were previously impossible for him.

*The individual attack.* The attack should be treated vigorously from the start by bronchodilator drugs. Many parents think they should attempt to 'harden' their children by withholding drugs but this is totally incorrect. Salbutamol is possibly the best drug for routine use and has the advantage over ephedrine of not producing tachycardia. Orciprenaline is also satis-factory in this respect.

Intravenous aminophylline is effective but must be used with great caution as it can cause cardiac arrest. It can be given more safely as a suppository but its administration by this route must be equally clearly recorded lest later intravenous aminophylline is considered. Subcutaneous adrenaline is effective but, being an injection, should be avoided as the patient may become dependent on injections. For the same reason inhalers are best avoided.

If the attack is preceded by allergic rhinitis this may be prevented by nasal inhalation of sodium cromoglycolate.

Antibiotics are indicated only if a definite infection is present. The mere finding of a rise in temperature in an asthmatic attack is not sufficient indication since the increased muscular activity alone may produce a fever.

As far as possible the child should be treated at home since, although the attack usually stops as soon as he is moved to hospital, the next time one occurs he may have additional fear from the possibility of being sent to hospital.

*Status asthmaticus.* Death from asthma can no longer be regarded as rare; when this does occur the child is usually in status asthmaticus. The major cause of death is bronchial plugging leading to acute anoxia, rather than infection. An ominous sign in status asthmaticus is an absence of wheezing since this is indicative of minimal air entry. Plugging of the bronchi is due to the thick viscid secretion, the cause of which is still unknown. To reduce the thickness of this secretion the inspired air should be moistened.

One of the reasons for the present increase in the number of deaths from status asthmaticus is that most children today have already received intensive therapy with antispasmodics, often by aerosol, before admission to hospital so that they may unwittingly be given lethal doses of these. The greatest danger comes from aminophylline which, if used correctly, is a most valuable drug but in high dosage is toxic. If there is no response to a full dose of aminophylline it must not be repeated. A combination of isoprenaline, adrenaline and ephedrine can be lethal. For the child at home in status asthmaticus, who is about to be moved to hospital, the safest and best drug to give is 50–100 mg hydrocortisone intramuscularly.

Children in status asthmaticus develop a respiratory acidosis. This must be recognized and corrected by intravenous therapy. It is essential that the child is kept fully hydrated. The use of a respirator giving intermittent positive pressure may be life saving.

*Steroids and ACTH in asthma.* There are few subjects which cause more heated arguments than the place of steroids in the management of children with asthma. The value of short-term steroids in the treatment of status asthmaticus is definite. The problem largely relates to their long-term prophylactic use and the side effects produced, particularly suppression of growth.

The advantage of corticotrophin over corticosteroids in this respect is discussed on p. 279, so that if this type of therapy is needed for long periods ACTH is the drug to use.

The selection of cases for long-term steroid therapy must be made with great care. The child who is having repeated attacks, developing increasing chest deformity and whose pulmonary ventilation studies show diminished function, is an obvious candidate if he is not responding to other measures, including physiotherapy. The change in such children, both physically and emotionally, is remarkable once steroids are given. The dose used is the lowest which will continue to control the disease. Physiotherapy must be continued while the child is on steroids.

### Bronchiectasis and pulmonary collapse

Bronchiectasis results from blockage of a bronchus; experiments have shown that dilatation of the wall occurs within a few hours of the onset of bronchial

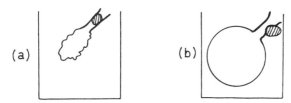

FIG. 107. The different results of complete and partial obstruction.
(a) Bronchus completely obstructed by a plug of mucus or foreign body. The air is then absorbed, leading to total collapse of the lobe beyond.
(b) Partial obstruction by tuberculous gland. Under these circumstances more air enters the lobe than is able to leave, resulting in obstructive emphysema.

obstruction. Once the bronchus has been obstructed no more air enters the segment of lung affected which therefore collapses from absorption of the air within (Fig. 107). Since the lungs are contained in the vacuum of the thorax something must dilate to take up the space formerly occupied by the collapsed portion of lung. This dilatation affects the bronchi leading to the collapsed lung. Provided the obstruction is removed rapidly the bronchi can return to their former size, but stasis leads to infection so that, if the obstruction persists, bronchial infection occurs, the dilatation then possibly becoming permanent.

Bronchial obstruction must be complete for the lung to collapse. Incomplete obstruction leads to obstructive emphysema since under these circumstances more air enters the lung on inspiration than comes out on expiration, the affected part becoming increasingly distended (Fig. 107b). This condition results mainly from obstruction outside the bronchus, particularly the pressure of tuberculous glands. When the obstruction is within the bronchus the obstructing object, which is most often a plug of mucus, is carried down to a point in the smaller bronchi where it completely fills the lumen. Obstruction by an irregularly shaped foreign body such as a peanut might not be expected to block the lumen completely, but this will soon occur from secondary oedema and inflammation of the wall around the obstruction. In such cases,

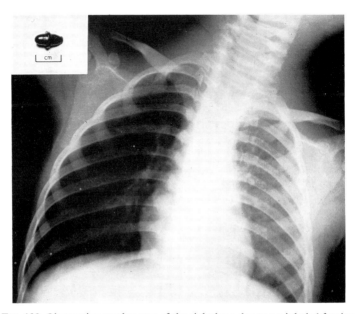

FIG. 108. Obstructive emphysema of the right lung due to an inhaled foreign body which was not radiopaque. The right lung is overfilled with air and therefore more translucent than the normal left lung. Inset shows the solitaire bead removed at bronchoscopy from the right main bronchus.

obstructive emphysema may be the first result (Fig. 108) but, if the foreign body is not removed at once, complete pulmonary collapse follows.

In addition, in the case of the peanut there is chemical irritation from the arachis oil. Peanuts should be forbidden to young children.

In children, the common causes of pulmonary collapse, and therefore of bronchiectasis, are sinobronchitis, ill-defined lower respiratory tract infections in infancy and the acute specific fevers, particularly whooping cough and measles; asthma is also a cause. In all these conditions the collapse results from blockage of the bronchus by a plug of mucus or mucopus. Another cause of blockage within a bronchus is a foreign body (Fig 109). Blockage from without results from enlarged mediastinal glands which in the majority of cases are tuberculous. Cystic fibrosis (p. 167) also causes bronchiectasis.

*Clinical features.* The symptoms of pulmonary collapse are largely those of the condition causing the collapse. Recession of soft parts is seldom apparent unless there is obstruction to a main bronchus causing a large part of the lung to be collapsed. Bronchiectasis should be suspected in all cases of persistent collapse, though a certain diagnosis can be made only by bronchography. The old-world picture of bronchiectasis causing a swinging fever, foul

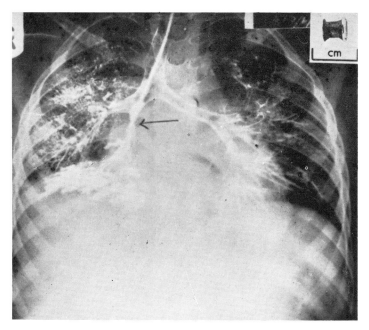

Fig. 109. Bronchogram in a boy aged 6 years showing stenosis of the right lower main branch of the right bronchus. There is collapse and bronchiectasis of the right middle and lower lobes. Inset shows the metal stud, coughed up a few weeks previously, which was presumably the cause of the stenosis.

sputum and clubbing is no longer true for the majority of affected children. The condition should be suspected in any child with a persistent and unexplained cough, especially in those with recurrent bronchitis and where râles are constantly audible in one site.

A bronchogram is necessary for the diagnosis of bronchiectasis but collapse is diagnosed from the plain X-ray (Fig. 104). In the radiological diagnosis of minor degrees of collapse particular attention should be paid to the line of the vascular markings. Normal vascular markings radiate progressively outwards from the hilum, whereas if the lung is collapsed they become closer together and even parallel. Lateral X-rays are unnecessary for localizing segmental collapse since Hodson (1956) has described a technique using the postero-anterior view. In this view the lesions seen can be localized if use is made of the interlobar septa and the outlines of the mediastinum, diaphragm and chest wall.

*Treatment.* The obstructed bronchus must be cleared as rapidly as possible and, if there is any possibility of a foreign body, bronchoscopy should be carried out as an emergency. The increased likelihood of a foreign body as a cause of bronchial obstruction in children must always be remembered. Fragments of peanuts or any object such as a marble which the child may have put in his mouth may be inhaled. The results of bronchoscopic suction of mucus and mucopus are not encouraging except when carried out early in post-operative cases. For the others it is a matter of very vigorous physiotherapy using postural drainage and breathing exercises. Postural drainage must be combined with percussion since the old method of merely leaving the child to sleep on a tipping board is relatively ineffective and is uncomfortable for the child.

The treatment of bronchiectasis is primarily preventive by the early diagnosis and treatment of collapse. Ideally, every child with whooping cough, measles or pneumonia should have an X-ray shortly after the infection to make sure there is no residual collapse. If bronchiectasis is present the first treatment is medical, consisting of intensive physiotherapy and antibiotics; by these means some or all of the dilated bronchi may be returned to their normal size. Surgery is indicated once the greatest improvement has been obtained by medical means, but when possible is postponed till after adolescence. Consequently, bronchograms are now carried out much less frequently and are largely only used once surgery is being contemplated in order to determine the extent of the disease. The operation is then one of selective lobulectomy rather than lobectomy.

**Idiopathic pulmonary haemosiderosis**
This is a rare condition, largely confined to children, which usually commences within the first 2 years of life. The underlying disorder is recurrent alveolar haemorrhage, followed by fibrosis. The condition is unrelated to generalized haemosiderosis. The cause is unknown, except that some of the children have associated symptoms of cow's milk allergy and recover completely when taken off milk.

The clinical picture is one of recurrent attacks of dyspnoea and cyanosis associated with cough, tachycardia and haemoptysis. Abdominal pain and vomiting are common; the vomit and the stools are likely to contain swallowed blood from the lungs. Each attack lasts several days and during this time the child develops increasing pallor and signs of right heart failure. Jaundice frequently develops before the end of the attack.

Between attacks the child fails to thrive but chest signs are minimal, in striking contrast to the usual finding in the chest X-ray. This shows scattered blotchy shadows which are transient and worse during an attack, slowly developing miliary reticulation in the middle and lower zones. The large acute shadows are multiple small haemorrhages, the reticulation resulting from the deposition of haemosiderin. Despite these findings it must be pointed out that the chest film may be normal when the patient is first seen.

*Treatment.* There is no satisfactory treatment though improvement has been reported with immuno-suppressive drugs (Steiner & Nabrady, 1965). This is worth a trial but the fact that spontaneous remissions occur makes assessment of its value difficult. The outlook is very bad, many of the children dying within 3 years of the onset.


## DISEASES OF THE PLEURA

### Pleurisy

In cases of pneumonia, the pleura overlying the area of lung involved is usually inflamed. This may cause pain in the chest on deep breathing or, if the diaphragmatic pleura is involved, the pain is referred to the shoulder on the same side. Dry pleurisy, as described in adults, is not a common condition in children and a pleural rub is rare. In most instances where a pleural rub is suspected the sound is due to a coarse inspiratory and expiratory rhonchus and can be differentiated by its clearance or alteration on coughing.


### Epidemic pleurodynia (epidemic myalgia, Bornholm disease)

This condition may affect children of any age after infancy and is due to a Group B Coxsackie virus. It usually occurs in epidemics, causing acute pain in the chest and abdomen associated with tenderness of the affected muscles, fever and often headache. Isolated cases may occur but diagnosis is not easy in the absence of an epidemic. Relapses are likely up to 2 weeks from the onset, this feature being of diagnostic value. Pleurisy is simulated and occasionally a pleural rub may be heard, though this is not usually a feature of the disease.

The condition may be complicated by other manifestations of Coxsackie infection such as aseptic meningitis (p. 404), pericarditis (p. 377) and orchitis (p. 645). It may also be the primary source of infection starting an epidemic of neonatal myocarditis in a maternity nursery (see p. 376).

*Treatment.* There is no specific therapy, but symptomatic treatment is required for the relief of pain. Complete recovery always occurs.

### Pleural effusion

A serous pleural effusion is uncommon in childhood, resulting in most cases from tuberculosis. It also occurs in association with the gross oedema of nephrosis and in severe cardiac failure. Very occasionally a pleural effusion occurs in cases of collagen disease.

The most valuable clinical feature is an impaired percussion note. Alteration of the breath sounds is very variable in childhood because they are so well conducted from the other side. Mediastinal shift will be obvious with a large collection of fluid. The diagnosis is made from the X-ray but the type of fluid can be determined only by pleural tap.

### Empyema

Purulent pleural effusion is more common than serous, occurring most often in association with pneumonia. This particularly occurs in staphylococcal pneumonia in young children (see p. 347) and may be present when the child is first seen. In others the empyema is a sequel to pneumonia.

Signs of an empyema are less clear cut than in adults, mediastinal shift seldom being obvious. The condition must be suspected in all children with pneumonia showing obvious impairment of percussion note, usually at the bases. Diminution or absence of breath sounds is usual but occasionally the breath sounds are bronchial. An X-ray will usually decide whether an effusion is present but only the diagnostic tap will determine that this is purulent. In all cases, whether the diagnosis is in doubt or not, an exploratory tap should be made, using a needle of a size sufficient to allow the passage of thick pus.

*Treatment.* This requires antibiotics and drainage. The pus should be sent for culture and bacterial sensitivity, though treatment should start without awaiting the results. Adequate drainage in children can usually be achieved through an intercostal tube, rib resection being seldom required. It is usual to instil penicillin into the empyema cavity, although its value is debated.

### Pneumothorax

In childhood this condition occurs most often in association with pneumonia especially staphylococcal, and is usually a pyo-pneumothorax. It is rare for tuberculosis to produce an empyema in childhood. Uncomplicated pneumothorax results from the rupture of an emphysematous bulla and may occur during whooping cough or an attack of asthma. Surgical emphysema may also occur under such circumstances. In infancy, a pneumothorax may result from damage to the lungs during a difficult delivery and it is being increasingly recognized in association with the respiratory distress syndrome of the new-born (p. 64).

Spontaneous pneumothorax is more common in the newborn that at any other period of life. It may occur not only in association with the respiratory distress syndrome but as a primary condition causing respiratory distress (p. 67), emphasizing again the need for routine chest films in all such cases. The cause of spontaneous pneumothorax is alveolar rupture in association with atelectasis; in newborn infants with atelectasis the diaphragm has sufficient mechanical advantage to cause higher pressures across those alveoli which are aerated.

In infants with respiratory distress the diagnosis is unlikely to be made until the routine chest film is taken, although the shift of the apex beat is a valuable clinical sign. In older children with pneumonia or empyema the primary condition will overshadow the signs of the pneumothorax.

*Treatment.* If much of the lung has been collapsed a needle should be in-serted without delay and the air aspirated. Drainage by means of an under-water seal should then be arranged in combination with continuous suction.

## COT DEATHS

Every year a number of young babies, mainly aged 1–6 months, are found dead in their cots. The inclusion of this subject in the section on respiratory disorders is only because some of them are found to have died of an over-whelming respiratory infection; this could explain the higher incidence during the winter. Sutton & Emery (1966) have shown a close correlation between the unexpected deaths in infancy in Sheffield during 1961–64 and the in-cidence of respiratory illness in the community, especially during epidemics of influenza. The cause in the majority of cases is not known; in a few a previously unrecognized congenital malformation of the heart is discovered at autopsy. Most newborn babies are obligatory nasal breathers. It is possible that sudden nasal obstruction from an upper respiratory infection could be the cause of death (Cross & Lewis, 1971). Poor environment plays a part since the condition occurs more often in overcrowded homes and in families who are at socio-economic disadvantage.

In the past, the cause of death was often ascribed to overlying, but it is no longer believed that a healthy baby can be suffocated in this way since he will always struggle successfully to achieve an airway.

There is a greater incidence of cot deaths among babies who are artificially fed as compared to breast fed. This could be because the mother who breast feeds her baby is likely to be a different type from the mother who immediately puts her baby on a bottle. Breast feeding is more commonly practised by the professional classes than by those in the lower social classes and cot deaths occur more often among the babies of poorer mothers. Another possibility put forward by Parish *et al.* (1960) is that some of the deaths in artificially fed infants are due to modified anaphylactic shock from aspiration of cow's milk regurgitated during sleep by infants sensitized to it. This theory is backed by experimental work in guinea-pigs but, since most infants fed on cow's milk develop antibodies to it, the significance is not yet clear.

The parents need special help in order relieve them as much as possible of their inevitable feelings of guilt. A full clinical history should be taken as for any other patient. In another room the doctor will make a complete clinical examination and take appropriate bacterial and viral specimens, including the cerebrospinal fluid. This is important for research and is also therapeutic for the parents, being very different from just referring them to the coroner's officer. Arrangements should be made for them to be seen the next day by the same doctor, ideally with a social worker experienced in this field who will provide on-going care.

## BIBLIOGRAPHY

CARPENTER R.G. & SHADDICK C.W. (1965) Role of infection, suffocation and breast feeding in cot death. *Brit. J. prev. soc. Med.*, **19**, 1.

COLLEY J.R.T., HOLLAND W.W. & CORKHILL R.T. (1974). Influence of passive smoking and parental phlegm on pneumonia and bronchitis in early childhood. *Lancet*, **2**, 1032.

COOKE R.T. & WELCH R.G. (1964) A study in cot death. *Brit. med. J.*, **2**, 1549.

CROSS K.W. & LEWIS S.R. (1971) Upper respiratory obstruction and cot death. *Arch. Dis. Childh.*, **46**, 211.

FROGGATT P., LYNAS M.A. & MACKENZIE G. (1971) Epidemiology of sudden unexpected death in infants ('Cot death') in Northern Ireland. *Brit. J. prev. soc. Med.*, **25**, 119.

GARDNER P.S., ELDERKIN F.M. & WALL A.H. (1964) Serological study of respiratory syncitial virus infections in infancy and childhood. *Brit. med. J.*, **2**, 1570.

HODSON C.J. (1956) The localization of pulmonary collapse-consolidation. *J. Fac. Radiol.* (Lond.), **8**, 41.

HOLZEL A., PARKER L., PATTERSON W.H., CARTMEL D., WHITE L.L.R., PURDY R., THOMPSON K.M. & TOBIN J.O'H. (1965) Virus isolations from throats of children admitted to hospital with respiratory and other diseases, Manchester, 1962–64. *Brit. med. J.*, **1**, 614.

HORN M.E.C. & GREGG I. (1973) Role of viral infection and host factors in acute episodes of asthma and chronic bronchitis. *Chest*, **63**, 44 S.

HUTCHINSON-SMITH B. (1970) The relationship between the weight of an infant and lower respiratory infection. *Medical Officer*, **123**, 257.

HUXTABLE K.A. & WEDGWOOD R.J. (1964) Staphylococcal pneumonia in childhood. *Amer. J. Dis. Child.*, **108**, 262.

JOHNSTONE J.M. & LARVY H.S. (1966) Role of infection in cot deaths. *Brit. med. J.*, **1**, 706.

JONES R.S. & BLACKHALL M.I. (1970) Role of disodium cromoglycate ('Intal') in treatment of childhood asthma. *Arch. Dis. Childh.*, **45**, 49.

MITCHELL R.G. & DAWSON B. (1973) Educational and social characteristics of children with asthma. *Arch. Dis. Childh.*, **48,** 467.

PARISH W.E., BARRETT A.M., COOMBS R.R.A., GUNTHER M. & CAMPS F.E. (1960) Hypersensitivity to milk and unexpected death. *Lancet*, **2,** 1106.

PINKERTON P. (1967) Correlating physiologic with psycho-dynamic data in the study and management of childhood asthma. *J. Psychosom. Res.*, **11,** 11.

RICHARDS W. & PATRICK J.R. (1965) Death from asthma in children. *Amer. J. Dis. Child.*, **110,** 4.

ROONEY J.C. & WILLIAMS H.E. (1971) The relationship between proved viral bronchiolitis and subsequent wheezing. *J. Ped.*, **79,** 744.

RUDHE U. & OZONOFF M.B. (1966) Pneumomediastinum and pneumothorax in the newborn. *Acta Radiol. Diagn.*, **4,** 193.

STEINER B. & NABRADY J. (1965) Immunoallergic lung purpura treated with azathioprine. *Lancet*, **1,** 140.

SUTTON R.N.P. & EMERY J.L. (1966) Sudden death in infancy: a microbiological and epidemiological study. *Arch. Dis. Childh.*, **41,** 674.

# CHAPTER 12

# DISORDERS OF THE CARDIOVASCULAR SYSTEM

## CONGENITAL MALFORMATIONS

These are discussed on p. 175 in the chapter on congenital malformations. The clinical picture of cardiac failure in infancy is described on p. 190.

## DISORDERS OF CARDIAC RATE AND RHYTHM

### Sinus arrhythmia

This indicates an acceleration of heart rate on inspiration. It is a normal physiological occurrence in children, disappearing when the heart rate increases with exercise.

### Extrasystoles

These occur less often in children than in adults and are of no significance provided there is no evidence of organic heart disease. They usually disappear with exercise and there should be no difficulty in differentiating auricular fibrillation; if necessary an electrocardiogram can be used. Most children are unaware of their occurrence even though they are sometimes frequent and persistent.

### Paroxysmal tachycardia

*Aetiology.* This may occur in children of any age but is uncommon, except in infancy. In most cases the heart is otherwise normal, although there may be an associated congenital heart lesion; the condition has also been described in infants with myocarditis and fibroelastosis. Some of the children, between attacks, show the electrocardiographic features of the Wolff-Parkinson-White syndrome in which there is a short P–R and a long QRS interval, the P–S being unaltered. Paroxysmal tachycardia may occur in rheumatic fever and occasionally in association with acute infections.

*Clinical features.* The onset is sudden, the child becoming pale and restless. Feeds are refused and vomiting may occur. The pulse rate is over 180 per minute, respirations are laboured and cyanosis develops. The rapid carotid pulse is visible in the neck so that mothers of children with repeated attacks sometimes come to recognize this as the first sign. The attack ends abruptly after a few seconds or several days but if it is prolonged, heart failure may develop, in which case there is rapid enlargement of the liver.

In infants, the clinical features simulate pneumonia and it is very easy at that age to overlook the diagnostic tachycardia. Enlargement of the liver is the important sign in paroxysmal tachycardia.

*Treatment.* Vagal stimulation by pressure over one carotid sinus or both eyeballs is sometimes successful in terminating an attack but may be danger-ous. Neostigmine can be tried but if it fails digitalis should be given in full dosage and is often successful; those who respond to digtalis must be main-tained on the drug for several months. For those who fail to respond to digitalis, electrical cardioversion is now preferred to quinidine. Assessment of the value of drugs is difficult owing to the paroxysmal nature of the condi-tion. If there is cardiac failure the management should be that outlined on p. 190, maintenance digitalis being continued for at least one month.

## Heart block

*Complete heart block* may be congenital in origin, in which case it persists throughout life; this condition is described on p. 183. Complete heart block may also occur in diphtheria, but if the child survives, the heart recovers its normal function.

*First degree heart block* indicates prolongation of the P–R interval and is associated with myocarditis. It is often seen in rheumatic fever but also occurs in diphtheria.

## Auricular fibrillation

This is a rare condition in children; most cases are of rheumatic origin but it may occur in any variety of myocarditis. Its presence during childhood indi-cates a severe cardiac lesion, the prognosis being very bad.

## Cardiac arrest

The prognosis in cases of cardiac arrest is dependent on the cause, but every case should receive immediate and energetic treatment in the hope that the condition is reversible. The success of therapy is directly related to the speed with which it is initiated. Every doctor and nurse should know what to do in this emergency and they should encourage non-medical members of the public to master the easily learnt technique.

*Treatment.* As soon as cardiac arrest is suspected, attempts should be made to confirm the diagnosis by the absence of the heart beat and respiratory movements and the fact that the pupils no longer respond to light. The airway is cleared, by suction if means are available, but otherwise by sweeping the finger round the back of the throat to remove mucus and other material. External cardiac massage has now replaced the open chest operation as the first method of treatment unless the chest is already open or there is evidence of intrathoracic haemorrhage. It is particularly effective in children since the softer thoracic cage make it possible for the heart to be massaged more efficiently than in adults. The patient must be lying on a firm surface; this can be rapidly achieved by placing a wooden tray at his back or putting him on the floor. The heel of the hand is then placed on the lower sternum and sufficient force used to depress the sternum about 2 cm. This movement is repeated rhythmically at a rate of about 100 per minute. The force must be short and sharp and is followed by relaxation to permit diastolic filling. Excessive force will damage the ribs or thoracic contents; the amount used should be just sufficient to maintain a good femoral pulse.

While cardiac massage is proceeding, an assistant should be giving mouth to mouth respiration at a rate of one breath every 4 seconds. The operator's mouth must be removed after each breath to permit expiration to take place. If no assistant is available cardiac massage should be interrupted every 30 seconds to allow the operator to ventilate the patient by 3–4 mouth to mouth breaths.

Cardiac arrest causes the rapid development of metabolic acidosis. This must be relieved by intravenous 8·4 per cent sodium bicarbonate (1 mEq/ml). In an emergency 5 ml/kg should be given at once without prior estimation of the base deficit. Further requirements determined by acid–base analysis are given according to the formula: ml bicarbonate = base deficit × wt (kg) × 0·3.

The first sign that the patient is responding to treatment is the return of responsiveness of the pupil. Cardiac massage can be effectively maintained for 1–2 hours. Endotracheal intubation and intermittent positive pressure ventilation should replace mouth to mouth respiration as soon as possible. Intravenous or intracardiac isoprenaline may be of value, particularly in order to bring about a fast rhythm when only a slow rate has been induced. Ventricular fibrillation can be corrected by an external defibrillator.

Patients who have been successfully resuscitated must be continuously monitored for 48 hours since they are particularly susceptible to cardiac arrhythmia.

## ENDOCARDITIS

*Aetiology*. Rheumatic fever, described on p. 649, is much the most common cause of endocarditis in children, which is then part of a pancarditis. Bacterial endocarditis is the next most frequent cause although it is now seen less often owing to the advent of antibiotics and cardiac surgery; it is rare under the age of 5 years. There are a number of rare forms of endocarditis of obscure aetiology, such as endocardial fibroelastosis and endomyocardial fibrosis.

## Bacterial endocarditis

Descriptions of this condition commonly refer to acute or subacute bacterial endocarditis, but today, with antibiotics, this separation has outlived its value; cases are better designated by the causal organism since this is the deciding factor in prognosis. The condition results from bacteraemia in a patient with existing heart disease and occurs at any age. The heart disease is either congenital or rheumatic, congenital being the more common. In about 80 per cent of cases the organism is *Streptococcus viridans* which is part of the normal flora of the upper respiratory tract, being particularly associated with dental sepsis. Staphylococcus, the next most common infecting organism, is found on the skin and in the upper respiratory tract of normal individuals, being particularly associated with skin sepsis.

The type of cardiac lesion most likely to be complicated by bacterial endocarditis is that in which a jet of blood, resulting from a deformed valve or a high-pressure gradient across a defect, is directed against one area of the endocardium. This area is liable to be damaged, leaving it more vulnerable to infection and the formation of vegetations. Of the congenital heart lesions Fallot's tetralogy is especially affected, but it also occurs in aortic and pulmonary stenosis, patent ductus, coarctation of the aorta and ventricular septal defect. An atrial septal defect is seldom complicated by bacterial endocarditis.

*Clinical features.* The onset is usually insidious and the commonest complaint is excessive tiredness. Fever, anorexia and loss of weight occur and there is increasing pallor from anaemia.

The more obvious signs result from minute arterial emboli which come from the vegetations and settle anywhere in the body. The skin is particularly involved, the emboli producing petechiae and Osler's nodes. These nodes are painful red areas about the size of a pea which occur particularly on the pads of the fingers and toes, remaining for 1–2 days. Splinter haemorrhages occur under the finger nails. Microscopic haematuria, resulting from renal emboli, is very significant. Emboli may enter any organ, it being particularly serious if the brain is affected. If the vegetations affect only the right side of the heart the emboli enter the lungs and there are no peripheral embolic manifestations. Small pulmonary emboli produce few signs and there may be little more than slight pain in the chest from pleurisy.

It must be emphasized that embolic phenomena are relatively late signs; the condition must be suspected before they develop. The onset of tiredness and pallor in a patient with a pre-existing cardiac lesion is very significant and the finding of microscopic haematuria makes the diagnosis almost certain. The character of the cardiac murmur may change and enlargement of the spleen is usual. A positive blood culture confirms the diagnosis and is essential for correct antibiotic therapy. Six blood samples should be tested before excluding the disease and sometimes the organism can be isolated only from the arterial blood or bone marrow. In coarctation of the aorta, blood should be collected from the foot rather than the arm.

*Treatment.* The objective in treatment is to eradicate the organism before it has time to damage the myocardium or the valves; therefore the correct antibiotics must be given in adequate dosage. For this reason therapy must not be started until the organism has been identified; the prognosis is less affected by the duration of symptoms before treatment than by failure to isolate the organism. If the infection is due to *Streptococcus viridans*, penicillin is the drug of choice, but it should always be combined with streptomycin. Very large doses of penicillin should be used, in the order of 100 million units a day, as an aqueous solution given intravenously every 3 hours. After a week the dose of penicillin can be reduced and be given by mouth. It must be continued for 4–6 weeks, checks being made that the blood culture is sterile. The streptomycin is given intramuscularly in usual dosage (40 mg/kg/ day) throughout the period of therapy.

If the organism is a staphylococcus the condition is much more serious and a combination of two or more antibiotics should be used. Iron and blood transfusions are required for anaemia. Surgical correction of the heart lesion, if this is possible, is carried out after the infection is controlled.

*Prognosis.* Before the introduction of antibiotics the condition was uniformly fatal whereas now the majority recover, the outlook for cases due to *Streptococcus viridans* being the best. The prognosis is better in cases of congenital heart disease where the myocardium has not been damaged than in rheumatic carditis.

*Prophylaxis.* Since the majority of cases follow dental extraction, causing *Streptococcus viridans* to enter the blood stream, penicillin must be given to cover all dental operations in children with known heart disease. 300,000 units each of penicillin G and procaine penicillin are given intramuscularly 1 hour before the operation, followed by the same dose 6–12 hours later. The penicillin should not be given 2 days prior to surgery since sensitive strains of *Streptococcus viridans* can become resistant within 2 days. The same precaution must be taken to cover any operative manipulation which might lead to bacteraemia, such as the removal of tonsils and adenoids and operations on the intestinal or genito-urinary tract.

The emphasis in children with cardiac lesions must not so much be placed on the correct management of dental extractions as on the correct precautions to prevent dental sepsis (p. 298).

### Endocardial fibroelastosis

This condition presents as heart failure in infancy. It is coming to be more frequently recognized although a definite diagnosis can be made only at post-mortem. The endocardium, particularly on the left side of the heart, is involved in a non-inflammatory process. There is an increase in the sub-endocardial fibrous and elastic tissue, producing thickening of the mural endocardium so that it is transformed into a uniformly dense, white glistening membrane. The affected valves are also thickened and become distorted. The heart enlarges and the ventricles, especially the left, hypertrophy.

The disorder starts during intrauterine life but its cause is unknown. It has been suggested that it is a developmental abnormality of the endocardium resulting from anoxia. In support of this theory is the fact that stagnation of blood in a vessel is followed by fibrous and elastic proliferation of the intima, this possibly being a factor in the closure of the ductus and hypogastric vessels after birth. Evidence that anoxia might be an aetiological factor is supported by the finding of associated congenital malformations which could cause anoxia, such as an anomalous coronary artery, valvular atresia or premature closure of the foramen ovale.

*Clinical features.* There is a sudden onset of dyspnoea and distressing cough in a previously healthy infant who is usually less than 6 months old. Cyanosis is variable and often there is no cardiac murmur. Enlargement of the liver is the chief evidence of cardiac failure and should lead to differentiation from pneumonia for which the condition is likely to be mistaken, since widespread râles are audible. Paroxysmal tachycardia has been reported in some patients. An X-ray shows the heart to be much enlarged and also differentiates the condition from pneumonia. Left ventricular strain may be seen in the electro-cardiogram.

*Treatment.* The prognosis is very bad but full doses of digitalis and other measures for cardiac failure in infancy (see p. 190) offer the only hope; a few children have survived.

### Endomyocardial fibrosis (EMF)

This is a totally different condition from endocardial fibroelastosis, there being no increase of intimal elastic tissue. It is found particularly in Africa, where it is common, but is exceptional in Europe; it may occur at any age.

The characteristic lesion is endomyocardial fibrosis affecting predominantly the apical portions of one or both ventricles, with a preference for the left.

Mitral incompetence, but not stenosis, results from thickening of the valve and shortening of the thickened chordae tendineae. Tricuspid incompetence may occur but the aortic and pulmonary valves are never involved. In late cases there is extensive fibrosis of the endocardium and myocardium of one or both ventricles, often with thrombus formation on the fibrosed endocardial surface. A pericardial effusion is common.

*Aetiology.* The cause is unknown but malnutrition is certainly a factor. Aschoff bodies have been found in the myocardium and also a non-specific type of myocardial inflammation. It has been suggested that EMF is the final common path for many different forms of assault on the myocardium, especially the anaemia, chronic infection and malnutrition which so many of these patients have suffered from birth. In some cases it is possible that rheumatic carditis is concerned in the process.

*Clinical features.* African patients usually present when heart failure has already developed so that ascites is the chief mode of presentation. Oedema of the legs is not common. There is usually a large pericardial effusion. The clinical picture varies according to which side of the heart is mainly involved; signs of mitral incompetence and pulmonary hypertension may predominate. The prognosis is very bad, and although treatment with digitalis and diuretics may prolong life the condition is irreversible.

### Muscle glycogen storage disease (Pompe's type)

The condition should be suspected when heart failure occurs in the early weeks of life in association with gross cardiac enlargement but no murmurs. It is discussed on p. 575.

## MYOCARDITIS

AETIOLOGY

The commonest cause of myocarditis in children is rheumatic fever (p. 649). Diphtheria, by the action of its toxin, may attack the myocardium and in so doing may involve the conducting bundles, causing arrhythmia or block. This lesion is reversible so that if the child recovers there is no residual cardiac damage.

Myocarditis may also be caused by toxoplasmosis and by a number of virus infections such as poliomyelitis, influenza, Group B Coxsackie, measles and probably by many other unidentified viruses.

### Neonatal myocarditis

In the newborn the disease is particularly caused by the Group B Coxsackie virus. It may occur in epidemic form in maternity nurseries, when the origin has sometimes been traced back to patients with Bornholm disease. The clinical picture is that of a fulminating infection with heart failure predominating, but in which encephalitis and hepatitis also occur. The heart is considerably enlarged, the electrocardiogram usually showing low voltage waves without evidence of a conduction defect.

*Treatment.* There is no specific therapy for the virus infection and a high proportion of the patients die from cardiac failure despite full treatment for that condition (see p. 191). Early diagnosis is essential for cases occurring in a nursery in order to ensure their isolation, thereby reducing the risk of spread to other babies.

## PERICARDITIS

AETIOLOGY

The commonest cause is rheumatic fever but the condition is occasionally seen in rheumatoid arthritis. Pyogenic pericarditis may occur by blood-stream spread from a focus of infection such as osteomyelitis or pneumonia, or by direct spread from pneumonia or a penetrating chest wound. Tuberculous pericarditis can occur from extension of a tuberculous lesion in the lung. Acute benign pericarditis (see p. 378) is due to infection with the Coxsackie B virus.

*Clinical features.* These vary with the primary condition whose other features may overshadow those of the pericarditis. Its onset will lead to a serious deterioration in the patient's condition with pallor, tachycardia and possibly heart failure. Precordial and abdominal pain may be felt, the signs depending on whether pericarditis has led to a pericardial effusion. If an effusion is present, the area of cardiac dullness is increased and the heart sounds are muffled. The apex beat is no longer visible or palpable and the neck veins are distended but do not pulsate. The cardiac shadow on X-ray is increased and globular. If there is no effusion, a to-and-fro friction rub may be heard which is very superficial, sounding like the creaking of an old door. A pericardial rub is uncommon in children, being reported, more often than it exists. In such cases the mistaken sound results from inspiratory and expiratory rhonchi; the error should not be made since a good cough will alter the sound of the rhonchi.

Confirmation of the diagnosis is made by a pericardial tap, the nature of the fluid aspirated usually indicating the cause of the peridarditis; the fluid should be cultured. The effusion in rheumatic fever and rheumatoid arthritis is usually serous whereas if tuberculous it is often bloodstained.

*Treatment.* This is directed to the underlying condition, but in all cases as much of the effusion as possible should be removed by aspiration. Pericardo-stomy may be required for purulent pericarditis.

### Acute benign pericarditis

This occurs at any age, is viral in origin and is most often due to infection with the Coxsackie B virus. The infection is confined to the pericardium, the illness is not severe and recovery is usual. This is in contradistinction to the same infection in the newborn, in whom immunity is limited and myocarditis and pericarditis occur as part of a fulminating and often fatal, generalized disease (see p. 376). Pain is the presenting feature and may often be referred to the abdomen rather than felt in the chest.

*Treatment.* No specific therapy is available and, since recovery is usual, aspiration of the pericardial fluid is unnecessary.

# CHAPTER 13

# DISORDERS OF THE URINARY TRACT

## General considerations

The diagnosis of urinary disease in childhood is more difficult than in adults, since symptoms such as frequency, pain on micturition and dysuria are less obvious. A baby in the napkin stage will need to have a very astute mother to recognize such symptoms. It is usual for young children to be incontinent of urine, especially at night, and children, particularly boys, are less able to hold their urine for long in the bladder. But because these difficulties exist, the doctor looking after children must be all the more on the alert lest he overlooks a urinary disease; he must be aware that symptoms such as anorexia, vomiting, vague abdominal pain and failure to thrive may well result from disease in the urinary tract.

The first investigation is the examination of the urine, but since collection is difficult the doctor is liable not to make the test. Many tricks can be used to assist in collecting a specimen: babies tend to pass urine on waking or feeding so that a sterile receiver should be ready on such occasions; in infancy, the bladder is more of an abdominal than a pelvic organ so that gentle suprapubic pressure may stimulate urinary flow; wiping the lower abdomen with an ether swab may also stimulate flow. If this fails, then in boys Paul's tubing should be strapped to the cleaned penis in preference to the traditional test-tube, which is far less comfortable. A knot is tied in the distal end and the urine when passed can be poured into the sterile specimen bottle. Alternatively, the urine can be left in the tube by tying a knot in the proximal end of the tubing after its removal from the penis. A specimen obtained in this manner can easily be brought back to the surgery if it is impractical for the mother to wait once the tubing has been applied. It is unnecessary to catheterize girls since satisfactory plastic bags are available for strapping round the vulva, after washing down. Similar bags can be used for boys instead of Paul's tubing and are especially suitable for small infants; their only disadvantage is greater expense. The certain method for procuring an uncontaminated specimen is to perform a suprapubic puncture.

Intravenous pyelography (IVP) is often required to exclude a congenital malformation of the renal tract. The common mistake is to use insufficient opaque media so that the pictures are unsatisfactory. The dose should be 10 ml plus 1 ml for each year of life so that a boy of 10 years receives the full adult dose of 20 ml. If the blood urea is raised more contrast medium will be required owing to lack of renal concentration. Gas shadows obscuring the kidneys are always a problem, but the use of an aerated drink such as Pepsi-Cola causes sufficient gaseous distension of the stomach to displace the intestine, allowing a clear view through the stomach. In infancy, if the intravenous route is impractical, the dye can be given subcutaneously with hyalase into the thighs. A micturating cystogram is required in order to determine whether or not there is reflux from the bladder up the ureters.

## Postural proteinuria (orthostatic albuminuria)

Some children excrete protein in their urine, only when standing up; it is therefore necessary to exclude this cause in every patient in whom proteinuria is discovered. They are usually lanky, with rounded shoulders and an exaggerated lordosis. It used to be thought to result from increased pressure on the renal veins but present evidence suggests that pooling of the blood in the extremities is the most important factor (Greiner & Henry, 1955). Renal blood flow is less in the erect position than when lying down. It is believed that this results from a reduction in cardiac output due to pooling of blood in the extremities. The reduced return of blood to the heart causes arterial vasoconstriction which is believed to be proportionately greater in the renal arteries. Peripheral vasodilatation is greater in hot conditions, thus explaining the greater frequency of postural proteinuria in hot climates. The question remains as to whether normal kidneys, subjected to this low renal blood flow, leak protein. The studies of Robinson et al. (1961, 1963) suggest that an abnormality in the glomerulus is unmasked by the low renal blood flow of the erect position. It should be remembered that the proteinuria associated with renal disease increases in the erect position.

Having found protein in an ordinary specimen of urine, the diagnosis of postural proteinuria is made by showing that none is present in a specimen of urine excreted while lying down. This is achieved by empting the bladder immediately before going to bed at night and passing urine immediately after getting out of bed in the morning.

No treatment is indicated and the parents should be told that this is a functional problem affecting the kidney which does not affect the child's health. The condition tends to disappear in adult life.

### 'PROTEINURIA' IN THE NEWBORN

It is sometimes stated that proteinuria often exists during the first 2 weeks of life as a physiological phenomenon. This has been shown to be incorrect

(Doxiadis *et al.*, 1952). The apparent positive test for protein is due to interference from the excessive excretion of urates in the first few days of life.

### Haematuria

Blood in the urine may originate from any part of the renal tract. It should always be regarded as a serious symptom necessitating full investigation. The amount will vary from the presence of red cells on microscopic examination only, to frank haematuria. Moderate quantities of blood alter the colour of the urine to a smoky colour; the amount of blood must be very considerable if the urine is to look obviously blood-stained.

There are three conditions in children which are liable to be mistaken for haematuria. A pink spot may be seen on the napkins of small infants due to uric acid crystals. It is found more often in boys since their stream of urine is directed on to one area of the napkin, causing a greater concentration of crystals. Secondly, the aniline dye in cheap sweets may be excreted in the urine. Finally, a number of individuals pass red urine after eating beetroot. This trait runs in families, being due to the presence in the urine of anthocyanin, the red pigment in beetroot. The urine turns yellow on the addition of sodium hydroxide.

AETIOLOGY

*Acute nephritis.* This is probably the most common cause of haematuria in children in temperate climates.

*Inflammation.* Pyelonephritis and cystitis may be associated with haematuria, but as this is usually microscopic only it is not a presenting feature. A meatal ulcer, which mainly occurs in circumcised male infants in association with ammoniacal dermatitis, causes bleeding during micturition, when the passage of urine removes the scab. Renal tuberculosis is an important cause although now less common. Bacterial endocarditis causes microscopic haematuria, this being of diagnostic value. In endemic areas schistosomiasis is a common cause of haematuria, the blood characteristically appearing at the end of micturition; it is much more common in boys, since they expose themselves to the infection more than girls.

*Trauma.* Injury to any part of the renal tract may result in haematuria. A blow or crush injury in the loins can cause profuse bleeding from the kidney. Penetrating wounds may affect any part of the tract, the male urethra being particularly liable to injury from falling astride a sharp object. Foreign bodies inserted into the urethra are not rare, causing damage to the urethral and bladder mucosa. Similar damage to the mucosa of the renal tract is caused by calculi but these are uncommon in childhood.

*Blood disorders.* Leukaemia, purpura and scurvy may cause haematuria. In the newborn, haemorrhagic disease very occasionally causes the symptom.

*Tumours.* Papillomata and angiomata occur anywhere in the renal tract and cause bleeding. Nephroblastoma occasionally causes severe haematuria.

*Congenital abnormalities.* Polycystic disease of the kidneys is the particular malformation likely to be associated with haematuria. Any malformation may lead to haematuria by predisposing the child to infection of the urinary tract.

## Glomerulonephritis

It is no longer possible to differentiate two types of nephritis, type 1 (acute nephritis) and type 2 (nephrosis), in the way that Ellis (1942) described, although at the time his classification was an advance on the previous confusion. It is now known that intermediate types occur; for example, a few cases of acute nephritis have such heavy proteinuria as to lead to the nephrotic syndrome. Anaphylactoid purpura can be complicated by nephritis giving the clinical picture of acute nephritis, nephrosis or chronic nephritis. Renal biopsy has altered the understanding of the disease in the sense that morphological changes are not associated with a standard clinical picture. More or less any combination of clinical features and histological abnormality can occur so that it is necessary to consider these aspects separately.

### ACUTE NEPHRITIS

This is an immunological disorder resulting from an infection which in about 85 per cent of cases is due to Lancefield's group A $\beta$-haemolytic streptococcus. In the United Kingdom the haemolytic streptococcus usually infects the throat but it may cause infection of the skin, often secondary to scabies. This has reached epidemic proportions in Trinidad (McDowall *et al.*, 1970; Svartman *et al.*, 1972). One particular variety of the haemolytic streptococcus—type 12—is the commonest cause of the throat infection leading to acute nephritis, but other types are involved if the skin is the primary site of infection.

The most frequent renal lesion found on biopsy is diffuse proliferative glomerulonephritis. The glomerular tufts are enlarged from proliferation of the endothelial and mesangial cells and there is associated polymorphonuclear infiltration. Electron microscopy shows deposits of immunoglobulin and $C_3$ component of complement causing 'bumps' at intervals along the basement membrane.

*Clinical features.* The illness, which particularly affects school-age children, occurs 1–2 weeks after the start of the streptococcal infection. This infection is likely still to be present unless antibiotic therapy has been given. The onset is acute with haematuria, making the urine smoky, and backache as the principal features. The backache is due to severe congestion within the tight renal capsule (this is so great that in autopsy specimens the renal substance overflows the cut edge of the capsule when the kidney is incised). The child feels unwell but is seldom seriously ill; in fact there is often remarkably little constitutional disturbance even when the blood urea is moderately raised. Headache may occur as a result of hypertension. Oedema sufficient to cause puffiness of the eyes is common but it is seldom severe or generalized. It is often noticeable only to those familiar with the child's usual facial appearance.

Evidence of the primary streptococcal infection is likely still to be present—most often as acute follicular tonsillitis with cervical adenitis—much less often as skin sepsis.

There are usually two distinct phases to the illness: oliguria followed by diuresis. The oligaemic phase is associated with hypertension and azotaemia. The amount of blood in the urine is variable; some cases develop gross haematuria but in others the red cells are seen only on microscopy. Proteinuria is usually moderate and there are white cells and casts—these are hyaline, cellular and, most significant of all, granular.

Occasionally the hypertension is sufficient to cause left ventricular heart failure with pulmonary oedema and raised venous pressure causing dyspnoea and vomiting. An additional factor leading to cardiac enlargement and embarrassment is the retention of salt and water, resulting from glomerular and tubular imbalance, producing reduced filtration and reabsorption. Hypertensive encephalopathy is an additional complication in a small number of cases leading to severe headache, restlessness, visual disturbances, convulsions and coma.

During this phase the $C_3$ component of complement is almost invariably lowered to at least half its normal value. The ASO titre is raised to 200 Todd units or more, except in those with a skin primary when it may remain normal.

The second phase is characterized by diuresis which occurs 1–2 weeks after the onset of renal symptoms. With this there is a return to normal of the sodium and blood urea levels and a subsidence of clinical features, although microscopic haematuria may persist for several months.

*Treatment.* All patients should receive a 10-day course of penicillin as soon as throat swabs (and skin if indicated) have been taken, without waiting for the results. During the oliguric phase, fluid should be restricted in accordance with the urinary output and the calculated needs. The diet at this stage should be high in carbohydrate and low in protein and salt. The fall in the daily weight readings is the best indication of the loss of oedema. Severe hypertension should be treated by hypotensive drugs such as reserpine, combined if necessary with hydrallazine, in order to prevent hypertensive encephalopathy.

The child should be isolated for the first week since the haemolytic streptococcus could infect other patients, but bed rest should be reduced to a minimum. Bed is only required during the oliguric and hypertensive stage and can be stopped when macroscopic haematuria disappears. The old plan of maintaining bed rest until microscopic haematuria had disappeared is quite unnecessary.

*Prognosis.* In at least 90 per cent of cases there is a complete return to normal even though microscopic haematuria may persist for months. Death in the acute stage is now rare but up to 10 per cent of children develop chronic nephritis with persistent proteinuria, haematuria and the presence of urinary casts. The persistence of a lowered $C_3$ complement for more than two months is a bad sign.

### 'FOCAL NEPHRITIS'

This term should no longer be used as a clinical description since its meaning differs with clinicians and pathologists. Clinically, it used to be applied to those cases of recurrent painless haematuria of unknown origin, unaccompanied by oedema, oliguria, hypertension or other evidence of renal impairment. This is a benign condition, and in those cases where a renal biopsy has been performed this has often been normal or the glomeruli have shown endothelial and mesangial proliferation.

It is correct to use the term histologically since renal biopsy in some cases of glomerulonephritis show focal, rather than diffuse, proliferation. In children, this is most often seen in cases of nephritis associated with anaphylactoid purpura.

### NEPHROTIC SYNDROME

This results whenever sufficient glomerular damage occurs to produce persistent severe proteinuria. It comprises gross oedema, low serum proteins and severe proteinuria. There are three varieties: congenital, idiopathic, and secondary.

### CONGENITAL NEPHROTIC SYNDROME

A rare familial condition associated sometimes with anatomical abnormalities of the nephron and almost always fatal within the first year of life. It occurs particularly in Finland.

IDIOPATHIC NEPHROTIC SYNDROME

This is the commonest variety of the syndrome, believed to be due to an immunological disorder. The cause of the antigen–antibody reaction is unknown, but it is likely to be a variety of infections including viral.

Renal biopsy in the majority of cases shows a 'minimal change' lesion. This term is now used in preference to 'normal glomeruli' since there is often slight hypercellularity or an increased number of mesangial fibres or both. There is no thickening of the basement membrane, but electron microscopy may reveal fusion of the foot processes—a non-specific and reversible change. Much less often the histology shows focal glomerulosclerosis or proliferative glomerulonephritis.

*Clinical features.* The onset is insidious, the child presenting with severe oedema, ascites and proteinuria. This oedema is periorbital unlike the oedema of adults which particularly affects the ankles; the difference is probably due to better tissue turgor in children. Pleural effusions are common.

The proteinuria is usually selective, indicating that it is composed of low molecular weight (small molecule) protein only—mainly albumen. Non-selective proteinuria indicates an escape of proteins of all molecular weights. There is hypoproteinaemia which correlates with the loss of protein in the urine and hyperlipaemia. Typically there is no hypertension and no azotaemia.

*Diagnosis.* The disorder must be differentiated from congenital and secondary nephrotic syndromes. The clinical picture in kwashiorkor may be similar because of oedema, but in such children proteinuria is absent or slight only. Other causes of generalized oedema such as beri-beri, hookworm disease or protein-losing enteropathy are excluded by the absence of proteinuria and the other signs of the diseases.

*Treatment.* The child with severe oedema is unlikely to wish to get up but he should be allowed to do so as soon as he wishes. The diet should be high in protein and low in sodium until there is no oedema or proteinuria, unless uraemia supervenes. Antibiotics should be used therapeutically rather than prophylactically, with careful bacteriological control.

The best diuretic for those who are sensitive is corticosteroid therapy. For those with a minimal change lesion, 95–100 per cent will respond and this is correlated with selective proteinuria so that a renal biopsy is not required before starting treatment. Prednisolone is a satisfactory form of the drug given in high dosage (60 mg daily) irrespective of the child's weight. It is continued for 6 weeks, being gradually tapered off after the first 2 weeks.

Corticotrophin can be given on alternate days by injection during the last 10 days of the course in order to counteract the suppressive effect of the therapy on the child's adrenal glands.

About half of those who respond to steroid therapy remain well after the first attack whereas the other half relapse but respond to a second course. For those who are steroid sensitive but who relapse frequently, an 8-week course of cyclophosphamide in a dose of 3 mg/kg reduces the liability to relapse. This is given while the child is receiving steroids and after a diuresis has been obtained. The steroid is tapered off and stopped after the course of cyclophosphamide has been completed. The mode of action of cyclophosphamide is unknown but it does not alter the renal biopsy changes. It may cause damage to the testicular germinal cells. Parents and child should be warned that it may cause baldness but the hair will quickly return once the drug is stopped. Meanwhile a wig can be worn if necessary. They should similarly be warned of the obesity caused by steroids.

Renal biopsy is indicated for those who fail to respond to this form of treatment. Other diuretics such as frusemide may be used in such cases. In steroid-resistant patients it is essential to check that there is no associated infection of the urinary tract. Renal biopsy is also indicated in those with non-selective proteinuria, hypertension, high blood urea, normal plasma lipids or a high ASO titre.

SECONDARY NEPHROTIC SYNDROME

This is a much less common cause of nephrosis except in the tropics where quartan malaria (*Plasmodium malariae*) is an important cause. This was first suggested in 1960 by Gilles and Hendrickse, and the association is now proven. Unfortunately, treatment of the malaria does not improve the nephrosis which is steroid resistant in about 80 per cent of cases.

Other causes of secondary nephrosis are allergic nephrosis from pollen, a bee sting or immunization; toxic nephrosis from heavy metal poisoning such as lead or mercury; renal vein thrombosis; collagen nephrosis causing anaphylactoid purpura, disseminated lupus erythematosus or polyarteritis nodosa; post-nephritic nephrosis when the condition follows acute nephritis— this is less common than nephrosis following anaphylactoid purpura.

**Chronic nephritis**

Both types of glomerulonephritis may progress to chronic nephritis. The clinical features may then be identical so that only a knowledge of the earlier history will permit a diagnosis of the primary condition. The children present a very variable picture of renal failure and in some there may be no symptoms for many years. Others tire easily, are more liable to infection and have anaemia, hypertension, convulsions and renal osteodystrophy. In the most severe cases drowsiness leads to coma, convulsions and death.

There is persistent proteinuria and urinary casts, the blood urea is raised and renal function tests show progressive impairment.

A few cases of chronic nephritis follow symptomless, progressive glomerulonephritis. ('Silent' nephritis—White, 1964.)

*Treatment.* This can be symptomatic only. Fluids should be unrestricted, a high-protein diet given and the children should be in bed only if absolutely necessary.

## Acute renal failure

This may develop during the course of acute nephritis or the nephrotic syndrome. It more often occurs from circulatory disturbances resulting from shock, dehydration, burns, septicaemia, accidental poisoning and incompatible transfusion. The haemolytic–uraemic syndrome (p. 612) is another cause of acute renal failure in children. Acute tubular damage results in oliguria or anuria and leads to uraemia; this causes vomiting, drowsiness and hypertension. Recovery is associated with the passage of large quantities of dilute urine from renal impairment, before normal urinary excretion returns.

*Treatment.* This must first be directed towards the cause, if this is apparent. Fluid intake is limited to the amount being lost from the body during the phase of oliguria in order to prevent pulmonary oedema and cardiac failure. The child must be weighed daily, a gain in weight indicating excessive fluid administration. No protein should be given, the minimal calorie requirements being provided by fat and carbohydrate. If vomiting prevents oral administration, carbohydrate should be given intravenously. In view of the high concentration of glucose required, which scleroses the small veins, a catheter in the inferior vena cava may be necessary; fructose is less liable than glucose to cause thrombosis. Frequent electrolyte estimations are essential and the acid–base imbalance corrected. Hypertension is treated with hypotensive drugs. These patients are very liable to die from secondary infection, therefore vigorous prophylactic antibiotic therapy should be given.

Hyperkalaemia is liable to develop and is an important cause of death; therefore, fruit juices, with their high level of potassium, must not be allowed. Insulin can be given with glucose in order to force the potassium into the cells. Some success in reducing the high level of serum potassium also results from ion exchange resins. If the biochemical disturbance cannot be controlled by conservative means, dialysis is indicated. Peritoneal dialysis is the method of choice for this.

### Acute pyelonephritis

The term 'pyelitis' should be discarded in favour of pyelonephritis since the lesion always involves the renal parenchyma as well as the pelvis. Even this is too limiting, it being more accurate to think of infection of the urinary tract as a whole. The commonest organisms are *Escherichia coli* first and *Streptococcus faecalis* second, both being normal inhabitants of the bowel. *Proteus vulgaris* and *Pseudomonas pyocyanea* are particularly found if there is an underlying congenital malformation of the renal tract. Staphylococcal infections are not common.

The route of infection is mainly by ascending the urinary tract. Blood stream spread occurs in staphylococcal cases but is much less common. During the neonatal period, boys are affected more than girls because of their greater incidence of congenital malformations causing obstruction to the lower renal tract. After early infancy there is a striking preponderance of girls, probably because their short urethra increases the chance of ascending infection. The condition may occur at any age but especially during the first year. It is common in the neonatal period though frequently missed because the symptoms at that age do not suggest a urinary origin. In young infants the condition presents as failure to thrive associated with anorexia and vomiting. Fever is common and may precipitate a convulsion, but it is not constant, especially in babies. Jaundice may develop in the neonatal period as with other infections at that age. In older children, abdominal pain is common, it is more often vague and generalized rather than localized to any one area. In these children frequency of micturition and dysuria may be noted and enuresis either by day or night may occur. Haematuria is uncommon but can occur in severe attacks, especially if a stone is present. Occasionally pyelonephritis is associated with the nephrotic syndrome.

*Investigations.* The diagnosis of urinary tract infection is difficult, particularly in babies. It is this which accounts for the difference of opinion regarding the frequency of the condition.

The most reliable test of urinary infection is the bacterial colony count. More than 100,000 organisms per ml of urine, provided it has been plated within 1 hour of being passed, is definite evidence of infection. If there are less than 10,000 organisms these can safely be regarded as contaminants. Between 10,000 and 100,000 the diagnosis is uncertain. Repeat cultures must be performed and the results of other investigations assessed. The technique of suprapubic bladder puncture is the best way to avoid contamination. The presence of any bacteria in a suprapubic sample indicates infection. It should therefore be used routinely in sick babies for whom an immediate diagnosis is essential. This method gets over a problem in girls in whom efflux of urine into the vagina before it enters the collecting bag can cause a rise in cells and bacteria. A new, simple and effective method of obtaining a quantitative bacterial count is the dip-inoculum technique ('dipslide') which can be used in the home or surgery as well as in hospital (Arneil et al., 1973).

The next best test is the number of white cells in the urine. Clean uncentrifuged urine, obtained as a mid-stream or catheter specimen, is examined; more than 10 white cells per $mm^3$ indicates an infection. There is no chemical test for pus cells and it is a waste of time to record the number of pus cells by such vague terms as 'few', 'moderate number' or 'many'—or as the number per high-powered field. Clinicians should insist on a service which provides accurate urinary white cell counts.

It must be emphasized that the presence or absence of proteinuria is of no value in the diagnosis of urinary infection.

*Investigations.* Every child who has a urinary tract infection should be investigated radiologically since half may be found to have anatomical or functional (i.e. 'reflux'—see below) abnormalities of the renal tract (Smellie et al., 1964).

The radiological investigations are an intravenous pyelogram (IVP) and a micturating cystogram. Both are required in every case under investigation since one only may be diagnostic. The IVP determines the presence of congenital malformations of the upper urinary tract and shows the size of the renal cortex and the shape of the calyces. 'Chronic pyelonephritis' is a radiological diagnosis made by finding a reduction in the overall size of the kidney and irregular coarse scarring causing localized thinning of the renal substance with flattening or clubbing of the corresponding calyx. Scarring particularly occurs at the upper poles; at this site the renal substance is normally thicker than in the middle of the kidney. A micturating cystogram outlines the bladder and urethra, shows any residual urine and determines whether there is reflux from the bladder up one or both ureters.

Cysto-urethroscopy may be required as an additional investigation to detect minor degrees of obstruction in the bladder neck and changes in the urethral mucosa; it is of less value than the other investigations.

The results of renal biopsy in the diagnosis of pyelonephritis in children are unsatisfactory because they are too variable, presumably because the inflammatory changes are patchily distributed in the kidney.

URETERIC REFLUX

Under normal circumstances reflux of urine from bladder to ureter is prevented by contraction of the bladder during micturition. This causes contraction of the intramural portion of the ureter—there is no actual sphincter. This portion passes obliquely through the bladder wall, thereby increasing the length of the ureter which is shut down during micturition. Reflux is most liable to occur towards the end of micturition since, the bladder being nearly empty, the intravesical pressure is high and the intramural ureter relatively short.

Whether reflux is a congenital anomaly or secondary to pyelonephritis is uncertain. Probably both occur, though a congenital origin is the more likely since reflux continues between attacks of pyuria. The diagnosis and management of reflux is an essential part of the treatment of urinary infection in childhood. There is a natural tendency for reflux to disappear since, as the child grows older, the bladder settles further into the pelvis thereby increasing the obliquity of the angle of entry of the ureters into the bladder.

The most damaging situation as far as the kidneys are concerned is the coexistence of reflux and urinary infection. This causes infected urine to return to the bladder after micturition has been completed. When micturition is next performed infected urine is forced up the ureters, causing perpetuation of the ascending infection.

Infection without reflux seldom causes scarring, whereas long-standing pyelonephritis is almost always associated with reflux, the worst situation being the combination of reflux and urinary obstruction. Coarse focal scarring in an adult indicates damage inflicted in childhood. Infection occurring during adult life causes general shrinkage without scarring. Infection in childhood can lead to scarring and generalized renal atrophy. Irreversible loss of parenchyma is serious at any stage but especially in children whose kidneys must grow. A normally growing kidney on X-ray is a normal kidney. Both kidneys grow at the same rate so that asymmetrical kidneys indicate failure of one side to grow, the difference in size being possibly exaggerated by compensatory hypertrophy of the normal side.

*Treatment.* In the cases where the diagnosis is certain, vigorous treatment is started at once. But in those cases where, despite all the investigations, the diagnosis is still uncertain, treatment should be withheld, the investigations being repeated after a further interval. It cannot be over-emphasized that keeping a doubtful case off treatment is the correct management, provided the child remains under close management and investigation. The worst thing possible is to start treatment when the diagnosis is still in doubt since this almost certainly precludes a correct diagnosis ever being made.

Sulphonamides are still the drug of choice: either sulphadimidine which is cheap, or sulphafurazole (Gantrisin). The total daily dose for children under 1 year is 0·25 g, for 1–5 years 0·5 g and over 5 years 1 g. It may be useful to make the urine alkaline, particularly when using sulphadimidine, but a high fluid intake is not required. Co-trimoxazole—a combination of trimethoprin and sulphamethoxazole—is a synergistic combination which interferes at different stages in bacterial folic acid metabolism.

Cases resistant to sulphonamides are usually best treated with nitro-furantoin in a dose of 2–4 mg per kg daily. Other drugs for use with organisms resistant to sulphonamides and nitrofurantoin are ampicillin, streptomycin, nalidixic acid and colistin.

The duration of therapy is debated. Some would treat with a short course of 10–14 days only, others would follow this with a low-dosage prophylactic therapy for at least 6 months. The decision between these two alternatives is not difficult since the one essential is for the urine to remain free of infection over a period of years. The rationale of treatment is to prevent reinfection of the urinary tract from below, not to suppress a persistent renal infection. If this can be achieved by a short course with regular urine checks at short intervals, there is no need for prolonged prophylactic therapy.

The risk of reinfection is much greater if there is reflux and such cases may well require long-term therapy to achieve continuous sterility of the urine. 'Triple micturition' will also help to keep the urine free of infection in those with reflux. By this means the child passes urine twice more at intervals of 1 minute after the completion of normal micturition. Ideally, he should do this each time he passes urine, but if told to do this he is likely not to do it at all. It is therefore wiser with most children merely to ask for triple micturition before going to bed, thereby reducing the possibility of infected urine passing up the ureters during the night.

The second criterion of adequate treatment is that the kidneys grow normally on serial IVP's. Provided the infection is controlled, the kidneys can grow normally in the presence of reflux, even if they are already scarred.

In most children this conservative regime will control the infection. Reflux may take as long as 4 years to disappear, but so long as the urine remains sterile nothing more is required.

In a few children the infection cannot be controlled by these measures. For these, surgery is necessary, the ureters being reimplanted into the bladder in such a way as to increase their intramural course.

### Cystitis

The bladder is resistant to infection so that acute cystitis rarely occurs as an isolated event, being more often seen as part of a generalized urinary infection with pyelonephritis.

Chronic cystitis occurs from obstruction of the lower urinary tract or in association with a neurogenic bladder. The bladder walls become thickened and fibrotic, the ureteric orifices gaping so that free reflux occurs. Removal of any obstruction is essential if treatment is to have a chance of success but if severe changes have already occurred in the bladder it will be impossible to clear the urine of pus cells.

## Calculi

Urinary calculi in children are still common in endemic areas in the world. In Europe and America the sporadic form is the one most often seen but this is uncommon.

### ENDEMIC CALCULI

This problem is now largely confined to the Middle East, though less in Negro races than others, males being affected considerably more often than females. The stones are usually composed of uric acid and urates, many factors being involved in their aetiology. The incidence is highest amongst those who are least well off, a dietary deficiency being important. Dehydration with consequent concentration of the urine is also a factor.

### SPORADIC CALCULI

The aetiology of these calculi differs from that of the previous group; a congenital malformation is the most important predisposing cause. Foreign bodies may be inserted into the bladder by the child, particularly a girl, and lead to the development of a surrounding calculus. The stones are usually composed of calcium phosphate, but if a urinary infection occurs there will also be deposition of ammonium phosphate.

Cystine stones are deposited in patients with cystinuria (see p. 564); calculi also occur in association with nephrocalcinosis.

*Nephrocalcinosis.* This only denotes the presence of calcium deposits in the renal parenchyma and does not indicate any particular disease process. Microscopic nephrocalcinosis, which cannot be detected radiologically, is common in and around the renal tubules in a considerable proportion of children dying from all causes. It is also found in certain disease states such as idiopathic hypercalcaemia (p. 564) and renal acidosis (p. 565), when it may be sufficient to show radiographically.

## Nephroblastoma (Wilms's tumour)

This is the only common renal tumour in children and is second only to neuroblastoma as the most common malignant tumour of childhood. It is of embryonic origin, arising within the substance of the kidney. Although it is predominantly composed of primitive blastema there is usually some differentiation of tubular and, less commonly, glomerular structures, as well as connective tissue and smooth muscle. Occasionally, differentiation of bone, cartilage and striated muscle occurs.

It occurs equally in both sexes, almost all cases developing during the first 4 years. It may be present at birth and is bilateral in about 10 per cent of cases (Jagasia *et al.*, 1964). A painless swelling of the abdomen is the most common presenting symptom, the mother often first feeling a lump while bathing the child. Haematuria is not uncommon, occasionally being the presenting symptom.

A plain film of the abdomen demonstrates a soft tissue swelling with displacement of the intestines. Calcification may be present in the tumour, but is seen less often than in a neuroblastoma. An IVP shows some excretion of the dye but the renal pelvis is distorted and displaced. A chest film must be taken to exclude secondary deposits since this tumour tends to invade the blood stream at an early stage, causing lung metastases. Occasionally, the secondaries are deposited in the liver but skeletal metastases are rare.

*Diagnosis.* A large hydronephrosis may simulate a nephroblastoma but is more likely to be painful. This may vary in size from day to day and can sometimes be transilluminated. An IVP usually shows complete lack of function on the affected side.

An adrenal neuroblastoma may be very difficult to differentiate, although it usually causes more constitutional disturbance and the children are more often anaemic. The mass occurs high up under the costal margin, is more likely to cross the midline and to protrude in the loin. It is fixed and hard whereas the nephroblastoma may be mobile. Radiological calcification is not uncommon and the IVP shows the renal pelvis to be displaced downwards. There is less distortion of the renal pelvis and it may be obvious from the outline that the kidney has been flattened and is lying underneath a large tumour (see Fig. 136b, p. 634). A neuroblastoma causes an increased urinary excretion of catecholamines and their metabolite vanillyl mandelic acid (VMA).

Polycystic disease of the kidney is bilateral but occasionally other forms of cysts occur in one kidney and can be differentiated only at operation. A retroperitoneal sarcoma produces a hard fixed abdominal mass which arises from the posterior abdominal wall and does not keep to one side only.

*Treatment.* Immediate nephrectomy should be performed as an emergency once the diagnosis has been established. All unnecessary palpation of the tumour must be prohibited in order to avoid the risk of dissemination. Once the tumour has been removed, irradiation is given at the earliest opportunity to most patients. No interference with wound healing has resulted. The presence of lung metastases is not a contraindication to nephrectomy, but the lungs also are irradiated. Chemotherapy using actinomycin D or vincristine, which is less toxic, either alone or in combination has greatly improved the prognosis. In a recent series 80 per cent of the children have survived for 2 years without evidence of recurrence (Martin & Rickham, 1974).

Unlike most malignant tumours of childhood which are more malignant the younger the child, the outlook with a Wilms's tumour is better for those under 2 years than over 2 years of age.

### Balano-posthitis

Inflammation of the glans (balanitis) and of the prepuce (posthitis) result from retention of smegma within the preputial sac. The condition is associated with phimosis, which is an acquired condition (see p. 203), and poor hygiene. Retraction of the foreskin is usually prevented by oedema and there is an offensive purulent discharge from the sac. The disorder must be differentiated from primary inflammation of the skin which is commonly the result of ammonia dermatitis.

*Treatment.* The infection clears rapidly with improved hygiene and frequent potassium permanganate baths. When the reduction in inflammation permits, the foreskin should, if possible, be retracted but this should not be undertaken if it causes pain. In most cases, circumcision must be performed when the inflammation has settled as the condition is likely to recur. A preliminary dorsal slit is required if retraction remains impossible, since drainage of the preputial sac is necessary before the condition will clear.

### Paraphimosis

This is produced by forcible retraction of the prepuce beyond the corona where it causes obstruction to the circulation in the glans; the consequent swelling prevents its return and causes great pain.

*Treatment.* Cold compresses should be applied and manual reduction performed if possible. Failing this, the injection of 1–2 ml of hyaluronidase into the swollen tissues usually causes sufficient shrinkage of the swelling to permit reduction. If this is unsuccessful a dorsal slit should be made and a later circumcision performed.

### Meatal ulcer

This condition is seen only in circumcised boys, usually in association with ammonia dermatitis (see p. 666). The ulcer is situated on the glans at the edge of the urethral meatus and a downward extension of the ulcer involves the urethral mucosa. Considerable pain is experienced every time urine is passed and healing is prevented by its repeated passage. Slow fibrosis occurs causing meatal stenosis and further impairment of healing.

*Treatment*. This is the same as that described for ammonia dermatitis but in addition an ointment containing benzalkonium chloride should be applied to the glans whenever the napkins are changed. The ointment must reach the urethral extension of the ulcer. This is best achieved by the use of a solid glass ophthalmic rod which is dipped into the ointment and then inserted into the meatus. This method also achieves dilatation of the stenosed meatus.

### Vulvo-vaginitis

Until recently the commonest infecting organism was the gonococcus acquired from the clothing or towels of infected individuals. This organism is now a rare cause, investigations usually showing a mixed collection of staphylococci, streptococci, diphtheroids and coliform organisms. An irritating offensive white discharge is present which is seldom profuse.

The standard of hygiene in the affected individuals is usually poor, but the debilitated patient of the older descriptions of the disease is seldom seen today. Before treatment is started it is necessary to exclude any underlying cause such as a vaginal foreign body which produces a foul smelling blood stained discharge, or the presence, in the stools, of threadworms which may enter the vagina. A rectal thermometer makes a convenient sound for the detection of a foreign body in the vagina. Masturbation may be a factor and such children sometimes show dilatation of the hymen.

*Treatment*. Specific therapy is dependent on the result of bacterial investigations. The most satisfactory local treatment is twice daily potassium permanganate sitz baths. Parents should be warned not to use the family bath for these, since the potassium permanganate causes unpleasant staining. If this should occur sodium thiosulphate helps to remove it.

Many of the children brought to the doctor for a vaginal discharge have nothing more than a combination of excess normal vaginal mucus and an anxious mother or an over-zealous and ignorant school matron. In boarding schools, such children are often put into strict isolation and it is therefore essential that an early correct diagnosis is made.

## BIBLIOGRAPHY

ADENIYI A., HENDRICKSE R.G. & HOUBA V. (1970) Selectivity of proteinuria and response to prednisolone or immunosuppressive drugs in children with malarial nephrosis. *Lancet*, **1**, 644.

ALLISON A.C., HOUBA V., HENDRICKSE R.G., DE PETRIS S., EDINGTON G.M. & ADENIYI A. (1969) Immune complexes in the nephrotic syndrome of African children. *Lancet*, **1**, 1232.

ARNEIL G.C., MCALLISTER T.A. & KAY P. (1973) Measurement of bacteriuria by plane dipslide culture. *Lancet*, **1**, 94.

BARRATT T.M., BERCOWSKY A., OSOFSKY S.G. & SOOTHILL J.F. (1975) Cyclophosphamide treatment in steroid-sensitive nephrotic syndrome of childhood. *Lancet*, **1**, 55.

BARRATT T.M., CAMERON J.S., CHANTLER C., OGG C.S. & SOOTHILL J.F. (1973) Comparative trial of 2 weeks and 8 weeks cyclophosphamide in steroid-sensitive relapsing nephrotic syndrome of childhood. *Arch. Dis. Childh.*, **48**, 286.

CAMERON J.S. & BLANDFORD G. (1966) The simple assessment of selectivity in heavy proteinuria. *Lancet*, **2**, 242.

DOXIADIS S.A., GOLDFINCH M.K. & COLE N. (1952) 'Proteinuria' in the newborn. *Lancet*, **2**, 1242.

ELLIS A. (1942) Natural history of Bright's disease. *Lancet*, **1**, 1.

GILLES H.M. & HENDRICKSE R.G. (1960) Possible aetiological role of *Plasmodium malariae* in nephrotic syndrome in Nigerian children. *Lancet*, **1**, 806.

GREINER T. & HENRY J.P. (1955) Mechanism of postural proteinuria. *J. Amer. med. Ass.*, **157**, 1373.

HODSON C.J. & WILSON S. (1965) Natural history of chronic pyelonephritic scarring. *Brit. med. J.*, **2**, 191.

JAGASIA K.H., THURMAN W.G., PICKETT E. & GRABSTALDT H. (1964) Bilateral Wilms' tumors in children. *J. Pediat.*, **65**, 371.

LINES D.R. (1969) Selectivity of proteinuria in childhood nephrotic syndrome. *Arch. Dis. Childh.*, **44**, 461.

MCDONALD J., MURPHY A.V. & ARNEIL G.C. (1974) Long-term assessment of cyclophosphamide therapy for nephrosis in children. *Lancet*, **2**, 980.

MCDOWALL M.F., RAMKISSOON R. & BASSETT D.C.J. (1970) Epidemic and endemic pattern of childhood nephritis. Pathogenesis, epidemiology and clinical course of outbreaks in Trinidad. *Clin. Ped.*, **9**, 580.

MACGREGOR M. (1970) Pyelonephritis lenta. Consideration of childhood urinary infection as the forerunner of renal insufficiency in later life. *Arch. Dis. Childh.*, **45**, 159.

MARTIN J. & RICKHAM P.P. (1974) Wilms's tumour—an improved prognosis. Report of 22 consecutive children seen from 1967–71. *Arch. Dis. Childh.*, **49**, 459.

MEADOW S.R., CAMERON J.S., OGG C.S. & SAXTON H.M. (1971) Children referred for acute dialysis. *Arch. Dis. Childh.*, **46**, 221.

PENSO J., LIPPE B., EHRLICH R. & SMITH F.G. (1974) Testicular function in prepubertal and pubertal male patients treated with cyclophosphamide for nephrotic syndrome. *J. Ped.*, **84**, 831.

ROBINSON R.R., ASHWORTH C.T., GLOVER S.N., PHILLIPPI P.J., LECOCQ F.R. & LANGELIER P.R. (1961) Fixed and reproducible orthostatic proteinuria. II. Electron microscopy of renal biopsy specimens from five cases. *Amer. J. Path.*, **39**, 405.

ROBINSON R.R., LECOCQ F.R., PHILLIPPI P.J. & GLENN W.G. (1963) Fixed and reproducible orthostatic proteinuria. III. Effect of induced renal hemodynamic alterations upon urinary protein excretion. *J. clin. Invest.*, **42**, 100.

SMELLIE J.M., HODSON C.J., EDWARDS D. & NORMAND I.C.S. (1964) Clinical and radiological features of urinary infection in childhood. *Brit. med. J.*, **2**, 1222.

SPITZER A., GORDILLO P.G., HOUSTON I.B. & TRAVIS L.B. (1974) Prospective, controlled trial of cyclophosphamide therapy in children with the nephrotic syndrome. Report of the International Study of Kidney Disease in Children. *Lancet*, **2**, 423.

SVARTMAN M., POTTER E.V., FINKLEA J.F. & POON-KING T. (1972) Epidemic scabies and acute glomerulonephritis in Trinidad. *Lancet*, **1**, 249.

WHITE R.H.R. (1964) 'Silent' nephritis. *Guy's Hosp. Rep.*, **113**, 190.
WHITE R.H.R., GLASGOW E.F. & MILLS R.J. (1970) Clinicopathological study of nephrotic syndrome in childhood. *Lancet*, **1**, 1353.
WITTIG H.J. & GOLDMAN A.S. (1970) Nephrotic syndrome associated with inhaled allergens. *Lancet*, **1**, 542.

# CHAPTER 14

# DISORDERS OF THE NERVOUS SYSTEM

**Pyogenic meningitis**

Pyogenic meningitis remains confined to the meninges, whereas virus infections are more likely to cause meningo-encephalitis. Meningitis is more common in winter than in summer, suggesting the importance of a previous respiratory infection. The infection usually arrives via the blood stream from some other septic focus, particularly the lung, middle ear (especially *Haemophilus influenzae*) or umbilicus. Direct infection of the meninges may occur through a myelocele (p. 213) or a congenital dermal sinus (p. 208). Such sinuses may exist at any point in the midline of the scalp or back and must be sought in all cases of meningitis, particularly if recurrent; in such patients the scalp should be shaved to facilitate the search.

Meningitis has been caused by every known bacterium, but in children the majority are due to the meningococcus, *Haemophilus influenzae*, pneumococcus and *Escherichia coli*; the latter is largely confined to infants (see p. 113). Tuberculous meningitis is considered separately (p. 522). All these infections produce an inflammatory exudate though its characteristics vary according to the organism involved. In meningococcal meningitis the exudate tends to be concentrated at the base of the brain somewhat similarly to tuberculous meningitis. In advanced cases it spreads upwards over the cerebral cortex along the middle and anterior cerebral arteries. In fulminating cases death may occur before the formation of pus; at autopsy there is only cerebral congestion with petechial haemorrhages scattered throughout the white and grey matter, especially in the subependymal regions of the lateral ventricles. In such cases the clinical picture is that of encephalitis with rapid development of coma.

The exudate of influenzal meningitis does not follow a fixed pattern. It is very thick, pockets of pus being found in the basal cisterns and in the sulci over the cortex. The organism has a tendency to produce arteritis and phlebitis, with consequent haemorrhage or abscess formation. In pneumococcal meningitis the exudate is thick and yellowish-green, mainly found over the vertex of the brain.

Although the organisms do not invade the brain it becomes swollen from oedema and congestion. This swelling is particularly serious since the skull limits the expansion of the brain; the consequent obstruction to venous drainage leads to further swelling and a vicious circle which may cause herniation of the brain. In infants whose sutures have not yet fused, there is more room for expansion.

*Clinical features.* The classical features of neck stiffness and head retraction as seen in the adult are late features in children and seldom seen in infants. Failure to appreciate this difference accounts for serious delays in diagnosis. In children, and especially in infants, the most frequent symptoms are irritability, vomiting and anorexia. An older child will complain of headache. Drowsiness is an early feature; the infant has a vacant expression with staring eyes and, in severe cases, may even present in coma. If the fontanelle is still open the tension may be sufficiently increased to cause bulging which is so obvious that the mother brings the child because of 'the bump on his head'. If the infant is dehydrated from vomiting or diarrhoea the increased tension of the fontanelle will be less obvious, but even then the tension is more than would be expected in a dehydrated baby.

The cry is high pitched ('meningeal'). Convulsions are common in infants, in whom they are often the presenting feature, although a history that the child has been off colour and refusing feeds for a few hours before is usually obtained. A squint is common. Petechial haemorrhages may be present in the early stages of a meningococcal infection; they occur less frequently in infection due to other causes. Papilloedema is not usual in children. Anaemia, which is often severe, is particularly likely to accompany *H. influenzae* meningitis.

The diagnosis is confirmed by an examination of the cerebrospinal fluid obtained from lumbar puncture. The fluid is opaque or frankly purulent, the cell count being increased as high as 15,000 the cells being polymorphs. The protein is raised and the sugar is low. The organism may be identified by smear or only by culture. *Haemophilus influenzae* are present in large numbers in the smear and are easily cultured, but meningococci are less easily seen and more difficult to culture. Consequently, the meningococcus is the most likely cause of purulent meningitis if no organisms are seen. An immediate diagnosis of meningococcal, pneumococcal and *H. influenzae* meningitis can be made by the latex test for the detection of specific antigen in the cerebrospinal fluid (Whittle *et al.*, 1974).

*Post-basic meningitis* is a chronic form of meningococcal meningitis occurring in infants. The exudate is largely confined to the basal cisterns since the soft infantile brain causes the sulci to be closed at an early stage of the disease. The clinical picture differs from the usual in that there is severe neck stiffness, head retraction and opisthotonos.

*Diagnosis.* In infants the clinical picture is that of an acute infection and the condition must be differentiated from all the other forms of sepsis. The increased fontanelle tension is most valuable in diagnosis. Children with meningitis dislike moving their heads and therefore lie still. But because delay in diagnosis is so serious a lumbar puncture must be carried out whenever the diagnosis is suspected. In the neonate the distinction between meningitis and intracranial haemorrhage can only be made by a lumbar puncture.

Virus meningo-encephalitis can be differentiated only by an examination of the cerebrospinal fluid although clinically there is less meningeal irritation and the state of consciousness remains more clear. The fluid is clear or at most opalescent, the rise of cells being seldom more than 1000 per mm$^3$. The cells may be polymorphonuclear at the onset but then become predominantly monocytic. The rise in protein is slight and the sugar is normal.

Subarachnoid haemorrhage is rare in childhood; it is more often due to an angioma than a ruptured aneurysm. The onset is acute, with intense headache and blood-stained cerebrospinal fluid. Differentiation from a bloody tap due to trauma sometimes causes diagnostic difficulties. In such cases, a comparative red cell count between the first and last tubes is helpful since the blood in a traumatic tap tends to clear.

*Meningismus* causes considerable diagnostic difficulties in children. This name is given to the neck stiffness which may accompany the onset of any acute infection in childhood, especially tonsillitis, otitis media, pneumonia and pyelonephritis. Its cause is unknown. Children with meningismus are alert and show signs of the primary infection, but an examination of the cerebrospinal fluid, which will be normal, may be essential to establish the correct diagnosis.

*Treatment.* Correct antibiotic therapy is dependent on the isolation of the causative organism, therefore it should never be given before the lumbar puncture. It is incorrect when writing to be dogmatic as to which antibiotic should be used for each organism since unexpected resistance may be encountered. For example, cases of ampicillin-resistant *H. influenzae* occasionally occur (Murray *et al.*, 1974). Meningococcal and pneumococcal meningitis are best treated with benzyl penicillin which is more active than ampicillin against these organisms. *Haemophilus influenzae* should be treated with ampicillin. *Escherichia coli* may be resistant to ampicillin, therefore gentamycin or kanamycin should be given in addition. If the organism cannot be identified the child should receive benzyl penicillin and gentamycin.

If the CSF is purulent, intrathecal ampicillin should be given except in the neonatal period when *E. coli* may be the cause. For this age group intrathecal gentamycin should be given. Continued intrathecal treatment is seldom needed since the majority of antibiotics cross the blood–brain barrier when it is inflamed. It should, however, be used in severe cases, especially those due to the pneumococcus in whom the prognosis is particularly poor, and where the cerebrospinal fluid is so thick that a spinal block is likely to develop.

For the first few days, until the child is well on the way to recovery, antibiotic therapy should be parenteral and preferably intravenous. This route is the most effective and, when given by drip, is the least painful. Antibiotic treatment should be continued for at least 2 weeks and should not be stopped until the CSF cell count is normal and a negative culture obtained. The lumbar puncture should be repeated after 48 hours to ensure that the organism has been destroyed and repeated at weekly intervals until a normal cell count is obtained.

The use of steroids is debated, but their use is wise if there is any danger of the development of a block. Intramuscular steroids are indicated if gram-negative shock develops. This is particularly liable to occur in the neonatal period and at any age in acute meningococcal septicaemia with or without meningitis. It also requires urgent treatment with intravenous fluids. Such patients are very liable to develop disseminated intravascular coagulation.

There is a close association between the occurrence of fits and the outcome of the disease. Each convulsion is liable to cause additional brain damage from anoxia and the exhaustion it produces is serious. Moreover, there is always the danger that vomit will be inhaled during the fit. Measures must therefore be taken to prevent fits by the routine administration of anti-convulsant drugs to all patients with meningitis. If the family doctor is reasonably certain of the diagnosis, he should administer the first dose in the home in order to reduce the chance of a fit from the extra disturbance during the journey to hospital. Phenobarbitone is suitable, the dose being suf-ficiently large to be effective. For most patients 30–60 mg is required, the first dose being given intramuscularly. A maintenance dose should be given every 6 hours during the acute phase of illness. If, despite phenobarbitone, a convulsion occurs the child should be given intravenous diazepam (0·3 mg/kg) or intramuscular paraldehyde (0·2 ml/kg).

Meningococcal meningitis is associated with a high carrier rate among contacts; for this reason prophylactic sulphadiazine should be given for 2 days to the other children in the house to reduce the risk of cross-infection. In view of the increased incidence of sulphonamide-resistant meningococci, sensitivity tests may show a need for penicillin instead. In the tropics it is associated with bad housing and overcrowding, but this does not appear to be the case in England; epidemics are particularly liable to occur in hot, dry countries.

### Complications of meningitis

Blockage of the flow of cerebrospinal fluid causes hydrocephalus. Any of the cranial nerves may be permanently damaged but the most frequent sequelae are deafness, and facial and ocular palsies. Deafness is such a common complication and delay in its diagnosis has such serious consequences, that all children who have had meningitis should be followed for long enough to ensure that they are not deaf. If deafness occurs, a hearing aid should be provided without delay. Severe cerebral damage leads to mental handicap and fits.

The frequency of sequelae, especially mental handicap, is greatest with pneumococcal infections and least with meningococcal. The younger the infant the higher the incidence of permanent damage; all patients must be followed up.

SUBDURAL EFFUSION

This is a common complication, especially in infants with severe meningitis and if untreated leads to serious sequelae from brain compression. It occurs most often with influenzal or pneumococcal meningitis, the effusion probably resulting from an abnormal permeability of the dural vessels. It is most often situated over the frontal or parietal region and is yellow with a high protein content. Although it may reabsorb spontaneously, the effusion tends to become encapsulated and then to increase in size, either as a result of osmotic action following the breakdown of protein within the sac, or because of abnormal permeability of the vessels in the wall. The effect of the effusion is to prevent the anticipated response to antibiotic therapy. The possibility of its existence must therefore be considered if the signs, particularly fever, fail to settle within 72 hours of the beginning of adequate therapy. An effusion must also be suspected if culture of the cerebrospinal fluid remains positive or if focal neurological signs develop.

*Diagnosis.* Daily measurement of the head circumference showing an unusual increase are suggestive of the condition but the only certain method is by subdural taps. The exploratory needles should be inserted in four places; at the two most lateral points of the anterior fontanelle and as far down the frontoparietal sutures as possible. Once the dura has been pierced the needle should be held to see if there is a flow of fluid. Before removal it should be gently turned through a full circle in case the position of the bevel affects the flow. Under normal circumstances only 1 or 2 drops of clear fluid are obtained.

*Treatment.* If an effusion is present it should be tapped daily but not more than 20–30 ml of fluid removed at one time. The condition is self-limiting provided the fluid is removed, but it is essential to prevent compression of the brain. If after daily tapping for 2 weeks there is no reduction in the amount of fluid obtained and the subdural space is large as determined by air studies, continuous drainage should be considered. This is achieved by inserting a tube between the subdural space and the pleural cavity on the same side. The tube is removed after a few weeks. Craniotomy in order to remove the membrane surrounding the effusion is seldom practised today.

ACUTE ADRENAL FAILURE (WATERHOUSE-FRIDERICHSEN SYNDROME)

This complication results from massive haemorrhage into both adrenal glands; it is usually caused by a fulminating meningococcal septicaemia. Less often it is due to other organisms, particularly *Pseudomonas pyocyanea*. The onset is so fulminating that the cerebrospinal fluid is seldom purulent by the time the symptoms develop, but becomes so if the child survives long enough. Within 2–3 hours of being perfectly well the child becomes collapsed with marked hypotension and massive blotchy, generalized purpura which can be seen to spread as the child is watched. This state of shock results from disseminated intravascular coagulation as well as adrenal failure. The mental state remains clear, in contrast to the collapse associated with fulminating encephalitis when coma develops early. The extremities are warm and flushed in comparison with most other causes of acute hypotension when they are cold and pale.

This is the most dramatic illness of childhood, death occurring within a few hours unless the child can be rescued by the immediate intravenous administration of hydrocortisone, antibiotics and fluids. Anti-coagulant therapy is also an urgent necessity if disseminated intravascular coagulation is taking place. The condition is one of the very few where every minute's delay is serious.

## Encephalitis

The majority of cases are of viral origin and the spinal cord is also frequently involved (encephalomyelitis). In many cases the meninges also are affected. Viruses show a predilection for certain areas of the central nervous system: poliomyelitis and most of the specific viruses of encephalitis favour the grey matter, whereas the reaction to the viruses of the specific fevers occurs mainly in the white matter.

VIRAL ENCEPHALITIS

The pathology and symptomatology in this group is similar, although some viruses show a special affinity for certain areas of the grey matter. These viruses may be neurotropic, that is they show an affinity for nervous tissue, or they may be viscerotropic, only occasionally attacking the nervous system. In the first group are a very large number of viruses such as poliomyelitis, Coxsackie, ECHO, rabies, lymphocytic choriomeningitis, epidemic encephalitis type A (encephalitis lethargica of von Economo). The different varieties of arthropod-borne epidemic encephalitis such as St Louis, equine encephalitis (both eastern and western forms), Japanese type B, Australian X disease and Murray Valley are also in this group.

In the second group are those viruses which seldom attack the nervous system but cause diseases in other organs; for example, infectious hepatitis, herpes simplex, virus pneumonia and infectious mononucleosis. Also in this group is mumps; this can attack the nervous system in two ways: first by direct involvement particularly of the meninges, producing the clinical picture of 'aseptic meningitis' (see below), secondly, by the production of a demyelinating encephalomyelitis of similar aetiology to that produced by the other specific fevers, as discussed below.

*Pathology.* If the meninges are involved they are infiltrated with mononuclear cells. The brain itself looks pink from dilatation of the capillaries immediately under the meninges and there may be areas of softening from necrosis. Microscopic examination shows cuffing of the perivascular spaces with mononuclear cells, and degeneration of the ganglion cells. The area of the nervous system principally involved varies with the different viruses: poliomyelitis affects mainly the anterior horn cells of the spinal ganglia; epidemic encephalitis type A the basal ganglia, mid-brain and pons; Australian X and Japanese type B usually involve the cerebellum.

*Clinical features.* If the meninges are involved the features are those of meningeal irritation to which the term 'aseptic meningitis' is applied (see below). If the brain itself is mainly involved the features of encephalitis predominate. Mental changes are common, speech may be affected and the state of consciousness may vary from drowsiness to coma. Involvement of the cerebellum causes ataxia, and of the brain stem cranial nerve palsies. The cerebrospinal fluid may show a rise of lymphocytes, but is often entirely normal.

*Treatment.* Specific antiviral therapy is still experimental. Sedation should be given as necessary. The prognosis varies with the different viruses.

SUBACUTE SCLEROSING PANENCEPHALITIS (SUBACUTE INCLUSION BODY ENCEPHALITIS: SUBACUTE SCLEROSING LEUCO-ENCEPHALITIS)

This condition is discussed on p. 495 since it is caused by measles.

ASEPTIC MENINGITIS

This is a syndrome produced by a number of different viruses and occasionally by other agents (see below) resulting in the same clinical picture. The condition is commoner in males, its highest incidence being from May to October.

The symptoms are those of meningeal irritation causing irritability and convulsions in small children, and headache and pain in the back in older children. Vomiting is common and there are no focal neurological signs. The cerebrospinal fluid shows a rise of mononuclear cells up to 3000 per $mm^3$; there may be a slight rise in protein. Complete recovery is the rule.

The virus of lymphocytic choriomeninigitis (LCM), transmitted from mice, is well known as a cause of this syndrome. Mumps virus produces the same condition and since it is not necessarily associated with parotitis, the clinical diagnosis must rest on evidence of contact with a known case of mumps. Poliomyelitis, Coxsackie (Groups A and B), herpes simplex and herpes zoster viruses may produce the same meningeal reaction; any of the viruses which cause encephalitis may also be responsible. The syndrome is also seen following scarlet fever and in leptospirosis and is produced by the toxic action of poisons such as lead or arsenic or the irritant effect of intrathecal injections of antibiotics, lipiodol or air.

*Diagnosis.* The condition must be differentiated from tuberculous meningitis on the findings in the cerebrospinal fluid. The cell count is of no help, but if the protein is over 100 mg per cent it is most unlikely to be aseptic meningitis. In tuberculous meningitis, the sugar is usually low (though a normal sugar does not exclude a tuberculous infection) but in aseptic meningitis it will be normal unless there has been much vomiting. In such cases the sugar in the cerebrospinal fluid will have fallen in common with the blood sugar, whereas in tuberculous meningitis the sugar in the cerebrospinal fluid is lower than the blood sugar. To avoid this fallacy the blood sugar should be taken at the same time as the cerebrospinal fluid.

Lesions within or near the central nervous system, such as a cerebral abscess or tumour, may cause a similar meningeal reaction and must be excluded.

### ACUTE DISSEMINATED ENCEPHALOMYELITIS

This condition may occur spontaneously but the majority of cases occur as a complication of the acute specific fevers, or of vaccination. The pathology is remarkably uniform in all types, differing from the forms of virus encephalitis already described in that demyelinization is the characteristic feature. The earliest change is lymphocytic infiltration of the walls of the veins. This is followed by demyelinization which occurs in patches that are often sharply demarcated and found in close relation to small and medium-sized veins. The lesions occur predominantly in the white matter of the brain and spinal cord. In severe cases the lesions are those of an acute haemorrhagic leuco-encephalitis, with haemorrhages related principally to capillaries and venules, and fibrinoid necrosis of their walls.

*Aetiology.* Although it is possible that the condition results from direct infection by the primary virus, this is unlikely since the condition is not contagious. The cerebral lesions differ from those already described in virus encephalitis and the virus has only occasionally been isolated. It now seems more likely that the condition represents a sensitization reaction to the infecting virus. A similar demyelinating effect has been produced in experimental animals by the injection of homologous or heterologous brain tissue. This theory would better explain the similarity of the condition despite the large differences in the primary virus infection, and the fact that it bears no relation to the severity of the original infection. It would also fit in better with the fact that the encephalitis usually comes on when the primary illness is subsiding and the virus no longer detectable. Such variations as there are in the clinical syndrome could be explained by the differing antigenic properties of the various viruses.

*Clinical features.* The onset is usually between the seventh and twelfth day of the disease, at a time when antibodies are being formed. The picture varies according to whether the involvement is principally of the brain (encephalitis), meninges (meningitis) or spinal cord (myelitis), any combination of these occurring. The child usually becomes irritable, drowsy and may lapse into coma. Convulsions are common and paralyses, more often of the cranial nerves particularly the facial, may occur. The cerebrospinal fluid may be entirely normal if the condition is one of encephalitis rather than meningo-encephalitis.

Measles is the most common cause, being especially liable to leave an intellectual defect. The mortality rate is appreciable and in some series has been as high as 20 per cent. Rubella is a rare cause but its mortality rate is about the same as measles. Varicella encephalitis differs in that the symptoms are predominantly cerebellar and the prognosis is much better than with measles and rubella, the fatality rate being about 5 per cent; few of the survivors have any neurological disability.

Mumps differs from the other three already discussed since, in the majority of cases, the cerebral symptoms are due to a true mumps meningitis caused by direct viral invasion of the meninges, so producing the syndrome of aseptic meningitis. However, cases of encephalitis, which are clinically and pathologically the same as the other three, occasionally follow mumps and can be presumed to have a similar aetiology. Particularly strong evidence is the fact that such cases occur without the meningeal symptoms or the lymphocytic pleocytosis which are cardinal features of the aseptic meningitis syndrome.

In assessing the question of encephalitis due to scarlet fever it is important to exclude such complications as bacterial meningitis and hypertensive encephalopathy. The syndrome of aseptic meningitis certainly occurs, though its aetiology is not clear. It may be due to a toxic or allergic effect and is quite different from the cases of true bacterial meningitis.

The neurological complications of pertussis differ both clinically and pathologically from those described for the other specific fevers. The cases usually occur during the first year of life, the period of greatest severity of pertussis but not of its greatest incidence. The onset is between the second and fourth week of the illness, the clinical picture being remarkably constant. There is a sudden onset of generalized convulsions and coma which may last for hours or days and is associated with a spastic paralysis which is usually symmetrical. The cerebrospinal fluid is usually normal. The mortality rate is about 30 per cent. About half the survivors are left with mental retardation, epilepsy or spastic paresis. Perivenous demyelinating encephalitis is not seen. The usual lesion is eosinophilic degeneration which is most marked in the pyramidal cells of the hippocampus and the Purkinje cells of the cerebellum. It is thought likely that anoxia is the basis of these lesions. A similar syndrome may follow pertussis immunization and is possibly a toxic or sensitization effect.

Post-vaccinial encephalomyelitis usually occurs 10–12 days after vaccination; the risk is least in young children during the second year of life. The clinical picture may be that of meningitis, encephalitis or myelitis, the histological picture of demyelinization being the same as that following the specific levers. The mortality rate may be as high as 50 per cent.

*Treatment.* This is symptomatic only as there is no specific therapy. It seemed reasonable to expect that steroids would be of value since the condition is a sensitization reaction, but these hopes were not realized; some patients have deteriorated when steroids have been given. Since there is viraemia in the case of mumps encephalomyelitis, steroids should never be given.

TOXOPLASMA ENCEPHALITIS (see p. 542)

## Poliomyelitis

This is a highly infectious disease which is caused by any of three different types of poliomyelitis virus (1, 2 and 3). Type 1 accounts for the majority of cases but there is no evidence that the incidence of paralysis varies with the different types. The incubation period is 7–12 days. The virus can be found in the throat after 36 hours and in the faeces after 72 hours. It persists in the throat for one week and in the faeces for up to 6 weeks or even longer.

The virus is spread by droplet infection and faecal contamination, reaching the alimentary tract of the host where it multiplies, then entering the blood stream for the phase of viraemia. From the blood it passes to the central nervous system (neural phase). This method of spread within the body accounts for the four stages of the disease, at any one of which it may be arrested; in only a minority of cases does it pass through all stages. These are:

1. *Silent infection.* The virus is in the alimentary phase.

2. *Abortive poliomyelitis.* The virus is in both the alimentary and viraemic phases, the result being an influenza-like illness.

3. *Non-paralytic poliomyelitis.* The virus is in the alimentary, viraemic and neural phase and an illness characterized by meningeal irritation occurs.

4. *Paralytic poliomyelitis.* The virus is in all three phases, its action on the neurone causing paralysis. In the majority of cases the paralysis affects the anterior horn cells of the spinal cord only, but in severe cases the cranial nerves and brain stem are also involved (bulbar poliomyelitis). Polioencephalitis indicates that there is also impairment of cerebral function. This occurs in fulminating cases which also involve the spine and brain stem.

### 1. SILENT INFECTION

The incidence of the silent infection alone is impossible to determine, but it is certainly very high, especially in communities where the standards of hygiene are poor. In some tropical countries it has been found that up to 95 per cent of the children have developed antibodies to all three types of virus by the age of 3 years, although few of these are known to have had a clinical infection and only a small proportion have gone on to develop paralysis. In such countries almost all the paralytic cases occur between the ages of 6 months and 3 years. The newborn infant is initially protected by transmitted maternal antibodies, but these diappear by the age of 6 months. In countries where the standards of hygiene are high the chances of early infection are much less and consequently paralytic cases occur at a later age. However, it is in these countries that the occasional case will be seen during the first 6 months, and even in the neonatal period, since the chance of maternal immunity is much less.

### 2. ABORTIVE POLIOMYELITIS

The true cause of the influenza-like illness will almost certainly be missed unless an epidemic of poliomyelitis is occurring, when a special watch for such cases will be kept. The fact that in temperate climates poliomyelitis occurs more often during the summer months may be of help since influenza occurs more often during the winter months. The illness is associated with fever, headache, vomiting, sore throat and sometimes with diarrhoea.

### 3. NON-PARALYTIC POLIOMYELITIS

An interval of 2–3 days occurs between stages two and three, so that the temperature which had fallen to normal, rises again to produce the second hump on the so-called 'dromedary' chart. The clinical features are those of meningeal irritation. Headache is a common presenting symptom and vomiting is frequent. Pain in the neck and back results from muscle stiffness and there may be similar pain in the limbs. Diagnosis depends on the demonstration of muscle spasm, since there is no paralysis. Neck stiffness can best be demonstrated by asking the child to sit up and kiss his knee. Stiffness in the back is seen by the child's characteristic 'tripod' position when asked to sit up, since in doing so he places his hands behind him on the bed to keep the spine rigid as he comes forward. (The 'tripod' is made up of the two hands and the buttocks.) An important diagnostic feature is the fact that though there are meningitic symptoms, the child is fully conscious.

The cerebrospinal fluid usually shows the early changes of pleocytosis (see below). Paralysis can be precipitated by lumbar puncture during the viraemic stage, but unless the clinical diagnosis is absolutely certain it is still essential to undertake the lumbar puncture lest the symptoms are due to bacterial meningitis. No intramuscular injections should be given in view of the risk of 'provocation' poliomyelitis (see below). Activity encourages the development of paralysis; therefore, strict bed rest is essential in this phase, the child being kept in bed until 1 week after all symptoms have disappeared.

### 4. PARALYTIC POLIOMYELITIS

Only a very small proportion of those infected develop paralysis. This may occur without any obvious antecedent illness, especially in infants. Alternatively, it develops some 12–72 hours after the onset of the meningeal phase. Pain and tenderness in the muscles is usually the first evidence that paralysis is developing, though this is less marked in children than in adults. The paralysis reaches its maximum extent within 48 hours of its onset. Fever indicates activity and the likelihood that the paralysis will extend, so that a fall in temperature is an encouraging sign. Fasciculation may occur in the affected muscles. A characteristic wobbly prefixation tremor of the eyes and retention of urine are common early features of the paralytic phase; a particular watch should be kept for distension of the bladder. The paralysis of limb mucles is flaccid and asymmetrical, with an early loss of tendon reflexes; paralysis seldom occurs in one limb only.

A close watch must be kept for early evidence of respiratory difficulty which, in most cases, results from pooling of saliva in the mouth owing to paralysis of swallowing or respiratory muscles. Involvement of the respiratory centre in bulbar poliomyelitis will also cause respiratory difficulty, but this is less common than the other two causes. Bulbar involvement is not necessarily severe and unilateral facial palsy, or isolated palatal paralysis, may be the only sign. A nasal voice or regurgitation of fluids through the nose without vomiting, indicates palatal weakness.

*Cerebrospinal fluid.* The fluid is clear, but in the meningeal stage there is a rise both in polymorphs and lymphocytes. The total figure is usually less than 500 per mm$^3$ but is occasionally as high as 1500; the higher the total cell count the greater is the percentage of polymorphs. There is a slight rise in protein and the sugar is normal. About a week later there are fewer cells and these are largely lymphocytes. The rise in protein may have continued, sometimes reaching 400 mg per cent. The cellular changes are equally abnormal in paralytic and non-paralytic cases but the rise in protein is more distinct in the paralytic cases. Occasionally the cerebrospinal fluid is normal.

*Diagnosis.* In the meningeal stage the condition simulates the 'aseptic meningitis' syndrome and only the isolation of virus from the throat, stool or cerebrospinal fluid, or the later finding of a rising antibody titre may make a definite diagnosis possible. But a careful history to determine any possible contact with other virus infections may give important clues. Lymphocytic choriomeningitis infection cannot be definitely differentiated without viral studies, but cell counts over 500 per mm$^3$ are unusual in poliomyelitis and usual in lymphocytic choriomeningitis.

Tuberculous meningitis causes a longer preliminary period of ill-health and, as in all forms of bacterial meningitis, the patient is likely to be confused and the eyes may be vacant, whereas in the meningeal phase of poliomyelitis, the child is fully conscious. Examination of the cerebrospinal fluid will complete the differentiation since the sugar is usually reduced and tubercle bacilli may be seen. In pyogenic meningitis the fluid is purulent and bacteria may be present.

Infective polyneuritis is not associated with meningeal symptoms, the paralysis is symmetrical, tending to progress over weeks and there are sensory disturbances. The cerebrospinal fluid contains no excess of cells but a high level of protein, though occasionally such a combination may be found in the later stages of poliomyelitis.

Painful lesions outside the nervous system accounting for refusal to move a limb must be excluded; these may occur in osteomyelitis, acute arthritis, rheumatic fever and scurvy. The arthralgia of undulant fever may simulate the pain of poliomyelitis; occasionally undulant fever causes pseudoparalysis.

*Prophylaxis.* Immunization (p. 485) has prevented the epidemics which used to occur in western countries. It should be universal throughout the world. Travellers to developing countries must ensure that their immunization against poliomyelitis is up to date.

*Treatment.* Strict bed rest in isolation is essential during the meningeal and acute paralytic phases of the disease, long ambulance journeys being avoided if possible. Pain should be relieved by sedatives; warm packs may have the same effect by reducing spasm. The extent of the paralysis should be accurately determined during the acute phase, but tests of muscle power must be short and infrequent to prevent any muscle exhaustion. Joints must be supported in the neutral position by simple splints and the use of a bed cradle. This avoids the development of deformities from the action of gravity or the pull of unparalysed muscles. But joint movement must be maintained by removing the splint and putting it through it full range of movement 2–3 times a day.

Once the acute phase has passed and the muscles have entered the period of recovery, which usually takes about 2 weeks, active exercise and physiotherapy should be performed to build up muscle strength. Recovery may continue for at least 6 months and possibly longer, but after 18 months any improvement in function is the result of hypertrophy of non-paralysed muscles.

Patients with respiratory difficulties require special management. In the first place it is essential to diagnose those in whom the difficulty results from pooling of the secretions in the back of the mouth, owing to paralysis of the muscles of swallowing. For these children a respirator is lethal since all the secretions are then sucked straight into the lungs. The immediate first-aid measure for such patients, which can be carried out in the home, is to turn them into the face-down position and raise the foot of the bed. Nursing is later maintained in the head-down position with repeated suction as required.

Patients with paralysis of the respiratory muscles will need respirator treatment but judgment is required to decide when this is necessary. Restlessness, which results from anoxia, is a definite indication and so is indrawing of the sternum. It is much better to err on the side of safety, putting the child early into the respirator, rather than to risk the vicious circle which develops in prolonged hypoxia. All patients with respiratory difficulties should be on prophylactic antibiotic therapy.

Isolation of patients is usually maintained for 3 weeks, but they may excrete the virus for a much longer period.

## PROVOCATION POLIOMYELITIS

Any intramuscular injection into a child who is incubating poliomyelitis is liable to precipitate paralysis in the injected muscles. This risk is greatest with certain immunizing agents, particularly those containing alum, or when combined antigens are being given. Pertussis carries a greater risk than other antigens in this respect. With modern vaccines the risk is much less than it used to be, and protection is afforded by previous poliomyelitis vaccination. It is therefore now regarded as safe to give alum-precipitated combined diphtheria and tetanus vaccine to a child who has already been protected against poliomyelitis.

### Acute infective polyneuritis (Guillain-Barré syndrome)

This condition may occur at any age. It is uncommon, but as a result of immunization it now occurs more often than poliomyelitis in the United Kingdom. The cause is unknown but a virus is the most likely, possibly the Epstein-Barr virus (Grose & Feorino, 1972). The onset is with a mild febrile illness, usually with evidence of an upper respiratory infection. Following this prodromal illness there is a latent period of a few days or even weeks before the onset of paralysis, which usually occurs quite suddenly. The limbs are symmetrically involved, the proximal muscles being more affected than the distal. Bulbar involvement is rare, except that bilateral facial paralysis is not infrequent. Subjective sensory symptoms are common, but objective sensory loss is often not detectable. The cerebrospinal fluid contains no excess of cells but the protein is much increased, even up to 1000 mg per cent; this dissociation is characteristic.

*Diagnosis.* Confusion with poliomyelitis is the main difficulty, but such patients are febrile when the paralysis appears; this develops more rapidly than in polyneuritis. In poliomyelitis, muscle involvement is asymmetrical, there are no sensory changes and in most cases there are meningeal symptoms with a rise of cells in the cerebrospinal fluid.

Other causes of polyneuritis must be excluded, such as diphtheria and other infections, lead poisoning and vitamin B deficiency.

*Treatment.* There is no specific therapy, the children being managed in the same way as in poliomyelitis. Corticosteroid therapy may be of benefit if given early in the illness.

## CONVULSIONS

*Aetiology.* In discussing the aetiology of convulsions in childhood it is usual to divide them into febrile convulsions, symptomatic convulsions (due to cerebral and metabolic disorders) and idiopathic epilepsy. However, with the newer knowledge derived from electroencephalographic, genetic and bio-chemical studies such as classification is unsatisfactory, though not enough is yet known to produce a satisfactory alternative. How, for example, should we classify the infant who has one febrile convulsion but an abnormal electro-encephalogram? Presumably such a case must be regarded as one of idio-pathic epilepsy in the absence of any obvious abnormality in the brain.

One of the difficulties is that we still do not know what causes a fit. Con-vulsions associated with a cerebral tumour cannot be directly produced by the tumour since otherwise the patient would be having them all the time. It is certain that genetic predisposition plays a large part, but its effect is by no means straightforward. The incidence of a family history of fits in children with febrile convulsions is far higher than in those with idiopathic epilepsy and yet, since those with idiopathic epilepsy do not require the trigger of fever, one might have expected them to have had the greater familial tendency. In patients with fits due to head injury or tumour there is no evidence of a familial predisposition to fits.

It is obvious that many factors must be involved. The greater incidence in young children can best be explained on the basis that the young brain is less stable than that of the older child and adult, but vascular and biochemical factors are also probably involved. In the absence of further knowledge, an open mind must be kept regarding the aetiology of fits and no satisfaction should be derived from the application of descriptive labels, even though these are required in order to discuss the subject. Above all, it should be realized that 'epilepsy' is not a diagnosis but a symptom whose cause must be determined.

### Febrile convulsions

These are common, affecting about 5 per cent of all children. They are almost confined to those between 1 and 5 years and particularly affect children aged 1–3 years. Under the age of 6 months the diagnosis should not be made since convulsions in young babies are usually due to a specific cause. The fit is usually very short lived so that some more serious underlying cause must be suspected if the fit lasts more than 10 minutes. However, a few children have no cause other than fever to account for fits lasting longer than this. Similarly, the attacks are seldom focal.

The fit usually occurs at the onset of a rapid rise in temperature associated with an intercurrent illness such as otitis media, tonsillitis, pneumonia, pyelonephritis and the infectious fevers. Genetic factors play a large part in the production of febrile convulsions and in some series a family history of fits has been found in as many as 45 per cent of the patients. It is striking that the families tend to run true to type and the age at which the convulsions have ceased in other members of the family gives a reasonable forecast as to what is likely to be in store for the patient.

The attack itself is a 'grand mal' convulsion and there is no means of distinguishing these attacks from those seen in idiopathic epilepsy, apart from the precipitating factor. The classic four stages as seen in the adult, namely aura, tonic phase, clonic phase and stupor, run more closely together in the child. In young children an aura can seldom be discerned though they may appear to be very frightened immediately before the fit starts. Stupor is characteristic and although it may be short lived, so that the child only appears temporarily confused, its occurrence is of diagnostic value when trying to determine from the mother's history whether a convulsion took place. Incontinence of urine may occur during the attack, but biting of the tongue or lip occurs less often than in an adult.

Most patients have an abnormal electroencephalogram during the convulsion but this has usually become normal by the next day if the child is not suffering from idiopathic epilepsy.

### Symptomatic convulsions

A large proportion of these are due to intracranial injury sustained at birth, anoxia being more often the cause than physical damage or haemorrhage. Infection of the brain, such as meningitis and encephalitis, accounts for a number of cases and a variety of intracranial disorders such as vascular accidents, congenital malformations, neoplasms and cerebral degeneration may cause fits. With any of these causes the fit is liable to be focal, although focal attacks are less common in infancy than in older patients. Hypoglycaemia (p. 640) is by far the most important metabolic cause and for this reason the level of sugar in the blood or cerebrospinal fluid should always be determined in the investigation of a child with fits. Hypocalcaemia in association with rickets used to be a common cause of fits, but is now rare; it can cause fits in hypoparathyroidism.

A deficiency of pyridoxine occasionally causes convulsions. This may occur in association with an obvious dietary deficiency, but also shortly after birth where there is no obvious deficiency—a condition termed 'vitamin $B_6$ or pyridoxine dependency'. This condition is sometimes familial and is possibly due to an inborn error of metabolism involving an enzyme defect. Such patients respond dramatically to the vitamin and a continuous electroencephalographic record during intravenous administration shows improvement within a few minutes. Delay in diagnosis leads to mental retardation so that a therapeutic test with vitamin $B_6$ is warranted in the absence of any cause to account for the convulsions.

Uraemia or poisoning from lead or iron are other metabolic causes of convulsions which must be considered. On no account should convulsions be ascribed to 'teething' or worms.

Residual paralysis may follow convulsions from any cause but is more likely to occur in those with a focal onset. In such cases the paralysis usually clears within a few hours (Todd's paralysis); if it persists the chance of a focal brain defect is greater. In some patients with a persistent paralysis, a vascular accident may have occurred at the time of the convulsion.

### Idiopathic epilepsy

A diagnosis of idiopathic epilepsy can be made only after the most detailed

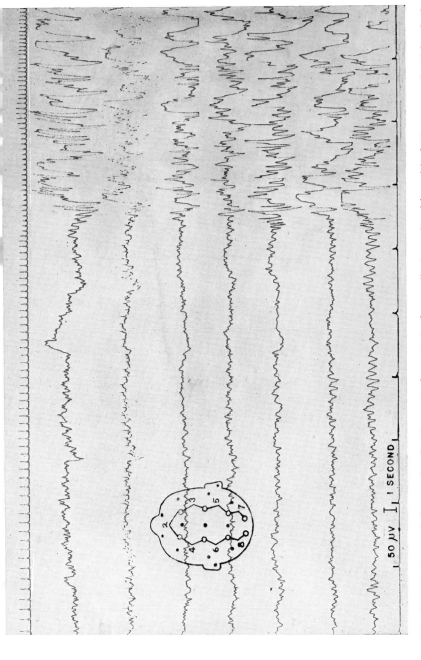

FIG. 110. Electroencephalogram showing the onset of an attack of generalized grand mal in a girl of 14 years, produced by photic stimulation at 11 cycles per second. High voltage spikes are seen to occur in all areas of the cortex. The frequency of the flash signal is recorded in the top channel.

search for an underlying cause; even if none has been found, the patient must be kept continually under review from this aspect. The attacks are most often of the *grand mal* type as described on p. 413. The electroencephalogram is helpful in diagnosis (Fig. 110), but there is no single characteristic picture in grand mal epilepsy; of more importance is the changing pattern of its abnormal features in subsequent records. The electroencephalographic record can be likened to a temperature chart in which a single abnormal reading gives only limited information, whereas an abnormal pattern seen over several days or weeks may be characteristic of a specific disease. It must also be interpreted in relation to the age of the patient. A normal newborn baby has waves which are slow, irregular, of low voltage and asynchronous. As the child grows older the waves become faster, of higher voltage and synchronization develops between the two ventricles.

*Status epilepticus* indicates a series of rapidly recurring grand mal attacks without any intervening return to consciousness. *Petit mal* (p. 420) is another form of idiopathic epilepsy. *Myoclonus* is a symptom indicating a sudden clonic spasm of a muscle or group of muscles. It may occur alone or in patients with perit mal or grand mal. Although typically occurring without loss of consciousness, this is not always so; but if it is lost the return to consciousness is immediate, unlike a grand mal attack which is followed by stupor.

An attack of epilepsy may be precipitated by psychological factors or by fever. It is often stated that psychological disturbances are common in the epileptic patient, but the more these are investigated, the more it is apparent that they are the result of the environment and the way the child is handled, rather than the fits themselves. Most children with epilepsy have normal personalities but their parents and some of their teachers find great difficulty in handling them in a normal balanced manner. Epilepsy is one of those conditions which may raise feelings of guilt in the minds of parents. Some parents try to hide the fact of the child's fits from their friends. This attitude is soon sensed by the child who may then feel guilty and try to avoid telling his parents when he has had a fit.

In only one type of epilepsy is abnormal behaviour common, namely *temporal lobe epilepsy*. In this condition abnormal discharges originate in the temporal lobe. The commonest cause is an area of scarring in Ammon's horn (mesial temporal sclerosis) which can be due to birth asphyxia. Convulsive anoxia during a febrile convulsion is another and most important cause of temporal lobe epilepsy, emphasizing the seriousness of such fits and the need to prevent and to shorten such attacks (Ounsted, 1971).

These fits may be preceded by a characteristic aura in which the child licks his lips, swallows and may have hallucinations of smell or taste. The serious consequences of temporal lobe epilepsy are hyperkinetic behaviour, bouts of cataclysmic rage and mental handicap.

*Diagnosis of grand mal.* The differentiation of febrile convulsions from true epilepsy may be impossible on clinical grounds; fever may precipitate a convulsion in an epileptic, while the muscular activity of any fit can cause a rise in temperature. A detailed history is essential; a febrile convulsion should be preceded by the child being unwell for at least one hour before the attack. A family history of febrile convulsions or of true epilepsy is helpful. Febrile convulsions occur only in young children and seldom last longer than a few minutes. An epileptic wave pattern in the electroencephalogram recorded after recovery from the illness is regarded as an indication of true epilepsy.

Convulsions must be differentiated from simple faints (p. 425); there is usually no difficulty if the doctor takes time to obtain a full history. Faints occur only when the child is standing up and there is no incontinence of urine and no biting of the lip or tongue; involuntary movements are rare in simple faints. The child becomes pale, slowly gliding to the floor. Sleep does not follow the attack.

Masturbation may produce a picture which is sometimes mistaken for convulsions. The child's attention is so absorbed in what he is doing that he looks vacant and is difficult to recall, but there is no loss of consciousness. The movements are slower than those due to fits and are rhythmic. They are also accompanied by flushing of the face and grunting. Breath-holding attacks (see p. 423) can be differentiated by a detailed history in which it becomes clear that the breath is always held before the fit occurs.

A diagnosis of idiopathic epilepsy must not be made until all the causes of symptomatic convulsions have been excluded; the possibility of hypoglycaemia must never be forgotten. Focal convulsions increase the likelihood that they are due to an actual brain lesion.

Patients with epilepsy sometimes present with bed-wetting if the convulsions occur only during sleep and have not been seen. Such children have usually become dry at night before their sudden incontinence develops; the disturbance caused to the bedclothes by the convulsive movements is helpful in diagnosis. In cases of doubt the electroencephalogram will decide the question. A lumbar puncture is usually required on the occasion of the first fit to exclude meningitis; the opportunity is then taken for the Wassermann reaction to be performed on the cerebrospinal fluid. The only occasion when a lumbar puncture need not be performed for a first fit is if the child has an obvious cause for the fever, has recovered completely from the convulsion and is under close observation. The skull should be X-rayed in case a calcified lesion is present.

### Treatment of grand mal

PREVENTION OF FEBRILE CONVULSIONS

It is impossible to be dogmatic about anticonvulsant treatment for children with febrile convulsions. There is general agreement that intermittent therapy given at the time of the fever is too late since it takes 2 days for therapeutic blood levels to be reached. Continuous phenobarbitone therapy is effective but unfortunately continuous phenytoin is not (Faerø et al., 1972). Moreover, the presence or absence of an abnormal electroencephalogram between fits should not be used as a guide to the need for anticonvulsant therapy.

The decision for continuous therapy would be much easier if phenytoin was effective since phenobarbitone is no longer recommended for children because it makes them irritable, inattentive and hyperactive. What is agreed is that all mothers should be aware of the immediate need to prevent a rapid rise of temperature in susceptible children. Immediate tepid sponging is essential and the child should be given an adult aspirin tablet. The room must be kept cool and the child unclothed until the temperature starts to fall.


PREVENTION OF GRAND MAL EPILEPSY

Anticonvulsant drugs are the basis of treatment. These must be given in sufficient dosage to be effective and for long enough to permit complete suppression; often too small a dose is given for too short a time. Because of the side effects of phenobarbitone, phenytoin is now the drug of choice for continuous anticonvulsant therapy. The dose is 5 mg/kg/day in one or two divided doses, but blood levels should be estimated at intervals in order to reduce the possibility of toxic effects. Hirsutes and gingival hyperplasia (Fig. 111) are common, though the latter should be prevented by good dental hygiene. Occasionally, gingivectomy is required to avoid dental damage from stasis of food under the hyperplastic gums. More serious are nystagmus, vomiting and ataxia which are dose dependent. Folic acid deficiency may develop, leading to megaloblastic anaemia which responds to folic acid therapy. Calcium metabolism can be disturbed, causing rickets from inactivation of vitamin D (p. 560).

If phenytoin alone fails to control the fits, it can be combined with phenobarbitone, provided side effects are avoided. Primidone can be given instead of the combination of phenytoin and phenobarbitone in a dose of 5–20 mg/kg/day in two divided doses. Abdominal pain and nausea may develop after the first few doses and for this reason it is wise to work up slowly to the full dose; these symptoms tend to pass off if treatment is continued. However, since primidone is also a barbiturate and it is partly metabolized in the liver into phenobarbitone, the same side effects may occur. If a child with epilepsy becomes hyperactive the first step must be to withdraw all barbiturate therapy.

If these medicines fail, some of the newer anticonvulsants should be tried such as sulthiamine, carbamazepine or clonazepam. Sodium valproate is another new medicine which is particularly effective in petit mal (p. 421) but is worth a trial in all forms of intractable epilepsey.

The same medicines are used in temporal lobe epilepsy. Surgical removal of the scarred area is occasionally performed.

It is essential that various combinations and doses of these drugs are tried until the fits are suppressed, but one month should be allowed for the trial of

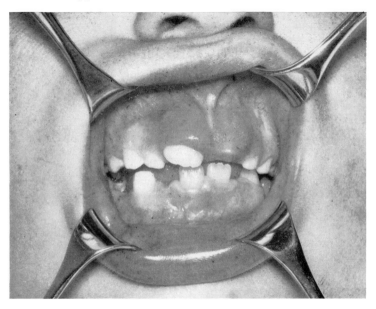

Fig. 111. Gingival hyperplasia from phenytoin.

each new drug or combination. If fits occur mainly at night the main dosage should be given to cover that period. Therapy should be continued for 3 years from the date of the last fit. The stopping of the drugs should be preceded by a period of gradual reduction in dose over a period of 6 months.

'Anticonvulsants' should not be referred to as 'drugs' when talking to parents. The word 'drug' carries the concept that the child may become addicted to it; this might cause some parents to avoid giving it.

MANAGEMENT OF A GRAND MAL ATTACK

Children seldom die during a convulsion and this only occurs if the airway becomes obstructed. The usual cause for this is the inhalation of vomit. Mothers need help not to panic by explaining that they should lie the child on his side on a bed or on the floor. On no account should the child be left in order to rush for a neighbour or to the telephone. Since children rarely bite their tongue or lips it is better not to force a gag into the mouth since greater trauma is liable to be caused.

The most useful drug for stopping a convulsion, including status epilepticus, is intravenous diazepam 0·3 mg/kg which does not cause respiratory depression. This has largely superseded paraldehyde which requires a glass syringe instead of a disposable one and can cause a sterile abscess when given intramuscularly. The doctor must not leave a convulsing child until he has stopped the attack. Status epilepticus increases the risk of subsequent brain damage owing to electrolyte imbalance and hypoglycaemia.

A child being transferred to hospital for the investigation of a recent fit should be given an anticonvulsant such as oral diazepam in order to prevent an attack during the journey. Not all children who have had a febrile convulsion need to be sent to hospital. If a child has recovered consciousness completely and close medical contact can be maintained with sensible parents it is safe for continued observation to take place at home.

GENERAL MANAGEMENT OF CHILDREN WITH EPILEPSY

Children with epilepsy must be treated as normal individuals and enjoy normal recreations. Cycling is the only activity which may need to be forbidden. Swimming is permissible provided someone is always with them, taking direct responsibility. No longer should they be sent to special schools. It is by these means that the child has the greatest chance of growing up to be normal. If fits are not controlled then the therapy is usually at fault.

PETIT MAL

In these attacks there is a transient loss of consciousness without appreciable convulsive movements. There is no preceding aura and no after-effect. The condition, which is often genetically determined, commonly starts between the ages of 3 and 9 years and rarely begins after the age of 15 years. The type of attack is usually constant for the same individual. The child may suddenly stop talking, remaining immobile, staring into space. After a few seconds he picks up his conversation where he left off, appearing in no way different. Transient pallor during the attack is common and a swaying movement of the upper part of the body may occur. In some children the head drops or the whole body bends forward. Patients rarely fall down during an attack although they may pass urine. Pyknolepsy is nothing more than repeated attacks of petit mal and should not be separately differentiated. Some patients may have hundreds of attacks in one day.

The attacks can usually be brought on by hyperventilation, a useful diagnostic aid. Some of the children can bring on their own attacks by photic stimulation; they produce a flickering light by hand movement or with the television, appearing to derive a compulsive form of pleasure from so doing. A fairly high proportion of the patients are mentally handicapped, but the condition is compatible with a high intelligence. Occasionally, children with petit mal have a sudden single muscular contraction in one part of the body which may cause them to drop to the ground (*myoclonic petit mal*). Many patients suffer grand mal attacks in addition to petit mal; the older the child the more likely is this association to occur.

Classically, the electroencephalogram in petit mal shows a 3 per second spike and wave discharge (Fig. 112) though this is found only in about half the cases. Other convulsive wave patterns are seen either alone or in association with the spike and wave. The abnormal wave pattern may be brought out by hyperventilation.

It is often stated that the prognosis for petit mal is good and that the child will grow out of it at puberty; this is incorrect. The majority of children still have the attacks when they reach adult life, although by then they have usually learnt to live with the condition and, to a large extent, are able to disregard the attacks. In some patients the petit mal attacks are replaced by grand mal.

*Treatment.* The majority of patients respond to ethosuximide in a dose of 20–50 mg/kg/day. For those who fail to respond, sodium valproate can be tried. This is a new anticonvulsant which is particularly effective in patients with petit mal showing a spike and wave pattern on the EEG (Jeavons & Clark, 1974). This drug may cause drowsiness, particularly if an intercurrent infection occurs. Troxidone and paramethadione are alternatives but these are toxic drugs. Skin rashes are not uncommon but the great risk with both these drugs is agranulocytosis. Even frequent white cell counts do not afford protection since the disaster may occur suddenly between blood tests. The patient must, therefore, be warned that a sore throat, fever or rash is an indication to stop the drug immediately and to call the doctor. Sulthiame is contraindicated in petit mal because it produces hyperventilation which might induce an attack.

Whichever drug is found to be effective should be continued for 2 years from the date of the last attack.

INFANTILE SPASMS (LIGHTNING FITS)

This is a less common form of epilepsy which usually starts about the age of 6 months and is rare after the age of 2 years. The infant suddenly drops his

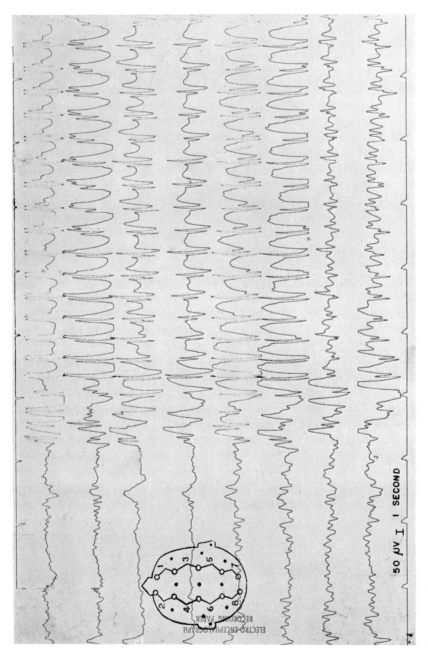

FIG. 112. Electroencephalogram showing the onset of generalized 3 cycles per second spike and wave discharges in a boy of 10 years suffering from petit mal. The interseizure record was normal.

head, the arms fly out and the legs are drawn up or extend. The attack only lasts a second and is often followed by a cry as though the child is in pain or very frightened. Runs of such attacks may follow in close sequence. Parents may describe their child as having 'colic', illustrating the need to get them to explain exactly what happens and the dangers which could result from the acceptance of a non-descriptive explanation.

A proportion of the patients have a recognizable cause for the brain damage such as perinatal birth injury, phenylketonuria, tuberose sclerosis and post-immunization encephalitis; these are termed symptomatic. The immunization risk is largely confined to pertussis (p. 484). In the remainder, termed cryptogenic, there is no obvious cause; such infants are mentally normal until the onset of the first attack when they develop severe mental regression; they are sometimes thought by their parents to have suddenly gone blind.

The electroencephalogram shows the pattern of 'hypsarrhythmia' in about half the cases and epilepsy in the remainder. By the term 'hypsarrhythmia' is meant an electroencephalographic record in which chaos has come to the normal electrical discharges. The waves are of high amplitude, these spikes discharging from different areas of the cortex each moment (Fig. 113).

It is usual for the attacks to die out between the ages of 3 and 6 years and for the electroencephalogram then to become much more normal. Unfortunately, there is no similar improvement in the mental state, most patients remaining hopelessly mentally handicapped, particularly those with an early history of brain damage. The mental outlook is best for those in the cryptogenic group and those following immunization (Jeavons et al., 1970).

The attacks do not respond to the usual anticonvulsant drugs and only steroid therapy, best given as ACTH, offers some hope. Such treatment, if begun early, will frequently stop the attacks and improve the electroencephalogram, relapses occurring when the treatment is stopped. Unfortunately, there has been little real mental improvement in such patients despite the remarkable reduction in their attacks. The action of steroids is unexplained; possibly it reduced the attacks by increasing the availability of pyridoxine to the brain, although there is no true deficiency of this substance. If ACTH fails to stop the fits nitrazepam should be tried.

### Breath-holding attacks

These mainly occur in the toddler age group and result from frustration in a self-determined child. An increased familial incidence is found. An association with anaemia has sometimes been found and this must be treated (Holowach & Thurston, 1963). The children are usually bright, reacting to being thwarted or to falls by breath-holding. They take a big breath as though they are going

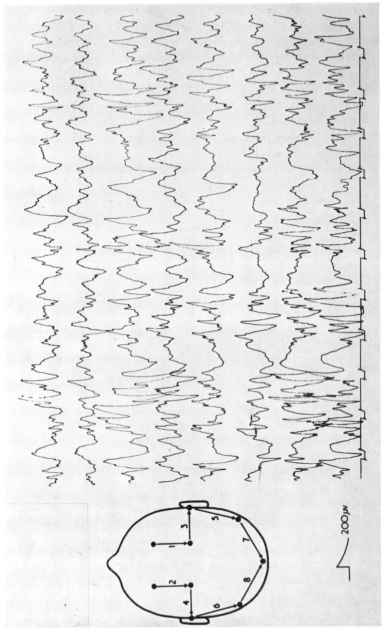

FIG. 113. Electroencephalogram in a girl of 15 months with hypsarrhythmia. The record is wildly abnormal; high voltage, random, slow waves mixed with spikes occur in all areas. The spikes vary from moment to moment in height, location and duration.

to cry louder than ever before but instead hold their breath and no cry emerges. Occasionally the child starts to cry and after a short spell of crying holds his breath. Cyanosis develops and if continued for long enough a convulsion occurs. A second group of children, less common than the cyanotic group described above but more alarming, become pale. There is a minimum of crying and the amount of breath-holding is less. Very often the child takes a single deep gasp before losing consciousness. In such cases cerebral anoxia results from circulatory failure secondary to asystole (Lombroso & Lerman, 1967).

By the time the mother consults the doctor she will almost certainly have tried slapping the child, or throwing cold water over him and found these to be ineffective in stopping an attack. The best treatment is for the mother to hook her index finger over the back of the tongue and then to draw it forwards, a manoeuvre which often makes the child start breathing again. This must be carried out the moment the child starts to hold his breath and before the teeth have clenched.

The prognosis is excellent in both types of attack, neither of which is related to epilepsy or mental handicap. The attacks cease spontaneously at or before school age. Anticonvulsant drugs have no place in treatment.

As far as possible the parents should avoid those situations which cause the child to hold his breath, though this can lead to behaviour problems if he is allowed to have his own way all the time. A wise balance must be adopted and if the finger in the mouth achieves its object the child will soon turn to other methods for the demonstration of his will-power.

### Simple faints

These are most common during the second half of childhood, especially in those who are growing fast. The child feels faint, thinks he is going to be sick, goes deathly white and sinks to the floor. Convulsive movements rarely occur and there is no incontinence. The immediate treatment is to loosen the collar, place the head between the knees and allow plenty of fresh air to reach the child.

The attacks occur only when standing up, particularly in crowded stuffy places. In England they most often occur during 'school assembly'. It would be difficult to imagine conditions more optimal for the production of faints since the children have just arrived at school early in the morning after a hurried breakfast and are left standing in a crowded hall. The prevention lies in allowing the children to sit down (on the floor if necessary).

## CEREBRAL PALSY

Cerebral palsy is a permanent disorder of movement and posture due to a defect or disease of the brain, appearing in the early years of life. The disease is not progressive although the manifestations may alter. Many of the patients also have sensory defects although these are not essential to the disorder. The title 'cerebral palsy' or 'spastic' has overemphasized the purely motor side of the disorder at the expense of overlooking the associated handicaps, such as those affecting hearing, speech and intellect.

*Aetiology.* Any condition which can cause death in the perinatal period may, by reason of lessened severity, cause cerebral palsy. It is not particularly rewarding to separate those causes operating in the prenatal period from those at the time of birth since they are often interdependent. Congenital malformation of the brain and infections transmitted from the mother during pregnancy are clearly of prenatal origin, but rhesus incompatibility, for which the stage is set during the prenatal period, produces cerebral palsy only if the degree of hyperbilirubinaemia developing after birth is sufficient to cause kernicterus. Birth injury, anoxia and low birth weight are the most important causes, often operating together in the same baby. Hypoglycaemia from any cause may result in cerebral palsy. Postnatal factors include intracranial infections such as meningitis and encephalitis, trauma and vascular accidents.

*Types.* Terms used in the definition of the different types of cerebral palsy must be clearly defined since there is no uniform classification.

## Spasticity

The word 'spastic' is used by the lay public to describe all forms of cerebral palsy but actually refers only to one group, although this is the largest. Spasticity is due to a pyramidal lesion, being diagnosed by an increase in muscle tone found only in one direction of joint movement, i.e. 'clasp-knife'. Rigidity is a different form of hypertonicity seen in cerebral palsy, being felt in both directions of joint movement, i.e. 'leadpipe'. Spasticity is associated with increased tendon reflexes, clonus and an extensor plantar response. Clonus can occasionally occur in normal individuals from nervous tension and in an ill-sustained form in normal infants, but in most cases is evidence of a pyramidal lesion. Spasticity is maintained during sleep. Spastic children with their slow movements are often overweight and feel the cold easily.

Spasticity affecting one limb only is probably an incorrect diagnosis. Detailed studies usually show the presence of hemiplegia if only one arm appears to be involved.

SPASTIC HEMIPLEGIA

The arm is more affected than the leg, being held close to the chest in a position of flexion. The leg is adducted at the hip, partially flexed at the knee and the foot is plantar flexed. The limbs on the affected side grow more slowly than those on the normal side. The face is seldom severely involved, more often being normal. Speech may be affected in right-sided hemiplegia of postnatal origin, but in congenital right-sided hemiplegia no speech defect occurs, presumably because the speech centre on the other side can take over at that age. Intelligence in this group is variable; it may be normal, the patients seldom being severely mentally handicapped. Convulsions are common.

The cause is obscure in a considerable proportion of cases, but the incidence of postnatal factors is higher than in the other groups.

*Acute infantile hemiplegia* is a condition in which convulsions suddenly develop in a previously healthy young child who, on recovery, is left with hemiplegia. It is always difficult to be certain that the child was normal before the episode. The majority of such cases are due to an acute vascular accident, particularly venous or arterial thrombosis, but in all cases it is necessary to exclude encephalitis or some other inflammatory cause.

SPASTIC DIPLEGIA

All four limbs are affected but the lower are more involved than the upper (Fig. 115a). The two halves of the body are affected symmetrically, this being important in the differentiation from double hemiplegia. Low birth weight, multiple birth and cerebral birth trauma are factors in the majority of cases and, as might be anticipated in view of such widespread damage, severe mental defect and convulsions are common.

SPASTIC DOUBLE HEMIPLEGIA

All four limbs are affected but the upper are more involved than the lower, as in single hemiplegia. Aetiological factors are the same as for other types of spasticity, mental handicap usually being severe.

Spastic diplegia and spastic double hemiplegia are sometimes classified under the common term of spastic tetraplegia or quadriplegia, but this does not reveal the differing distribution of the lesion in the two groups. However, because these children are often mentally retarded, it may be very difficult in severely handicapped patients to determine whether the arms or the legs are the more severely affected.

**Athetosis**

This condition is characterized by bizarre involuntary movements which may be slow and writhing, or jerky as in chorea. The movements are always absent in sleep and may not be present when the patient is relaxed. They are always grossly exaggerated as soon as voluntary movement is attempted. Athetosis may sometimes be associated with severe muscle tension which possibly represents a voluntary attempt to prevent the involuntary movements. These cases may be very difficult to distinguish from spastic diplegia until the child relaxes and the athetoid movements come through.

A large proportion of cases are due to kernicterus from severe neonatal jaundice (see p. 129); in these the basal ganglia are involved. Asphyxia, often associated with low birth weight, is another important cause and it is believed that the abnormality in the corpus striatum known as 'état marbré', found at autopsy in some cases of athetosis, is a sequel of neonatal asphyxia.

The neonatal symptoms of kernicterus disappear by the end of the second week and thereafter the usual picture is one of hypotonicity; this is one cause of the 'floppy infant' (see p. 684). In a smaller proportion, the picture is that of a hypertonic baby with relaxation during sleep but only occasionally at other times. Involuntary movements seldom appear during the first year and may be delayed as late as $3\frac{1}{2}$ years, but before then an experienced observer will be able to detect evidence of motor abnormality in about half the cases. As a general rule the longer the hypotonic stage, the worse the prognosis. Attacks in which the baby suddenly develops opisthotonos may occur and occasional respiratory stridor is not uncommon. Persistence of the Moro and tonic neck reflexes is common. The tonic neck reflexes (p. 273) may remain throughout life so that the patient finds it necessary to look the other way in order to pick up an object with his hand.

The patients are often of good intelligence though dysarthria, which commonly accompanies the condition, and the involuntary movements combine to make the child appear mentally handicapped; intelligence testing must be skilled.

Athetoids are usually very thin as a result of the excessive movement, in comparison with spastic children who are often fat. They are courageous individuals with a great sense of humour in comparison with the more dour and stolid spastic child. Many athetoids have high tone deafness. Convulsions are not common.

**Ataxia**

This condition, sometimes of hereditary origin, due to a defect in the cerebellum or its connections, or to cortical sensory impairment, affects only a small number of children. It may affect the arms, interfering with the precision of their movement, or the legs, causing an unsteady tremulous gait. In some cases all limbs are involved, in which case the legs are usually more severely affected than the arms. Occasionally, the ataxia is central so that the child is ataxic when sitting. There is nystagmus and an intention tremor. Incordination from abnormalities of muscle tone or athetosis must be excluded.

These children have a natural tendency to improve as they grow older.

## Flaccidity

The majority of cases of cerebral palsy associated with hypotonia will later develop the features of one of the types already described. Athetoids are more often hypotonic at first than are spastics, in whom hypertonicity can usually be detected early. A small proportion of patients remain with flaccidity all their life, evidence of a pyramidal lesion being found in these by the presence of increased tendon reflexes.

## Mixed types

The majority of patients fall into one category, but mixed types exist. These result from extensive brain lesions and are less common since they are not so likely to survive. Care should be taken not to regard the increased tone of a tension athetoid as being due to spasticity, mistakenly classifying the case as a mixed type.

### EARLY DIAGNOSIS

Cerebral palsy must be diagnosed early if treatment is to be successful and deformities prevented. Often a mother's first suspicion that all is not well is quelled by an ignorant doctor who either attempts to reassure her, or says it is too early to tell, asking to see the child when older. Many infants with cerebral palsy have feeding difficulties; sometimes the mother complains that when holding him, he does not 'feel right'. The reactions of the suspected child must constantly be compared with the normal. An intimate knowledge of normal development is essential if a diagnosis of cerebral palsy is to be made before the age of 6 months.

The risk of missing these patients in the early stages can be reduced by careful surveillance of all those who are 'at risk' (p. 91). Into this category fall all those babies who, by reason of their early history are more likely to develop cerebral palsy. Those with a family history of cerebral palsy should also be followed since the condition is sometimes genetically determined.

The diagnostic sign is poverty of movement so that the child should be given every opportunity to kick and perform. Asymmetry of movement, posture or of reflex response, as in eliciting the Moro reflex, are of great importance. The Moro, grasp and tonic neck reflexes (pp. 272, 273) should have disappeared by the age of 3 months but they persist for longer in cerebral palsy. The movements of a normal baby become totally symmetrical by the age of 4 months, since the asymmetrical reflexes have disappeared. It is the asymmetrical movements of the child with cerebral palsy which are diagnostically so important.

Stiffness of the limbs is less easily detected by passive movement in the early stages since the normal tone of a baby is relatively increased. The difference is exaggerated if the baby is held up so that the trunk lies parallel to the ground. In this position it will be seen that the normal baby, even by the age of 1 month, has developed some head control, the arms and legs being slightly flexed. The baby with cerebral palsy is either so hypotonic that the head, arms and legs hang down (Fig. 114) or so hypertonic that the legs remain straight out, almost in line with the rest of the body. Increased tone in the legs is best seen when the baby is held upright. In this position the legs are extended and may cross each other ('scissors position') whereas the normal baby will flex the hips and knees. While still held upright the feet should be made to touch a flat surface, when a stepping reflex (p. 272) can be elicited in a normal baby for the first 2 months of life, but not if there is cerebral palsy. In doubtful cases the child should be bounced on his feet, a manoeuvre which increases the tone, thereby making spasticity more obvious.

Head control is further tested by slowly pulling the child up from the supine position by the hands. By the age of 1 month, the head should maintain a normal relationship with the trunk for the first part of the movement instead of falling back. The hands should open loosely at times, a serious sign being when the thumb is persistently flexed across the palm after the first month of life (see p. 272). Increased tone in the tendo Achillis prevents full dorsiflexion of the ankles and may cause a brisk ankle jerk, though these reflexes are often brisk in the normal baby; sometimes the increased tone prevents the jerk from being elicited.

Once the child is old enough to reach for objects the movement of the hand should be observed. A child with cerebral palsy moves the hand in one piece like a mechanical grabber, instead of using normal finger movement. Failure to swing one or both arms, or the asymmetrical wearing out of shoes at a faster rate than normal may be evidence of cerebral palsy. In testing the hands it is useful to flap the hands rapidly, since this exaggerates the diminished movement of spasticity, or to ask the child to make rapid tapping movements with both hands alternately.

Associated abnormalities such as nystagmus, strabismus and abnormal head shape may be present and hearing must be tested in all cases. Impairment of hearing occurs almost exclusively in those with athetosis.

Testing for sensory defects is often not practicable in babies, though it must be remembered that many of the difficulties of the child with cerebral palsy result from a loss of discriminative sense and an absence of the normal body image, so that the child does not realize the position of his limbs in space.

The greatest difficulty lies in the early differentiation of cerebral palsy from mental retardation, particularly since the two may co-exist. This can be achieved only by finding an abnormality of motor development. Pneumo-encephalography has no place in the routine investigation of the child with cerebral palsy and although this may show evidence of cerebral atrophy, it does not differentiate mental from motor defect.

## TREATMENT

Early treatment is essential for the prevention of deformities (especially sub-luxation of the hip) and the provision of experiences required for normal development but denied to the child with cerebral palsy. The secret of success lies as much in the successful handling of the mother as of the child. She must be taught how to manage her baby so that with the utmost patience and understanding she helps him to do things for himself thereby attaining a more normal emotional adjustment. At no time, by reason of pity or guilt feelings, must she overprotect him.

In the early months, special emphasis must be placed on assisting the normal experiences to take place which are denied to him because of his motor (and possibly sensory) defect. For example, a developing infant learns about his mouth by exploring it with his fingers; the child with cerebral palsy should have his paralysed fingers moved round his mouth for him, in order to obtain similar experiences.

Splints and other appliances are being increasingly discarded. The funda-mental treatment is to teach the child how to balance so as to obtain good function, if necessary at the expense of a good cosmetic result. Treatment varies according to the type of cerebral palsy but the principles are the same. In a spastic child the abnormal patterns of posture and movement resulting from increased tone must be inhibited while normal patterns are facilitated. In an athetoid child where there is excessive movement, inhibition in order to reduce the amount of movement can help him to stabilize, thereby improving the quality of his movements. A floppy child requires pressure and support in order to increase muscle tone so as to increase his stability. In this way his active movements become more effective (Finnie, 1974).

The methods used in a spastic child are illustrated in Fig. 115. During half an hour's treatment the physiotherapist has been inhibiting the increased tone by holding the child in the reverse position from that adopted as a result of spasticity. The child is thereby helped to relax so that she can maintain this more normal posture on her own for a short time. By daily repetition of the technique this period increases. All the affected muscles must be considered together so that treatment is directed to the whole child rather than to a single limb, or even a single joint. Failure to do so causes an alteration in the equilibrium between the two dominant patterns of flexion and extension, thereby giving a false impression of spasticity being shifted from one group of muscles to another. Failure to consider all the muscles together accounts for the harmful effect of splints.

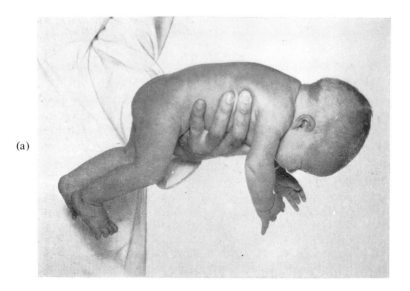

(a)

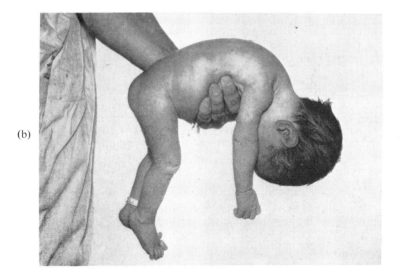

(b)

FIG. 114. Early diagnosis of probable cerebral palsy.
(a) Normal baby aged 2 days. Some degree of head control is already present and the limbs are partially flexed.
(b) Baby aged 6 days who suffered severe cerebral birth trauma at birth, showing the early signs of cerebral palsy. The infant is hypotonic, the head droops and the limbs hang limply down.

In training the child to walk the same order must be applied as in normal development. Head control must first be learnt, this being followed by sitting, kneeling, crawling, creeping, standing and finally walking, in that order. It is useless to try to get a child to stand if he has not yet learnt head control, this common error accounting for many of the bad results of physiotherapy.

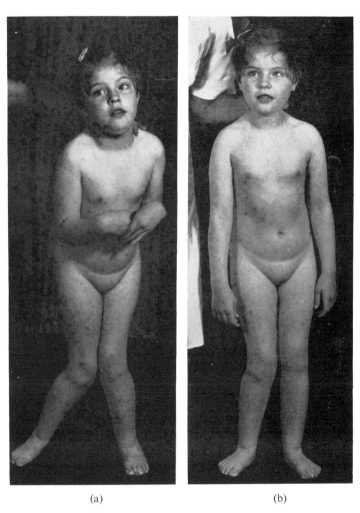

(a) (b)

FIG. 115. Spastic diplegia.
(a) Characteristic posture, the arms are flexed and the legs abducted.
(b) Same child half an hour later. In the interval she had been treated with postural physiotherapy to inhibit the increased tone.

A form of standing may be achieved without head control but reasonable function can never then be attained. These facts must also be emphasized to parents who may otherwise try to take short cuts in the normal sequence of development.

Mothers can easily be taught these new methods of physiotherapy; thereby, not only are they assisting in their child's treatment, but they have the satisfaction of feeling they are doing something positive. They are saved the appalling frustration which comes to those mothers who are told that nothing can be done in the early months of life.

As early as possible the child should be helped to become independent. To make this easier, crockery, eating implements and clothes should be suitably modified. Spastic children must not be allowed to get too fat. Physiotherapy has its major part to play in the pre-school years. Thereafter, the emphasis must be on education rather than physiotherapy. Whenever possible, children with cerebral palsy should attend a normal school, though severe cases will be helped by attending a special school where all the staff are conscious of the patients' particular needs, and where they can receive physiotherapy.

Numerous drugs have been tried in treatment, particularly those which cause muscle relaxation, but unfortunately these have been of little benefit. Surgery has little part to play during childhood; tendon lengthening reduces the final efficiency of muscles taught normal balance. Whenever possible, surgical measures should be delayed until after adolescence, so that growth has ceased.

## THE CLUMSY CHILD

Children vary in their natural skill in motor activities but a few are pathologically clumsy. Such children are often incorrectly regarded as mentally handicapped. The exact cause is unknown, but since the defect persists it cannot be ascribed to a simple delay in maturition. It is probably due to a defect in cerebral organization, bringing it into line with developmental aphasia (p. 478). This defect could be due to a minor degree of brain damage, especially since there is a greater than average association with intrauterine complications. These complications are more often long term rather than complications of labour. For example, there is an association of clumsiness with low birth weight, smoking, lower social class and high parity.

The child is awkward in all motor activities and has great difficulty in dressing, especially with buttons and laces, ball catching and writing. He is hyperactive and gets blamed at school for fidgetting. He trips over the smallest object and is constantly having accidents.

Many of the children have perceptual disabilities and are confused between their right and left. Spatial relationships and the concept of their body image may be disturbed.

It is unsatisfactory to term this 'minimal brain damage' since there is no evidence for this and the label may cause parents and teachers to feel that nothing can be done to help because part of the brain is missing. 'Cerebral dysfunction' is another unsatisfactory term but 'child dysfunction' might be useful.

These children require infinite patience from everyone around them. Specialised teaching can be very rewarding. At first it may help if new skills are broken down into simple parts so that they can be taught separately and then recombined into the whole. Verbal ability is usually much better than motor skills and every opportunity for developing this skill should be taken. The essential need is to reduce the level of outside stimuli so that the child is less distracted and helped to move more slowly. Drugs such as methylphenidate may help.

## INTRACRANIAL TUMOURS

The central nervous system and the urinary tract are the most common sites for neoplastic disease in childhood, accounting for about three-quarters of the cases. The majority of intracranial tumours are subtentorial, whereas in adults they are usually supratentorial.

*Clinical features.* These depend on the site rather than on the type of tumour and the classical features of headache, vomiting and papilloedema are modified by age. In the infant, where the skull bones have not yet fused, raised intracranial pressure is largely prevented by the expansion of the head. Consequently, although the tension of the fontanelle is increased, vomiting is a late sign. The possibility of an intracranial tumour must therefore be suspected in every case of hydrocephalus.

In older children vomiting is the most suggestive symptom and occurs particularly on getting up in the morning. It is not preceded by nausea, nor is it related to meals. Headache, though often present, is a less striking symptom than in the adult; however, since headaches are uncommon in young children, the possibility of an intracranial tumour as their cause must always be considered. Pain and stiffness in the back of the neck and across the shoulders are quite common. Ataxia is a most important sign and must be carefully sought; it occurs early in cerebellar tumours but may also be produced by a rise in intracranial pressure alone. Young children may be irritable, but raised intracranial pressure leads to lethargy and drowsiness as the pressure rises.

Papilloedema occurs early in subtentorial tumours and is therefore often seen. However, it is less easily recognized in children since the edge of the normal disc is frequently indistinct. The important feature is whether the vessels go out of focus at any point. In addition, oedema of the disc is usually accompanied by corroborative signs, particularly fullness of the vessels and flecks of haemorrhage on or near the disc. The colour of the disc is also often misinterpreted in children since there is a wide range of colours in the normal; a disc of such pallor as to indicate optic atrophy in an adult can be normal in a child.

Convulsions seldom accompany an intracranial tumour in childhood, but their sudden onset, for no obvious reason, must always raise this possibility. Nystagmus, which occurs in association with cerebellar tumours, and cranial nerve palsies are useful localizing signs. However, paralysis of the sixth nerve has little localizing value as it usually results from compression of the nerve by stretched blood vessels. These are due to raised intracranial pressure resulting from blockage of the fourth ventricle. Hemiparesis, from involvement of the pyramidal tract, is an early sign of a supratentorial tumour and may first be noticed by clumsiness of one hand or dragging of one leg.

A valuable sign of raised intracranial pressure in children is the 'cracked pot' note obtained by percussion of the skull. Radiographic evidence of raised pressure is shown by separation of the sutures and increased convolutional markings on the vault. It must be remembered that the skull film of a normal child always shows more convolutional markings than the adult because of pressure from the growing brain. If the brain is not growing, as in mentally handicapped children following birth injury, the skull is 'atrophic' from lack of convolutional markings and thickening of the skull vault (p. 447). The clinoid processes may be eroded by tumours in the pituitary region. Calcification within the tumour may take place, this feature being almost always present in a craniopharyngioma.

Lumbar puncture shows the pressure of cerebrospinal fluid to be increased if the fourth ventricle is obstructed, but otherwise the fluid is often normal, although a slight rise in protein and cells may occur. Air studies, cerebral angiography and isotopic scanning help in the localization of tumours. The electroencephalogram is valuable since the record is usually abnormal in tumours of the cerebral hemispheres. Echoencephalography is also used.

## TYPES

### 1. Glial tumours

The majority of intracranial tumours are gliomata, these varying from the highly malignant medulloblastoma to the slow-growing, localized astrocytoma.

## MEDULLOBLASTOMA

This tumour is derived from embryonic glial cells, occurring most often in the vermis of the cerebellum. Since it originates in the midline, it causes non-lateralized ataxia on walking and a tendency to fall backwards; in the early stages it is therefore impossible to detect any ataxia of the limbs when the child is lying down. These signs are followed by evidence of raised intracranial pressure from fourth ventricular obstruction.

The tumour occurs at any age and is more common in boys. It grows very rapidly but, as it is highly radiosensitive, radiotherapy in high doses is a more successful treatment than attempts at radical surgery. Survival up to 12 years has been achieved by this means, though the majority die sooner. The medulloblastoma has a particular tendency to extend to the meninges and to metastasize elsewhere in the central nervous system, especially along the spinal cord.

## ASTROCYTOMA

This benign tumour is derived from adult glial cells and occurs mainly in the cerebellum. The majority are localized but a diffuse variety occurs, particularly in the pons.

*Cerebellar astrocytoma.* This tumour, which is often cystic, always arises in the midline and grows slowly, so that obstruction of the fourth ventricle and cerebellar dysfunction usually occur at the same time. Consequently, headache and vomiting are associated with progressive unilateral limb weakness and ataxia. Nystagmus occurs, being more marked towards the affected side.

*Diffuse astrocytoma of pons.* This tumour arises from adult astrocytes which undergo a diffuse neoplastic change. It grows only slowly but its vital site and the occurrence of haemorrhage into the growth cause death within a year of the onset. The features are ataxia, vomiting, hemiplegia and multiple cranial nerve palsies which are unilateral. The occurrence of cranial nerve palsies before the development of raised intracranial pressure helps to differentiate this tumour from the two already described. No form of treatment is possible.

## DIENCEPHALIC SYNDROME OF CHILDHOOD

This condition, affecting young children, is almost always due to an astrocytoma involving the anterior hypothalamus. The patients seldom show signs of raised intracranial pressure but present with failure to thrive. Vomiting is not marked and they may have a good appetite. Despite their cachectic appearance from loss of fat, the children are often bright, alert and hyperactive.

It seems likely that the clinical picture results partly from hormonal side effects related to the site of the tumour.

## 2. Non-glial tumours

The non-glial tumours are represented by the craniopharyngioma, meningioma and choroid papilloma.

### CRANIOPHARYNGIOMA

These tumours arise from Rathke's pouch and comprise about 10 per cent of the intracranial neoplasms of childhood. They are almost invariably cystic, the cysts making up the greater part of the tumour.

The earliest symptoms are headache and vomiting. Visual disturbances from involvement of the optic chiasma occur later, whereas in adults these are usually the presenting symptom. In view of the site there are usually both pituitary and hypothalamic disturbances; arrest of skeletal development is common. Sexual infantilism results from severe anterior pituitary deficiency, but occasionally sexual precocity occurs if the hypothalamus is damaged and the pituitary left intact (see p. 285). Diabetes insipidus is fairly common but Fröhlich's syndrome of obesity, stunted growth and sexual infantilism is rare.

The diagnosis can usually be made on radiographic evidence from the presence of calcification; this is usually above the sella turcica but is occasionally intrasellar. The sella turcica is widened or the clinoid processes eroded in a large proportion of cases.

Although the tumour is benign, its site may render complete surgical removal impossible; surgery must then be combined with radiotherapy.

*Differential diagnosis.* Whenever an intracranial space-occupying lesion is diagnosed the possibility of a cerebral abscess must be considered. This will be more likely if there is a primary source of infection elsewhere, especially otitis media or bronchiectasis. A cerebellar abscess differs from a cerebellar neoplasm in that it arises in the periphery close to the dura. Consequently, it produces early unilateral cerebellar limb signs; obstruction of the fourth ventricle, with consequent raised intracranial pressure, occurs late. The cerebrospinal fluid may show a rise in protein and lymphocytes in consequence of the aseptic meningitis syndrome (see p. 404). Diagnostic needling of the brain should be performed in all doubtful cases.

Equally vital is the differentiation of a tuberculoma: other tuberculous lesions are usually present, the tuberculin skin test is positive, and the cerebrospinal fluid shows a greater rise in protein and cells than is usual with an intracranial tumour. The sugar in the cerebrospinal fluid is usually low if tuberculous meningitis is also present.

### Retinoblastoma

This is not an intracranial tumour but is considered here for convenience. It is by far the most common ocular tumour of childhood, is bilateral in one-third of cases and is sometimes familial. It is a disease of young children only, since it is a congenital tumour arising from embryonic tissue. The usual age of onset is about 2 years. The growth starts as a yellow nodule on the retina which eventually fills the vitreous producing a bright yellow light reflex easily visible to the naked eye. A squint is common and is often the presenting symptom, therefore the early diagnosis of the cause of every squint is essential.

## DEGENERATIVE DISORDERS OF THE NERVOUS SYSTEM

Sufficient progress has now been made in the aetiology of the degenerative disorders of the nervous system in children for the term 'Schilder's disease' to be discarded. This term was used to describe a condition of progressive mental and physical deterioration resulting from diffuse demyelination and sclerosis of white matter. It is now realized that a large number of different conditions were included in this definition and, although much more clarification is required, a broad classification is possible.

### Diffuse sclerosis

LEUCODYSTROPHIES

These are now known to be disorders of lipid storage. Included in the group are *Metachromatic leucodystrophy*, *Krabbe's disease*, and *Pelizaeus-Merz-bacher disease*. There are discussed on pp. 479–480.

CEREBRAL SCLEROSIS (SCHILDER'S CEREBRAL SCLEROSIS)

In this condition there are large areas of diffuse sclerosis, but also small plaques which are identical with those seen in multiple sclerosis. It is probable that the two disorders are the same, the apparent differences being due to the different reactions of the young brain to the unknown aetiological agent. The disease occurs at any age in childhood; the clinical features may be identical with those described for the leucodystrophies, except for the fact that cerebral sclerosis is not familial.

SUBACUTE SCLEROSING PANENCEPHALITIS (SUBACUTE INCLUSION BODY ENCEPHALITIS: SUBACUTE SCLEROSING LEUCO-ENCEPHALITIS)

This condition is now known to be due to measles and is discussed on p. 495.

### Friedreich's ataxia

This is an hereditary, degenerative disease of the spinocerebellar and pyramidal tracts and the posterior columns of the spinal cord. The onset is in early childhood. Ataxia occurs together with the unusual combination of a loss of tendon reflexes in the lower legs and extensor plantar responses. The characteristic deformity is that of pes cavus associated with hammer toes; scoliosis is common. Speech becomes explosive and indistinct; cardiac enlargement is not uncommon. The disease is slowly progressive so that after 10–20 years the patient is severely deformed, bed-ridden and demented.

'Formes frustes' of the condition may occur so that other members of the family may be found with only one aspect of the disorder, such as pes cavus.

### Peroneal muscular atrophy (Charcot-Marie-Tooth disease)

This is another hereditary disorder which is characterized by degeneration of peripheral nerves with consequent atrophy of certain muscle groups. Mainly the lower limbs are involved, particularly the peroneal group, so that the leg comes to look like an inverted club, being thick proximally and thin distally. The hands may be affected by wasting of the intrinsic muscles, whilst the feet and hands may develop a claw deformity. The disease is slowly progressive, but the majority of patients can still get about even late in life.

### Tuberose sclerosis (epiloia)

This is a familial disorder, of unknown cause, characterized by sclerotic patches in the cerebral hemispheres. It is inherited as an autosomal dominant character but about 80 per cent of cases are due to fresh mutations. The convolutions of the brain become firm and distorted so that some are smaller and others broader than normal, giving the typical 'peeled walnut' appearance (Fig. 116). Hard lumps, like marbles, may be felt in the brain. Convulsions are common and may be the presenting feature; they sometimes take the form of 'infantile spasms' (p. 421). Mental defect is usual but often develops slowly so that the intelligence may still be normal in childhood.

*Adenoma sebaceum*, a very characteristic skin rash appears on the face and is often the first manifestation of tuberose sclerosis. It is inappropriately named since it has nothing to do with the sebaceous glands and it is not adenomatous; the eruption is due to a mixture of vascular and fibromatous overgrowth. It may lead to the correct diagnosis in a child previously thought to have idiopathic epilepsy. The individual lesions are brown, flat-topped, polygonal papules first seen at the junction of the nostril and cheek, then spreading across the cheeks and nasal bridge in a butterfly distribution. White areas of vitiligo and café-au-lait patches are often present on the trunk; small white tumours, termed 'phakomata', may be seen in the retina. Rhabdomyomata may be found in the heart and adenomata in the kidneys.

The cerebral lesions may calcify, this being one of the reasons for taking a routine skull film in all cases of convulsions.

The disease is slowly progressive, no specific treatment being available. The parents should be examined for minor manifestations of the disorder such as adenoma sebaceum, vitiligo, café-au-lait patches and subungual fibromata.

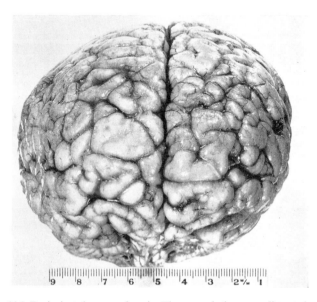

FIG. 116. Brain in tuberose sclerosis. The convolutions are distorted, some being smaller and others broader than normal, giving the 'peeled walnut' appearance.

## FAMILIAL DYSAUTONOMIA (RILEY-DAY SYNDROME)

This disease of the autonomic system is largely confined to Jews, being inherited as an autosomal recessive trait.

*Clinical features.* The patients may present in many different ways since there are disturbances affecting both the sensory and the motor systems. In infancy the impaired swallowing reflex causes difficulty in feeding, vomiting and excessive dribbling; this increases the likelihood of aspiration, the children commonly having recurrent respiratory infections. It is characteristic that crying does not produce tears and that there is excessive sweating. Vasomotor changes cause blotching of the skin, the extremities becoming blue and cold.

In the toddler age group periodic attacks of vomiting may become a feature. The children are excessively irritable and breath-holding attacks are common. In later childhood the degree of emotional instability increases with an exaggerated response to emotional stress. Postural hypotension may be so severe as to cause fainting on rising in the morning.

There is a relative indifference to pain; impairment of normal sensation leads to excessive trauma with consequent bruising and abrasions. Defective lacrimation causes corneal ulceration. Poor motor co-ordination results from disturbed proprioceptive function and the deep tendon reflexes are absent. This is another factor leading to excessive injury; it also leads to ortho-paedic abnormalities such as scoliosis. Most children also exhibit paroxysmal hypertension. Bouts of unexplained fever are common, and the degree of fever in response to infection is exaggerated.

*Diagnosis.* In the early weeks of life the condition is likely to be mistaken for other causes of feeding difficulty, but it should be apparent that the infant has an actual difficulty in swallowing rather than a dislike of food. Recurrent respiratory infections may suggest cystic fibrosis. Pink disease (p. 718) is strongly simulated by the cold blue extremities, excessive sweating, misery and lack of tendon reflexes. The periodic syndrome (p. 469) may be suggested by a history of recurrent vomiting.

*Prognosis and treatment.* The long-term prognosis is as yet uncertain, but a considerable proportion of the patients die in childhood from respiratory infections. In those who survive, growth is retarded. The motor defect may be considerable and, because of their emotional disability, the children have great difficulty in adapting to this. The psychological handicap becomes an increasing problem, psychiatric treatment being necessary to assist the children and their parents to adapt to the situation.

## BIBLIOGRAPHY

BOBATH B. (1967) The very early treatment of cerebral palsy. *Develop. Med. Child Neurol.*, **9**, 373.

BODIAN M. & LAWSON D. (1953) The intracranial neoplastic diseases of childhood. *Brit. J. Surg.*, **40**, 368.

BODIAN M. & LAKE, B.D. (1963) The rectal approach to neuropathology. *Brit. J. Surg.*, **50**, 702.

COOPER J.E. (1965) Epilepsy in a longitudinal study of 5,000 children. *Brit. med. J.*, **1**, 1020.

FAERØ O., KASTRUP K.W., LYKKEGAARD-NIELSEN E., MELCHIOR J.C. & THORN I. (1972) Successful prophylaxis of febrile convulsions with phenobarbital. *Epilepsia*, **13**, 279.

FINNIE N.R. (1974) Handling the young cerebral palsied child at home. Heinemann Medical, London.

FOLEY J. (1968) Deterioration in the EEG in children with cerebral palsy. *Develop. Med. Child Neurol.*, **10**, 287.

GIBBS F.A., GIBBS E.L., PERLSTEIN M.A. & RICH C.L. (1963) Electroencephalographic and clinical aspects of cerebral palsy. *Pediatrics*, **32**, 73.

GROSE C. & FEORINO P.M. (1972) Epstein–Barr virus and Guillain-Barré syndrome. *Lancet* **2**, 1285.

HOLOWACH J. & THURSTON D.L. (1963) Breath-holding spells and anemia. *New Eng. J. Med.*, **268**, 21.

JEAVONS P.M. & BOWER B.D. (1964) Infantile Spasms. *Clinics in Developmental Medicine* No. 15. Spastics Society/Heinemann Medical, London.

JEAVONS P.M., HARPER J.R. & BOWER B.D. (1970) Long-term prognosis in infantile spasms: A follow-up report on 112 cases. *Develop. Med. Child Neurol.*, **12**, 413.

JEAVONS P.M. & CLARK J.E. (1974) Sodium valproate in treatment of epilepsy. *Brit. med. J.*, **2**, 584.

LOMBROSO C.T. & LERMAN P. (1967) Breathholding spells (cyanotic and pallid infant syncope). *Pediatrics*, **39**, 563.

MURRAY J.D., FLEMING P., WEBER J., HSUEN J., BANNATYNE R. & ANGLIN C. (1974) The continuing problem of purulent meningitis in infants and children. *Ped. Clin. N.A.*, **21**, 967.

OUNSTED C. (1971) Some aspects of seizure disorders. In *Recent Advances in Paediatrics*. Ed. Gairdner, D. & Hull, D. Churchill, London.

RUSSELL A. (1951) A diencephalic syndrome of emaciation in infancy and childhood. *Arch. Dis. Childh.*, **26**, 274.

SMITH K.R., WEINBURG W.A. & McALISTER W.H. (1965) Failure to thrive: the diencephalic syndrome of infancy and childhood. *J. Neurosurg.*, **23**, 348.

TILL K. (1968) Subdural haematoma and effusion in infancy. *Brit. med. J.* **3**, 400.

WHITTLE H.C., TUGWELL P., EGLER L.J. & GREENWOOD B.M. (1974). Rapid bacteriological diagnosis of pyogenic meningitis by Latex agglutination. *Lancet*, **2**, 619.

CHAPTER 15

# MENTAL HANDICAP

The old term 'mental retardation' has been replaced by the title 'mental subnormality'. This is still an unsatisfactory term; it would be better replaced by 'mental handicap', thereby bringing it in line with 'physical handicap'. The Mental Health Act of 1959 amended the classes of subnormality and did away with the old terms: idiots, imbeciles and feeble-minded persons. There are now two classes: subnormality and severe subnormality. The severely subnormal child is defined as being 'incapable of living an independent life or of guarding himself against serious exploitations'. The subnormal child is in 'a state of arrested or incomplete development of mind not amounting to severe subnormality'. In general, subnormality is equivalent to the old term feeble-minded, with an IQ range of 50–70, while severe subnormality is equivalent to the former imbecile and idiot grades, the IQ being anything below 50. In practice, the boundaries cannot be so exact. The term 'educationally subnormal' is not a category of mental subnormality but an administrative label for educational convenience. It describes those children whose educational performance is below normal and for whom special educational facilities must be provided. The majority of these children will be intellectually retarded, coming from the subnormal class of mental handicap but some will be of normal intelligence, although educationally retarded.

### Aetiology

In the majority of cases no specific cause can be determined. This is particularly true for the large number of ESN children coming from the lower social classes. In such children, environmental factors are more important than genetic as a cause of mental handicap. Their homes are more overcrowded and there are fewer opportunities for learning, since their parents are often less interested in education. Additional factors are more frequent illnesses and less parental understanding of the child's emotional problems. A child who is emotionally disturbed performs less well intellectually.

Another very important and preventable cause of mental handicap is malnutrition during pregnancy and the first 3 years of life. Human beings, unlike many other animal species, have their brain growth spurt from mid-pregnancy to the third year of life. It is during this period that the brain is particularly vulnerable to lack of nutrition since its normal growth is thereby restricted. 'Catch-up' growth is incomplete in the brain, therefore malnutrition during this time produces lasting effects, particularly a defect in later intelligence. (Winick, 1969; Hertzig *et al.*, 1972; Dobbing, 1974). It is relative malnutrition which accounts for the intellectual achievements of the lighter of twins being less than that of the heavier one.

*Prenatal.* There are many varieties of congenital malformation of the brain some of which have been discussed in chapter 6. These include hydrocephaly, microcephaly, anencephaly and hypertelorism. In some of these malformations genetic factors are involved.

Three categories of genetically determined mental subnormality can be distinguished:

1. Conditions resulting from an abnormality of a single gene, such as those due to inborn errors of metabolism, discussed on p. 568; these include such disorders as phenylketonuria and galactosaemia. Though numerically not a large group the importance of these metabolic causes lies in the prevention of mental handicap by early diagnosis and treatment of cases, and by genetic counselling.

2. Chromosome anomalies, particularly Down's syndrome.

3. Familial mental handicap due to polygenic inheritance. This is a large and important group but reasons have already been given for believing the cause to be multifactorial and that environment probably plays a greater part than do genetic abnormalities.

Infections acquired *in utero* are a prenatal cause of mental handicap; these include rubella, syphilis, toxoplasmosis and cytomegalic inclusion disease. Intrauterine irradiation and certain drugs given during pregnancy may also cause mental handicap.

*Perinatal.* Birth trauma, particularly anoxia, accounts for a large proportion of those cases of mental handicap where the cause is known or suspected; it is an important cause of the backwardness associated with low birth weight. However, it is not always possible to be certain whether apparent cerebral agenesis has resulted from a primary malformation of the brain or from birth trauma. A brain which is severely damaged at birth fails to grow, presenting later as microcephaly.

Hyperbilirubinaemia and hypoglycaemia are the major causes of mental handicap acting after birth but during the first week of life.

*Postnatal.* Severe infection of the central nervous system and cerebral trauma are the major postnatal causes of mental handicap. Vascular accidents, such as cerebral thrombosis which may be associated with severe dehydration, are a less common cause. Idiopathic hypoglycaemia is a rare cause in young children; poisonings may occur at any age. Subclinical lead poisoning may be an important cause of mental handicap (p. 717).

Thyroid deficiency in the child is another factor operating after birth. The cretin lacks thyroid hormone but at birth is still receiving considerable supplies from his mother. Only after birth does severe thyroid deficiency and subsequent mental handicap occur (see p. 623).

Epilepsy is often associated with mental handicap since both may be due to the same cause; only rarely will convulsions actually cause mental handicap, though this can happen from anoxia, electrolyte disorders and hypoglycaemia during status epilepticus.

### Diagnosis

The diagnosis of mental handicap is made from a detailed knowledge of normal mental development (see p. 250) and the knowledge that the particular child's development is outside the variation of normal. It is this variation of normal which accounts for the unnecessary anxiety of many parents for their child's development. Parents often make the error of expecting one child to progress at exactly the same rate as his siblings or friends.

The correct diagnosis may immediately be obvious but in some cases it requires skilled and repeated testing at intervals in order to assess the rate of progress. Special attention should be paid to responsiveness, alertness, interest in surroundings, concentration and the use of hands. The mentally retarded child is backward in all fields, though this is more obvious in speech and less obvious in motor development. In view of this, no child is mentally handicapped who is backward in only one field of development.

Diagnosis is particularly difficult if there are associated defects such as cerebral palsy. In cerebral palsy the cerebral mechanism of speech or the muscles producing speech may cause the child to seem mentally handicapped; in the past many such children were incorrectly placed in institutions for the mentally handicapped. Similarly, the delay in motor development of the cerebral palsied child may suggest mental retardation alone. On the other-hand, the two conditions may co-exist.

A number of conditions may lead to a false impression of mental retardation; these must be excluded in every case. They include visual and auditory defects, emotional disorders, speech disorders (p. 476), autism (p. 453), developmental aphasia (p. 478) and the syndrome of the clumsy child (p. 434).

Deafness must be excluded as a cause of the symptoms. Congenital deafness causes a child to appear mentally handicapped; if it is overlooked he will become a deaf-mute.

Emotional factors can retard the development of a normal child and can increase the defect in one who is mentally handicapped; these must be assessed in every case. A child who has been deprived of his mother from an early age, as may occur if he has been in hospital for a long time, may develop only slowly until he receives the close individual care and love of his mother.

The early signs suggesting mental handicap are a lack of interest, and failure to smile or to recognize mother by the expected age. The baby may seem to sleep all the time or may be excessively irritable and hyperactive. He does not respond to sounds by watching with his eyes; normal eye contact at a few weeks of age is an important sign of normal development. Failure to start lifting his head off the pillow by 2–3 months is serious; it must be differentiated from a motor defect alone occurring in some cases of cerebral palsy, from other neurological defects such as infantile spinal muscular atrophy, and from disorders of muscle alone such as muscular dystrophy. Babies who are still unable to raise the head at 4–6 months of age will be found to have less hair than normal over the occiput.

Retardation of development will be diagnosed from the parents' history and from a careful examination of the baby. The examination may show an obvious cause for delay such as Down's syndrome (mongolism) or microcephaly. Even when the cause for mental handicap is obvious the examination must still be meticulous. This is necessary for the exclusion of associated handicaps and to be in a better position to help the parents. The doctor who has made an immediate diagnosis of Down's syndrome after a cursory examination will have greater difficulty in discussing the situation with the parents than one who has been seen to complete a full examination.

Careful measurement of the head circumference should be made since failure of the head to grow at the correct rate is often associated with mental handicap. The microcephalic child is often erroneously regarded as suffering from a congenitally malformed brain whereas the majority of children with a small head have sustained anoxia at birth. This cerebral damage prevents normal brain growth; consequently the head is small since its size is determined by brain growth. Lack of normal brain growth shows on the skull X-ray as lack of convolutional markings and thickening of the skull vault.

Every mentally handicapped child must be investigated to determine whether there is an underlying metabolic defect. This group is described in chapter 20, p. 568; the cause is an enzyme defect affecting aminoacid, carbohydrate, lipid or mineral metabolism. Although small, it is the most important group of all since treatment may be available to prevent mental retardation in cases diagnosed early and managed correctly. Mental retardation results from the accumulation of abnormal substances or of normal substances in abnormal quantities. Backwardness is not present at birth but may occur early, as in phenylketonuria, or late, as in Wilson's disease. Diagnosis is made largely by demonstration of the abnormal urinary excretion of amino-acids or sugars. Aminoaciduria can also be detected in the plasma. Liver biopsy can be used in those conditions where the abnormal substances are deposited in the liver, as in the lipidoses. A rectal biopsy for histological and enzyme studies is a valuable diagnostic test.

Sometimes there are associated physical findings which suggest the diag-nosis, such as fair hair in phenylketonuria, or cataracts in galactosaemia, but in the majority there are no specific physical features. The urine may have a characteristic smell, being musty in phenylketonuria and like maple-syrup in maple syrup disease.

It is probable that all these conditions are genetically determined, so that the chances of their occurrence are much higher if the parents are related. The carrier state can be detected by biochemical tests in phenylketonuria and galactosaemia. It is likely that this will soon be possible for most of the conditions. A special watch must be kept on babies born into families known to be affected with any of these disorders, so that there is no delay in diagnosis and treatment.

### Management

Early detection of mental handicap is important, not only for the rare treat-able cases but also for the others so that the parents may be given the maxi-mum help at a time when possibly they need it most. Reasons have already been stated (p. 220) for the belief that parents of mongols should be told the diagnosis as early as is practicable. The same arguments hold for the parents of all mentally handicapped children once the diagnosis is certain. However, whereas diagnosis is an easy matter in mongolism and in a few other specific disorders, it is difficult in the majority of mentally handicapped children. For these, a period of prolonged observation may be necessary, although increas-ing skill in the early detection of delayed development should shorten this period. For the parents of such children, the approach will vary with the type of parents; but even here an early explanation is preferable. In the past, doctors have tended to keep their suspicions to themselves; only when certain of the diagnosis have they communicated them to the parents, often thereby appearing to the parents to be suddenly forcing a diagnosis of mental handi-cap on them. Today's parents want to be taken into the doctor's confidence and are able to accept that a doctor is not infallible. Reasons have been given (p. 92) for the belief that parents are not made more anxious by the special observations provided for those at risk of handicapping conditions. In the same way the majority of parents are able to understand that suggestive early signs of mental handicap may or may not turn out to be well founded; they would prefer to hear the doctor's true opinion rather than be fobbed off by unwarranted 'reassurance'. Worst of all is the comment that it is too early to tell or that the child is just lazy. It is really a question of approach; if the doctor takes time and is honest in what he says, parents are able to appreciate the limitations of diagnostic certainty in young babies. It goes without saying that the premature diagnosis of mental handicap must be avoided at all costs.

Once it is obvious that the child is mentally handicapped, the choice of words used when talking to the parents is vital. Expressions such as 'slow developer' mean very little by themselves. Some parents will assume from this that a catch-up period in mental development will occur later. However, if the child is really mentally handicapped, such 'catch-up' is impossible unless he has a treatable disorder, since it would require faster than normal mental development, thereby suddenly transferring him to genius class.

Other parents told that their child is mentally handicapped will believe this means a standstill in further development. The use of a simple graphic

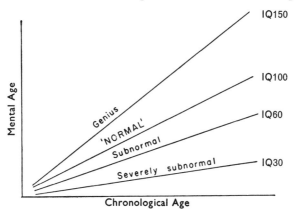

FIG. 117. Simple graphic description for parents, showing that even the most severely mentally handicapped child makes some progress each year.

description (Fig. 117) will be helpful to explain that all children progress to some extent each year, though the rate varies with the intelligence quotient. From the fact that even the lowest of the lines is sloping upwards the parents can understand that over a long period, such as a year, they will appreciate some development, even though slight.

There are few mentally handicapped children who fail to walk in the end; in fact, the amount of motor agility achieved by severely subnormal children is often surprising. A low IQ affects speech much more than walking.

Much time will be needed to persuade the parents of the true situation once the diagnosis is certain. It is essential that parents are helped to accept this since otherwise they will divert their energy into attempts to prove to themselves and others that their child is normal; the resulting emotional problems only make it worse for the child. Parental reaction to the diagnosis will vary from aggressive rejection to pathological attachment associated with feelings of guilt. Once they have accepted the fact that their child is backward, they are in a position to work out with the doctor the best ways to help their child.

It is best for mentally handicapped children to be brought up in their own homes, since no one can replace the mother or give as much individual attention to the child as she can. A handicapped child suffers from the absence of a normal home as much as the normal child. Residential accommodation is recommended only for the needs of parents or siblings, not for the patient. Many parents are given the impression that the child will be better off in a residential home because he will learn quicker if in expert hands; this is incorrect. Residential care may be recommended because the parents are suffering such emotional and physical strain that they decide to have no further children when there is no genetic cause for the condition and it is obvious that they are longing for another child. It may also be recommended if the siblings are suffering from lack of parental love and attention or if they are too ashamed of the backward child to bring their friends home; such a situation indicates earlier mishandling of the normal siblings.

Apart from those rare conditions where specific therapy is available, parents of mentally handicapped children must be told that no specific treatment is available. In saying this the doctor must not suggest that nothing can be done to help. A great deal can be done to help parents to help their child by understanding his needs and providing play situations to stimulate his development. Group therapy sessions with other mentally handicapped children and their parents are often beneficial, especially if they are run by an occupational therapist or physiotherapist as well as a social worker who are well experienced in the problem. This approach, coupled with the removal of suffocating emotional reactions which can increase the retardation, will permit the child to develop to the utmost of his capabilities.

The mentally handicapped child has the mind of one much younger than himself. He should therefore be handled in a manner appropriate to his mental age rather than to his chronological age. When parents can understand this, they will be able to give him the extra patience which the care of such a child demands and will be more able to accept his slower rate of progress.

A check should be kept on weight gain since these children are often overweight, making their motor activity still more difficult. This excessive weight gain is partly related to lack of exercise and partly to overfeeding. Since the child's normal responses to affection are lacking, parents often overfeed as a subconscious way of showing their love. Parental guilt feelings are to some extent appeased by providing excessive food.

A mentally handicapped child may cause marital rift but more often the parents draw closer together, withdrawing from society. It is in this connection that associations for the parents of mentally handicapped children can be particularly helpful; the realization that other parents have similar problems makes a world of difference. The doctor in charge should give the address of the local association as well as providing the parents with the titles of suitable books on the subject of mental handicap.

Educational needs will be determined by the Local Authority after formal assessment and the determination of the intelligence quotient (IQ), though too much stress must not be placed on the IQ figure. Most children whose IQ lies between 50 to 70 will be better educated in a special school for the educationally subnormal. When told of this decision, many parents may do their utmost to prevent the child leaving the ordinary school. Provided the doctor handles such patients with tact and patience, he will usually have little difficulty in persuading the parents of the advantages to their child in attending such a school where he will be taught by teachers specializing in the education of mentally handicapped children. The classes are smaller than in an ordinary school and the teachers are specially trained. The child is in a situation where he has a chance of shining amongst his peers rather than always being bottom of the class, gaining little from his education.

One of the major fears experienced by such parents is lest the other retarded children pass on bad habits to their child, dragging him down even lower. This is an understandable reaction and needs talking out. It is a possibility, but the children in an ordinary school may similarly pass on bad habits. Once parents realize that this is a common reaction, particularly when they meet other parents in a similar situation with whom they can talk, the problem falls into perspective. The retarded child is likely to be happier in a special school since his needs are better catered for and he is no longer the the subject of teasing for his slow learning or unusual appearance.

Another parental reaction to the recommendation of an ESN school is that of a personal slur against themselves. This can largely be prevented by a full discussion, at an early stage, of the aetiological factors in their child's mental handicap, particular attention being paid to the removal of guilt feelings. The reaction will be lessened by attendance at an ESN class in an ordinary school where the child can mix for some activities with children of a normal IQ. This is good for both groups of children, while there are obvious advantages both for teachers and parents of ESN children. Unnecessary segregation of the mentally handicapped child from the rest of the community must be avoided whenever possible.

Children whose IQ is less than 50 are no longer deemed ineducable in the United Kingdom. They may not be able to be taught to read or write, but there is much else to be learnt and even the most severely mentally handicapped child has the capacity to learn something. The change of nomenclature and staff for the severely mentally handicapped reflects this approach. At first such children were sent to an Occupation Centre, the children being occupied in order to keep them out of mischief. Then the name was changed to Training Centre with the idea that they could be trained in their new behaviour. Now it is a School for the Severely Subnormal, being run by specialist teachers.

For the dull child as for the average child, environment is supremely important. For the parents to achieve a suitable environment it is often necessary for them to receive help from the medical, educational and particularly the social services. Mothers are often frightened and uncertain what to do, and are hindered by relatives and friends who express ignorance because their own children were all normal. They should be told simple points, such as that immunization will be required just as for any other child, that he may take longer to get on to solids but by persevering he will learn to chew. The child should be given pocket money, being allowed, whenever possible, to go out without his parents to spend it.

More should be done to equip the home with practical aids so that the child can do more for himself, gaining satisfaction thereby and lightening his parents' task. The possibilities are enormous, including such items as simplified clothing to make dressing easier, modified cutlery, and handrails for lavatories and stairs. The Local Authority through its welfare department can assist in this direction, particularly with more major modifications such as the widening of doors and fixing of ramps to enable a wheelchair to be brought into the home.

Psychotherapy has an important place, though unfortunately this is often regarded as inappropriate for the mentally handicapped child who is mistakenly believed to be without insight regarding his intellectual and social failure. The high proportion of such children who show emotional disturbances indicates the size of the problem. Advice to parents on behaviour modification is helpful. Many have unknowingly reached the point where they respond only to their child's 'bad' behaviour. For example, unless he cries they take no notice of his requests for help. Small wonder, therefore, that he cries so much. Once parents are helped to understand what is happening and to respond to good behaviour rather than negative behaviour, the child's performance improves.

*Genetic counselling* must be given to the parents of all mentally handicapped children. Some who do not ask for advice on this subject are unwilling, from fear, to face up to its implications, though the number of genetically determined causes of mental handicap is very few. The advice given must be accurate, so that reference to a genetic clinic is often wise. If the cause of the mental handicap is unknown, an empirical risk of 3–4 per cent for future pregnancies should be given. The risk of mental handicap for any random pregnancy is 1 per cent. The role of the clinician is to indicate the risks as to the likelihood of a recurrence in future pregnancies, leaving the parents to make their own deicison; it is not his task to tell parents whether or not they should have further children. The way in which this information is presented will depend on knowing the family.

## PRADER-WILLI SYNDROME

This disorder comprises hypotonia, obesity, mental handicap and hypogonadism. Marked hypotonia at birth is constant but obesity, which seldom responds to diet, does not develop until the second or third year. The diagnosis can be made before this by the characteristic facies comprising a tall cranial vault of relatively small circumference associated with a prominent forehead and pronounced nasal bridge. The eyes are small but the cheek bones and jaw are prominent.

Boys have a small penis, a hypoplastic scrotum and undescended testes. No abnormalities of the female genitalia have been noted and it is this difference between the sexes which probably accounts for the male preponderance in published reports.

Feeding difficulties are common in infancy. Motor development as well as mental development is delayed, but the children eventually walk. Height is stunted, bone age retarded and growth hormone levels reduced. There is an increased incidence of diabetes and others may show a prediabetic glucose tolerance curve. Puberty is delayed and secondary sex characteristics poorly developed.

## AUTISM

Autism is a form of psychosis occurring in children which is poorly understood. It is probable that the basic defect is a developmental disorder which particularly affects the comprehension of speech. Autism is not a variety of schizophrenia as used to be thought because the differences between the two conditions are too great. For example, delusions and hallucinations are a feature of schizophrenia but not of adults with autism who might be expected to describe such disturbances if they were occurring. Moreover, schizophrenia is episodic, whereas autism does not show such fluctuations.

The disorder may date from birth but some of the features may occur in a transient form during periods of emotional or even organic illness. There is no single underlying pathological process and in many patients there has been no evidence of brain disease. In others, the syndrome has occurred in association with organic brain disease, as in some children who are blind, deaf or severely mentally handicapped. It has also occurred in children who have suffered severe emotional deprivation.

Autism is not a variety of mental subnormality. It occurs at all levels of intelligence and some of the children have a normal IQ. If a mentally handicapped child is autistic, brain disease or injury is almost certainly the cause of both conditions. It is uncertain whether this is also true for autistic children with a normal IQ. The symptom pattern varies with the level of intelligence. Similarly, environmental factors modify the symptoms but are not the primary cause of the condition.

Affected children are unable to develop normal relationships with other individuals; they fail to react to situations in the expected manner. Lacking the normal emotional response they appear to be without affection, treating people as though they were pieces of furniture. They are quite unable to be cuddled and will seldom sit on their mother's lap. They are withdrawn, seeming to live in a world of their own. But this withdrawal is never complete, so that the child may be entirely withdrawn from all except one person in his environment or be partially withdrawn from the whole of his environment.

The children are often thought to be mentally handicapped or deaf but this is not the case unless a child with either of these conditions develops secondary autistic features. Autism differs from mental subnormality in that the true potentiality exists but is masked. Islands of normal or even exceptional ability may remain to shine through the bizarre behaviour pattern. Moreover, instead of looking dull like a defective their initial appearance suggests they are bright; their movements are well co-ordinated and graceful.

In the consulting room, the child will wander around, taking no notice of the doctor. An obsession with water is common so that he is likely to make straight for the hand basin. He may smile on inappropriate occasions and is negativistic so that any attempts to make contact will almost certainly fail. Some degree of mutism is usual, but he may copy a word he hears without understanding its meaning, repeating it again and again. Repetition of speech is termed 'perserveration'; the children may also repeat actions, spending hours on end carrying out the same movement. This tendency to repeat can sometimes be demonstrated by turning the child round with a hand placed on the head, the child then whirling round for some time, as though involuntarily.

Other characteristic features are an obsessive ritual behaviour and an excessive anxiety for which there is no obvious explanation. Speech may fail to develop altogether or fail to mature; some children who have started to speak may lose the power of speech. About two-thirds of the children develop an oral language which is highly individualized. Most of them learn to understand speech.

Many of the parents seem to be unusually intelligent. There is an impression in England of a higher than average incidence amongst the immigrant population from developing countries. If this is the case, it could be due to the emotional stresses placed on such children from being brought up in a world of conflicting cultures and to the burdens facing their parents. Such immigrant mothers may be profoundly depressed by the strange environment which is often combined with having to leave some of their children in their own homeland.

*Management.* Early diagnosis is important for the child in order to make contact with him and for the parents in order that they may accept advice. Parents are less receptive if, for a long time, they have been told the child is normal or that nothing can be done for him.

Many different educational techniques are being tried; as yet it is unknown which is best. The essential need is to establish contact with the child so as to prevent him from sliding into complete isolation. They are best managed in small special groups by those with experience in the condition; on no account should they be relegated to schools for the mentally subnormal. The teacher will need to speak to the child in his own vocabulary; the teaching of words and articulation is not helpful. The best prognosis lies with those children who seek to communicate.

## BIBLIOGRAPHY

CREAK E.M. (1963) Childhood psychosis. *Brit. J. Psychiat.*, **109**, 84.

CREAK E.M. (1965) Problems of subnormal children studied in the thousand family survey. *Lancet*, **2**, 282.

DOBBING J. (1974) The later development of the brain and its vulnerability. In *Scientific Foundations of Paediatrics.* Ed. Davis J.A. & Dobbing J. Heinemann Medical, London.

HERTZIG M.E., BIRCH H.G., RICHARDSON S.A. & TIZARD J. (1972) Intellectual levels of school children severely malnourished during the first two years of life. *Pediatrics*, **49**, 814.

TIZARD J. (1964) *Community Services for the Mentally Handicapped.* Oxford University Press, London.

WALTON J.N., ELLIS E. & COURT S.D.M. (1962) Clumsy children; developmental apraxia and agnosia. *Brain.*, **85**, 603.

WING L. (1970) The syndrome of early childhood autism. *Brit. J. Hosp. Med.*, **4**, 381.

WINICK M. (1969) Malnutrition and brain development. *J. Pediat.*, **74**, 667.

WORKING PARTY REPORT (1961) Schizophrenic syndrome in childhood. *Brit. med. J.*, **2**, 889.

WORKING PARTY PROGRESS REPORT (1964) Schizophrenic syndrome in childhood. *Develop. Med. Child. Neurol.*, **6**, 530.

# CHAPTER 16

# EMOTIONAL AND BEHAVIOURAL
# DISORDERS

## Normal emotional development

To understand the mechanism and management of problems affecting the emotion and behaviour of a child, a knowledge of normal emotional maturation is required. During the early weeks of life the baby's needs are food, warmth and comfort. The mother, or mother-substitute, in satisfying these demands becomes the object to whom the young baby attaches himself. So close is the attachment that the baby becomes a barometer of the mother's feelings. If she is happy and relaxed her baby will be peaceful and content, whereas if she is anxious her baby is likely to reflect this anxiety and to cry excessively. The use of the word 'colic' as a 'diagnosis' for this crying only makes it more difficult for a mother to understand the real reason why her baby is crying.

This first 'love' of the infant is therefore purely material and selfish. Once his needs have been satisfied the baby falls asleep, having no further interest in the outside world. The satisfaction felt by the infant is also felt, though in a different manner, by the mother, whose natural instinct is to feed and protect her young baby. As with all normal instincts it may become disturbed; for example, the mother who over-protects her child may also overfeed him.

At about the age of 6 months the baby becomes aware of his mother as an individual, deriving pleasure from her attentions additional to those involving feeding. At this stage his desire for maternal affection has become as great as his need for food, warmth and comfort. Normal emotional maturation requires the development of this close bond between the child and his mother. If this is prevented, the child is unable to make future, solid and lasting relationships with other people. Children who have been 'deprived' of normal maternal affection are likely to produce the same problem in their own children since, having never known a close maternal bond, they are unable to create it for their offspring. This mechanism became clear during the last war when many children from the cities were evacuated from their homes, being made to live with strangers in the country. The insecurity this produced caused many of the children to react aggressively, often resulting in their being moved to another home. Some of these, now grown up with families of their own, are producing children with similar problems of deprivation. A serious reflection on our ignorance at that time is that children from the same family were often evacuated to different homes.

The bond between mother and child is so close that once it has developed, the young infant, usually of toddler age, is at first frightened to leave his mother. He will become prepared to do so only when he is certain that, in leaving his mother, he is sure to find her again when he wants to do so. The toddler who insists on clinging to his mother's skirts must not be pushed away; his needs are for more affection. The amount of affection demanded by different children varies greatly but the golden rule is to give as much as they demand. The child who demands most is the least secure, being in need of extra affection. This point is often not understood by mothers who, despite a maternal instinct to cuddle their children, fear it would be wrong and that they would be 'spoiling' the child.

The arrival of a new baby is bound to disturb the balance of the relationship which has developed between an older child and his mother. Great skill is required in preparing the child for the event, it being emphasized that the new baby will be for him. It is a mistake for the older child first to meet the new baby being cuddled in his mother's arms. Some children react to the arrival of a sibling by a return to babyish habits such as bed-wetting or soiling their pants.

Whether a situation is stressful for a child depends on the stage of development he has reached. The very young baby is less affected than the toddler by the sudden disappearance of his mother into hospital. Adverse events are particularly harmful to children when they create more anxiety than the child can cope with.

Parents must therefore learn to look for the need behind their child's disturbed behaviour. They must also know that emotional development does not take place equally in all aspects at the same time. For example, a child may be advanced in one direction, such as social relationships, but delayed in another, such as the expression of speech.

It used to be thought that childhood was free of sexuality and that the sex instinct was not normally aroused until adolescence. However, the work of Freud has demonstrated the existence of an infantile sexuality. The act of suckling not only gives the infant pleasure by appeasing his hunger but also by stimulating his oral sensations. The mouth is the first of the special areas of the body to provide this pleasurable stimulation. The child therefore soon learns to satisfy this pleasure, at times other than feeds, by sucking his thumb. Moreover, as soon as he is physically capable he puts all new objects into his mouth. This period Freud termed the 'oral phase'.

From about the age of 18 months the anal area takes over from the oral as the zone of pleasurable interest. This is the 'anal phase'. During this time the child enjoys playing with his excreta and with play substances which resemble faecal material. He has now become as absorbed in what is often described as 'dirty' play as he was previously in thumb-sucking. The extent of his interest in his bowels will depend to a large extent on the approach of those caring for him. Excessive pot training and concern about regular bowel habits engenders excessive bowel consciousness.

Between the ages of 3 and 4 years the child's interest moves to the genitalia. In this 'phallic phase' the boy is particularly interested in the penis, this being the time when he finds that handling it leads to pleasure and erection. Girls derive similar pleasure from the clitoris but those whose circumstances make them aware of their anatomical differences from boys are likely to be envious of the boy's penis. It is during this phase that the central sexual activity for both sexes is masturbation. Between the ages of 5 to 10 years the sex instinct remains more or less dormant, becoming aroused again shortly before adolescence.

Looked at in the light of normal emotional development, it becomes obvious that thumb-sucking and masturbation are normal occurrences. Other pleasurable activities coming within the same field are nail-biting and nose-picking.

**Aetiology**

The causes of a child's emotional and behavioural problems lie usually with the parents rather than with the child. Faulty parental handling is due often to ignorance of normal emotional development. If parents describe their child as 'highly strung' they are usually attempting to provide an explanation for the problems, thereby relieving themselves of their responsibility.

Many of the problems are simply a perpetuation of infantile behaviour to an age at which it is no longer appropriate; prolonged thumb-sucking is an obvious example. Insecurity and maternal deprivation are causes of serious emotional disorders. This may result from marital discord, a broken home or death of one or both parents. In other cases the parents may, by their behaviour, have set a bad example to their children who then copy them, growing up with a false set of values.

Problems can also result from mishandling a child's fears. A child is helped to master his fears by being made to feel bigger than the fear. Thus, if he cannot sleep because he is frightened of the dark, the dark should be made less terrifying by a night light or by leaving the bedroom door open. It also helps if the child knows that other children have similar fears. The wrong way of dealing with it is to tell the child that he is stupid to be frightened and that he should face up to it 'like a man'. This only increases his fears.

Many of the fears of childhood can be relieved if parents will only give their child a chance to explain his feelings. The first time a child overhears his parents quarrelling may cause him serious anxiety. This may be the occasion, which faces every child, when his parents suddenly have to be taken off the pedestal on which he has placed them because he discovers they are no longer the god-like figures he had imagined. Moreover, he may suddenly be frightened lest his parents are going to separate since, having never heard them argue before, he can think of no other solution, particularly if any of his friends come from a broken home.

A child's fears are sometimes based on a chance remark, perhaps made many weeks before, which has remained in his memory.

*Charles aged* 4 *years suddenly went into a panic when he saw his mother put on a coat to go out shopping. Several days before, in a moment of anger, she had said she would leave him if ever he did something naughty again; now he thought that moment had arrived.*

Functional symptoms in children with organic disease often result from unnatural fears about the disease; these can be relieved if the situation is discovered and an explanation given. A child with heart disease may overhear a remark relating to heart failure and then develop understandable anxieties relating to his own heart. For this reason, doctors and nurses must be particularly careful not to discuss a child's illness within his hearing.

A common mistake made by parents, and one which may lead to behaviour disorders, is an inconsistency of disciplinary measures; as far as possible both parents should apply the same methods. If the child is spoilt by one parent and thrashed by the other he will soon learn how to conduct his business so that within a short time he has driven a wedge between his parents. Physical punishment is always a mistake; children should not learn aggression from their parents but it is normal for them to learn about it by their interactions with other children. A safe and more effective punishment is the removal of a privilege, sweet or pocket money. Whatever method is adopted, to be effective, it must be one which can be applied immediately. On no account should children be sent to bed as a punishment. Bed is a child's castle where he feels snug and secure at night; it cannot serve the dual function of prison cell in the daytime and castle at night.

Parental knowledge of normal development is essential if they are to understand how to discipline their children. They must know what can be expected of a child at different ages before applying punishment for a supposed error. Increasing understanding of child development is the probable reason why the later children in a family are punished less. The punishment pattern adopted by parents is largely determined by their own experiences as children. The parent who had a rigid upbringing is likely to use the same methods on his own children. Parents from the lower social classes use more physical punishment whereas those from the higher classes use more words and gestures.

Driving a wedge between parents and exploiting their differences is one of the delights of the young child, although it may lead to disasters if the parents fail to have insight into the situation.

*Susan aged 3 years suddenly started to wake up crying in the middle of the night. Initially she would respond to the comfortings of her mother who came to her room, but after a time she insisted on being brought into her parents' double bed. Her next step was to cry unless her mother got out of the double bed and into her bed; her parents being frightened of the neighbours' complaints of noise and the possibility that they might be turned out of their flat acceded to her increased demands. The nightly ritual therefore began whereby Susan cried in the early hours, this being the signal for her mother to change beds with her. The next step in wedge-driving was Susan's refusal to eat off her own plate and her insistence that she ate off her father's plate. Even then, with Susan allied to her father against her mother, the parents remained oblivious of the way the situation was developing. Only when they were on the brink of divorce did they appeal for advice.*

Many problems result from incorrect training methods, especially the creation of rigid rules which evoke a negativistic response from the child. Negativism occurs particularly in relation to meals, bowel-habits and going to sleep. Rules which are so rigid that the child is almost certain to break them, are bound to lead to a situation in which the child either learns to flout parental authority or is always punished.

When one child is emotionally disturbed it is likely that others in the same family are affected to some extent. The doctor must discover why the particular child was brought to him for treatment. Individual treatment of a disturbed child will have repercussions on the rest of the family, though this will be appreciated only if the whole family is studied. For this reason, as far as possible, only one doctor should treat the family. In treating such children, doctors must avoid becoming 'pro' the child and 'anti' the parents. They must particularly avoid taking over the child, thereby antagonizing the parents.

In the management of physical problems, prevention and treatment is well defined, whereas it is far from clear in the management of emotional problems. Many of the children with emotional disorders come from 'problem families'. In managing problem families it is clear that social services are no substitute for the material needs of the families. Special observation of children 'at risk' of physical handicaps has already been stressed (p. 91). A similar approach is needed for those 'at emotional risk'. Included in this category is the child of an aggressive parent, the child of a depressed mother or a mother who keeps asking seemingly irrelevant questions (Howells, 1966).

Although this chapter is involved with functional disorders, it must be emphasized that emotional factors influence the clinical pattern of every organic disease. The child who is surrounded by anxious and fussy relatives produces a different behavioural pattern from the child whose relatives are able to keep their own emotions under control. Parents are often surprised at the early age at which a child can be made anxious by those around him. The mother of a newborn baby who is herself on edge will soon affect the feeding and sleeping habits of her baby. The child of anxious parents gets more colds and other infections than the average. This is partly due to parental concern, causing more notice to be taken, but such children do also seem to pick up infections more easily.

It is always necessary to check that the child is physically well before diagnosing an emotional disorder, since any chronic disease may produce alterations in behaviour. Mental retardation must also be excluded, though on the whole the children who exhibit behavioural problems have a good intelligence.

Today, many more children with emotional problems are being brought to the doctor. This results partly from the increased tensions of life today and partly because parents are demanding to understand the emotional problems of their children more than did their grandparents. The doctor whose work brings him into contact with families must be trained to deal with these problems. In their management he must look beyond the presenting symptom, studying the whole family. The more one listens to parents and explains the problems underlying a child's behaviour the less one prescribes, particularly sedatives.

### Thumb-sucking

It is normal for a child of about 6 months of age to suck this thumb. By this age he has discovered the delight of possessing a mouth; everything he handles is put there. This oral phase normally lasts a few months only and, as the child develops, so the habit of thumb-sucking is lost. On the other hand if the child feels insecure, for example when he goes to bed or is frightened, then he may revert to the habit. If his parents understand the mechanism they will not attempt to remove his thumb from his mouth but will do what they can to relieve his fears. Thumb-sucking is sometimes due to sheer boredom so that if the child is suitably amused the thumb soon drops out of the mouth. It is at this stage that some infants acquire the habit of insisting on chewing an old blanket or cloth when going to sleep. Such children, if admitted to hospital, should be permitted to keep their cloth, since if it is needed to give security at home, much more is it needed in the strange surrounding of a hospital.

Perpetual thumb-sucking can adversely affect the alignment of the teeth. Such deformity is not serious up to the age of 6 years since only the primary dentition is involved. If the habit persists after that age the permanent teeth can be affected, the deformity remaining throughout life unless treated by an orthodontist. It is sometimes possible to fit the thumb into the position in which it is perpetually sucked, thereby determining the exact mechanism of the deformity. Children are occasionally seen who have developed the habit of sucking the forearm, a practice which results in serious deformities of the teeth.

The disadvantage of a dummy is not that it is unhygienic, since it is no dirtier than a thumb, but that it acts like a plug stopping fingers and toys going in and noises coming out. It is normal for a child to use his mouth to explore objects and he should not be stopped unless the object is dangerous.

### Masturbation

After discovering his mouth, the developing child, as already explained (p. 457), reaches the age at which he discovers that handling his genitalia gives him greater pleasure than any other part of the body. This phase is common to all children but if parents are unaware that this is normal, they may have intense reactions to the situation. Such a reaction increases the child's interest in the area, causing him to carry on the practice more often when his parents are not present; in this way masturbation develops. Parents must therefore be educated to understand that handling genitalia is a normal phase of development, just as much as thumb-sucking. It is only perpetuated if they draw attention to the situation, thereby increasing their child's interest.

Masturbation in young children is usually achieved by rubbing the thighs together and sometimes by rocking the body. During the act the child may appear to be in a trance, going red in the face with audible breathing; this is sometimes mistaken for a convulsion (see p. 417). Masturbation in older children is more common in boys than girls, particularly between the ages of 10 and 15 years.

The incidence of masturbation is always likely to be high, but earlier sex education and the removal of guilt about the habit reduces its frequency. More parental instruction is required so that the subject can be discussed openly; parents should be informed that there is no risk that the practice will cause their child to become a sex pervert.

## Nail-biting

This habit usually results from increased nervous tension; it is this which should be relieved rather than any direct attack on the nails. The painting of bitter substances on the nails is useless since it can be wiped off, thereby creating a situation in which parental authority can easily be flouted.

A simple device which is often useful in a girl who bites her nails is to get her mother to buy her a bottle of colourless nail varnish. The child will be delighted that she is permitted nail varnish and will wish to demonstrate this fact to her friends, but she will not do so until her nails have grown. The school teacher should be informed that this is 'medical nail varnish' in order to obtain her co-operation.

## Head-rolling and head-banging

These movements commonly start as a child's method of rocking himself to sleep; like any simple repetitive movement they help to induce sleep by relaxation, in the same way as the counting of sheep by adults. The movement may be pleasurable, being sometimes combined with masturbation if the whole trunk is being rocked.

The habits usually start around 9 months and they are serious because they indicate the child's need to provide his own comfort. The underlying problem is a break in the normal mother/child relationship, causing a loss in the child's security and in his natural curiosity. On no account should such a mother be fobbed off with advice suggesting this is just a harmless passing phase and that her child will 'grow out of it'. It is essential for her to play more with her child. In this way he may no longer need these repetitive habits which are so wasteful of his time since they restrict his natural opportunities for learning.

Parents are extremely alarmed by head-banging for fear of causing brain damage. They can be assured this does not occur, but it is a simple matter also to pad the end of the cot. If the child has learnt the trick of making the cot move round the room, the cot can be fixed to the floor with a right-angled metal strut.

### SPASMUS NUTANS

This term is used to describe those infants who have acquired the habit of head nodding associated with tilting of the head and nystagmus. The condition is more common in those with poor social conditions. It is self-limiting, usually disappearing by the age of 3 years.

It is now much rarer and it seems likely that the condition is comparable to head banging and related to boredom and lack of stimulation.

## Sleeplessness

This is one of the commonest complaints made by parents about their children. The problem commonly starts around 9 months of age when the child becomes conscious of being left alone and is frightened lest his mother disappears for ever. Parental anxiety is increased by the misconception, held by many parents and encouraged by some books on child care, that children require a specific number of hours of sleep according to their age. This leads to a belief that the child will be harmed by failure to sleep the requisite amount. A common misconception is that the brain will 'tire' if sleep is inadequate.

In fact, the sleep needs of children vary enormously, the bright active infant often sleeping less than the more placid one. Such bright children commonly wake early in the morning, wishing to be played with. There is no way of making them go to sleep again—nor would one want to do so since their development is being stimulated through play. The parents of such children can only hope to obtain peace for themselves by surrounding the child with toys and colouring books to occupy him in the early morning. By the age of about 3 years the child can understand that he can play as much as he likes provided he does not wake his parents by creating a noise. If play is allowed, the child, not being bored, makes less noise; he is also more likely to fall asleep again.

Parental anxiety about a child's lack of sleep is soon sensed by the child, who may become worried that he cannot get to sleep. Therefore, the first step in management is to ensure the parents are aware that no harm will come to the child from lack of sleep. The only reason for trying to get a child to sleep is to give his parents their well-earned rest. An air of nonchalance about the subject will do much to relieve the child's anxiety, thereby helping him to stop 'trying' to get to sleep. If a child calls his parents to say he cannot get to sleep, an offer of 10 pence if he can stay awake all night will usually find him asleep within 5 minutes!

Habit has an important part to play in assisting sleep. The child who knows he cannot call his mother back after being tucked up in bed is much more likely to go straight to sleep than the one who can get his mother back every time he calls out. On no account should children be brought into their parents' bed when they cannot sleep as this will soon develop into a habit. Equally, children should not be bribed by presents or special activities in order to cajole them into going to sleep.

Noise may prevent children from sleeping, this being more of a problem in the overcrowded homes of today. But much of this relates to earlier training methods. If the parental approach to noise has been one of 'Hush! You'll wake the baby' the child is more likely to be kept awake by noise when he is older. The baby should be expected to sleep through the normal noise of the household, this pattern being set from the start.

Ideally, the child, from a baby, should have his own bedroom. Although this is often impossible, much can be done to achieve a separate room at night by moving the child to the living room or kitchen when his parents go to bed. A landing makes an adequate and independent 'bedroom' if the baby has been conditioned to noise from an early age.

Other measures should be adopted in order to make it more easy for sleep to come. A child cannot be expected to go straight to sleep when he has just left an exciting game or a cowboy film. A period of 'unwinding' is essential, the time-honoured bed-time story having much to commend it. In light summer evenings it is more difficult for a child to go to sleep but fear that he will have insufficient sleep is often the reason for putting him to bed too early. It is better that a child should go to bed later and so fall asleep sooner, than spend hours trying to get to sleep. If children are overclothed and thereby too hot, they may find it difficult to sleep.

A long sleep in the middle of the day renders it less easy for a child to go to sleep in the evening. This rest period should therefore be shortened and then cut out to suit the mother's convenience.

Sedatives have little or no place in the management of sleeplessness in childhood.

### Night terrors

Some children wake up screaming and panic-stricken in the night. For a time they may seem semiconscious only and it may be some minutes before they can be comforted and brought back to reality. The episode is due to a severe nightmare, usually in children having a vivid imagination. The measures already recommended to induce sleep should reduce this problem, especially giving the child a period to unwind before going to bed. Sleep-walking is a still more vidid form of the same problem in which the child actually takes part in the act he is imagining. Parents will naturally be worried lest their child harms himself but, fortunately, this seldom occurs though appropriate safety bolts should be fixed to doors and windows. Care should be taken to ensure that none of these fears are transferred to the child.

### Refusal to eat

Much of what has been said about sleeplessness applies to the problem of refusal to eat. The subject is discussed on p. 88.

### Pica

Children who develop this habit acquire a perverted taste, choosing to eat dirt, coal, paper, hair and portions of their toys; they are usually toddlers. There is a risk that their abnormal eating habits may lead them to chew objects containing lead, so causing lead poisoning. The children usually have an iron deficiency anaemia; possibly the lack of iron causes a perverted appetitite in an attempt to satisfy the body's demands for iron. Whatever the explanation, the habit usually disappears when the anaemia is corrected by iron therapy, but permanent cure is dependent on the maintenance of adequate haemoglobin levels (McDonald & Marshall, 1964).

**Enuresis**

A doctor's first responsibility when faced with a child who wets the bed is to ensure there is no underlying disorder of the renal tract, such as infection or a congenital malformation. An organic cause is unlikely if the child, though wet from birth, has achieved even only one dry night in his life. The majority of the patients will be found to be normal. If a child has achieved control but then starts to wet the bed again the cause may be organic such as a urinary infection, diabetes mellitus or diastematomyelia. Alternatively it may be due to a sudden emotional disturbance such as starting school.

It used to be said that spina bifida occulta was a cause of enuresis in other-wise healthy children, but this was incorrect. The disorder leads to enuresis only in the very rare case where neurological signs are present. Many mentally handicapped children are enuretic but these will usually be brought to see the doctor because they are backward and not because they wet the bed.

Increasing age is of over-riding importance in achieving nocturnal control of micturition. This, together with the frequency of a family history of the condition, supports the concept that enuresis is due to delayed development of bladder control (Bakwin, 1961; Barbour et al., 1963). Most of the children are psychologically normal. For this reason parents should wait until the child is 4 years old before seeking special treatment. Early training is of value provided parents do not expect too much of their child, making the situation worse by unreasonable demands.

There is a small group of children whose enuresis is associated with encopresis. These children are usually suffering from severe emotional stresses.

*Treatment.* This is aimed at encouraging the development of normal control and removing any contributory emotional factors. A mother must avoid scolding or chastising her child when he is wet. Praise for dry nights and no comment for wet ones is required. Often the child has been reprimanded for his wet beds so that by the time he is brought for advice much harm has been done, although by then his mother has usually realized that repri-mands only make him worse.

The patient is more often a boy than a girl since a boy's bladder capacity is possibly smaller than a girl's; for this reason one aspect of the treatment is 'day-clock training' in order to accustom the bladder to hold urine for longer periods. A mother is better able to understand what is being attempted if she is told that it is to 'stretch the bladder'. She must ensure that her child passes his urine every hour on the hour. An alarm clock is required, a mother accompanying her child to ensure that he actually passes urine. The interval is then steadily increased each day by hourly or half-hourly periods. By the time a child has been trained to hold his urine for 6 hours during the day it will be found that he has become dry at night.

The child should go to bed with an empty bladder, being lifted again when the parents are themselves ready for bed, which must be as late as possible, preferably midnight. If he is ever wet at this time he should also be lifted as often as necessary in the interval before his parents go to bed. When lifted the child should use the pot which is kept in the bedroom. For some unexplained reason parents are often told that their child must go to the lavatory, an instruction which often meets with antagonism in the middle of the night. All that is required is that the child should empty his bladder into the pot. Many children will achieve this, without seeming to wake up, as soon as the rim of the pot touches the thighs. It is unnecessary to force the child to wake up fully, as many parents and some doctors believe; attempts to do so only cause unnecessary battles often resulting in a refusal to pass urine. For obvious reasons the child must use the pot on the floor, not on the bed.

A prize should be awarded for success, being given for each dry night rather than when a final dry state is achieved. Parents sometimes promise a bicycle or other major prize to be given when their child is finally dry but they might as well promise the moon for all the effect it has. A penny for each dry night is a reasonable and very successful bribe, but the way in which it is given is important. The mother should place the penny beside a money box away from the bed immediately before she tucks her child for the night. While doing so, she discusses with him what he is going to buy with his prize money; by this means his last waking thoughts are of the treasures which lie ahead for him, if only he can be dry. In the morning, as soon as he wakes, the child uses the pot which is kept under the bed, then putting the penny in the box. If he is wet, no comment is made by his mother who removes the penny during the day but resets the trap in the same manner the next night.

Jealousy could develop between brothers and sisters who have already achieved dry beds and are thereby denied the extra income available to the wet one. This problem is easily avoided, and can be turned to advantage, if the dry children also receive a penny every time the wet one is dry. This not only removes the chance of jealousy but enhances the reputation of the wet child who receives added incentives from the other members of his family standing to benefit.

If the parents wake before their child, they should immediately pot him as their noise may disturb the child so that, in a half-wakeful state, he wets the bed. It is unnecessary to restrict fluids after 5 o'clock in the evening as is commonly recommended; this practice only causes discomfort and may make it more difficult for a child to go to sleep.

The child should have an outside source of praise for his successful nights and there is no one better to give this than the doctor. A simple method is to ask the child to make a calendar to be known as 'Dr ——'s calendar' on which he rings in red the dates of every dry night. The pride with which the children bring this calendar to the doctor is evidence of its value.

These measures are usually most effective, provided sufficient time is given to the mother and child on the first visit. In this condition success breeds success; the child and his parents are so delighted with the improvement that the whole house becomes less tense, thus increasing the chances of further improvement. A mother may have been afraid lest the kidneys were seriously wrong and that her child would never be dry, but once he starts to have dry nights her confidence returns.

Drugs such as amphetamine for deep sleepers or ephedrine to relax the bladder muscle are of little value. They are poor substitutes for the doctor who is prepared to spend time and, by his own enthusiasm, help the child to a lasting cure. The use of the tricyclic antidepressants is highly dangerous owing to the risk of poisoning (Goel & Shanks, 1974). Most mothers are unaware that such drugs are lethal to their children if taken in excess.

If enuresis persists, particularly in older children, the electric buzzer is a useful method of treatment (Wickes, 1958). Two metal pads are placed in the child's bed causing an alarm to ring when the bed becomes wet. The response to the alarm is unconscious, micturition stopping before the child is fully awake. It is believed that it works by strengthening an inhibitory reflex (Gillison & Skinner, 1958).

### Encopresis

This is defined as incontinence of stools of non-organic origin although some authors use the term incorrectly to describe psychogenic incontinence only. The vast majority of children who soil do so as a result of chronic constipation which in most instances is of psychogenic origin. This problem is discussed on page 304.

A small group of children with faecal incontinence do not have chronic constipation. These are usually emotionally disturbed and they may also be enuretic.

## Habit spasm (tic)

These are common in nervous children, often starting by the perpetuation of a simple habit. For example, a lock of hair which falls in front of one eye may be tossed back by a movement of the head and this can become a habit. The head and shoulders are principally involved, the abnormal movements including blinking, wrinkling of the forehead, grimacing, head shaking and shrugging of the shoulders.

The movements must not be mistaken for chorea. They are repetitive and can be repeated on request, whereas in chorea they are always changing. A habit spasm can be controlled for a time when asked, whereas choreic movements become exaggerated by such a request.

*Treatment.* The reason for the increased tension must be discovered, no attention being drawn to the symptom. The child must never be told to stop making the movement, but he should be told it is not his fault and that it will disappear.

## Recurrent abdominal pain

In Chapter 8 (p. 308) stress has been laid on the frequency with which recurrent abdominal pain in childhood is due to emotional causes. Reference has been made to the two major clinical patterns which emerge: in one the pain is part of the 'periodic syndrome'; in the other it is one of the 'recurrent pains of childhood'.

### THE PERIODIC SYNDROME

In this syndrome the child complains of central abdominal pain, the onset usually being acute. Feeds are refused, he becomes pale and within 2–3 hours begins to vomit. Having emptied his stomach, repeated vomiting produces only a little bile-stained fluid, this persisting for about a day. The stools remain normal but fever may occur. In a severe attack the child shows evidence of dehydration, the breath smells of acetone, and ketone bodies are present in the urine. The abdomen remains soft on palpation. The attack is usually over in 2 days, the child then rapidly returning to normal.

*Aetiology.* In the past these attacks were often referred to as 'acidosis' but this is biochemically incorrect and adds nothing to the diagnosis, therefore the term should be dropped. The exact cause is unknown but the absence of organic disease and the obvious emotional factors leave no doubt that the disorder is of emotional origin. The children are frequently described by their parents as 'highly-strung' or 'over-sensitive' and the parents themselves are often nervous and over-protective. These children are more subject than the average to travel sickness. The condition tends to improve as the child grows older, although a proportion of them still show nervous symptoms in adult life, especially headaches which may be typical of migraine. A history of a similar illness in childhood may be obtained about other members of the family or the parents, indicating a family pattern of reaction to emotional stress. The association with migraine in adults has led to the use of the term 'abdominal migraine' to describe the syndrome. But the word migraine, meaning half a head, should not be applied to this disorder. An association with epilepsy has been claimed by some writers but controlled electroencephalographic studies have shown no such relationship (Apley *et al.*, 1956). The term 'cyclical vomiting' is sometimes used as an alternative. This has the merit that it is purely descriptive, but it is too limiting a term since vomiting does not occur in every attack.

*Diagnosis.* All organic causes of abdominal pain must be excluded before the diagnosis is made. Important among these are renal causes, especially pyelonephritis and hydronephrosis, and intestinal causes, particularly recurrent intussusception and Hirschsprung's disease. Some children who are subject to recurrent upper respiratory infections have abdominal pain with each attack. This may be due to associated mesenteric adenitis but is sometimes due to the constipation which accompanies the fever. An intracranial tumour and lead poisoning may cause similar symptoms.

Parents usually think first of the possibility of appendicitis but this condition does not produce the same recurrent picture. Obviously, children who are subject to the periodic syndrome may develop acute appendicitis just like any other child, so that this diagnosis can be excluded only by examination. Parents also worry about tuberculosis as a cause, but if this were sufficiently severe to be causing abdominal pain it would also cause chronic ill-health, whereas children with the periodic syndrome are perfectly well between attacks.

*Treatment.* The first step is to reassure the parents that there is no organic disease. This alone will do much to reduce the symptoms, since the parents' anxiety about the possibility of an operation, especially appendicectomy, has so often been conveyed to the child. Small quantities of glucose fluids should be given frequently. The attacks in some children can be prevented by giving a glucose drink last thing at night. The long-term problem in therapy is to determine the underlying emotional factors and to attempt to correct them.

RECURRENT PAINS OF CHILDHOOD

Recurrent pain in the abdomen, limbs or head is a common symptom in childhood, being usually the result of an emotional disorder. The children and their parents show the same features as those described for the periodic syndrome. The children are usually tense and anxious and, like their parents, are often over-conscientious. The pattern of symptoms usually remains remarkably constant for each child, the pain being felt most often in one site only.

### Abdominal pain

This is the commonest site in young children; it is usually central and not associated with vomiting. It may occur at any time of the day, though especially before meals, sometimes waking the child at night. It may be brought on by fear or anxiety, such as when it occurs just before the child goes off to school. The pain may sometimes be very severe, so that the degree of pain is of no value in differentiating this condition from organic disease. It is never possible to differentiate functional from organic pain on the basis of severity.

*Diagnosis.* The possible organic causes of abdominal pain which must be differentiated are the same as those already given for the periodic syndrome on p. 470. Organic pain is usually more localized than functional pain. Constipation is often given as a cause for this type of pain but pain is not a feature of this problem (p. 305). It is true that the passage of a large hard stool may cause local pain, though even this is exaggerated by the feelings of the parents as they watch their child straining *to hold on* but interpret his distress as due to straining to let go. If a child with constipation does complain of abdominal pain it is usually because his parents have made him so worried about the problem and its supposed harmful effects.

*Treatment.* The first essential is that the child and his parents should be made aware that the doctor knows he feels the pain. Almost certainly someone will have suggested that the child is making it up, or exaggerating the pain or doing it for attention. Pain is subjective and only the individual concerned can say whether he is feeling pain. If he were making it up he would be a malingerer—a condition I have never met in childhood.

The exclusion of organic disease and the reassurance of the parents on this fact goes a long way towards successful treatment. These children are more easy to help than those with the periodic syndrome. By the use of a diagram and simple explanation it is possible to convey to a child that the pains he feels result from the normal workings of his 'tummy'. Peristaltic waves are described, the child being told that these waves may be felt either because the threshold for pain is lowered, as in someone who is worried, or because the waves are stronger than usual, as occurs before a meal. When the child has grasped these facts, which can be put across in a very simple manner, he is no longer frightened by the pain, realizing that they indicate that his stomach is working normally.

Many parents have little understanding of gastric physiology. They can be helped in this if told the classic experiments of Beaumont, an army surgeon, on Alexis St Martin in 1833. This man suffered an accidental gunshot wound leaving a gastric fistula and exposed gastric mucosa. Beaumont persuaded Alexis to let him study him and on one occasion purposely made him extremely angry. This caused the pink mucosa to change to red and then to purple as it swelled up. Small wonder that anger and stress can lead to a gastric erosion and bleeding, or that healthy children sometimes feel pain in the abdomen.

## Limb pains

These are felt in the muscles and not in the joints. They occur mainly in the calves and thighs and usually come on in the evening when the child is tired, sometimes waking the child at night. They have nothing to do with growth, which is not a painful process; therefore the term 'growing pains', which so often leads parents to think of rheumatic fever, should be discarded.

The explanation for the pains is difficult. Probably, as the child roars around while playing he jars his muscles and ligaments just like anyone else. The resulting aches are not complained of by most people but if a child and his parents are anxious, and particularly if this unexplained pain comes on at night, it is liable to be alarming.

*Treatment.* The parents and child are reassured about organic disease and particularly that 'rheumatism' is not the cause. The child is told that if he wishes he can sit down and rub his legs when he gets the pain, but that he will come to no harm by going on playing. During the night the pain can be relieved by rubbing but for a time he may need this to be done by his mother.

## Head pains

These are usually frontal; they occur at any time of the day and are not associated with vomiting. They must be differentiated from those due to an intracranial tumour, in which case the headache usually occurs on getting up in the morning and is associated with vomiting.

It is sometimes helpful to enquire whether the headache is more a pain or an uncomfortable feeling since a child with emotional pain will often refer to it as an uncomfortable feeling when asked in this way. It may be informative that the child looks to his mother before answering the question or that she answers first.

The blood pressure must be measured in all children with headaches in order to avoid missing the rare case of hypertension.

### General management of recurrent pains

Having excluded organic disease, an emotional disorder must be diagnosed and the factors underlying it determined by considering the family and the whole of the child's environment. The therapeutic approach must be positive rather than the negative one of merely excluding organic disease; the greatest care is needed to ensure that in explaining the absence of organic disease the idea is not left that the pain is imaginary. Parents must understand that whether a pain is organic or functional makes no difference to the pain itself, only to its mode of treatment.

With all three types of pain it is often helpful to suggest to the child that he should not tell his mother that he has the pain until it has left him.

## Recurrent fever

The same emotional tensions which lead to recurrent pains in some children may produce recurrent fever in others; any individual may develop a rise in temperature when anxious. An emotional basis may also account for a persistence of fever after an infection has cleared. In the absence of physical signs such children should be allowed up and temperature recordings stopped. When in doubt a normal sedimentation rate is useful in excluding an organic cause for the fever.

## Depression

Children who are depressed often present with headache. The condition should be obvious from the look of the child whose facial appearance gives away his flat affect. However, it is often missed because of an unawareness that depression is common in older children.

These children are subject to mood changes and may be aggressive at times. They have few friends, having withdrawn from social contacts, and are often frightened of going to school. Sleep disturbances are common and various somatic complaints are made.

## Hysteria

This is not a common symptom in childhood; it usually takes the form of an hysterical paralysis or limp and, less often, a glove or stocking type of anaesthesia. Occasionally fits, choking or an inability to speak occur.

Diagnosis is usually obvious; for example, paralysis, which has often followed a trivial injury, is bizarre, the patient being remarkably complacent about his apparently serious symptom. But hysteria must always be regarded as a dangerous diagnosis to make in childhood because of the risk of overlooking a serious disorder such as a cerebral abscess. Bizarre symptoms may well be caused by organic disease.

*Treatment.* These children are highly responsive to suggestion so that treatment is often easy.

## School Phobia

The term indicates an irrational fear of going to school. A preferable term is 'school refusal' since the phobia may not consciously be expressed (Michell, 1966). The degree of fear varies from mild apprehension on a Monday morning, to uncontrollable panic resulting in tachycardia, a dry mouth and a complete inability to go to school. The child is unable to explain the reason for his fear, though he may project it on to some specific aspect of school, such as the meals or lavatories. Somatic manifestations, such as vomiting or abdominal pain, may occur.

Boys are affected more than girls; the commonest ages are the early years when just starting school and 10–12 years. The onset is usually acute, though a deeper search frequently uncovers a poor school attendance record. The child may have found difficulty in changing schools previously. The earlier academic record is usually good.

The acute distress disappears with the arrival of school holidays or when absence from school is accepted.

*Treatment.* School phobia must not be regarded as a clinical entity but as one reaction to stress involving the whole family. The basis of the problem is the child's fear of separation from his mother with whom he feels a strong bond, whereas commonly the bond with father is weak. Separation anxiety may be shared mutually by mother and child. The mother may have been similarly torn as a child.

It is important to consider the family as a functional unit which has reached equilibrium through the child's problem. For this reason the family must be successfully treated before the child is got back to school, otherwise his return to school may precipitate another family breakdown.

## School Truancy

This disturbance of behaviour is quite different from school phobia, being closely related to delinquency. The child may also lie and steal. A similar age group is affected but the child is likely to have a lower intelligence. The thought of school does not produce panic reactions and, whereas the child with school phobia stays at home, the school truant may leave home as well as school. By deceit he may play off the school against the home so that the school believes he has good reason to be absent whereas his parents think he is at school.

Most truants are lonely insecure boys who are unable to make stable friendships at school. They are incapable of finding emotional or social satisfaction at home or at school. Their truant behaviour represents an attempt to escape from an intolerable world of failure and boredom into a fantasy world represented for them by the cinema, television or a football match.

Their family background is poor, houses being overcrowded and parents having similar problems; they may have truanted as children and are now unhappily married. These parents make little contact with the school and make it obvious to the child that they do not value education and learning. Such problem families are extremely difficult to help, especially as they are often resentful of any assistance from the Social Services.

## Stealing

All children steal. It may be meaningless, such as an infant picking up a toy belonging to someone else before he realizes fully that he does not own everything around him or it may be a sign of disturbance.

Stealing to be found out is a powerful way of asking for help and must be recognized. Some children steal sweets and other trivial objects which they give away as a means of buying affection. Some steal in order to own something, having no belongings of their own. Being given pocket money may help such children.

## BIBLIOGRAPHY

APLEY J. (1975) The Child with Abdominal Pains. 2nd Ed. Blackwell Scientific Publications, Oxford.

APLEY J., LLOYD J. & TURTON C. (1956) Electro-encephalography in children with recurrent abdominal pain. *Lancet*, **1**, 264.

BAKWIN H. (1961) Enuresis in children. *J. Pediat.*, **58**, 806.

BARBOUR R.F., BORLAND E.M., BOYD M.M., MILLER A. & OPPÉ T.E. (1963) Enuresis as a disorder of development. *Brit. med. J.*, **2**, 787.

GILLISON T.H. & SKINNER J.L. (1958) Treatment of nocturnal enuresis by the electric alarm. *Brit. med. J.*, **2**, 1268.

GOEL K.M. & SHANKS R.A. (1974) Amitriptyline and Imipramine poisoning in children. *Brit. med. J.*, **1**, 261.

HOWELLS J.G. (1963) *Family Psychiatry*. Charles C. Thomas, Illinois.

HOWELLS, J.G. (1966) Personal communication.

JOLLY H. (1966) Put the child to bed. *Lancet*, **2**, 541.

MCDONALD R. & MARSHALL S.R. (1964) The value of iron therapy in pica. *Pediatrics*, **34**, 558.

MICHELL E.P.G. (1966) Personal communication.

SENN M.J.E. (1962) School phobias: the role of the paediatrician in their prevention and management. *Proc. Roy. Soc. Med.*, **55**, 975.

WICKES, I.G. (1958) Treatment of persistent enuresis with the electric buzzer. *Arch. Dis. Childh.*, **33**, 160.

# CHAPTER 17

# SPEECH DISORDERS

There is considerable variation in the age at which normal children speak; possibly the most common reason for apparent delay is physiological late development of speech, the child speaking normally in the end. Some children, whose mothers are able to interpret their every grunt, are slow to talk because they have little incentive to do so. Others develop a grunt language as a negativistic reaction to parental concern that they should speak well. These soon learn to speak when they mix with other children to whom their noises are unintelligible. Mothers of such children should compromise between the extremes of interpreting every sound and insisting on words before they respond.

Mothers should be taught the importance of vocal play in the development of speech during the early years of life (p. 252). This play should not be interrupted but its value can be enhanced by repeating to the baby those sounds which have meaning. If this repetition is combined with pointing at the relevant object, the child is taught the meaning of words.

## AETIOLOGY

Much remains to be discovered of the cause of some speech disorders but a simple aetiological classification makes the problem more easily understood:

> Mental handicap
> Deafness
> Lack of learning opportunities
> Developmental aphasia, including developmental dyslexia
> Infantile autism
> Dysarthria
> Stuttering
> Lisping

**Mental handicap** (see chapter 15, p. 444)

Apart from physiological late development of speech this is the most common cause of delayed speech, but the evidence must be complete before accepting this diagnosis. Inevitably, children who cannot speak seem to be mentally handicapped but, if the diagnosis is wrong, incorrect treatment is given and the chances of normal speech development are lessened.

## Deafness

Normal speech depends on normal hearing. High-tone deafness is particularly liable to be overlooked as the cause of delayed speech since the child can obviously hear some sounds and so may mistakenly be thought to hear them all. Consonants are carried on the high frequencies and are more distinctive in character than vowels; they must be heard if words are to be intelligible. High-tone deafness may not delay the onset of speech very much, but will seriously impede its development; the disability may not be appreciated until the child enters school.

## Lack of learning opportunities

During the first crucial year of life, the child's ability to develop speech is dependent on the close instruction and encouragement that can adequately be given only by his mother. A child deprived of his mother at this stage receives fewer opportunities to learn than one with a normal mother–child relationship. In the most severe case, the maternally deprived child remains apathetic and silent.

Maternal deprivation can occur without physical separation from the mother. Many West Indian mothers fail to understand normal child development and the importance of play in order to learn, since they were not played with as children. A child who is left on his own shows little impairment of motor function but is retarded in language and in the personal and social areas of behaviour. It is the attainment of language which is particularly affected so that although the child can understand, he can only express himself poorly. Lack of cuddling and play causes a child to have a weak sense of his own identity.

Physical restriction in infancy reduces the amount of learning opportunities so that children who have to have their limbs restricted for therapeutic reasons must be given every opportunity to move about.

The acquisition of speech may also be delayed by over-anxious parents who, considering their child should be speaking more, repeatedly try to make him say words. By producing anxiety and self-consciousness in the child, this has the reverse of the desired effect. Very often there is a family history of speech problems. It is this which has made the father or mother to be particularly concerned about speech development. Such parents are helped by an understanding of the normal variation in the acquisition of all new skills.

## Developmental aphasia

This is a complex group of disorders which is not yet fully understood, nor is terminology uniform. The children are brought because they are late in talking but they are mentally normal. The lack of speech results from an inability to comprehend the spoken word (congenital auditory imperception or word deafness), or is associated with failure to understand the written word (developmental dyslexia or word blindness). It is sometimes ascribed to a lag in the maturation of the responsible brain centres, but some of the patients never acquire these skills. It is more probable that there is a defect in cerebral organization, as is believed to be present in some 'clumsy children' (p. 434). Such a defect could be due to minimal brain damage. The condition is commoner in males and may be familial.

The patients often develop emotional disorders as a result of their difficulties. Such emotional problems, being more easily diagnosed, are often regarded as the cause instead of the result of the speech difficulty.

### CONGENITAL AUDITORY IMPERCEPTION (WORD DEAFNESS)

In these children, not only is there a defect in the understanding of the spoken word, but also a failure of perception of the significance of other sounds in the early years. After a number of years without speech the children eventually develop a vocabulary of their own (idioglossia).

The condition is rare and diagnosis difficult, but modern audiological techniques will show that there is a response to sound. It must not be confused with high-tone deafness, for which a hearing-aid is indicated, since children with congenital auditory imperception are disturbed by the magnified sounds received through the aid.

### DEVELOPMENTAL DYSLEXIA (WORD BLINDNESS)

Not all patients with this condition have retarded speech development, though late speech and imperfect articulation are common concomitants. The significance of 'crossed laterality' in these children is uncertain. In the normal individual one cerebral hemisphere is dominant so that the eye and hand on one side, usually the right, dominate the other. In individuals with 'crossed laterality' the dominant eye is on the opposite side from the dominant hand. Such individuals show a confusion in differentiating their right from their left and may show mirror-writing (some of the characters are the mirror image of normal). Although many children with developmental dyslexia show crossed laterality and all have some confusion of right and left, its significance as an aetiological factor is now thought to have been exaggerated. It is more likely that the lack of strong laterality and the difficulties with reading and writing result from a similar, though as yet undetermined, disturbance of cerebral function. Such children often have difficulties with spatial orientation as well. Visual disorders must be excluded.

Dyslexia is unrelated to intellect or social class but the problem is more obvious in intelligent children. Moreover, parents in the higher social classes are likely to be more aware of the problem as well as knowing how to hunt out the relatively rare therapeutic resources.

A correct diagnosis of developmental dyslexia is needed since those affected can be helped by special training. The child should remain in his own class, provided he has a sympathetic teacher, but receive a number of additional, individual, remedial lessons each week from a specially trained teacher. It is important to emphasize to the dyslexic child, as to all children, that writing is their speech on paper and not a mass of symbols which they must decipher as though it were a code.

If left untreated, even those with normal speech will go through life oblivious of the meaning of the written word, with all the problems that such a disability brings. In view of the normal dominance of one cerebral hemisphere, it is wiser that the child who naturally writes with the left hand should not be forced to change to the right since this causes him considerable confusion.

### Infantile autism (see p. 453)

These children are psychotic, living in a world of their own and developing their own language. They fail to show a normal response to people or situations, giving a false impression of being mentally handicapped, deaf or dumb.

### Dysarthria

Cerebral palsy, by affecting the muscles involved in speech, causes dysarthria. In spastics the increased tone prevents normal muscle action and in athetoids the involuntary movements have a similar effect. Cleft palate causes a characteristic nasal voice from inability to close the oral cavity.

### Stuttering

Stuttering, the term now preferred to stammering, usually begins between the ages of 2 and 6 years. It is more common in boys than girls, although this difference is less marked in early childhood than in later life because the prognosis is better in girls. A family history of the condition is frequent, probably because such parents are particularly concerned that their child should speak perfectly and they correct him during the normal babbling stage of learning to speak. Associated emotional disturbances often occur. It is interesting that stuttering seldom occurs when singing.

It is often stated that affected children have a high intelligence. However, Andrews and Harris (1964) found the disorder to be commoner in those with low intelligence, although those who attended for treatment were of above average intelligence. They thought the probable explanation for this difference lay in the increased importance placed on the handicap among the intelligent, and the ready availability of treatment for them.

The disorder occurs in two stages. In the primary or clonic stage there is excessive repetition of syllables. This is nothing more than a persistence and exaggeration of the infant's normal babbling stage which occurs during the acquisition of speech. At this stage, the child is often unconscious of what he is doing. On no account should attention be drawn to the problem as it will probably correct itself. If an over-anxious parent makes the mistake of trying to correct the child's speech, he will become conscious of the problem and move into the more serious second stage.

In the secondary or tonic stage the child has become aware of what he is doing and, fearful of his mistakes, tries to correct them by voluntary effort. This results in tonic spasms of the muscles involved in speech, especially those of the lips, throat, larynx and diaphragm. Speech becomes entirely blocked and the child may perform accessory actions such as clenching the fists, closing the eyes, whistling and contortions.

*Treatment.* In the primary stage no attention should be paid to speech but emotional tensions should be relieved. Once the secondary stage has started, the help of a speech therapist is required without delay.

### Lisping

This is due to faulty action of the tongue. It may occur in children of normal intelligence who fail to give up the habits and speech appropriate to a baby. It may also occur with mechanical defects, such as a cleft palate.

## BIBLIOGRAPHY

ANDREWS G. & HARRIS M. (1964) The syndrome of stuttering. *Clinics in Developmental Medicine*, No. 17. Spastics Society/Heinemann Medical, London.
RENFREW C. & MURPHY K. Ed. (1964) The child who does not talk. *Clinics in Developmental Medicine*, No. 13. Spastics Society/Heinemann Medical, London.

# CHAPTER 18

# INFECTIOUS FEVERS

## PHYSIOLOGY OF IMMUNE RESPONSES

When an antigen enters the body two different immune responses may occur.

### 1. Humoral immunity

The antigen stimulates the formation of humoral antibody which circulates freely in the blood and tissue fluid. Antibodies combine specifically with the antigen which stimulated their production. The antibodies produced are the immunoglobulins of which there are a number of types (see below).

### 2. Cellular immunity

This is effected by specifically sensitized lymphocytes which carry the antibody on their surface—'cell-bound immunity'.

The small lymphocyte is fundamental to both forms. Two types of this cell exist:

*β lymphocytes*—so named because in birds these cells are dependent for their maturation on the Bursa of Fabricius. This is the hind-gut lymphoid organ which in mammals is equivalent to the lymphoid tissue associated with the gut, such as the tonsils, Peyer's patches and the appendix. These cells develop into plasma cells which synthesize circulating antibodies.

*T lymphocytes*—so named because they are dependent on the presence of a thymus gland for their maturation. These become transformed into lymphoblasts which are responsible for cell mediated immunity.

### The immunoglobulins

There are 5 major types: IgG, IgA, IgM, IgD and IgE, each with distinct physical properties.

IgG is the only one capable of crossing the placenta. At birth its level in the blood of a full-term baby is the same as that in the maternal serum. Consequently it provides a major defence against infection in the first few weeks of life. The level relates directly to gestational age so that a preterm baby is deficient of its full supply. IgG comprises 85–90 per cent of all immunoglobulins in the adult. It is distributed widely throughout the extra-cellular fluid as well as the blood.

Colostrum contains a higher level of IgA than maternal serum and it also provides some IgM but little IgG. Breast fed infants are therefore at an advantage compared with those fed on cow's milk.

The synthesis of antibodies belonging to the different classes proceeds at different rates. IgG and IgM can be formed by the fetus from the 20th week of gestation, but during a normal pregnancy small amounts only are synthesized. IgA and IgD synthesis starts immediately after birth. From then on the production of all types gradually increases, though the build-up of IgG is slow and does not reach adult levels till about 7 years of age.

The placenta is not a complete barrier against infection. Rubella, herpes simplex, toxoplasmosis, cytomegalovirus and syphilis are especially liable to cross. Fetal infection with these organisms can cause raised fetal IgM particularly, but also IgA. Increased cord levels of IgM may also follow maternal respiratory tract infections. Clearly, therefore, the fetal lymphoid system is not as immature as previously thought. The levels of immuno-globulins, other than transferred IgG reflect a lack of stimulus by appropriate antigens because the placenta has remained a barrier to these. Animals reared under sterile conditions from birth show a persistence of the immature lymphoid system.

### Primary immunodeficiency

Examples of a deficiency of each cell type have now been identified. Deficiency of $\beta$ lymphocytes causes hypogammaglobulinaemia (Bruton) (p. 614). Deficiency of T lymphocytes causes thymic hypoplasia (Di George). A severe combined deficiency is caused by failure of the stem cell (Swiss type).

## ACTIVE IMMUNIZATION

### General considerations

Active immunization can be induced by three methods using different agents:

1. An attenuated living organism, e.g. BCG vaccine.
2. A killed organism, e.g. pertussis vaccine, inactivated poliomyelitis vaccine.
3. A modified product of an organism, e.g. tetanus toxoid.

No standard immunization programme is suitable for all the children in one community and even less so for those in different countries, but the principles governing the choice of schemes remain the same. Three considerations are of particular importance:

1. The greatest protection possible should be provided against each disease.

2. The least possible number of injections should be given.

3. There should be the least possible risk of inducing reactions and complications, especially provocation poliomyelitis (see p. 411).

To some extent these considerations are incompatible. To give the greatest protection a start should be made early in life in order to cover early infections. But in the early months of life the mechanism for antibody formation is immature; it is probably not fully developed until 6 to 9 months of age. Moreover, it is inhibited by maternally transmitted antibodies which gradually disappear during the first 6 months of life. A disease like pertussis in which the fatalities largely occur in the first year, especially in the first 6 months, requires a very early start, whereas the risk of diphtheria and tetanus occurs later. Therefore, there are advantages in delaying the start of immunization against diphtheria and tetanus for the first few months in order to obtain the maximum response at the optimum time. Consequently, if maximum protection is to be achieved against pertussis the vaccine must be given separately, thus increasing the number of injections. Moreover, the risk of severe reactions to pertussis is greater at 3 months of age than in those over 6 months old.

The risk of provocation poliomyelitis is greatest with alum-precipitated toxoids, though these are antigenically superior, thereby producing a greater antibody response. Mixed antigens, even without alum, carry a greater risk than single antigens, pertussis being the most liable to produce this complication. However, the widespread use of poliomyelitis immunization has reduced this complication to a minimum, particularly since protection against poliomyelitis can be given at the same time as the potentially provoking agent (p. 486).

Early immunization programmes find the mother at her most receptive and the baby at his least antagonistic. On the other hand, if the baby thereby has to have a larger number of injections the mother may fail to attend. The resolution of all these different points of view is essentially a compromise and any immunization scheme will need to consider them in the light of local conditions, facilities for giving injections and funds available. A record card of all immunizations given should be kept by the parents.

**Pertussis**

Pertussis immunization is most conveniently combined with diphtheria and tetanus as a triple vaccine, given by deep subcutaneous or intramuscular injection. To achieve the maximum antibody response it is now recommended that the vaccine is given at the ages of 6, 8 and 12 months. The increasingly long intervals between the injections produces a better antibody response than the previous schedule which allowed one month only between each of the injections.

There is small risk of encephalopathy following pertussis vaccination. Fits due to the vaccine occur within 12 hours of its administration, those occurring later being 'febrile' (p. 413). The possibility that pertussis vaccine has been responsible for some cases of infantile spasms has been raised (Jeavons & Bower, 1964) but is not proven. In view of these possible cerebral complications, pertussis vaccine must not be given to infants with brain damage, those who have had neonatal hypoglycaemia or those who have had convulsions. Any reaction to the first or second triple injections, such as fever, or the child going off colour or prolonged screaming is a definite indication that pertussis vaccine must be omitted from subsequent inoculations; the immunization course is completed with diphtheria–tetanus vaccine. In view of the possible risks from pertussis immunization and the publicity these have received, some parents will wish their child to be given diphtheria and tetanus vaccine only. This is obviously preferable to a complete omission of this immunization as has sometimes occurred.

It has been usual to give a booster dose of the triple vaccine during the second year and again at school entry when the child is 5 years old. However, it is better to omit the pertussis component from these boosters in view of its possible risks and the fact that pertussis is less of a hazard in the older child.

The possibility that pertussis immunization is contraindicated in children with a history of infantile eczema or asthma has been raised (Butler & Benson, 1965). Experience has shown that eczema, even if active, is not a contraindication to pertussis immunization and that it is safe to give pertussis vaccine to an asthmatic child provided he is not wheezing at the time. A family history of allergy is not a contraindication to pertussis immunization.

### Diphtheria

Immunization against diphtheria is most conveniently given with tetanus and pertussis, unless pertussis vaccine has been given earlier. It is given at 6, 8 and 12 months of age with a booster on school entry at the age of 5 years.

The widespread use of diphtheria immunization has had dramatic results in Great Britain, deaths from diphtheria having almost vanished. Recently there has been anxiety that fewer mothers have sought protection for their children as they are no longer frightened of the disease. However, the situation has been saved by giving poliomyelitis immunization at the same time, since mothers are still extremely frightened of poliomyelitis and very anxious to seek this protection for their children.

## Tetanus

Parents are still insufficiently aware of the risk of tetanus. Tetanus toxoid is highly effective and its use should be universal. It can be given combined with diphtheria alone or in the triple vaccine. Quite apart from the protection given, tetanus immunization affords the advantage that prophylactic anti-tetanic serum (ATS) is unnecessary when the child receives a potentially infected injury. A booster dose of tetanus toxoid is given instead, thus avoiding the common serum reactions.

If the injured child has not previously been immunized he can be given ATS and active immunization started. The risk of sensitization from ATS has always to be considered. If the risk of tetanus is considered to be slight, a decision to give prophylactic penicillin only may be taken. Whenever it is available, antitetanus immunoglobulin should be given instead of ATS.

It used to be necessary to delay the start of active immunization until 6 weeks after giving ATS owing to interference with antibody formation; many patients failed to return for this. However, the new adsorbed tetanus toxoid can be given at the same time as ATS and, 6 weeks later, only one further dose is required. A reinforcing dose should be given 6–12 months after this primary course and again 5 years later. A problem arises as to how to be certain that an injured child has received tetanus immunization since the information is often not available at the time. A small tattoo mark produced by the intra-dermal injection of a dye and made on completion of immunization is probably the best answer.

In countries where there is a risk of neonatal tetanus, the disease can be prevented by full immunization of the mother during pregnancy. Babies born to mothers who have not been immunized, if seen in the first 10 days of life, should receive 1500 units of prophylactic ATS. In the same countries tetanus may occur in children as a complication of otitis media. In these areas it is wise for prophylactic ATS to be given to unprotected children with otitis media.

## Poliomyelitis

The live attenuated vaccine (Sabin) is preferable to the killed vaccine (Salk). It has many advantages: it is easier to administer, being given by mouth instead of intramuscularly; by inhibiting virus excretion in those who have been immunized it helps to eliminate wild poliovirus from the community.

This results from virus interference within the intestine and can be used during epidemics to limit the spread of wild virus.

Oral vaccine has a further advantage by causing secondary infection of others; such spread is not dangerous since virulence is not increased by this passage. In mass immunization campaigns, spread through the community increases the number immunized, although persistence of the virus in the community lasts only 2–3 months. Oral vaccine causes a more consistent and durable response than the intramuscular vaccine.

For the successful elimination of poliomyelitis an on-going programme is essential. All infants should be immunized during their first year, both for their own protection and because it is they who are largely responsible for transmitting the infection within the community. A trivalent oral preparation is used which can be given at the same time as triple immunization, both for the initial and the booster doses.

### Measles

Active immunization during the second year is now recommended for all children apart from the few contraindictions given below. An overall protection of at least 83·7 per cent has been recorded in one large sample (Warin *et al.*, 1972). A single dose of a freeze-dried preparation containing living attenuated measles virus is given subcutaneously or intramuscularly. In a substantial proportion of the children mild febrile reactions lasting 24–48 hours and transient rashes will occur. Children who develop these rashes are not infectious.

Febrile convulsions occasionally occur. The risk of convulsions after live vaccine is much less than with a natural attack of measles (M.R.C. Committee Report, 1966). This finding supports that of Gibbs & Rosenthal (1962) who found a very low incidence of electroencephalographic changes in children receiving live attenuated measles, compared with the high incidence in children with natural measles (see p. 493). It is therefore extremely unlikely that this vaccine will cause encephalitis.

It is wise not to vaccinate infants with a history of convulsions. Measles vaccination is also contraindicated if the child is receiving drugs, such as steroids or immuno-suppressive treatment, which would affect the antibody response. Children with leukaemia, Hodgkin's disease or hypogamma-globulinaemia should not be vaccinated. Pregnant women should not be vaccinated since, on theoretical grounds, there is a risk that the virus could damage the fetus as is known to occur with vaccinia (see below).

Passive immunization with gammaglobulin should be given to babies and debilitated children who have been in contact with measles. The dose given (see p. 494) is that which will produce an attenuated attack with consequent full immunity, rather than complete suppression and no lasting immunity.

## Rubella

In the United Kingdom vaccination against rubella is offered routinely to all girls between their 11th and 14th birthdays. Unlike the measles vaccination campaign, whose aim is the elimination of the disease, this campaign is solely to prevent the risk to the fetus from a woman catching rubella when pregnant. Because of diagnostic difficulties a previous history of rubella does not justify withholding the vaccine. The preparation is a live attenuated vaccine, one dose being given subcutaneously or intramuscularly. The same contraindications operate as for measles. The vaccine may cause mild fever and rashes. It sometimes also causes arthralgia in adult women.

## Smallpox

An artificially acquired attack of vaccinia by vaccination produces active immunity against variola. In view of the slight risk of post-vaccinial encephalitis, and the improved world control of smallpox, routine vaccination of babies is no longer recommended in the United Kingdom. Vaccination can safely be left until it is required for travel, since there is now no appreciably greater risk of complications in an adult as compared with a child. Moreover, it is likely that as world control improves, an increasing number of countries will be able to remove smallpox vaccination from being a condition of entry. In countries where smallpox is endemic, vaccination should be performed at 6 months. Vaccination is performed by the single linear scratch or the multiple pressure technique, using freshly prepared calf lymph or a freeze-dried preparation. No alcohol should be used in the preparation of the skin; ether or soap and water are suitable substitutes. No blood should be drawn during the process and the lymph must be allowed to dry before the clothes are replaced. A dressing should be applied when the vesicle appears.

If successful, a flush appears at the vaccination site on the third day. This becomes a papule on the fourth day and a vesicle on the fifth. Pustulation occurs from the eighth to tenth day and the regional lymph glands become enlarged. A scab forms which separates after 2–3 weeks, leaving a scar. A variable degree of disturbance, which is more severe in older patients, occurs during the vesicular and pustular stages. The production of a vesicle is required if protection is to be conferred but the size of the vesicle is unrelated to the degree of protection.

Re-vaccination should be carried out every 5 years. Two different reactions may result: the *accelerated reaction* occurs in those with partial immunity, the lesion going through the same stages as the primary reaction already described, but at a greater speed; there is very little constitutional disturbance. The *immediate reaction* consists of erythema and induration occurring within 8–72 hours. This is an allergic reaction and is no proof of immunity; vaccination should therefore be repeated.

### COMPLICATIONS OF VACCINATION

*Generalized vaccinia.* The primary site heals normally and, 6–14 days after vaccination, similar but more rapidly evolving lesions occur on the body, resulting from dissemination of the virus by the blood stream. The majority

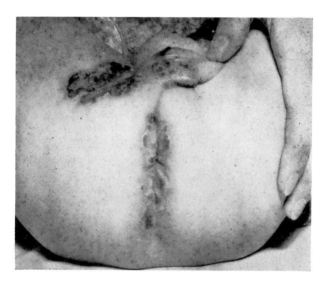

Fig. 118. Accidental vaccinia. The child was infected by sitting on the mother's recently vaccinated thigh. A typical umbilicated papule is visible in the upper part of the left-hand lesion.

of patients survive, but a few fatalities have been reported in association with hypogammaglobulinaemia when the lesions persist for many weeks. Anti-vaccinia immunoglobulin should be given to all cases. Methisazone which is active both prophylactically and therapeutically against viruses of the vaccinia–variola group should also be used.

*Eczema vaccinatum.* Patients with eczema are particularly susceptible to infection of the eczematous skin with vaccinia, either following primary vaccination of the patient or contamination from a recently vaccinated individual. This is an extremely serious condition, often being fatal. Treatment is the same as for generalized vaccinia.

*Accidental vaccinia.* Accidental inoculation of the virus and development of vaccinia may occur through an abrasion or septic lesion by direct contact with a recently vaccinated individual (Fig. 118).

*Progressive vaccinia.* In these patients the original vaccinial lesion continues to spread locally. There is no interval as in the phase of viraemia which occurs in generalized vaccinia.

*Post-vaccinial encephalitis.* The risk is slight and is less in young children than in older children or adults (see p. 407).

*Vaccinial osteomyelitis.* This arises insidiously and joint swelling or temporary weakness of the limb may be the only indication. It is believed to be due to the virus itself.

CONTRAINDICATIONS TO VACCINATION

1. Infantile eczema is an absolute contraindication in view of the risk of eczema vaccinatum. Moreover, any child with eczema must be rigidly isolated from any recently vaccinated person for at least 3 weeks. For this reason, before an individual is vaccinated, specific enquiry should be made whether anyone in the house has eczema.

2. Children with any skin complaint, particularly septic lesions, burns and severe napkin rashes.

3. Children recently exposed to any infectious fever and those who are not thriving.

4. Children on steroid therapy.

5. Hypogammaglobulinaemia.

6. Pregnant women. Vaccination of the mother has been followed by fetal vaccinia. The risk is greatest in the early weeks of pregnancy but has been reported as late as the sixth month (Green *et al.*, 1966). Vaccination during the first 3 months has been associated with an increased abortion rate.

If for some clear reason vaccination has to be given to those with contraindications, it should be accompanied by the simultaneous administration of antivaccinia immunoglobulin and methisazone.

## Tuberculosis

BCG vaccination is discussed on p. 528.

## Mumps

This vaccine is widely used in the United States although it is not routinely given in the United Kingdom. A single subcutaneous injection of a live attenuated virus can be given at any time after the first year of life. It is particularly useful for children approaching puberty who have not yet had the infection since it will reduce the loss of time caused by the disease and the possible discomfort from the complication of orchitis.

## PASSIVE IMMUNIZATION

Whereas active immunization produces an immunity after a few days which may be lifelong, passive immunization provides protection within a few minutes but only lasts only a few weeks.

Only human gammaglobulin is used, this having a half-life of 2–3 weeks. Two preparations are available:

1. Normal gammaglobulin prepared from pools of human plasma and used against measles, rubella and infective hepatitis.

2. Immunoglobulin prepared against a specific agent from the plasma of convalescent or hyperimmunized individuals, for example, antivaccinia immunoglobulin.

## VIRUS INFECTIONS

### Rubella (German measles)

This mild illness is caused by a virus which has been isolated from the mouth one week before the rash, persisting there for up to 3 weeks after the onset of the rash. Epidemics may occur, especially during the spring, but the disease, which is spread by droplet infection, is not as infectious as measles or chickenpox. It attacks older children and adolescents rather than young children and, although one attack usually confers lasting immunity, second attacks may occur since the immunity is less solid than with measles.

The incubation period is 14–21 days. The prodromal symptoms of generalized aches and pains and mild catarrhal symptoms may be so slight that the rash, which usually appears within the first 24 hours, becomes the first sign. The rash lasts only for 1–2 days, starts behind the ears and on the forehead, spreading to the face, trunk and limbs. It consists of discrete pink macules which are most profuse on the trunk where they may become confluent. Fever is mild or absent. The characteristic feature of the disease is the discrete enlargement of the occipital glands, which may be tender. These appear shortly before the rash, often remaining enlarged for many weeks after the illness is over.

The blood picture is characteristic: there is an initial neutropenia and lymphopenia with an almost regular occurrence of Türk and plasma cells which persist to the tenth day.

Complications are rare but thrombocytopenic purpura may occur. This is possibly not as infrequent as is supposed since it has been found that asymptomatic thrombocytopenia and increased capillary fragility are not rare, bearing no relationship to the severity of the rubella.

Encephalitis is an extremely rare complication, and although complete recovery is usual, the condition may prove fatal (see p. 406).

*Treatment.* No specific treatment is required. The patients recover within 3–4 days but should be isolated for a week from the appearance of the rash.

## CONGENITAL RUBELLA

The most sinister effect of rubella is on the fetus of a mother infected with the disease (see p. 140). If the virus strikes the fetus before organ differentiation is complete, damage occurs particularly to the eye, ear, heart and brain. The commonest lesions are retinopathy, cataract, nerve deafness and congenital heart disorders, especially patent ductus arteriosus; mental defect may occur. The retinopathy consists of patchy black pigmentation. This does not affect vision but it is probably the commonest ocular manifestation of congenital rubella, occurring in about half the cases. It is therefore very useful diagnostically. The cornea may be cloudy and the eye itself small.

More widespread defects have also been found, indicating a continuous systemic infection of the fetus with the rubella virus (Korones *et al.*, 1965; Lindquist *et al.*, 1965; Plotkin *et al.*, 1965). Many of these children are retarded in growth at birth. This cannot be explained by a severe congenital heart lesion and is believed to be due both to placental insufficiency resulting from its infection with the virus and to the generalized viral invasion of the baby. Widespread purpura associated with thrombocytopenia occurs, being a grave symptom with a high mortality. Hepatomegaly may be present, as well as unusual changes in the long bones; these comprise small radiolucent areas in the metaphysis.

Prenatal rubella infection causes a rise of IgM in the baby. The diagnosis of congenital rubella is confirmed by finding rubella specific IgM in the infant's blood during the first 3 months of life. This immunoglobulin cannot cross the placenta, therefore its presence in the blood of a newborn baby can only be due to intrauterine infection. The mother's blood should also be tested since if she had no rubella antibody it would be unlikely that her child had congenital rubella.

Affected infants are often found to be excreting virus at birth and may continue to do so for some months, especially those most severely affected. Virus has persisted in a lens for 3 years (Menser *et al.*, 1967). Consequently, precautions must be taken to prevent spread of infection from such infants. To explain the anomaly of persistent virus in the presence of antibody it is postulated that the antibody limits the spread of virus through the extracellular fluids but is unable to influence its presence within cells.

**Measles (morbilli)**

This is a highly infective condition caused by a virus and is much more serious than rubella. In poor communities it is an important cause of death. The disease is spread by droplet infection, mainly affecting children between the ages of 1 and 6 years. Such fatalities as occur are usually in those aged less than 3 years. The disease is endemic throughout the world. In the United Kingdom, prior to the introduction of immunization, epidemics occurred every second year since the attack rate was so high that a large proportion of the susceptible population was affected. Consequently, a new generation of the susceptible toddler age group had to appear for the disease to flourish in epidemic proportions again, this taking 2 years. Patients develop a solid immunity so that second attacks are exceptional. Mothers who have had an attack confer passive immunity on their babies. This prevents the disease for the first 3 months of life and causes any attack in the next 6 months to be mild from the attenuating effect of this passive immunity.

The incubation period is 10–15 days, the prodromal symptoms consisting of fever up to 39·5° C (103° F), anorexia, lethargy, vomiting, nasal discharge and rashes. Prodromal rashes are scarlatiniform or morbilliform and are characteristically fleeting. The prodromal illness usually lasts 1–2 days only but sometimes continues as a mild illness throughout the incubation period. In some patients there is a distinct 'illness of infection' in which the symptoms are the same as in the prodromal illness but the temperature falls, the child returning to normal for an interval of 2–3 days before the main illness. It is suggested that an initial viraemia accounts for the first rise in temperature, the virus then settling in the reticulo-endothelial system and multiplying before producing the second viraemia responsible for the main illness.

The first evidence of the main illness is the catarrhal stage with runny nose and conjunctivitis. The injected eyes, barking cough and miserable appearance of the child are very characteristic at this stage and the diagnosis can be confirmed before the eruption of the main rash by finding Koplik's spots. These appear on the anterior portion of the buccal mucous membrane, looking like minute grains of salt on a red base; they are much more easily seen in daylight than artificial light. They are sometimes confused with milk flakes or thrush, but these are huge in comparison and are haphazardly arranged, in comparison with the regular distribution of Koplik's spots. The tonsils are inflamed and the tongue is furred.

Although the rash usually appears on the third to fifth day it is often later than this and may even be delayed until the sixteenth day. It starts behind the ears, spreads to the face, chest and abdomen and finally to the extremities. The individual lesions are macules or maculo-papules which are dark red (in contrast to the pink colour of rubella) and soon become confluent to form irregular blotches. When this occurs the child begins to feel better. As they fade they leave a light-brown pigmentation ('measles-staining') and a branny desquamation, both of which are valuable in retrospective diagnosis. In coloured children the colour of the rash is not apparent but the skin looks granular in the early stages. This is best seen over the front of the shoulders when viewed from above and behind; in the later stages the typical desquamation is very helpful. If the child is first seen after the Koplik's spots have faded, the appearance of the buccal mucous membrane is still of value since it is never normal, being usually red and granular.

Leucopenia is present from the onset of fever but is replaced by leucocytosis if bacterial complications occur.

*Diagnosis.* The main difficulty is to differentiate measles from rubella, but the premonitory symptoms are much more severe in measles. Red eyes are characteristic and Koplik's spots diagnostic. The rash of measles is much more profuse, a darker colour and becomes more confluent, whereas the enlarged occipital glands of rubella are very characteristic. The widespread desquamation which follows the rash of measles is very different from the slight desquamation which may follow rubella and does not affect the palms or soles.

*Complications.* Measles involves the respiratory tract in all cases so that secondary bacterial respiratory infections are common; pneumonia accounts for almost all the deaths, which may be as high as 5 per cent in developing countries. In these countries, measles may be the forerunner of kwashiorkor due to the lowered plasma albumin which occurs in measles (Poskitt, 1971). Loss of protein in the stools from diarrhoea is a factor. Diarrhoea is such a common symptom in severe measles that gastroenteritis can hardly be called a complication, but it is an additional factor causing death. Diarrhoea occurs particularly during the stage of skin desquamation when comparable changes are involving the intestinal epithelium. These debilitated children are liable to develop tuberculosis and some may acquire cancrum oris from mouth sepsis and poor oral hygiene.

Otitis media is a common complication though it is interesting that this was not the case in a study of Nigerian children (Cobban, 1963). This could be because such children, even though ill, still spent much of the time upright on their mothers' backs. If treatment is inadequate and hygiene poor, severe conjunctivitis may lead to corneal ulceration and panophthalmitis; measles is an important cause of blindness in developing countries.

A demyelinating encephalitis (p. 405) is the outstanding complication and, in countries where medical facilities are good and the risks of bronchopneumonia less, this is the most serious complication. The incidence has been assessed at one in 1000–1500 cases, but the frequency of electroencephalographic changes (Gibbs & Rosenthal, 1962; Pampiglione, 1964) suggests that subclinical encephalitis is common. Of all the infectious fevers of childhood, measles is by far the most likely to be followed by encephalitis. The symptoms usually develop when the rash is beginning to fade and the onset is either abrupt with convulsions followed by coma, or more gradual with headache, vomiting and irritability followed after a few hours by stupor. Paralysis, involuntary movements and retention of urine may occur. The cerebrospinal fluid may show a rise of lymphocytes up to 300 per mm$^3$ and increased protein. Relapses do not occur but the incidence of long-lasting or permanent sequelae is high. The special sequelae are deterioration of emotional and intellectual ability; residual paralysis is less common. A tendency to convulsions may persist and it is possible that some cases of so-called 'idiopathic epilepsy' have resulted from unsuspected measles encephalitis. Convulsions may occur at the onset of measles in association with a high fever, but these are not due to encephalitis, this occurring later in the course of the illness. Steroid therapy has been used in the treatment of encephalitis but the results are not encouraging and it may make the condition worse.

Thrombocytopenic purpura may follow measles, just as it follows rubella. It is due to increased capillary fragility as well as to a low platelet count. It is probable that these changes occur more often than is realized without causing purpura.

A serious long-term problem is the development of bronchiectasis from pulmonary collapse as a result of blockage of the small bronchi with mucus. Steps must be taken to ensure that the lungs are fully expanded before the child leaves medical care.

*Treatment.* The dangers of respiratory complications are so great that immediate antibiotic therapy must be given for any secondary bacterial infection. However, there is no evidence that routine prophylactic antibiotics are of value. Close attention must be paid to the eyes, which should be bathed or irrigated with saline. Chloramphenicol eye ointment should be used if there is any indication of secondary infection. Patients should be isolated for 10 days from the appearance of the rash.

ATTENUATED MEASLES

Measles can be attenuated or suppressed in contacts by the administration of gammaglobulin, this being used to protect babies and debilitated children (see p. 486). An attenuated attack has the advantage that it confers the same lasting immunity as a natural attack. To suppress the attack 250 mg gammaglobulin is given during the first year and 500 mg for infants aged 1–3 years. Half these doses are used if attenuation rather than suppression is desired.

The incubation period of attenuated measles is somewhat longer than that of natural measles. The clinical features are similar but very mild, the rash resembling rubella. Koplik's spots are inconstant and complications do not occur. It should be remembered that these patients are just as infectious as those with natural measles.

SUBACUTE SCLEROSING PANENCEPHALITIS (SUBACUTE INCLUSION BODY ENCEPHALITIS: SUBACUTE SCLEROSING LEUCO-ENCEPHALITIS)

This rare form of encephalitis is now believed to be caused by the measles virus. Measles antibody levels are invariably high and the virus has been isolated from brain tissue. The disease does not occur at the same time as the attack of measles but averages $6\frac{1}{2}$ years after the original infection (Dick, 1973). The commonest age for the condition is therefore 6–12 years.

The disorder affects both the grey and white matter. The onset is insidious with intellectual deterioration and personality changes as the usual first signs. These progress to profound dementia. Characteristic sudden movements of the arms occur, these being raised to shoulder level where they remain 'hung up' for a few seconds.

The CSF usually shows a Lange curve of paretic type. The EEG is diagnostic, comprising runs of slow, high-voltage complexes which commonly correspond in time with the involuntary arm movements.

The disease is universally fatal, often within one year of the onset. Symptomatic treatment only is available.

### Roseola infantum (exanthema subitum, sixth disease)

This condition is practically confined to the first 3 years of life. There is an abrupt fever, lasting 3–4 days, without a preceding prodromal illness. The characteristic feature is the appearance of the rash when the temperature has fallen to normal. The rash is composed of small pink macules resembling rubella rather than measles. Leucopenia with relative lymphocytosis is usual after the first day.

Infectivity is slight, though occasional isolated outbreaks have been reported. There are no complications apart from the risk of convulsions in association with the fever. No specific treatment is required. It is probable that the condition occurs more often than diagnosed owing to its mild nature.

### Mumps (epidemic parotitis)

This virus is now regarded as a generalized infection with a predilection for the salivary glands but also a tendency to involve other glands, especially the testicles, and the nervous system. Previously, it was considered an epidemic disease of the salivary glands which occasionally also affected the gonads. In children, the disease is most common from the age of 5 years upwards; it is rare in infancy. There is no difference in sex incidence but, since the risk of orchitis is much greater than the risk of oophoritis, it must be regarded as a more serious disease in males.

The disease is transmitted by droplet infection but it is not highly infectious. It is common for it to occur for the first time in adults who have been repeatedly exposed to it as children. The incubation period may range from 12–28 days but in most cases is 17–18 days. A short prodomal period of 1–2 days of fever and malaise may occur, though more often a swollen tender parotid gland is the first manifestation. Usually one gland is affected before the other and sometimes the disease remains confined to one side. The other salivary glands may also be involved. The ability to open the mouth is limited by the swollen glands and biting may be very painful. The openings of Stensen's ducts are often red.

### ADDITIONAL MANIFESTATIONS

*Orchitis.* This is usually unilateral and occurs at or after puberty. It most often occurs about a week after the onset of the parotid swelling, there being a return of fever. The testicle is enlarged, tender and firm; atrophy may follow though sterility is uncommon. Mumps orchitis may occur without preceding parotid involvement.

*Meningo-encephalitis.* This complication probably occurs more often than is realized. It usually develops about 10 days after the onset of symptoms, but it is now realized that it may occur as an isolated manifestation of the disease. The condition is most often a true meningitis rather than encephalitis (p. 406). The onset is sudden with signs of meningeal irritation. Paralysis is uncommon though modern methods of investigation show that some cases, which on clinical grounds resemble paralytic poliomyelitis, have had a recent infection with the virus of mumps. The cerebrospinal fluid shows a lymphocytic pleocytosis with a slight rise in protein. Complete recovery is the rule.

*Pancreatitis.* This is a less common complication which causes persistent vomiting and central abdominal pain for a few days. It is followed very rarely by diabetes mellitus.

*Oophoritis.* This may occur after puberty but is much less common than orchitis.

*Nerve deafness.* This is a common sequel, being due probably to labyrinthitis occurring as an extension of the infection from the meninges via the eighth nerve. The deafness is usually total, though fortunately it is unilateral in about three-quarters of the cases. It usually develops during the first 2 weeks of the illness and, although it may be associated with mumps meningitis, it may occur as an isolated neurological incident.

The blood picture usually shows leucopenia with relative lymphocytosis. A complement fixation test has been developed which gives evidence of recent mumps infection. A high serum amylase level has been reported in cases of recent infection. The importance of these tests lies in the diagnosis of meningo-encephalitis and orchitis unaccompanied by parotitis.

DIAGNOSIS

Swelling of the lymphatic glands in the region of the angle of the jaw is sometimes mistaken for mumps, but the parotid swelling also extends over the ramus of the mandible. The only real difficulty is in cases of recurrent parotitis (see p. 297) where the infection is bacterial and often associated with sialectasis. Such cases are always regarded as mumps on the first occasion but the same mistake should not be made the second time.

TREATMENT

Pain should be relieved by analgesics, warm cotton wool also giving considerable relief. Food must be of a fluid nature until the mouth can be opened properly. During this phase special attention must be paid to oral hygiene; food particles may remain in the mouth and lack of saliva causes drying of the buccal mucous membrane. The patient should be isolated for 7 days from the disappearance of the swelling.

## Varicella (chickenpox)

This is a highly infectious virus disease which causes a very mild illness. The majority of patients are under 10 years and, although it occurs throughout the year, there is a peak of incidence in the autumn and winter. The incubation period is 11–21 days, the usual being 14–15 days. The disease is spread by droplet infection since it is primarily an infection of the upper respiratory tract. Patients are infectious from 24 hours before the eruption until 7 days afterwards; the scabs are not infectious since, unlike smallpox, they do not contain the virus.

Chickenpox and herpes zoster are caused by the same virus, the varicella-zoster (V-Z) virus which is a member of the herpes group. Chickenpox results from the individual's first exposure to the virus while zoster is due to reactivation of a latent virus, there now being an additional sensitization element.

The prodromal illness of malaise and slight fever for a day is often so slight that the rash is usually the first sign of the disease. The lesions, which appear in crops, start as dark pink macules which become papular and, in a few hours, are transformed into vesicles. These look like drops of water on a slightly red base and are characteristically elliptical. They are extremely fragile and easily broken by the clothes so that not many will be seen at any one time, especially as they appear in crops. They are converted to pustules which become crusted, then drying to form scabs. These drop off about 10 days after the onset, leaving shallow pink scars which in time become white.

The earliest lesions appear in the mouth and scalp, spreading to the trunk and finally to the extremities. The distribution is centripetal so that the majority of lesions are on the trunk with the back affected most, the minority being on the face and extremities. The lesions on the limbs are more profuse near the trunk, the hands and feet being least affected. It is characteristic that unexposed sites such as the axillae are particularly involved.

Cropping causes lesions in all stages of development to be visible at any one time after the first few days. Those in the papular and pustular stage cause intense irritation, scratching increasing the amount of secondary infection.

VARICELLA HAEMORRHAGICA

Very occasionally the lesions become haemorrhagic; bleeding occurs into the vesicles and into the unaffected portions of the skin as purpura, and also from the mucous membranes. Steroid therapy has increased the importance of this rare form, since varicella in patients receiving steroids is more likely to be severe and may take this serious and usually fatal form.

COMPLICATIONS

Encephalitis is a rare complication occurring between the fourth and tenth day after the appearance of the rash. Cerebellar involvement with ataxia and nystagmus usually predominates; the majority recover completely (see p. 406).

DIAGNOSIS

*Variola (smallpox)*. Successful vaccination within the last 7 years excludes variola. In variola there is a prodromal illness of 2–4 days which is severe. The lesions do not crop so that all will be found at the same stage; their evolution takes much longer than in varicella. The vesicles are circular rather than elliptical. The distribution is centrifugal so that the periphery of the body is most affected.

*Papular urticaria (lichen urticatus)*. This is often difficult, but the lesions are distributed in a haphazard manner; they have a larger area of erythema, whereas the papule, surmounted by its tiny vesicle, is small. Lesions do not occur in the mouth or on the head and there have usually been many previous attacks.

*Scabies*. The secondarily infected vesicles may be confused with varicella but the distribution differs. Lesions may be profuse on the fingers and fronts of wrists but do not occur on the face or in the mouth. Typical burrows may be visible.

## TREATMENT

No specific treatment is available and most patients do not feel ill enough to go to bed. Children should not return to school for 14 days from the appearance of the rash. Steps should be taken to reduce secondary infection by relieving the irritation, which may be intense. Potassium permanganate baths give considerable relief, helping to dry the lesions, though the mother must be warned that this will temporarily stain the skin brown. A collodion spray may be useful in forming a seal and reducing infection. Oral antibiotics should be given if there is much secondary infection.

In view of the risk of severe varicella in those on steroid therapy, such contacts should be given hyperimmune varicella gammaglobulin.

## Variola (smallpox)

This occurs throughout the world, its age incidence being determined by the vaccination state of the community. The disease is the most infectious of all the specific fevers, being spread by droplet infection from the upper respiratory tract and by the virus contained in the scabs. These remain infectious until they disappear.

The disease exists in a number of forms:

### VARIOLA MAJOR

This is the classical severe form of the disease. The usual incubation period is 12 days to the onset of symptoms, or 14 days to the onset of the rash which can be more accurately determined. The prodromal symptoms are very severe. The onset of fever is acute, is associated with headache and a characteristically severe backache. There may be intense prostration and a purpuric or petechial rash may be visible in the flexures, especially the groins. These symptoms last for 2 days, the typical rash then developing. The earliest lesions are macular, occurring in the mouth and on the face. The spread is then to the arms and trunk so that the legs are the last part to be affected. The macules change to papules; these are in the skin rather than on it so that they feel spotty. By the fourth day of the rash, the papules change to grey vesicles with an umbilicated surface. These gradually become pustular, a change which is associated with a secondary rise in temperature. The pustules dry up to form a scab which falls off about the fourteenth day, leaving a pitted scar.

The rash is symmetrical, has a centrifugal distribution and affects particularly those areas which are exposed to friction and the air. Thus it is most severe on the face and hands and on the upper part of the back, whereas the flanks, abdomen and axillae, being less subject to friction, are less severely affected. Because some days may elapse between the appearance of the rash on the face and that on the legs, the maturity of the lesions will vary, but within any one region all the lesions will be similar.

VARIOLA MINOR (ALASTRIM)

This is the mild form of the disease due to a less virulent strain; the patient is usually unvaccinated. The incubation period is longer than in variola major and may be as long as 17 days. The prodromal period is usually mild; the lesions appear more slowly but pass through the different stages more rapidly. The most important point is that despite these differences, which may cause the individual lesions to be similar to varicella, the distribution is the same as variola major.

VARIOLOID (MODIFIED VARIOLA)

The modified form of the disease resulting from partial immunity in a vaccinated individual whose immunity has lapsed, usually due to time. Consequently, the picture may be variable but the distribution of the lesions remains constant. The disease may be indistinguishable from variola minor.

*Complications.* In severe cases a *haemorrhagic form* may occur in which bleeding occurs into the rash and elsewhere into the skin, as well as from the mucous membranes. *Encephalomyelitis* is a rare complication.

*Osteomyelitis variolosa* is an unusual complication. It develops insidiously, producing joint swellings which are often bilateral and symmetrical, appearing about 1-4 weeks from the onset of the illness. The elbow is especially liable to be involved (Cockshott & MacGregor, 1959).

*Diagnosis.* The great problem is to differentiate the condition from varicella. In variola minor and varioloid this may be very difficult since the patient may not be severely ill. The essential difference lies in the distribution rather than in the character of individual lesions. Cropping in varicella causes lesions of different maturity to be seen within the same region. Varicella lesions are elliptical and superficial, whereas variola lesions are in the skin and are umbilicated, though umbilication is not constant. Successful vaccination within the last 3 years almost certainly excludes variola.

*Treatment.* Methisazone, though more effective prophylactically against smallpox, has a therapeutic action and should be given, as should anti-vaccinia immunoglobulin. Antibiotics will be needed for the pustular stage and the highest possible standard of nursing skill is required.

**Glandular fever (infectious mononucleosis)**

This disease is due to the Epstein-Barr virus (EBV), a member of the herpes group. The incubation period is unknown but is probably 30–50 days. Infection causes a rise of EBV antibody and a high state of immunity. The pattern of distribution of EBV is similar to poliomyelitis, there being passive transfer from mother to fetus followed by a high incidence of the disease in those living in poor socio-economic circumstances. In most cases in children the infection is mild, unlike the disease in young adults. This clinical difference may relate to the mode of transfer. The cases in children probably result from transfer of small amounts of virus via the fingers. The infection in young adults probably results from the transfer of large quantities of infected saliva, especially during a heavy petting session.

Mild cases may be overlooked but in the more severe the onset is usually acute, with malaise, fever and sore throat. Severe tonsillitis occurs, being associated with a white exudate and often ulceration. The cervical glands are much enlarged and other glands are affected, though less than those in the neck. The spleen is palpable in about half the cases. A petechial eruption, lasting about 3 days, may appear at the junction of the soft and hard palate from the third to seventh day of the illness. This is not diagnostic for glandular fever and may be seen in other acute infections. It must also be differentiated from the traumatic petechiae which can be produced by a spatula.

Hepatic involvement shown by hepatomegaly and jaundice is not uncommon; liver-function tests suggest that the liver is affected in the majority of patients, although only a proportion have detectable jaundice. The central nervous system is less often involved but encephalitis may occur, causing headache, neck stiffness and sometimes convulsions (see p. 404). The cerebrospinal fluid may be normal or show a rise in protein and mononuclear cells. Skin rashes are common, especially in those given ampicillin. In fact, this frequent association is regarded as an indication of the diagnosis. The rashes are very variable but the macular, papular and morbilliform varieties are the most common, the trunk being mainly affected. Haemorrhagic manifestations sometimes occur; nephritis is an occasional complication and its prognosis is good.

*Investigations.* The diagnosis should be made only if one of two tests is positive: the presence of atypical mononuclear cells in the peripheral blood; or the Paul–Bunnell test. A raised titre to EB virus confirms the diagnosis. The abnormal cells, which vary in size and shape, are thought now to be derived from the lymphoid series. The cytoplasm is bluish grey and may contain azure granules; the nucleus is oval or horse-shoe shaped and its chromatin may be arranged in coarse clumps. These cells are not specific for glandular fever and may be seen in other virus infections such as rubella, measles, infective hepatitis and virus pneumonia. But they are more common in glandular fever and may comprise 60–70 per cent of the total leucocytes.

Polymorphonuclear leucocytosis is common at the onset of the infection. Thrombocytopenia occasionally occurs and may be sufficient to cause purpura.

The Paul–Bunnell test is a heterophile antibody reaction using sheep's red cells. A titre of one in sixty-four or over is positive, being usually reached during the first week. This antibody is not the same as the EBV antibody. It is a transient phenomenon of unknown cause which lasts for about 3 months whereas the rise in EBV antibody persists for years.

*Diagnosis.* The common error which causes the disease to be over-diagnosed is to regard non-specific cervical lymphadenopathy as glandular fever, but the severe tonsillitis and the large size of the glands in glandular fever should make it possible for a correct clinical diagnosis to be made in most cases. Splenomegaly is of no assistance in diagnosis since the spleen enlarges easily in any infection in childhood. Acquired toxoplasmosis causes a similar glandular disorder but the Paul–Bunnell test is always negative.

*Course and treatment.* No specific treatment is available but antibiotic therapy is indicated for the severe tonsillitis. Steroid therapy should be reserved for children with thrombocytopenia. Recovery is often slow (the child and particularly a young adult remaining tired for weeks) but complete.

### Influenza

Apart from epidemics, when the condition is in no doubt, this is an unsatisfactory diagnosis since it is so easily made and so difficult to prove. A number of different viruses are responsible. At present the diagnosis must be largely retrospective and based on a rising antibody titre to a specific virus. Secondary bacterial infection accounts for much of the clinical picture.

Children are less severely affected than adults and present with coryza, fever, malaise and generalized or abdominal pains. There may be severe prostration. Respiratory or gastrointestinal symptoms may predominate, the clinical picture tending to remain constant in any one epidemic. Epistaxis is common and there is infection of the throat and conjunctivae. Complications may affect the upper or lower respiratory tract, bronchopneumonia, with blood-stained sputum, occurring in the most virulent varieties.

*Treatment.* There is no specific therapy but intensive treatment with wide spectrum antibiotics should be given for the secondary infection.

## BACTERIAL INFECTIONS

### Scarlet fever

This infection, comprising pharyngitis and a rash, is due to the haemolytic streptococcus. The rash results from an erythrogenic toxin possessed by some strains of the streptococcus which are otherwise the same as nonerythrogenic strains. Consequently, from the practical point of view, scarlet fever and streptococcal sore throat do not differ, the course of the disease and the complications being the same in both.

The incubation period is 2–5 days, the onset being abrupt with fever and loss of appetite. Vomiting is common and the young child is more likely to complain of abdominal pain than a sore throat since, for some unexplained reason, children are much less sensitive than adults to pain in the throat. The abdominal pain probably results from associated mesenteric adenitis. A white exudate is present on the inflamed tonsils; the faucial pillars and uvula are red and swollen, producing an arch of erythema around the fauces. Petechial haemorrhages may be visible on the palate. The tongue is furred at the onset, the fur then peeling off to leave it clean and red with prominent papillae ('strawberry' tongue). Considerable enlargement of the anterior cervical glands occurs.

The rash usually appears on the second day and is a punctate erythema, that is, an underlying flush on which minute intensely red spots are super-imposed. The rash is due to hyperaemia and fades on pressure. There is no punctate erythema on the face but it is uniformly flushed, except in the circumoral region where pallor is striking. The rash first appears as a facial flush, then punctate erythema develops on the neck, chest and abdomen and finally on the extremities. It is most marked in the flexures and punctate haemorrhages may be present in the elbow flexures (Pastia's sign). At the end of the first week the skin desquamates to form flakes which have a character-istic pin-hole from denudation of epithelium at the site of the intense red spot. The hands and feet are the last to desquamate and in these areas it may be severe. The desquamated epithelium contains no organisms and is not infectious.

The blood count shows a polymorphonuclear leucocytosis. Haemolytic streptococci are grown from the throat and there is a rise in the anti-streptolysin O titre.

*Complications.* Otitis media is very common and cervical adenitis may lead to suppuration. Septicaemia can occur and lead to distant complications, such as osteomyelitis, meningitis, peritonitis or suppurative pericarditis. Rheumatic fever or acute nephritis may develop some 2 weeks after the onset, being due to hypersensitivity to the haemolytic streptococcus. Thrombocyto-penic purpura may occur, being possibly due to hypersensitivity also.

*Diagnosis.* The appearance of the throat must be differentiated from diphtheria; this is discussed on p. 504.

*Treatment.* All patients should be treated with penicillin or sulphonamides and, if the child is vomiting, intramuscular penicillin is the drug of choice. They should be isolated for 7 days and, if possible, a throat swab should be examined at the end of treatment to ensure that the haemolytic streptococcus has been eradicated since some patients become carriers.

## Diphtheria

This is due to infection by a virulent strain of *Corynebacterium diphtheriae*, a Gram-positive pleomorphic rod, which produces its effects from its toxin. The disease is transmitted by droplet infection, affecting patients of any age but especially during the first 10 years of life. It is now rare in Great Britain as a result of the routine immunization of infants.

The incubation period is 2–5 days, the clinical features depending on the site and extent of the characteristic membrane. This membrane is produced by the bacilli and consists of fibrin, necrotic epithelial cells, leucocytes, granular debris and organisms. When seen in the throat it is dirty grey and present over a part or the whole of the tonsils. It may spread over the faucial pillars and on to the palate. The membrane is adherent, though if forcibly removed bleeding occurs. If it is confined to the throat the only local symptom is a sore throat. In nasal diphtheria the membrane is confined to the nose and a serosanguinous discharge results, excoriating the upper lip. Laryngeal diphtheria is the most serious form, since the membrane causes laryngeal obstruction; diagnosis is more difficult as it cannot be seen without laryngoscopy. Less commonly, diphtheria may involve the skin, conjunctiva or female genital tract. This is particularly seen in hot climates where secondary diphtheritic infection of tropical sores occurs.

Fetor is characteristic of diphtheria; cervical adenitis and periadenitis are often so great as to produce serious brawny oedema of the neck. Fever is not prominent, in contradistinction to infection with the haemolytic streptococcus. The most obvious feature is toxaemia, the severity of which depends on the extent of the membrane. The child looks ill and pale, the pallor being severe if cardiac failure is imminent. The pulse is rapid and soft, the extremities cold and the blood pressure low. Respiratory obstruction will be added to this picture if a laryngeal membrane is present.

The white cell count is normal or slightly raised and proteinuria is common. Diphtheria bacilli are found in swabs from the membrane; they grow on Loeffler's membrane but treatment is dependent on a clinical diagnosis and must not wait for laboratory confirmation.

### COMPLICATIONS

*Myocarditis.* This is due to the direct action of the toxin and may occur during the first week. Early circulatory failure is probably due to the action of the toxin on all the organs so that changes in the electrocardiogram are slight or absent. In the second week the action of the toxin on the heart alone may be more obvious, the electrocardiogram showing changes from myocarditis and conduction defects. Restlessness and vomiting at this stage are serious and may indicate cardiac failure. Death from this cause may occur during the second or third week but, if the child survives, the heart returns to normal.

*Neuritis.* Nerve involvement usually occurs at the same stage of the disease as the myocarditis, the order of nerves affected being usually the same in all cases developing neuritis. Paralyses are more obvious than sensory changes, but the damage is not permanent. The first muscle to be affected is the palate; this occurs during the third week, causing regurgitation of food through the nose and a nasal twang to the voice. Ocular palsies occur during the fifth week and are usually intrinsic. The most common is paralysis of accommodation, causing blurred vision. Paralysis of the pharynx, larynx and diaphragm occur during the seventh week and peripheral neuritis during the seventh to tenth week.

DIAGNOSIS

*Faucial diphtheria* must be differentiated from acute follicular tonsillitis which produces a white follicular exudate confined to the tonsils, differing from the dirty-grey confluent membrane of diphtheria which may extend beyond the tonsils. The fauces and posterior palate are red and swollen in follicular tonsillitis and a high temperature occurs, whereas in diphtheria the temperature may not even be raised. The toxaemia of diphtheria and the bull-neck are distinctive features.

*Post-tonsillectomy sloughs* look very similar to faucial diphtheria but do not spread beyond the site of operation. There are none of the other features of diphtheria, the absence of toxaemia being particularly important.

*Vincent's angina* may cause a membranous lesion on the tonsil but ulceration is also present, whereas this is not a feature of diphtheria. The lesions often involve the gums and fetor is much more unpleasant than in diphtheria. Toxaemia is not a feature of Vincent's angina. The presence of the spirochaete *Treponema vincenti* and the fusiform bacillus in a direct smear support the diagnosis.

*Glandular fever* may be associated with a tonsillar membrane, but this is less confluent and whiter than the diphtheritic membrane; there may also be ulceration. The patients are not so ill as they would be with the same amount of membrane in diphtheria and the temperature is higher. Cervical adenitis is not associated with the extensive periadenitis seen in diphtheria; other groups of glands in the body are also involved. Atypical monocytes in the blood film, a positive Paul–Bunnell test and a raised EB virus titre confirm the diagnosis.

*Laryngeal diphtheria* must be differentiated from other causes of laryngeal obstruction and particularly from acute laryngitis. Toxaemia is a feature of diphtheria but not of acute laryngitis; however, since a diphtheritic membrane sufficient to cause laryngeal obstruction may not be extensive, toxaemia is not necessarily severe. A high temperature may occur in acute laryngitis but not in diphtheria. The only certain method of differentiation is laryngoscopy to see the membrane; this should be performed in all doubtful cases.

*Treatment.* This must not wait for laboratory confirmation, antitoxin being given without delay in all doubtful cases. If treatment is delayed, the toxin becomes fixed to the tissues and can no longer be neutralized by the antitoxin. The dose depends on the severity of the disease, varying from 15,000–100,000 units. The estimated quantity should be given at one time; if it is more than 40,000 units it should be given by slow intravenous injection. Smaller doses are given by intramuscular injection.

Oxygen is needed for cardiac failure but digitalis is dangerous in view of heart block. Tracheostomy may be necessary for laryngeal obstruction; restlessness is an important indication of anoxia. Intramuscular penicillin should be given to eliminate secondary infection and to reduce the risk of carrier state; it has no effect on the toxaemia.

The children should be nursed strictly in bed for the first 4 weeks in view of the risks of sudden cardiac failure. Activity is cut down to the minimum, the child being fed and bathed. Normal activity is then resumed very gradually.

An attack of diphtheria does not confer lasting immunity so that active immunization should be started as soon as the child has recovered. Any susceptible child contacts should be given 1500 units of antitoxin prophylactically, followed 1 month later by active immunization.

Contacts should be excluded from school for a minimum of 7 days, being allowed to return then only if nose and throat swabs are negative.

### Pertussis (whooping cough)

During infancy, this is the most deadly of all the infectious fevers. Almost all the deaths occur within the first year of life, although its maximum incidence is between 1 and 4 years of age. It is due to *Bordetella pertussis*, a highly infectious. Gram-negative cocco-bacillus. Pertussis differs from the other contagious diseases of childhood in that little or no immunity is transferred from the mother to the newborn. This accounts for the finding that 40 per cent of all deaths from the disease occur in the first 4 months of life. The reason is that pertussis antibody is not carried on the IgG fraction which crosses the placenta (p. 481), thereby differing from the other infectious fevers. It is probably carried on the IgA fraction. Colostrum may transfer immunity since IgA antibodies are secreted in this (p. 482). A small proportion of cases of clinical pertussis are due to adenovirus infection or to the respiratory syncitial virus.

Prompt diagnosis and isolation of cases is essential for the safety of the community; the number of deaths could be reduced by earlier treatment. Early recognition is made more difficult by the modifying effects of vaccination but, although the disease in the partially immune patient is less serious, the infectivity for others is just as high.

The usual incubation period is 7–10 days, the patient being infectious during the last 4 days of this period, although clinically well. Cough is usually the first symptom and is often regarded as the start of a cold, though in half the cases there is no nasal discharge. If a nasal discharge is present it is watery and mucoid rather than thick and purulent as in acute coryza. After 7–14 days the cough becomes paroxysmal, but only in older children does a whoop occur. In bronchitis and other conditions causing a cough, the patient feels the need to cough and takes a breath in anticipation. In pertussis he is caught unawares, his chest tightens and the air is expelled in a sharp rapid stutter. 'Whooping' is a knack which children acquire in order to replace the air in their lungs as rapidly as possible. The noise is made by the sharp blast of air through the glottis which is still only half open. Young infants fail to acquire this skill, being consequently more distressed by the paroxysms; in such cases the diagnosis is easily missed. It would be better to drop the title 'whooping cough' in preference to 'pertussis' in order to emphasize the fact that whooping is unnecessary for the diagnosis and not usual in infants.

Diagnosis is made by the fact that the cough is paroxysmal and associated with vomiting, a most significant feature. Examination of the chest is surprising since, despite the serious cough and general symptoms, the lungs are often found to be clear, especially after a severe coughing paroxysm when vomiting has forced out the secretions.

Paroxysms are often started by disturbing the child, being very likely to occur as soon as he is picked up to be fed. During a paroxysm, cyanosis develops and the congestion may be so great as to cause conjunctival haemorrhage, while the anoxia may precipitate a convulsion. Persistent coughing causes puffiness just below the eyes and both epistaxis and haemoptysis may occur. Reference is often made to a sublingual ulcer in those who have cut their lower incisors, but this is not common.

Infectivity lasts 28 days and the child should be isolated for that time, though paroxysms and whooping often continue far longer. These are often perpetuated as a habit; even when they have ceased the child may whoop when he next has an illness causing a cough. Such cases account for a number of those who are alleged to have had pertussis twice. A small number of such patients have an infection with *Bordetella parapertussis*, but this accounts only for about 1 per cent of patients with clinical pertussis. Its differentiation from pertussis is impossible without bacteriological investigation, though it usually produces only a mild illness.

*Investigations.* Isolation of the organism is difficult, but the most successful method is to obtain a specimen of fresh laryngeal mucus by means of a supralaryngeal swab. The mother sits the child on her lap facing the doctor, holding him tight with his head well back. The swab is placed just above the glottis and the child asked to cough or, if this is impractical, made to cough by touching the throat with a spatula. Cough plates are a much less practical method and are now seldom used.

Leucopenia is present in the early stages; it is succeeded by leucocytosis with a relative lymphocytosis when the paroxysms commence.

*Complications.* Bronchopneumonia is a serious complication and accounts for the majority of deaths. Otitis media is common because infective material is forcibly injected along the Eustachian tube during a paroxysm. Encephalitis is a very serious complication and is possibly due to anoxia. Convulsions, coma and paralyses occur and the prognosis is bad (see p. 407).

Blockage of the small bronchi and bronchioles leads to pulmonary collapse and infection; if this is not cleared bronchiectasis will follow (see p. 362).

*Diagnosis.* In the early stages pertussis is likely to be mistaken for a common cold. In a cold the nasal discharge becomes thick and mucopurulent, whereas in pertussis it is thin and watery or there is none. A history of contact with pertussis should always be sought; it is a valuable confirmation of the diagnosis.

Once the cough has developed, an incorrect diagnosis of bronchitis is likely to be made. Such patients are sometimes admitted to a general ward instead of being isolated, causing infectious havoc. The mistake should be avoided because in bronchitis moist sounds will always be heard in the chest and wheezing is common, whereas in pertussis the lungs are often clear, especially in the early stages, and there is no wheezing. The difficulties of diagnosis are increased in children who have been immunized, the illness being less severe; but, although whooping may not take place, the characteristic paroxysmal type of cough remains.

*Treatment.* Tetracycline being safer than chloramphenicol is the drug of choice. The most valuable aspect of antibiotic therapy is the prevention of secondary infection, therefore it is wise to give penicillin in addition although it has no action on *Bordetella pertussis*. Skilled nursing has possibly the largest part to play in recovery. Infants under 1 year frequently require oxygen and in case of doubt it is safer to place the child in an oxygen tent. Sleep is essential, chloral or amylobarbitone being given if necessary. Linctuses have little effect on the paroxysms but atropine methyl nitrate (Eumydrin) may help; it is used as a 0·6 per cent alcoholic solution, 1 drop for each year of age being given on a sugar lump at 4-hourly intervals. Pertussis immune globulin may be of value.

Feeding is a problem because the patients are so liable to vomit, but if the child is refed immediately after a vomit he is likely to retain it. Feeds should be given often and should always be small to reduce the risk of vomiting.

Fresh air is important and in good weather the children should, if possible, be nursed in the garden. At the end of the illness, a chest X-ray should be carried out on every child in order to check that there is no residual collapse of the lungs. If collapse is present, vigorous physiotherapy must be performed until expansion is complete in order to prevent bronchiectasis.

### Brucellosis (Undulant fever)

This is caused by the ingestion of one of the three main strains of *Brucella* organisms. *B. abortus* from cow's milk and *B. melitensis* from goat's milk may occur in children, but *B. suis*, from handling the carcases of infected pigs, is unlikely to occur in children. The disease is named undulant on account of the alternating periods of febrile and afebrile periods.

The disease usually starts in the autumn or winter, the incubation period being about 2 weeks. The onset is usually insidious with anorexia, tiredness, headache and chronic abdominal pain. Constipation is common and epistaxis may occur. Intermittent fever is characteristic, each bout lasting about 2 weeks and being accompanied by sweating. The apyrexial periods last about 10 days. Enlargement of the liver, spleen or lymph glands and transient arthritis are not uncommon. A systolic cardiac murmur is audible in a considerable proportion of cases.

*Investigations.* Slight anaemia is usual and leucopenia is present with a marked diminution in the number of polymorphonuclear neutrophils. The erythrocyte sedimentation rate is often surprisingly low.

The serum agglutination test against a suspension of killed organisms is positive if present in a titre of one in eighty or over; a rising titre is the most definite indication of the disease. An intradermal sensitivity test with brucellin is available but, like the Mantoux test for tuberculosis, a positive result merely indicates that the patient has had the infection at some time, not proving that the present illness is undulant fever.

*Diagnosis.* The indefinite nature of the symptoms makes diagnosis difficult, but the possibility of undulant fever must be remembered in every case of obscure fever, abdominal pain and arthritis. Poliomyelitis must be differentiated (see p. 410). The vagueness of the symptoms sometimes results in a diagnosis of psychoneurosis being made in the first instance.

*Prophylaxis.* The disease should be eradicated from cattle; the present drive is to produce abortus-free herds in the same way as TB-free herds. All milk should be pasteurized, thereby destroying the organism.

*Treatment.* Tetracycline and streptomycin are the most effective antibiotics. Tetracycline can be given alone for 3 weeks or in combination with streptomycin.

## Salmonella infections

The clinical manifestations from the *Salmonella* organisms fall into two types:

*Enteric fever.* This is caused by *S. typhi* and *S. paratyphi* A, B and C. The incubation period is up to 2 weeks.

*Food poisoning.* This is caused by *S. typhimurium, S. enteriditis* and *S. choleraesius.* The incubation period is a few hours only.

### ENTERIC FEVER (TYPHOID AND PARATYPHOID)

These infections may occur at any age, though on the whole, except for infants, they are less serious in children than in adults. Paratyphoid is usually milder than typhoid. Infection results from ingestion of milk, water or food which has been contaminated by sewage or by a carrier. The incubation period is usually 12–14 days, this being followed by invasion of the blood stream.

The clinical picture is extremely variable in children. In infants the features are those of acute gastroenteritis, the correct diagnosis being made only by bacteriological investigation. In older children the onset is more gradual, though an acute onset with meningismus and convulsions may occur. Although diarrhoea is usual in infants, constipation is more common at the onset in older children, the motions becoming loose during the second week. Abdominal distension is usually marked, abdominal pain is present and the spleen palpable. The illness may be dominated by bronchopneumonia so that the gastrointestinal symptoms are obscured. Rose-coloured spots, which appear from the beginning of the second week, are seen more often in paratyphoid than typhoid, occurring less frequently in children than in adults. Proteinuria is common.

*Investigations.* The blood picture shows a leucopenia at the onset, the fall being in neutrophils and eosinophils. Positive cultures may be obtained from the blood, stool or urine during the first 2 weeks. Cultures from the bone marrow have been found to be positive more often than those from the peripheral blood. The Widal test becomes positive from the tenth day onwards.

*Complications.* There are fewer complications in children than in adults, although relapses are more frequent. As a result of the early septicaemic stage, the organisms may become localized in any part of the body and meningitis, osteomyelitis, arthritis, pyelonephitis and appendicitis may occur. Perforation and haemorrhage are rare.

*Treatment.* Chloramphenicol is the drug of choice and the greatest nursing skill is required. Parenteral fluids may be required for dehydration, and tepid sponging for high fever.

FOOD POISONING

Contamination of food with *S. typhimurium, S. enteritidis* and *S. choleraesius* usually comes from a human source, either as an active infection or from a carrier. After an incubation period of a few hours the symptoms of acute gastroenteritis develop (see p. 299).

*Diagnosis.* The other major bacterial cause of food poisoning is the staphylococcus. During preparation the food becomes contaminated with a strain of staphylococci which produces an exotoxin. The usual foods to be affected are creams and custards. The onset is very acute; it may occur as soon as 1 hour after taking the food and always within 6 hours. There is severe nausea, vomiting, abdominal pain and diarrhoea, the patient becoming rapidly prostrate. Recovery occurs within 12–24 hours.

Staphylococcal food poisoning is more dramatic in its symptoms than *Salmonella* food poisoning. It is likely to affect a larger number of people very suddenly since all those eating the infected food usually develop symptoms. Recovery is more rapid. Bacterial investigations will complete the differentiation.

## Isolation

The majority of infectious fevers occur during childhood since their infectivity

TABLE 8. Incubation and isolation of the common infectious fevers

| Disease | Incubation period (days) | Period of isolation |
|---------|-------------------------|---------------------|
| *Short incubation* | | |
| Diphtheria | 2–5 | Until clinically well and swabs negative. |
| Scarlet fever | 2–5 | 7 days, provided free of discharges. |
| Influenza | 1–3 | During pyrexia. |
| *Medium* | | |
| Measles | 10–15 | 10 days from appearance of rash. |
| Pertussis | 7–10 | 3 weeks from onset of cough. |
| Variola | 10–13 | Until scabs dry and healed. |
| Enteric | 12–14 | Until two consecutively negative stools and urine. |
| *Long* | | |
| Mumps | 12–28 | 7 days from disappearance of swelling. |
| Varicella | 11–21 | 14 days from appearance of rash. |
| Rubella | 14–21 | 7 days from appearance of rash. |

is high and passive immunity from the mother soon lost. They are particularly likely to be caught at school when large numbers of susceptible individuals are in close contact. The exclusion from school of contacts, by means of quarantine regulations, has in the past caused much loss of schooling but made little difference to the amount of infection. For this reason, most authorities no longer insist on exclusion for contacts of patients with pertussis, rubella, measles, varicella, scarlet fever or mumps. The situation with diphtheria is different since this disease is now rare in Great Britain.

## BIBLIOGRAPHY

BUTLER N.R. & BENSON P.F. (1965) Immunization in general practice. *Brit. med. J.*, **1**, 841.

COBBAN K. (1963) Measles in Nigerian children. *W. African Med. J.*, **1**, 18.

COCKSHOTT P. & MACGREGOR M. (1959) The natural history of osteomyelitis variolosa. *J. Fac. Radiol.*, **10**, 57.

DICK G. (1973) Register of cases of subacute sclerosing parencephalitis. *Brit. med. J.*, **2**, 359.

GIBBS F.A. & ROSENTHAL I.M. (1962) Electroencephalography in natural and attenuated measles. *Amer. J. Dis. Child.*, **103**, 395.

GREEN D.M., REID S.M. & RHANEY K. (1966) Generalized vaccinia in the human foetus. *Lancet*, **1**, 1296.

JEAVONS P.M. & BOWER B.D. (1964) Infantile Spasms. *Clinics in Developmental Medicine* No. 15. Spastics Society/Heinemann Medical, London.

KORONES S.B., AINGER L.E., MONIF G.R.G., ROANE J., SEVER J.L. & FUSTE F. (1965) Congenital rubella syndrome: new clinical aspects with recovery of virus from affected infants. *J. Pediat.*, **67**, 166.

LINDQUIST J.M., PLOTKIN S.A., SHAW L., GILDEN R.V. & WILLIAMS M.L. (1965) Congenital rubella syndrome as a systemic infection. Studies of affected infants born in Philadelphia, U.S.A. *Brit. med. J.*, **2**, 1401.

MENSER M.A., HARLEY J.D., HERTZBERG R., DORMAN D.C. & MURPHY A.M. (1967) Persistence of virus in lens for three years after prenatal rubella. *Lancet*, **2**, 387.

MRC COMMITTEE REPORT (1966) Vaccination against measles: a clinical trial of live measles vaccine given alone and live vaccine preceded by killed vaccine. *Brit. med. J.*, **1**, 441.

PAMPIGLIONE G. (1964) Prodromal phase of measles: some neurophysiological studies. *Brit. med. J.*, **2**, 1296.

PLOTKIN S.A., OSKI F.A., HARTNETT E.M., HERVADA A.R., FRIEDMAN S. & GOWING J. (1965) Some recently recognized manifestations of the rubella syndrome. *J. Pediat.*, **67**, 182.

POSKITT E.M.E. (1971) Effect of measles on plasma-albumin levels in Ugandan village children. *Lancet*, **2**, 68.

WARIN J.F., HARKER P. & MAYON-WHITE R.T. (1972) Measles in vaccinated children in Oxford 1971. *Lancet*, **2**, 810.

WOOD C.B.S. (1972) The development of immunity in fetal life and childhood. *J. Roy. Coll. Phys. Lond.*, **6**, 246.

# CHAPTER 19

# TUBERCULOSIS, LEPROSY, SYPHILIS, TOXO-PLASMOSIS AND HISTOPLASMOSIS

## TUBERCULOSIS

The successful reduction in the incidence of tuberculosis in childhood in the United Kingdom has led to the possibility of the disease being forgotten by doctors, especially those who have never worked in developing countries, where it is still rife. In the U.K. now the danger is from the adult, often elderly, who has TB and infects his family. Such a patient may have associated lung disease, especially carcinoma, which has lit up an old TB focus.

### NATURAL HISTORY

The same two factors influence the response of an individual to infection with the tubercle bacillus as occurs in any other form of infection. In the first place there is the question of resistance. This is of two types: natural and acquired. Natural resistance is present at birth. It is mainly dependent on race but to a lesser extent on familial and individual variations. Acquired resistance is due to the development of immunity from a previous infection. The second factor is the size of the infecting dose; the greater the concentration of tubercle bacilli, the more likely is the individual to contract the disease.

**Tuberculin test**

The likely response of an individual to infection with tuberculosis can be determined by his response to the tuberculin test. Six weeks after first infection the patient develops a positive tuberculin test. This is a specific reaction to the intradermal injection of tuberculin protein, indicating a state of allergy but not immunity. A positive test shows that the individual has at some time been infected with tubercle bacilli, unless he has previously received BCG vaccination, which has the same effect. It gives no indication when the infection occurred, except that it must have been at least 6 weeks previously, though it might have been 60 years or more. This can be determined only by knowing when the test was previously negative and, therefore, when conversion to positive could have taken place. Nor does it give any indication whether the patient is now suffering from active tuberculosis. One individual with a positive test might, by reason of natural and acquired resistance, be immune to the disease; another might be dying from it owing to lack of immunity. The test cannot differentiate between human and bovine infection. Malnutrition may delay, reduce or, in severe cases, prevent the development of tuberculin sensitivity, the patient thereby being tuberculin negative despite earlier infection. Children who are very ill with TB, especially after measles, may similarly give a negative response.

It is probable that in most individuals with a positive test, living tubercle bacilli are present in the body. Surveys planned to determine the tuberculosis attack rate in those whose tuberculin state was previously known, have shown that the highest morbidity is now in those already positive, whereas until recently the reverse was the case. This emphasizes the error of regarding a tuberculin positive state from a natural infection as a form of protection, and underlines the need to follow all such children through adolescence when their risk of adult tuberculosis is greatest.

To undertake the test a number of methods are available. Patch and jelly tuberculin tests would seem to be ideal for children, since they avoid the pain of an intradermal injection but, unfortunately, they are too liable to give false results to be recommended. For this reason, either a Mantoux or a Heaf test should be used. The Mantoux test is available in three dilutions and the following doses can be given:

1. 0·1 ml of 1/10,000 old tuberculin (1 unit).
2. 0·1 ml of 1/1000 old tuberculin (10 units).
3. 0·1 ml of 1/100 old tuberculin (100 units).

For routine use the 1/1000 solution should be used, 0·1 ml being injected intradermally into the flexor surface of the left forearm. The same site should always be used for ease of reading. The test should be read in 72 hours, a positive result being indicated by an area of induration more than 6 mm across. The reaction must be palpable, erythema alone being insufficient. The only occasion the 1/10,000 solution is necessary is in cases of erythema nodosum, when a positive reaction may be so strong as to cause local ulceration. The 1/100 solution is seldom used since, at that strength, non-specific reactions are liable to occur.

The Heaf test uses a special gun whose multiple needles simultaneously pierce the skin for the correct distance. It has the advantage of ease, accuracy and absence of pain. The method was designed for use in Africa, the result being much more easy to read on black skin than the single Mantoux mark. Moreover, being still positive after 1 week it is ideal for communities where mothers only come to the big city on the weekly market day. The solution used is tuberculin PPD (purified protein derivative) containing 100,000 units per ml. The test is not a quantitative one but is considered to be equivalent to the 1/100 Mantoux test. It is most important that the correct solution is used, this being more viscous than that used for a Mantoux test. A small drop of this solution is placed on the skin using a sterile platinum loop. The end plate of the Heaf gun must be held at right angles to the skin, being pressed firmly on the centre of the film of tuberculin solution. The needles are sterilized by flaming the head end after dipping it in spirit; sufficient time must be allowed for it to cool. Multiple heads are available to ease the problem of sterilization when large numbers of tests are being made. The result is read in 72 hours but can be delayed up to 7 days. A positive result is indicated by the development of palpable induration at the site of at least four of the puncture points. Confluent induration is not a positive result but is due to a burn.

The 'tine' tuberculin test uses a similar principle to the Heaf method. Its advantage is that the needles (tines) are already covered with dried tuberculin and each unit, comprising 4 tines, is sterile and disposable. However, it is more expensive and painful than the Heaf method while being less reliable.

When infection with tubercle bacilli occurs, one of two different reactions takes place depending on the patient's immunity. A primary infection finds the patient without immunity and causes the 'non-immune or productive reaction'. An infection in an individual who has undergone a primary infection and thereby developed some immunity, causes the 'immune or exudative reaction', also termed the 'adult infection'.

The clinical reaction of the individual infected with tuberculosis, as with any other infection, depends on the size and strength of the invading organisms and the resistance of the host. However, in the case of TB (and leprosy) there is the additional element of the development of sensitivity which shows itself histologically by an aggregation of lymphocytes and clinically by fever and malaise. Sensitivity is the commonest cause of the acute inflammatory component of the tissue reaction, whereas caseation and destruction of tissue without inflammatory response occur when 'resistance' is low. Resistance and sensitivity can vary independently, but it is usual for resistance to be high when sensitivity is high and vice versa (Miller, 1970).

These facts explain the differing clinical pictures seen in children of varying ages and varying states of nutrition and also the reduced or absent tuberculin test in the malnourished child and in the very ill child. Sensitivity is less in young children and those who are malnourished. Therefore, erythema nodosum (p. 518) and phlyctenular conjunctivitis (p. 519) being hypersensitivity states are uncommon in young children anywhere. They are also uncommon at any age in developing countries whereas in the U.K. they are not rare in the older child. A tuberculous pleural effusion is also an index of hypersensitivity so its age and geographical distribution is identical to that just described. Moreover, the amount of fluid in any effusion is related to the degree of sensitivity, high sensitivity causing large effusions. For the same reasons large caseous glands are often seen in the necks and axillae of children in developing countries whereas these are small in children in the U.K.

### The non-immune or productive reaction (primary infection)

Primary infection results in a lesion with two components which together are known as the 'primary complex'; these components bear the same relationship to each other wherever the site of the lesion. One is the parenchymal component or tubercle, whose site is dependent on the route of infection. The other component is glandular, resulting from lymphatic spread to the glands draining the parenchymal lesion. There are two types of infection: human and bovine. Human infection is now by far the more important, usually occurring by droplet spread from a patient with open pulmonary tuberculosis. Bovine tuberculosis reaches the body by the ingestion of infected milk; this disease is now uncommon in Great Britain as tuberculosis amongst cattle has been largely eradicated. Since the major route of infection is droplet, the most common site for the primary complex is the lung. Ingestion of bacilli causes a primary lesion in the intestine; direct contact, often associated with local trauma, causes a lesion on the skin or, less commonly, in the mouth.

The primary focus in the lung is sometimes known as the Ghon lesion after the Prague pathologist who gave the first description. This lesion lies immediately under the pleura; it may occur anywhere in the lungs but is most often in the right upper lobe. The glandular element involves the mediastinal glands. In the abdomen, the parenchymal lesion is in the intestine, the mesenteric glands being involved. The tonsils are sometimes the primary site, the tonsillar glands then comprising the second component of the primary complex. They become infected by droplets from an open case or by the ingestion of infected milk. It is also probable that they are sometimes infected from bronchial secretions in cases of primary intrathoracic tuberculosis. When tonsillectomy has been required in such cases, the tonsils have sometimes been found to be tuberculous, although cervical adenitis is not present. Involvement of the skin or mouth causes a similar enlargement of the appropriate regional glands.

Although the primary complex is usually single, multiple simultaneous primary infections may occur. Abdominal tuberculosis is now more often an additional primary infection caused by ingestion of tubercle bacilli from a primary lung infection.

Both components of the primary complex may heal or extend and undergo caseation. However, extension and caseation is far more likely to occur in the glandular component than in the parenchymal. Involvement of the glands accounts for the majority of the clinical features of the primary complex, their effect varying greatly according to the site. Enlarged cervical glands cause no trouble from pressure, but similar enlargement in the mediastinum results in serious bronchial damage. Healing takes place by fibrosis and later calcification is common. Calcification in the neck causes little disturbance but in the chest may cause bronchial stenosis. Even though healing has proceeded to calcification, living tubercle bacilli may remain in the lesion for many years. Extension may occur from either of the components, taking place by local spread or via the bronchi, blood or lymphatics.

If direct or bronchial spread of the primary infection occurs, it usually does so within a few months of the original infection. Lymphatic spread to the group of glands draining the primary gland usually appears within a year, but may be delayed as long as 7 years. Blood-stream spread results from erosion of a blood vessel and, if it occurs, is likely to be very soon after the onset of the primary infection, often before this has been detected. This liability continues with diminishing frequency for about 2 years, being very rare after that time. Haematogenous spread, causing miliary tuberculosis or meningitis, occurs earlier than spread to bone or kidneys which often takes place during the second year after the primary infection. Part of this longer interval may be due to the fact that bone and kidney lesions take longer to manifest themselves. Needle biopsy of the liver has shown evidence of hepatic spread in a significant proportion of cases of primary tuberculosis, although there are no symptoms referable to the liver in these cases. There is no enlargement of the regional glands from a haematogenous deposit.

The age at first infection is important in deciding the subsequent clinical pattern. Active tuberculosis is far more likely to follow infection in infancy than in older children, the type of lesion being affected by the age at which first infection occurs. The younger the child, the larger is the lymph gland component and the more often does the disease become disseminated. The older the child, the more often does a pleural effusion occur. Pleural effusions may result from blood-stream spread or from direct involvement of the pleura; they usually occur about 6 months after the primary infection. In older children and adolescents the risk that the adult type of the disease will supervene is much greater than in young children.

### The immune or exudative reaction (adult infection)

The entry of tubercle bacilli into a patient who has already developed some immunity as the result of a primary infection is much more violent, but remains local; it is known as the adult type of the disease. The local reaction is one of acute inflammation and may be sufficiently intense to proceed to caseation and necrosis with consequent cavity formation. Cavitation is common with this type of reaction; it is uncommon in a primary complex. Alternatively, depending on the degree of resistance and the size of the infecting dose, it may resolve completely with or without fibrosis. Unlike the primary lesion, which may occur anywhere in the lungs, this lesion is most often posterior, either in the subapical region of the upper lobe or, less commonly, in a similar position in the lower lobe. There is no enlargement of the regional lymph glands and haematogenous spread is rare.

It is still uncertain whether this secondary form of tuberculosis is the result of spread from the primary complex or reinfection from outside. The balance of evidence, including the constant site of the lesion, favours a bronchogenic spread from breakdown of the primary lesion.


## PRIMARY TUBERCULOSIS

Before describing the clinical features of primary tuberculosis it is necessary to consider erythema nodosum and phlyctenular conjunctivitis. These are hypersensitivity states which represent an allergic reaction to infection with the tubercle bacilli or the haemolytic streptococcus. Their recognition is therefore of paramount importance since they may be the only indication of primary tuberculosis. Both conditions are very rare in the first 2 years of life. They differ in that erythema nodosum is seen only in the early phase of the primary complex and, if of tuberculous origin, occurs once only, whereas phlyctenular conjunctivitis may occur during all stages of activity of the primary complex and has a tendency to relapse. When erythema nodosum is of streptococcal origin, repeated attacks may occur.


### Erythema nodosum

Tender mauve nodules appear on the front of the shins and occasionally on the extensor aspects of the forearm. They have a similar appearance to that produced by a positive Mantoux test and are exactly comparable, except that they have occurred spontaneously. The lesions always disappear in about 2 weeks, going through the colour changes of a fading bruise; unfortunately parents may mistake them for this, thereby not calling the doctor.

Usually there is insufficient pain to warrant local therapy but if this is required, a lead lotion compress is soothing. No other treatment is necessary, though a full investigation for tuberculosis is indicated. If the significance of this exceedingly important condition is missed, it may be many months before the effects of the primary infection become detectable once again; in the interval much harm may have been done.

The frequency of a tuberculous origin of erythema nodosum is declining in England, but it is still in the order of 40 per cent; under the age of 5 years tuberculosis is still by far the commoner cause.

### Phlyctenular conjunctivitis

A phlyctenule is a minute vesicle or ulcerated nodule found on the cornea or conjunctiva. It is best seen by examining the eye obliquely, when a granular surface can be observed. The lesion occurs most often at the corneoscleral junction, its site being clearly marked by a triangular leash of blood vessels whose apex lies at the site of the phlyctenule (Fig. 119).

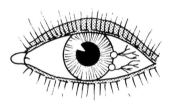

Fig. 119. The appearance in phlyctenular conjunctivitis. Two vesicles are present on either side of the corneoscleral junction, from which injected blood vessels radiate.

Lacrimation and photophobia occur if corneal ulceration has taken place, but in many cases the condition is quite mild, its serious relationship to tuberculosis not being appreciated. Cortisone eye drops relieve the local symptoms but if corneal ulceration has occurred, healing leaves an opacity.

### Intrathoracic primary tuberculosis

Most often an uncomplicated primary infection passes unnoticed, having either produced no symptoms or only a period of vague ill-health which may have been regarded as 'influenza'. It cannot be emphasized too strongly that night sweats, haemoptysis and a severe illness, as seen in adults with tuberculosis, are not features of a primary infection and that loss of appetite and tiredness are the main presenting symptoms. Pain in the limb muscles sometimes occurs which may be acribed to 'growing pains'; occasionally pain may be felt in the joints. In an uncomplicated case there are no physical signs in the chest.

Cough is not a prominent feature unless there is pressure on a bronchus by enlarged hilar glands; then it is likely to be 'brassy'. Physical signs in the chest may not be obvious. It is thereby surprising how large a shadow on the X-ray can be unassociated with clinical signs, emphasizing the need for radiography in all suspected cases.

The most common complication of the primary complex is the segmental lesion which occurs more often in younger patients. This is often ascribed to pulmonary collapse, but studies of specimens removed at thoracotomy have shown that the affected portion of lung has always been consolidated from

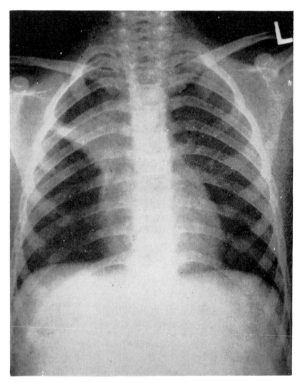

Fig. 120. Primary tuberculosis. The segmental opacity in the right upper zone comprises enlarged hilar glands together with consolidation and collapse in the upper lobe.

pneumonia, collapse being usually only a minor element. The lesion is an aspiration tuberculous pneumonia, with or without caseation, which has resulted from the perforation of a caseous lymph gland through the bronchial wall. The X-ray shadow is composed of the enlarged glands and the pulmonary lesion. It is seldom possible to determine their respective limits (Fig. 120). Caseous lymph glands often contain large numbers of tubercle bacilli and it is understandable that simple collapse rarely, if ever, occurs. Consequently, clearing of the opacity results from resolution of the tuberculous exudate and not from simple reaeration of a collapsed lobe. The term 'epituberculosis' was used in the past to describe these shadows, but should now be discarded in view of the more detailed pathology available. The primary complex occurs more often on the right, and a right-sided lesion is more liable to extend than one on the left.

Although cavitation of a primary lung lesion is rare in comparison with that in adult-type tuberculosis, intensive investigation, particularly the use of tomography, has shown that this complication occurs more often than was previously supposed. Similarly, the more frequent use of bronchoscopy has shown the high proportion of children with a radiological primary lesion in whom endobronchial tuberculosis is present. In the light of this information it becomes surprising that tuberculous bronchopneumonia is such a relatively rare complication, but it explains the frequency of bronchiectasis.

Obstructive emphysema is a serious complication which is not rare but is easily missed. Partial obstruction of the bronchus by an eroding gland permits more air to enter the lung than can come out, the lobe becoming over-distended (Figs. 106, 107). Wheezing may occur and diminished movement and air entry on the affected side are detectable. An inspiratory film may show no difference between the two sides but, on expiration, the diseased lung, remaining aerated, appears clearer than the normal side. Later, the gland entirely blocks the lumen, causing complete collapse of the lung with the complications of tuberculous pneumonia and bronchiectasis.

### Abdominal primary tuberculosis

With the reduction in bovine tuberculosis, this is now an uncommon condition in Great Britain; more cases are now of human than bovine origin. Those of human origin result from the transfer of infection from a pulmonary lesion in the same patient or from the swallowing of organisms introduced from outside. Tuberculous mesenteric adenitis is one of those conditions which is overdiagnosed, many children with abdominal pain being referred to hospital with this mistaken diagnosis. A complaint of abdominal pain is seldom due to this condition. In many cases the condition is discovered only when the abdomen is X-rayed for some other condition and calcified glands are found.

A small proportion of patients develops tuberculous peritonitis. This is a severe illness with much wasting, associated with abdominal distension and often severe colicky abdominal pain from partial intestinal obstruction. The loops of intestine may become so matted together that complete obstruction develops.

## Cervical adenitis

The primary source of this infection is most often in the tonsil but may be in the adenoids, middle ear or teeth. The tonsils may look diseased but are just as likely to look entirely normal. It is impossible to be definite as to whether the infection is more often human or bovine in origin, although many dogmatic and conflicting statements exist in the literature. The difficulty is that although tubercle bacilli are seen in the pus from caseous glands, they are seldom living, this being a prerequisite for their differentiation. Evidence points to a human infection being more common than bovine.

The glands cause no pain and no systemic illness, being therefore often disregarded until the condition is far advanced. So long as the infection in the gland is purely tuberculous the gland remains discrete and mobile, not being fixed from periadenitis. Caseation is common, as shown by the incidence of radiological calcification, but not all those glands which caseate develop clinical abscesses. The development of an abscess appears to be determined by size, being likely to occur once the diameter of the gland is greater than 2 cm.

A mixture of tuberculous and streptococcal infections in the gland is common. The tuberculous infection progresses steadily, but the streptococcal infection waxes and wanes. A mixed infection causes periadenitis and, once this has occurred, the skin is likely to break down. The first evidence of this is the gland becoming tethered to the overlying skin. The skin becomes pink and then mauve and thinned; this is followed by the discharge of caseous material, an indolent discharging ulcer remaining.

Generalized lymphadenitis is uncommon in England but it seen quite frequently in older children in Africa. In such cases the enlargement of the axillary lymph nodes is usually greater than any of the other groups.

## Tuberculous meningitis

Although headache, vomiting and constipation are commonly given as the classical symptoms, all but vomiting are relatively late. The rapidity with which the symptoms develop varies with the age of the child, the onset being most insidious in infants unless they present with convulsions. The first sign in a child is most often a change in temperament associated with loss of appetitite. From being a normal, placid individual the child becomes irritable, wanting to be left alone. He may sit on his own for long periods, making little fuss provided no one disturbs him. Abdominal pain may be a prominent feature; it has sometimes been so severe as to lead to the removal of the appendix before the correct diagnosis has been realized. Sleep rhythm may be disturbed so that he tends to be awake at night, sleeping by day. A change in the level of consciousness is important. This varies from merely being less alert than normal to obvious drowsiness or even coma. Symptoms of an upper respiratory infection are common, sometimes obscuring the early evidence of tuberculous meningitis.

Examination in the early stages shows an irritable feverish child with neck stiffness which can be best detected, if the child is able to co-operate, by asking him to kiss his knee (see Fig. 4). At the same time it must be emphasized that in young children, as in those with pyogenic meningitis, there may be no signs of meningism. If still open, the fontanelle is tense. Photophobia is not common in children. The child is seldom fully alert and is often apathetic so that normal contact cannot be made. Examination of the fundi may confirm the diagnosis by showing choroidal tubercles if there has been a miliary spread. The inflammatory exudate in tuberculous meningitis remains around the base of the brain, being very liable to involve the cranial nerves thus causing paralyses in the later stages. Head retraction and Kernig's sign are unreliable signs in children, occurring only late in the disease.

The cerebrospinal fluid is colourless and under increased pressure, though pressure readings are invalidated if the child is crying. The fluid has a fine ground-glass turbidity when held to the light and slowly moved from the vertical to the horizontal position. A spider-web clot may develop. The initial cell count is usually 200–400 per $mm^3$, a higher level than this being in favour of pyogenic meningitis. The majority of the cells are lymphocytes but in the early stages, particularly in those cases of acute onset, about 20 per cent may be polymorphs. The protein is raised to over 100 mg per cent but is of little diagnostic value. Far more important is the sugar level which is below 50 mg per cent in most cases; if the level is over 50 mg per cent the diagnosis should be seriously questioned. However, a normal sugar does not rule out tuberculous meningitis. In doubtful cases daily examinations of the cerebrospinal fluid should be made, a steady fall in the sugar level being of great significance. The finding of tubercle bacilli in a centrifuged specimen is conclusive. The level of chlorides falls but this is variable and of little diagnostic value.

## Miliary tuberculosis

The disease is so named because the parenchymal lesions disseminated throughout the organs of the body resemble millet seeds. The patient is often described as presenting with dyspnoea and cyanosis, but more often these children are picked up with the same story of vague ill-health which leads to a chest X-ray in the usual case of primary intrathoracic tuberculosis. A careful search will reveal that choroidal tubercles are often present; because of the magnification provided by the ophthalmoscope, these may be visible before there is radiographic evidence of miliary dissemination.

### Visible primary lesions

The primary focus occurs in a visible situation more often than is appreciated. The majority of such lesions occur on the skin, but they may be found in the eye or mouth, either on the buccal mucous membrane or, more often, on the gum. There is often a history of trauma causing a break in the continuity of the epithelium which allows the entrance of the tubercle bacilli; in all cases there is enlargement of the regional glands. The appearance of the lesions is very variable but all are indolent and indurated, ulceration being common. In some cases 'apple jelly' nodules are seen in the edge of the lesion. The possibility of a tuberculous skin infection must be considered in any child whose skin wound has healed and then breaks down, and where painless enlargement of the regional lymph glands also exists.

### Bone and joint tuberculosis

The most common sites in children are the spine (Pott's disease) and hip; tuberculous dactylitis is a rare manifestation. Trauma is an aetiological factor, influencing the localization of the disease. Synovial lesions usually present earlier than bone lesions; their course is more rapid so that they may simulate acute suppurative arthritis or rheumatic fever.

SPINAL TUBERCULOSIS

The disease most often affects the lower thoracic spine, causing limitation of movement and local pain, although this may sometimes be referred to the abdomen. Spasm of the muscles causes the affected area of the spine to be held rigid. Paraplegia occurs in a considerable proportion of the patients and may be the presenting feature. It is due to pressure from tuberculous granulations and caseous material rather than to the collapse of the vertebrae. A psoas abscess, which is 'cold', may develop and if this presents externally, it appears immediately above the inguinal ligament; less often a lumbar abscess develops. These abscesses may be the first manifestation of the disease. X-rays may show one or more vertebrae to be involved; these will be decalcified and have often collapsed, causing considerable deformity.

TUBERCULOSIS OF THE HIP

These patients are usually under 5 years of age and present with a limp or pain in the hip, though this is sometimes referred to the knee. Examination reveals wasting of the hip muscles and limitation of joint movement. The X-ray shows rarefaction of the bone around the joint.

### Renal tuberculosis

This is much less common in children than in adults, rarely occurring under the age of 10 years. It results from haematogenous spread, usually from a pulmonary lesion and often produces no clinical features. The fact that the kidney is involved may be discovered only on routine urinary examination in a child with tuberculosis, or at autopsy. The possibility must always be considered in cases of sterile pyuria.

### Metastatic abscesses

These abscesses are haematogenous in origin, forming in the subcutaneous tissue. They are usually painless and slowly involve the overlying skin to produce one or more discharging sinuses from which indolent ulcers develop. Healing eventually takes place, a puckered, tethered scar remaining.

### Congenital tuberculosis

A rare condition of generalized tuberculosis resulting from intrauterine infection in a case of maternal tuberculosis. There are two possible routes of infection: haematogenous from the placenta and oral from aspiration of infected amniotic fluid. Contrary to expectation the Mantoux test is not necessarily positive, so that if the mother is known to have active tuberculosis and the child has an unexplained illness, treatment for tuberculosis should be given as the condition is often fatal. There is enlargement of the liver and spleen. Tubercle bacilli may be obtained from gastric washings.

## DIAGNOSIS OF TUBERCULOSIS IN CHILDREN

### History

A history of tuberculosis in a contact of the patient is strong evidence in favour of the diagnosis. In all cases a wide search for possible contacts should be made as discussed on p. 527.

A recent history of infection or trauma immediately before the onset of tuberculosis is often obtained. This factor sometimes causes a delay in diagnosis, since the symptoms of tuberculosis are wrongly attributed to the previous infection or trauma. Measles is the most common infection to act in this way, doing so by lowering the resistance and allowing the tubercle bacilli to gain a foothold. This sequence occurs particularly in malnourished children, being a serious complication of measles in the tropics. Pertussis is a less common antecedent infection. Trauma, which includes surgical operations, plays its part by causing the effected organ to become a nidus in which the infection can settle.

### Direct smear

The only certain proof that a patient is suffering from tuberculosis is the finding of tubercle bacilli. Sputum is seldom available from children since they tend to swallow the material they cough up, but this can be obtained from gastric washings. Where the urine is to be examined, a 24-hour collection should be made so as to have a large quantity. In common with all fluids to be examined for the bacilli it is spun down so that only a concentrated deposit is searched. As renal tuberculosis often causes no symptoms, a periodic urinary check should be made in all cases of tuberculosis. Tuberculous pus, if thoroughly searched, will be found to contain the bacilli in a high proportion of cases.

### Culture and guinea-pig

A concentrate of any material obtained is cultured on Löwenstein's medium and also inoculated into a guinea-pig. The results are not available for 4–6 weeks and therefore have no influence on therapy; they give retrospective evidence of infection. These tests are positive much less often than the direct smear, since the bacilli seen are usually dead.

### Tuberculin test

The significance of a positive tuberculin test has been discussed (p. 513). A negative test is strong evidence against the diagnosis of tuberculosis, unless the lesion is so early that there has been insufficient time for conversion to positive. Some children with severe kwashiorkor and associated tuberculosis give a negative result because of their malnourished and anergic state; for this reason the chest should always be X-rayed in such children. To save time in the diagnosis of tuberculous meningitis, it is useful to use the 1/100 Mantoux solution without going through the previous dilutions which may produce negative results. This will cause more severe reactions in some patients, but the achievement of earlier diagnosis amply compensates for this.

### Radiography

Wherever the site of suspected tuberculosis, the chest should be X-rayed since the majority of non-pulmonary lesions have resulted from pulmonary tuberculosis. Miliary tuberculosis can be diagnosed on sight by its typical 'snow-storm' appearance but none of the other pulmonary shadows are diagnostic.

### Biopsy

This may involve the removal of an enlarged regional gland or a portion of skin. In bone and joint tuberculosis a biopsy of the synovial membrane is made or, occasionally, of a portion of bone.

# PROPHYLAXIS

## Case hunting

The prevention of tuberculosis in children lies in the eradication of disease in adults. This can be achieved only by the continued hunt for unsuspected cases and the correct isolation and treatment of those known to have the disease. Mass radiography is one method of tracing patients but, although it has brought to light many unsuspected cases, it is relatively expensive in time and money for the number of new cases discovered. Moreover, the patient who suspects he has the disease often avoids X-rays in case his worst fears are realized. Its use lies particularly in the regular checking of susceptibles such as miners, certain factory-workers and those working in contact with tuberculous patients. Education of the public to the fact that tuberculosis can now be cured and to the risks for children, is an essential part of any prophylactic campaign. By these means patients can be persuaded to report the earliest suspicious symptoms, the element of fear having been reduced.

In addition to these general sweeps, a more concentrated hunt centres round the contacts of any case, whether adult or child. If the patient is an adult, the search is to discover those to whom he has given the disease. If the patient is a child, it is a matter of discovering from whom he has caught it. A positive tuberculin test in a child, despite the absence of activity, should still stimulate a hunt for contacts. The wider the net is cast, the greater the chance of success and it must go far outside the immediate relatives. The school teacher and the lodger should be suspect and, in view of their close contact with children, school teachers should be required to have regular X-rays. The younger the child with tuberculosis, the greater the chance that the primary source of infection will be discovered because the number of contacts is less and the intimacy of contact greater. When the patient is under 1 year of age it is usual for a contact to be found in over 90 per cent of cases. Very detailed information of the child's recent movements must be obtained; sitting on the bed of an unsuspected patient for half an hour is long enough for infection to occur.

## Milk

All the herds in Great Britain have now reached the tuberculin tested (TT) standard. Testing of cattle continues and the occasional reactor is discovered. In 1974, 0·034 per cent of those tested were positive. Tuberculosis in cattle has not, therefore, been totally eradicated so that milk should still be pastuerized. Milk for feeds should also be boiled until the child is 1 year old in case other bacteria have been introduced in the home.

**BCG vaccination**

Bacille Calmette-Guérin is a strain of tubercle bacillus which was attenuated by Calmette and Guérin by growth on a special medium until it became avirulent. Vaccination with this material protects against infection from human and bovine tuberculosis.

When the tuberculosis rate in a country is high, as in most tropical countries, all newborn babies should be vaccinated. If the tuberculosis rate is low, vaccination is given in later childhood to those whose tuberculin test is negative. BCG can be safely given to those who are tuberculin positive, but preliminary testing is useful for its epidemiological information. Late BCG vaccination avoids its higher complication rate in infancy and maintains the tuberculin test as an epidemiological tool. The most practical age for this vaccination is 11 years, thus ensuring protection before the higher risk period of adolescence. BCG should also be given to those at special risk, such as diabetics, hospital workers and contacts, who are found to be tuberculin negative. In view of the high incidence of TB among immigrants it is wise to regard all their children as contacts to whom BCG should be given. When vaccination is undertaken during infancy no preliminary tuberculin testing is required.

A freeze-dried vaccine is now available which maintains its activity for a year, if kept in a refrigerator, and obviates the problem of the short life of the liquid preparations. The vaccine is injected intradermally. It is wise to keep the right arm for BCG vaccination since no other injections should be given into the arm for 6 months in order to reduce the risk of axillary adenitis. Moreover, international use of the right arm for BCG and the left arm for smallpox vaccination allows immediate identification of past vaccination procedures. After 3–6 weeks a small red papule appears which, in most cases, breaks down to a shallow ulcer after 4 weeks. Healing is slow and may take as long as a year, leaving a small puckered scar. Occasionally, painless axillary adenitis develops which may break down to form an abscess. These abscesses should not be incised as they are liable to leave a discharging sinus. Even aspiration should be undertaken only if they are very large; usually they are best left alone. If an indolent ulcer develops, para-aminosalicylic acid ointment will hasten healing.

Provided a highly effective vaccine is used, the degree of immunity conferred by BCG vaccination is not dependent on the degree of sensitivity produced by the vaccine (Hart et al., 1967). Such a vaccine produces a high degree of protection—in the order of 80 per cent. It is therefore unnecessary to test for tuberculin sensitivity after vaccination, and revaccination after sensitivity has waned is also probably unnecessary.

An isoniazid-resistant BCG has now been developed which is of great value in countries where breast feeding is essential for the survival of newborn infants. By this means the baby of a mother with open tuberculosis can be protected with ioniazid (INH) and INH-resistant BCG, and breast feeding permitted. The ioniazid (INH) should be given to the baby from birth and he should be vaccinated as soon as possible with INH-resistant BCG. The mother should receive full anti-tuberculous treatment, the baby being isolated from her for the first 48 hours to allow the protective blood level of INH to be reached. Thereafter, feeding at the breast is permitted, INH being continued until Mantoux conversion has occurred. In some developing countries INH-resistant BCG is still not available. Where this is the situation, and because in such countries it is essential to maintain breast feeding, the baby should be given INH by mouth until the mother's TB has healed. The baby should then be vaccinated with ordinary BCG.

It must be emphasized that BCG vaccination cannot produce complete immunity to tuberculosis any more than can a subclinical infection. It is only one weapon in the fight against tuberculosis and should be used only in combination with all the other measures. Antagonism to routine BCG vaccination exists in some quarters where fears are expressed that this might lead to loss of emphasis on case control and preventive measures, but there is no reason for this to occur.

## TREATMENT

### Specific

For regular use three drugs are available for the treatment of tuberculosis:

*Streptomycin.* Dosage 40 mg per kg (20 mg per lb) intramuscularly in one dose daily (maximum 1 g daily). Dihydrostreptomycin should never be used as it is too toxic to the auditory system.

*Isoniazid* (INH). Dosage 20 mg per kg (10 mg per lb) by mouth per day, preferably in one dose since this has been shown in adults to be more effective than half the same dose given twice daily. Maximum 400 mg daily. The drug may cause peripheral neuritis. This complication is commoner in adults than in children; to reduce its risk pyridoxine should be given as well.

*Sodium para-aminosalicylate* (PAS). Dosage 200 mg per kg (100 mg per lb) per day in three to four doses. Maximum 12 g.

Not less than two drugs in combination should be used owing to the risk that resistant strains of tubercle bacilli will emerge. The chief function of PAS is to reduce this risk, having little therapeutic value on its own. PAS is very liable to cause nausea and vomiting. For this reason the dosage given above is a little lower than is sometimes recommended, but it is still effective. INH should always be one of the drugs in any combination since its action is more rapid than either of the other two. The dosage of 20 mg per kg given above is higher than is sometimes recommended, but this is because it is such an effective drug and is relatively non-toxic. In children, the present tendency is to increase the amount of INH and to reduce the amount of PAS.

The direct effect of PAS and INH on the primary lesion is limited, but they hasten the rate of healing to some extent, relieve the systemic symptoms and return the child to his normal vigour. Their unique ability is the prevention of haematogenous dissemination. As the risk of haematogenous dissemination from a primary complex occurs during the first 2 years, PAS and INH should be given to all cases of primary tuberculosis for 2 years. A problem arises where a child is found to have a positive tuberculin test but a normal chest X-ray and no other evidence of active tuberculosis. For such cases no dogmatic advice can be given, but the physician must attempt to assess the risk of possible haematogenous dissemination. If the patient is under 2 years of age, the chance that this is a recent infection is great and it is best to give PAS and INH for a year and to repeat the chest X-ray at intervals. If he is a child of 10 years, it is probable that the infection took place some time previously, prophylactic therapy being unnecessary. However, in such a case routine chest films should be taken during a long follow-up period which covers adolescence.

Streptomycin should be given in addition to PAS and INH in all cases of miliary tuberculosis and meningitis and in any other severe cases of renal, bone or joint involvement. The duration of streptomycin therapy varies with the individual case but 3 months is usually sufficient. Before INH was available, streptomycin was also given intrathecally but this is no longer necessary.

Steroid therapy, in combination with the other three drugs, is often used in cases of tuberculous meningitis during the early weeks. It reduces the inflammatory reaction and exudate, thereby lessening the chance of a blockage of cerebrospinal fluid. Steroids may be used as an adjuvant in the treatment of a tuberculous pleural effusion in order to reduce the incidence of adhesions. The therapeutic role of steroid therapy in the management of primary intrathoracic tuberculosis is still unproven.

A number of new drugs have been developed and these are available for use in cases where resistance to the standard three agents has developed. Rifampicin is an alternative to streptomycin and has the advantage that it is given by mouth. Its disadvantages are its greater expense and a degree of hepatic toxicity. Thiacetazone can be used as an alternative to PAS and has the great advantage for developing countries of being much cheaper. Its dose is critical, the therapeutic dose being near the toxic level. Ethambutol is another alternative to PAS and is less liable to cause nausea and vomiting. Other drugs include viomycin, cycloserine, pyrazinamide and ethionamide. Viomycin is toxic and must never be used in combination with streptomycin owing to the greatly increased danger of damage to the eighth nerve.

Of particular importance in developing countries is the need, at the start of treatment, to correct any anaemia present and to eradicate any intestinal parasites.

## General management

Since tuberculosis in children is entirely different from the disease in adults, it is wrong to apply uncritically the same methods of therapy. This applies particularly to the question of bed rest which may be of value in adult tuberculosis but there is no evidence that such is the case with children. The modern approach to the question of bed in the management of any sick child is that if the child feels well enough to get up, there must be some positive reason for making him stay in bed. In primary tuberculosis a child should be allowed up as soon as he feels like it. In Nigeria, where almost all cases are treated as out-patients, the speed of recovery is remarkable and many more children in Great Britain could be treated in the same way. Good food and good home conditions are ideal, but intensive research in Madras (*Lancet*, 1961) has shown that tuberculosis can be treated effectively by chemotherapy alone, even when the patient remains undernourished.

Another difference from adults is the duration of surveillance. It is reasonable to say of an adult that if his disease has been quiescent for 5 years he has 'recovered'; to do the same for a child could be extremely dangerous. To stop supervising a child of 11 years because his disease has been quiescent for 5 years entirely disregards the fact that he is just about to start his puberty growth spurt and run the risk of developing adult tuberculosis. All children with a positive test from a natural infection should be followed through adolescence.

A further difference in emphasis is that, whereas in adults the aim is towards radiographic improvement and negative sputum, in children improved methods of treatment will show their greatest effect by a reduction in the expected rate of haematogenous complications. Apart from the absence of complications, progress under treatment is assessed by the general health of the child as determined by his appearance, energy and weight, as well as by radiographic improvement. The sedimentation rate is of little or no value.

A constant problem is whether children in hospital with primary tuberculosis should be isolated (which they dislike) because of the risk of infection to others. In practice, these children are not infectious and large surveys of the hospital contacts of such patients have failed to show any transfer of infection. This is in line with the observation that a child with primary tuberculosis does not infect other members of his family. Despite these facts, many physicians prefer to isolate the children because of the theoretical risk of transfer of infection from a child with positive gastric washings. However, in hospital a far greater risk is the possibility that one of the parents visiting the child is the primary source of his infection, thereby putting the whole ward in danger. It should therefore be the rule to check that the parents are free of tuberculosis before permitting them to come into the ward.

### Regional treatment

INTRATHORACIC PRIMARY TUBERCULOSIS

The place of surgery in the early management of primary intrathoracic tuberculosis has diminished. Earlier work (Thomas, 1952) was carried out when only streptomycin and PAS were available. Long-term therapy with INH has now enhanced enormously the power of chemotherapy. Surgery should be considered in all cases of stridor or obstructive emphysema. Chemotherapy alone may be given for a few weeks in case there is a dramatic response, but bronchial and parenchymal damage will be permanent if the bronchial obstruction is allowed to remain for long.

In the later management of the disease, surgery is required for some cases of bronchiectasis following bronchial obstruction. The upper lobe is the common site of tuberculous bronchiectasis and, in this position, is usually asymptomatic because of drainage by gravity. Bronchiectasis in the middle and lower lobes, though less common, causes much more trouble. Broncho-scopy should be used as a diagnostic rather than a therapeutic weapon. Although the removal of caseous material and granulations blocking the lumen is sometimes performed by bronchoscopic suction, it is a waste of time, having no lasting effect.

CERVICAL ADENITIS

In view of the frequency of a primary tonsillar infection, most workers recommend tonsillectomy for patients with cervical adenitis. With chemo-therapy the glands may heal without tonsillectomy but the focus in the tonsil is liable to light up the glands later, particularly if a superadded streptococcal infection occurs. Adenoidectomy should be combined with tonsillectomy since the adenoids may be involved, though less often than the tonsils.

Block dissection of the glands is no longer practised, but surgery still has a place. Chemotherapy is given first to obtain maximal reduction in their size. The largest glands and their neighbours are then removed by careful dis-section. Since the largest gland is likely to be the primary node, chemotherapy should control the remainder. If the gland has already broken down when the child is first seen, it should be evacuated as thoroughly as possible through an incision.

## MENINGITIS

Early diagnosis is required in all forms of tuberculosis but in meningitis it is vital if treatment is to have the full chance of success. The most important prognostic factor is the degree of mental impairment at the start of therapy; if the child is unconscious when treatment is started there is a serious risk of residual brain damage. With early modern treatment the chances of full recovery are excellent, thus the cured but mentally defective and often para-lysed patient should be a figure of the past. The prognosis does not appear to be made worse by coincident miliary infection.

## MILIARY TUBERCULOSIS

Generalized miliary tuberculosis unassociated with TB meningitis is fortun-ately now a rare disease. The diagnosis is made by the characteristic snowstorm appearance of the chest X-ray and the presence of choroidal tubercles. These may be visible before the X-ray changes (p. 523).

With the introduction of antituberculous drugs, and especially since the start of INH therapy, the virtual 100 per cent mortality has been transformed to a virtual 100 per cent recovery (Lorber, 1966).

## SPINAL TUBERCULOSIS

One of the remarkable discoveries in Nigeria, born of necessity, is that with chemotherapy the results of treatment in uncomplicated cases are just as good if the child is ambulant as if he is put to bed for months on traction (Konstam, 1963; Konstam & Blesovsky, 1962). The fears that such treatment would lead to collapse of the vertebrae and paraplegia have not been realized, the final deformity being possibly less than that seen in patients treated along orthodox lines. In children with paraplegia the caseous material should be evacuated after removal of the vertebral transverse process and adjoining portion of rib. Such children are left in plaster for a month, by which time their paraplegia has improved; they are then started on ambulant therapy.

The application of these lessons to other forms of bone and joint tubercu-losis have still to be learnt, but they suggest that prolonged bed treatment is not required for pure bone lesions, and prolonged traction may not be needed in joint cases.

## Anonymous mycobacteria

In recent years attention has been focused on a group of anonymous (atypical) acid fast mycobacteria, previously regarded as non-pathogenic. These are a common cause of weakly positive tuberculin sensitivity but are neither a human nor a bovine strain. Separation is made on the basis of differential skin testing and on their cultural and biochemical characteristics. Patients with this form of tuberculin sensitivity have increased resistance to tuberculosis, indicating that the anonymous mycobacteria provide some protection against tuberculosis (Rees, 1969).

These anonymous mycobacteria are a common cause of mycobacterial cervical adenitis, indistinguishable clinically from that due to human or bovine tuberculosis. MacKellar *et al.* (1967) described 30 children under 8 years of age with superficial mycobacterial lymphadenitis, seen over a period of 7 years in Western Australia. Twenty-eight of these were infected with anonymous strains of mycobacteria and only 2 with *M. tuberculosis*. The organisms are resistant to anti-tuberculous drugs, treatment being surgical excision of the affected glands.

Man to man transmission of anonymous mycobacterial infection is very rare. Similarly, they seldom cause metastatic infection. Uncommonly they may cause a primary pulmonary complex, erythema nodosum and chronic bone disease (Krieger *et al.*, 1964).

## LEPROSY

This chronic disease is widespread in Africa and India. It particularly affects children, since they are more easily infected than adults. The disease is due to *Mycobacterium leprae* (Hansen's bacillus) which is difficult to study because it cannot be cultured and has only recently been successfully inoculated into animals, using the mouse foot pad.

Prolonged and intimate contact is necessary for the transfer of infection so that congenital leprosy does not occur. The incubation period is usually 2–4 years. It used to be thought that the infection was transmitted by direct person to person skin contact, but recent studies have shown that insignificant numbers of the bacilli are shed from the intact skin of lepromatous patients whereas large numbers are shed from the nose. The main source of infection is therefore the nose and not the skin (Rees & Meade, 1974).

Unfortunately, there is no skin test comparable to the tuberculin test to indicate susceptibility or previous infection. The lepromin test indicates potential resistance to the antigen; this is prepared from macerated tissue containing large numbers of bacilli. The test is negative in lepromatous leprosy and positive in the tuberculoid type.

### Types

The earliest variety is called *indeterminate leprosy*. Thereafter, the type of disease is determined by the body's resistance and therefore its reaction to the bacilli. If resistance is low there is free multiplication of the organisms with widespread dissemination causing *lepromatous leprosy*. If resistance is high there is intense cellular activity with minimal spread of bacteria resulting in *tuberculoid leprosy*. Cases of *borderline leprosy* exist between these two extremes. These types can be summarized:

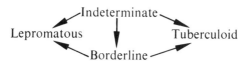

INDETERMINATE LEPROSY

These early signs occur anywhere on the skin. The lesions are slightly hypopigmented macules which sometimes correspond to an area where paraesthesiae are felt. There is no impairment of sensation.

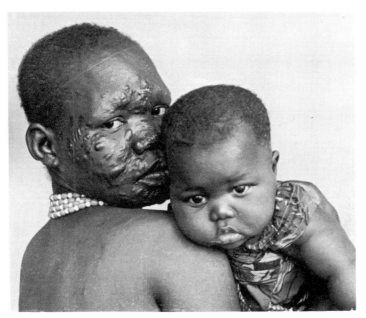

FIG. 121. Lepromatous leprosy. Numerous nodules present on the mother's face. The right ear is also involved. The baby is clinically unaffected, but the mother's milk contained large numbers of leprosy bacilli.

LEPROMATOUS LEPROSY (Fig. 121)

The early skin lesions are ill-defined, smooth, hypopigmented macules mainly over the trunk. Skin snips show these to be teeming with bacilli.

Infiltration is the feature of this type and it is this which leads to the production of nodules, especially on the face and earlobes, eventually creating the 'leonine facies'. There is generalized involvement of nerves but this is minimal in the early stages, in contrast to the tuberculoid type, so that anaesthesia is slight. Later there is increasing nerve involvement with enlargement and hardening of nerves which can be felt under the skin, and loss of function. Destruction of the autonomic pathways leads to loss of sweating. The mucosa of the nose, throat and eyes is frequently involved.

The bacilli pass rapidly to the lymph nodes and then by the blood stream to the eyes and testes, and to the liver, spleen and bone marrow.

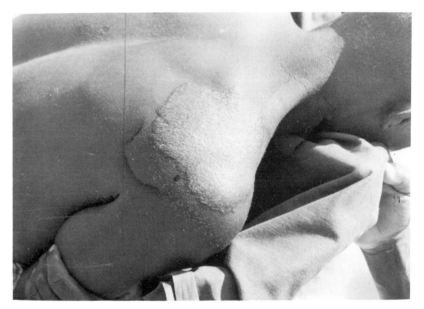

FIG. 122. Tuberculoid leprosy. Clearly demarcated hypopigmented lesion with raised border. The surface is rough and dry. No sweating occurred in the affected area which was also anaesthetic. This was the only skin lesion present.

## TUBERCULOID LEPROSY (Fig. 122)

The term 'tuberculoid' refers to the histological tubercles which are present in most lesions. Skin and nerves only are involved. The skin lesions are clearly demarcated, hypopigmented, anaesthetic areas with a raised border and saucer-like centre. The surface is often rough. The skin snip is negative for bacilli.

Nerves are involved early, becoming large and hard from the intense fibrous reaction and leading to paralysis of muscles and deformities, trophic changes and extensive anaesthesia.

BORDERLINE LEPROSY
This is an unstable form of the disease with skin lesions of both the main types present at the same time. The lepromin test may be positive or negative and may later reverse. Skin snips are always positive.

## Reactions in leprosy
It is these which cause the severe constitutional disturbances in patients with leprosy who otherwise remain reasonably fit. They occur more often in lepromatous leprosy, affecting over half the patients. This is due to the fact that bacilli are always multiplying and dying, thereby precipitating the antigen–antibody reaction. A reaction is often heralded by erythema nodosum.

In severe reactions the skin and eyes (especially iridocyclitis) become acutely inflamed and the nerves become swollen. Nerve damage is due much more to neuritis from reactions than from the bacilli themselves. Reactions in tuberculoid leprosy cause death of the nerve and the bacilli but reactions in lepromatous leprosy while causing death of nerve tissue allow the organisms to proliferate.

Reactions are caused by stress, hunger, alcohol, intercurrent infection and over-treatment.

## Diagnosis
*Tinea versicolor and Tinea circinata.* These cause itching and therefore scratch marks may be seen. It must be remembered that the patients who catch leprosy may not have the linguistic ability to differentiate itching from paraesthesiae which do not cause scratching. Scrapings will show the fungus.

*Vitiligo.* This may be difficult in the early stages. The patches are usually paler and may contain white hairs. There is no anaesthesia.

*Prophylaxis.* The availability of treatment has reversed the old policy of segregation which in any case was ineffective because persons with the early disease who were highly infectious often went into hiding. It was the improved socio-economic conditions which brought about the virtual disappearance of the disease from western countries, therefore these changes together with public education about the disease are required in those areas where the infection still occurs. Chemoprophylaxis with dapsone and BCG vaccination are additional weapons. The effectiveness of BCG varies in different areas, an 80 per cent protection being achieved in Uganda, 56 per cent in Papua New Guinea and zero in Burma (Browne, 1970).

*Treatment.* Patients should be isolated in hospital for the first few weeks. Dapsone is the best drug for individual and mass treatment, being relatively non-toxic and very cheap. It can be given by mouth, though an intramuscular preparation is also available. Lepromatous leprosy should be treated for life whereas the tuberculoid and borderline types are curable. Lepromatous skin lesions heal equally throughout the lesion whereas tuberculoid lesions heal from the centre.

Clofazimine is a new drug which is particularly useful in reactions since it suppresses these and is antibacterial. It is valuable for cases with dapsone resistant *M. leprae* and for severe lepromatous leprosy. Light-skinned patients should be warned that the drug may cause their skin to become reddish or violet. This is reversible, disappearing when the drug is stopped. Their urine and sweat may also become red. It is much more expensive than dapsone.

The treatment of reactions requires great skill. Mild reactions are handled by eliminating the precipitating factors and reducing the dose of drugs. Symptomatic treatment with analgesics and antihistamines are also used. Severe reactions require steroid therapy. A change to clofazimine will also help.


## CONGENITAL SYPHILIS

Recognition and treatment of syphilitic mothers in the antenatal period has now rendered congenital syphilis a rare disease. It is due to a spirochaete, *Treponema pallidum*, the mother herself always being infected. The infection of the fetus is acquired by placental transfer, occurring mainly during the second half of pregnancy; before then the relationship of placenta and fetus is insufficiently intimate to allow the infection to get across. In its most severe form the disease causes the infant to be stillborn.

The manifestations of congenital syphilis can be divided into the early signs, which occur during the first 3 months and correspond to secondary syphilis, and the later signs (juvenile congenital syphilis) which correspond to tertiary syphilis.

The more recent the mother's infection the worse the baby's disease— abortion, stillbirth or early congenital syphilis. On the other hand, if an untreated mother had a baby 2–5 years after her original infection, her baby would develop late congenital syphilis.

## Early congenital syphilis

The infant is commonly born prematurely, usually appearing normal at birth. The signs of infection develop from the age of 2 weeks to 3 months. The earlier the onset of signs the worse the prognosis. The child fails to thrive, the most obvious changes being oedema and a skin rash. The rash shows the typical characteristics of a secondary syphilitic lesion, being symmetrical, non-irritating and copper coloured. The lesions may be maculo-papular, bullous (pemphigus) or ulcerative; desquamation may occur on the palms and soles. Fissures occur round the mouth which, on healing, leave radiating scars termed 'rhagades'. Ulceration of the buccal mucous membrane may occur, whilst ulceration of the nasal mucous membrane causes the characteristic 'snuffles', subsequently leading to the saddle-shaped deformity of the nasal bridge from erosion of the cartilage. Condylomata may appear round the anus and vulva.

The effect on the liver is to produce a fine pericellular cirrhosis with consequent hepatomegaly and jaundice. The jaundice is not very deep but is characteristic of the disease. Splenomegaly occurs in almost all cases. Orchitis is occasionally found. Pneumonia alba occurs in the lungs of those stillborn or dying soon after birth.

The bone lesions are very typical so that the condition can sometimes be diagnosed by X-ray before clinical signs appear. There is widespread and usually symmetrical periostitis causing new bone formation and a double contour to the shaft. Parrot's nodes are bosses on the parietal bones resulting from periostitis. Osteochondritis results from erosion of the bone and occurs mainly at the ends of the long bones, the metaphysis being the chief seat of the changes. The upper limbs are more often affected than the lower and the associated tenderness may prevent the baby from moving the arm ('syphilitic pseudo-paralysis'). X-rays show a clear band of decalcification in the metaphysis near the end of the shaft, with a narrow dense line between this and the epiphysis. The epiphysis may be widened. Wimberger's sign is the symmetrical 'bite' out of the medial aspect of the upper end of the tibiae which can be seen on X-ray. It is due to an area of decalcification. Syphilitic dactylitis may occur, causing a painless fusiform swelling of one of the fingers or toes. Eye involvement is less common in early congenital syphilis than in the juvenile form, but disseminated choroiditis, iritis and optic neuritis occasionally occur. A moderate anaemia is found and numerous circulating erythroblasts are present.

Involvement of the central nervous system occurs early, so that a rise in cells and protein in the cerebrospinal fluid is common. Clinical manifestations of meningitis are less common; they indicate a very serious prognosis if present.

### Late congenital syphilis

The child is undersized, poorly nourished and with a sallow complexion. Stigmata of the early lesions, such as the depressed nasal bridge, rhagades and bossing may be present but do not necessarily indicate active disease. 'Hutchinson's teeth' are diagnostic and indicate the characteristic peg-shaped deformity of the upper central incisors of the permanent dentition. The tooth is wider at the alveolar margin than at the cutting edge and the crown may be notched. The first permanent molar may have multiple cusps (mulberry molar). The teeth in the first dentition may be poorly developed but show no specific change.

The destructive bone lesions of infancy have disappeared and the typical lesion is the 'sabre tibia' which occurs at any time after the third year. This is a smooth, fusiform cortical thickening of uniform density affecting a considerable length of the shaft, resulting from periosteal new bone formation and causing pain, particularly at night. Perforation of the palate or nasal septum may occur. The commonest joint affection is a painless symmetrical effusion into the knee joints (Clutton's joints).

Gummata may develop in the skin, liver, lungs or long bones. The spleen may be enlarged and nephritis may occur.

Interstitial keratitis is one of the more common lesions; it is often bilateral. It usually develops between the ages of 6 and 12 years, the first sign being clouding of the cornea associated with conjunctivitis and ciliary injection. Lacrimation and photophobia are intense. The cornea may become completely opaque, resulting in total blindness.

Involvement of the central nervous system is common, being due to meningo-vascular syphilis. The disease spreads slowly causing mental retardation, convulsions, paralyses, hydrocephalus and optic atrophy. The cerebrospinal fluid shows a rise in cells and protein. The serological reactions are positive and there is a paretic colloidal gold curve. Deafness is due either to disease of the nerve or to compression of the nerve from temporal bone disease. The heart and blood vessels are seldom affected in children.

*Diagnosis.* Material from skin or mucous membrane lesions should be examined for *Treponema*. Wassermann, Kahn and *Treponema* immobilization tests should be performed on the infant's blood, but a negative test at birth does not exclude the disease since the test may remain negative for up to 6 months. After 6 months of age it is always positive in untreated cases. A positive test at birth does not necessarily mean that the child has syphilis, since antibodies are transferred across the placenta from the mother and may remain in the child's circulation for about 3 months. The infant must therefore be reviewed in the light of the mother's serological tests. Provided the baby looks well at birth he should be kept under close supervision without treatment. If he remains well and his test is negative at 6 months no treatment will be required. The characteristic X-ray changes are seen in most of the infantile cases.

*Treatment.* Early treatment is essential, intramuscular penicillin being the drug of choice. 250,000 units 6-hourly for 8 days is effective and routine surveillance and serological tests should be carried out for the next 2 years.

## TOXOPLASMOSIS

This disease is due to a unicellular protozoan, *Toxoplasma gondii*, which has a wide geographical distribution and a remarkably wide host range. It is capable of infecting all mammals, many birds and some reptiles; probably the same species of *Toxoplasma* is responsible in all instances. Serological tests in this country suggest that between 20 and 40 per cent of the population have been infected and yet, despite this quite extraordinarily high incidence, clinical manifestations of the disease are rare because the toxoplasma seldom does harm. The fetus is the most susceptible to the disease, therefore the congenital form is the most easily recognized and the most dangerous.

### Congenital toxoplasmosis

Infection is transmitted from the mother who must herself have been very recently infected, since otherwise she would have developed sufficient antibodies to protect the fetus. It appears likely that maternal infection must occur during the second half of pregnancy when the parasites can get through the placenta—as in the case of congenital syphilis. It is exceptional for the mother to have shown any symptoms suggestive of a primary infection. Antibodies remain in her circulation but there is no risk of infection of the fetus in subsequent pregnancies. The incidence of the infection as a cause of stillbirth is not known, but it may be an important cause.

*Clinical features.* Signs of the disease may be present but may be delayed for up to 6 weeks. The brain and the eye are principally affected. Widespread areas of necrosis develop within the brain which is sometimes converted to a necrotic gelatinous mass. Suppuration does not occur but the necrotic areas eventually calcify. Hydrocephalus is very common and, though some of the patients are microcephalic, internal hydrocephalus is present even in these. Convulsions are frequent and spastic paralysis may develop. Cerebral calcification occurs in multiple linear specks which may be present at birth. The cerebrospinal fluid is characteristically yellow with a very high protein content but few leucocytes.

Bilateral choroidoretinitis is the most common ocular feature and, since this particularly affects the macular region, vision is defective or absent. The eye is small and abnormally retracted into the orbit; there is often nystagmus and squint.

Involvement of the brain and eye overshadows the effects on the other organs, but jaundice from pericellular fibrosis of the liver is common and may be associated with slight enlargement of the spleen. A haemorrhagic diathesis is frequent and purpura may be the presenting symptom. Myocarditis may also be present.

The infants may die shortly after birth or survive for many years, in which case they are very likely to be mentally defective as well as blind, and to have epilepsy. The effects of the disease are very similar to those of cytomegalic inclusion disease (p. 117) from which it must be differentiated.

### Acquired toxoplasmosis

Despite the fact that serological investigations demonstrate the widespread nature of the disease, its mode of transmission is still unknown. Domestic animals may be one source, toxoplasma having been found in their faeces, urine and saliva, but cases occur without any animal contact. Meat from sheep and pigs may be infected but would have to be eaten raw if the disease were to be transmitted. Toxoplasma has been found in the saliva of a patient and possibly this may turn out to be an important source of infection.

In the majority, the infection passes unrecognized but a number of clinical types can be recognized.

### Glandular toxoplasmosis

This is the commonest type of the disease, simulating glandular fever. It has the same age incidence, affecting mainly older children and young adults. Enlargement of the cervical glands is usually the first symptom, sore throat not being a prominent feature. Fatigue may be severe and there may be headache, limb pains and abdominal pains. An erythematous maculo-papular eruption may occur and the blood picture with atypical monocytes can be identical with glandular fever. The spleen is seldom enlarged. The Paul-Bunnell test is always negative and the patient makes a complete recovery. In view of their similarity to glandular fever, it is advisable to perform tests for toxoplasmosis and cytomegalovirus on all patients with suspected glandular fever where the Paul-Bunnell test is negative.

### Meningo-encephalitis

This form of the disease occurs particularly in late childhood, presenting with headache, vomiting and often convulsions so that an intracranial tumour may be suspected. Enlargement of the lymph glands and spleen may occur.

There may be a rise of monocytes in the cerebrospinal fluid and toxoplasma has been found in the fluid.

In adults an acute typhus-like illness has been seen, associated with rigors and a maculo-papular rash; also a form of chronic encephalitis.

*Investigations.* During life toxoplasma has very rarely been demonstrated in the cerebrospinal fluid, but at post-mortem it may be found in direct smears and sections or by animal inoculation. The Sabin-Feldman dye test and a complement fixation test are two serological investigations which are available. They are often negative in the first few months of life, despite the presence of disease. A positive test may be due to passive maternal transfer. The interpretation of the test in the newborn requires the same considerations as the serological reactions in congenital syphilis. A toxoplasmin skin test is available but is used as an epidemiological tool rather than for diagnosis.

*Treatment.* Sulphadimidine and pyrimethamine should be used in combination. Sulphadimidine is given in full dosage (see p. 738) for 3–4 weeks. Pyrimethamine is given daily for 2 weeks in a dose of 10 mg for children under 8 years and 25–50 mg for those over 8 years.

## HISTOPLASMOSIS

This disease is caused by the fungus *Histoplasma capsulatum* and, although Europe appears to be free of the infection, it is prevalent in the Americas, particularly in the east-central area of the United States. The fungus has been isolated from a number of different animals, especially dogs and rodents, and also from the soil.

It enters the body through the mouth or nose to reach the intestines or lungs, or through the skin; an ulcerative lesion is produced at the site of entry. Once in the body the fungus has the unusual characteristic of becoming intracellular within the reticulo-endothelial system.

*Clinical features.* The most common form of the disease is the *benign form*. The patients are usually symptom-free, the diagnosis being made by a positive histoplasmin skin test. As in tuberculosis the patients with a positive test frequently give no history to suggest when the primary infection occurred, although they may show multiple small calcified shadows in the lungs and mediastinal glands. Scattered pulmonary infiltrations may be found in some patients with minimal or no symptoms; at a later date these areas of infiltration calcify, the patient remaining well.

The *fulminating form* of the disease principally affects young children, being often fatal. The onset is gradual, the child developing a febrile illness associated with loss of weight and anaemia. Since the fungus attacks the reticulo-endothelial system there is enlargement of the liver, spleen and lymph glands. Ulcerative lesions may develop in the mouth and intestines so that diarrhoea is a frequent symptom. Pulmonary infiltrations may be present. Leucopenia with a relative lymphocytosis is usual.

*Intermediate forms* of the disease are now being recognized. These consist either of ulceration of the skin or mucous membranes associated with lymph-gland enlargement, or pulmonary infiltration and enlarged mediastinal glands. Splenomegaly is usually present.

*Diagnosis.* In the benign form the diagnosis is made by a positive histo-plasmin skin test, especially in the presence of calcified shadows in the lungs. Calcification in tuberculosis is seldom generalized, but differentiation from the miliary calcification which is occasionally seen in tuberculosis can be made for certain only by the additional finding of a negative tuberculin test.

In the fulminating form the skin test will be negative in the early stages; a change to positive during the course of the illness is highly significant. The fungus may be visible within monocytes in blood and marrow smears or in biopsy material from lymph gland, liver, spleen or marrow. Alternatively it may be cultured from material from these sites.

*Treatment.* No treatment is required for the benign form of the disease. For the fulminating and intermediate cases, amphotericin B has been used with success. Unfortunately the drug has unpleasant side effects and must be continued for several weeks. In view of the response of some cases to sulphonamides (Tesh *et al.*, 1964), these drugs should be tried first.

## BIBLIOGRAPHY

BROWNE S.G. (1970) Leprosy: epidemiology and control. *Brit. J. Hosp. Med.*, **4**, 39.

GRIFFITH A.H., MARKS J. & RICHARDS M. (1963) Low-grade sensitivity to tuberculin in school children. *Tubercle, Lond.*, **44**, 135.

HART P.D'A., SUTHERLAND I. & THOMAS J. (1967). The immunity conferred by effective BCG and vole bacillus vaccines, in relation to individual variations in induced tuber-culin sensitivity and to technical variations in the vaccines. *Tubercle, Lond.*, **48**, 201.

KING M. (1966) Ed. *Medical care in developing countries.* Oxford University Press, Nairobi.

KONSTAM P.G. (1963) Spinal tuberculosis in Nigeria. *Ann. Roy. Coll. Surg. Engl.*, **32**, 99.

KONSTAM P.G. & BLESOVSKY A. (1962) The ambulant treatment of spinal tuberculosis. *Brit. J. Surg.*, **50**, 26.

KRIEGER I., HAHNE O.H. & WHITTEN C.F. (1964) Atypical mycobacteria as a probable cause of chronic bone disease. *J. Pediat.*, **65**, 340.

*Lancet* (1961) The Madras experiment. *Lancet* **2**, 532.

LORBER J. (1966) The long-term prognosis of generalised miliary tuberculosis in childhood. *Lancet*, **2**, 1447.

MACKELLAR A., HILTON H.B. & MASTERS P.L. (1967) Mycobacterial lymphadenitis in childhood. *Arch. Dis. Childh.*, **42**, 70.

MARSDEN H.B. & HYDE W.A. (1962) Anonymous mycobacteria in cervical adenitis. *Lancet*, **1**, 249.

MASTERS P.L. & SMYTH J.T. (1965) A double Mantoux test applied to screening children for mycobacterial infections: its value in distinguishing infections by anonymous strains. *Aust. Paed. J.*, **1**, 166.

MILLER F.J.W. (1970) Tuberculosis in children. In *Pediatric problems in developing countries*. Ed. Rao, P.T. Orient Longman's Ltd., Madras.

MILLER F.J.W., SEAL R.M.E. & TAYLOR M.D. (1963) *Tuberculosis in Children*. Churchill, London.

NYBOE J. (1960) The efficacy of the tuberculin test. *Bull. Wld. Hlth. Org.*, **22**, 5.

REES R.J.W. (1969) BCG vaccination in mycobacterial infections. *Brit. med. Bull.*, **25**, 183.

REES, R.J.W. & MEADE T.W. (1974) Comparison of the modes of spread and the incidence of tuberculosis and leprosy. *Lancet* **1**, 47.

TESH R.B., SHACKLETTE M.H., DIERCKS F.H. & HIRSCHL D. (1964) Histoplasmosis in children. *Pediatrics*, **33**, 894.

THOMAS D. (1952) Discussion on the fate of the tuberculous primary complex. *Proc. roy. Soc. Med.*, **45**, 743.

# CHAPTER 20

# DEFICIENCY DISEASES AND METABOLIC DISORDERS

## PROTEIN–CALORIE MALNUTRITION

The clinical picture resulting from starvation varies with the type of food deficiency. A diet lacking principally in calories, though also in protein, causes nutritional marasmus whereas a lack of protein alone causes kwashiorkor. These two disorders lie at opposite ends of the spectrum of malnutrition with intermediate cases—marasmic kwashiorkor—falling in between. The least severe form of malnutrition causes the child to be underweight with associated retardation of growth but without additional features. Oedema is universally present in kwashiorkor and serves to separate the types when taken with the weight loss. A simple classification has been suggested (*Lancet*, 1970).

*Underweight*: 60–80 per cent of expected weight. No oedema.

*Marasmus*: less than 60 per cent of expected weight. No oedema.

*Marasmic kwashiorkor*: less than 60 per cent of expected weight. Oedema present.

*Kwashiorkor*: 60–80 per cent of expected weight. Oedema present.

### Nutritional marasmus

This is much commoner than kwashiorkor although it has received less attention. It also carries a worse prognosis. It results from a constant pattern of early weaning, dirty and nutritionally unsound artificial feeding often compounded by starvation therapy for the frequent bouts of gastroenteritis. The harmful effects of 'resting' the gastrointestinal tract while diarrhoea persists has long been recognized, but doctors as well as grandmothers still prescribe rice water, barley water or weak tea for long periods, unaware of the dangers.

*Clinical features.* The children look like little old men, being grossly underweight and stunted in height. There is marked wasting of muscles and loss of subcutaneous fat so that the skin hangs in folds, though it is otherwise normal. In contrast with the apathy and anorexia of kwashiorkor, the marasmic child is alert and often anxious, and is also extremely hungry. The children are younger than those with kwashiorkor, being in their first year and often around 6 months. Anaemia is less than in kwashiorkor and hair changes are fewer.

### Kwashiorkor

This disorder was first described by Dr Cicely Williams in 1933 while working in the Gold Coast (Ghana) where she found it was already known in the vernacular as 'kwashiorkor', a Ga word meaning 'the deposed one'. This describes the effect on a child of the arrival of a new baby who deposes him both from his mother's breast and from her intimate affection. It is interesting that on the other side of Africa the Baganda people of Uganda call the same disease 'obwosi', meaning 'the disease your child gets when you become pregnant'.

The development of kwashiorkor is strongly connected with cultural patterns which vary greatly among different tribes. One almost constant feature is the belief that breast milk is harmful to the baby when a lactating woman becomes pregnant. So strong is this belief that a mother with plenty of milk is quite unable to put her starving, crying baby to her breast.

Kwashiorkor is not seen during the first 6 months of life when the baby is on the breast and there is sufficient milk. It is rare during the second 6 months of life since, although there may be insufficient breast milk and not enough supplements, there is usually sufficient to prevent kwashiorkor and the child is still secure in his mother's affection. Whether the disease develops during the second, third or fourth year depends to a considerable extent on local custom. For example, in some parts of East Africa children are sent away to stay with relatives when they are about a year old so that they are suddenly weaned and deprived of maternal affection. Such children develop kwashiorkor during their second year of life. On the other hand, in Nigeria, where children are not sent away and a gap of 2 years is left between the birth of subsequent children, the disease is often not seen until the age of 3–4 years. Urbanization is altering some of these traditional patterns causing kwashiorkor to occur earlier.

The onset of kwashiorkor is precipitated by a number of causes, particularly infection; measles, gastroenteritis and tuberculosis are the most important. Maternal deprivation removes not only the source of breast milk but also causes a psychological disorder, an understanding of which is essential for the prevention and treatment of the disease. The child becomes apathetic, losing the desire for food just at the time when he is expected to start feeding himself, so that a vicious circle is set up.

### Clinical features (Fig. 123)

The child is miserable, oedematous and with flaking, discoloured skin.

Retardation of growth may be partly obscured by the oedema. Misery and apathy predominate so that the child may sit all day with no interest in food or in his surroundings. Oedema from hypoalbuminaemia is most marked in the legs, feet and hands; ascites is less common. The moon-shaped face is a reflection of a rise in cortisol.

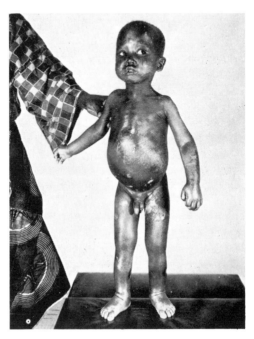

FIG. 123. Kwashiorkor. The child has generalized oedema and is apathetic. The skin is dry and flaky, showing areas of hyper- and hypopigmentation. The hair is scanty.

The skin becomes dry and flaky so that it peels, and there are areas of hyper- and hypopigmentation. These occur particularly on the legs and in the napkin area. If kwashiorkor has been precipitated by measles, skin involvement is more generalized, the desquamation of measles blending with the changes of kwashiorkor. If the amount of carbohydrate in the diet is very high, there is generalized puffiness but no skin changes; such children have been termed 'sugar babies' and have particularly low albumin levels.

The hair becomes brittle and is easily pulled out. It loses its normal lustre, becoming a lighter colour and sometimes red, although the incidence of red hair in kwashiorkor has been exaggerated. Some mothers, being worried by the light coloured hair dye it black. This could lead to diagnostic difficulties if other signs were not noted.

Diarrhoea is almost constant and often torrential. This is more chemical than infective. Villous atrophy in the jejunum causes a secondary disaccharidase deficiency, especially lactase. Lactose and sucrose cannot be split and therefore they remain in the intestinal lumen causing a severe osmotic diarrhoea with the appearance of lactic acid and sugar in the stools. Pancreatic atrophy is also a feature of kwashiorkor and increases the problem of malabsorption.

Fatty infiltration of the liver is a constant feature causing impaired carbohydrate metabolism and hepatic enlargement. Moderate hypoglycaemia is common but of little clinical significance provided the blood sugar remains above 20 mg per cent. Profound hypoglycaemia is a rare complication, but a very serious one occurring in association with hypothermia and severe infection when it is universally fatal (Wharton, 1970). Hypothermia is always a danger in these children since their metabolic rate is below normal so that they cannot respond to a fall in environmental temperature. Such a fall is particularly likely to occur on the first night in hospital when the child is no longer being warmed by his mother's body.

A common and unexplained feature is a non-specific swelling of the parotid glands. A bright red tongue and angular stomatitis indicate an associated deficiency of riboflavine and nicotinic acid. Secondary lack of these vitamins may account for some of the skin changes.

The serum proteins are low and there is a disproportionate loss of albumin. The fall in serum albumin triggers the many metabolic abnormalities which are a feature of severe kwashiorkor. The crucial figure for albumin is 3·0 g per cent. Once this is reached, insulin falls below normal whereas in the earlier stage it has been raised. Cortisol rises and moon face develops, followed by a rise in growth hormone. The pattern of serum aminoacids is altered and there is a fall in serum $\beta$-lipoprotein which is believed to be the primary cause of the fatty liver (Whitehead et al., 1973).

Normally a rise in growth hormone causes an increased urinary excretion of hydroxyproline but in kwashiorkor this falls from a lack of raw materials. The blood urea, serum cholesterol and potassium are reduced while sodium is retained.

Anaemia is always present but the haemoglobin does not fall appreciably until the serum albumin has reached 3·0 g per cent. Purpura in association with thrombocytopenia is a serious sign.

*Diagnosis.* There is usually no difficulty in making the diagnosis, the only condition likely to cause confusion being nephrosis because of the oedema. The difference is obvious once the urine is tested since it is loaded with protein in nephrosis, whereas in kwashiorkor proteinuria is never more than slight. Skin changes are not found in nephrosis and ascites is uncommon in kwashiorkor.

Severe hookworm infestation may be associated with oedema from gross anaemia, but the severity of the anaemia should lead to a correct diagnosis, although both conditions may be present.

## PREVENTION OF MALNUTRITION

Marasmus is on the increase as the scourge of bottle-feeding in the developing world takes increasing hold, leading to early weaning or no attempt at breast-feeding. The barrage of advertisements from the milk manufacturers are powerful. In one teaching hospital in Africa the staff permitted each mother on discharge to be given a baby's bottle and a packet of the donor's milk. The fall in breast-feeding among the educated classes is convincing the poorer classes that the advertisements are right and bottle-feeding is best.

On the other hand, kwashiorkor which is related to a more traditional way of life is becoming less common. The prevention of these two disorders does not require money but education. An increasing sense of responsibility is required from the educated classes, both native and expatriate, who by their own actions could do so much to influence a trend back to breast-feeding. This particularly applies to the prevention of marasmus. The approach to the prevention of kwashiorkor must be more subtle and requires great understanding of the people and their culture. The mother of the child with kwashiorkor becomes angry when told she has not been feeding her child properly, because in her mind the disease is not related to eating. Eating is required to satisfy hunger and her child has not gone hungry. He has always stopped crying after she has given him a meal of cassava or steamed plantain (matoke), and she is unaware of the meaning of the low protein content of these two widely used foods which have been the traditional basis of feeding for generations. She believes that so long as her child's stomach is full of food it does not matter what sort this is.

Beliefs exist in some countries that eggs, fish, chicken or mutton are harmful. These beliefs must be changed and education must involve both parents so that they choose to grow high-protein foods such as beans. In addition, the emotional aspects of the disorder must be explained in the hope that the custom of removing children from their homes will stop.

Failure of growth is an important indicator of impending malnutrition. For years Morley (1973) has been encouraging the use of simple growth charts which the mother keeps in a cellophane envelope, bringing it with her to the clinic on each visit.

TREATMENT OF MALNUTRITION

This not only involves recovery for the child but also a new understanding of nutrition by the mother so that her child does not relapse. Whenever possible the child should be treated as an outpatient in a nutrition unit. Admission to the ward and treatment with western 'medicines' only convinces a mother, particularly one whose child has kwashiorkor, that her child has a disease. Whereas if her child gets better as a result entirely of her own new methods of feeding she is much less likely to let him relapse, especially if she has learnt all this with a group of mothers whose children are similarly affected. Nutrition rehabilitation is group therapy in which the mothers of recovering children become the teachers of the new arrivals.

The child with marasmus does not have the metabolic disorder of kwashiorkor therefore his treatment is more straightforward. All children with kwashiorkor must be regarded as in potential danger from heart failure, resulting from fluid retention causing an increased load on an already weakened myocardium in the face of diminished oxygen carrying capacity of the blood due to haemodilation and anaemia. An injudicious intake of sodium may be sufficient to tip the balance. For this reason the intake of sodium should be limited to that in breast-milk—1 ml per kg. Transfusion of malnourished children should be avoided whenever possible since this increases the work load of the heart. Morever, the kidneys are unable to respond with an increased glomerular filtration rate.

The basis of treatment is a diet containing sufficient high-class protein and calories in order to restart growth, together with the correction of other deficiencies particularly potassium, magnesium (Cadell, 1965, 1967) folic acid and vitamin A. In addition, any associated infection must be diagnosed and treated. Initial feeds must be small since kwashiorkor causes a delay in gastric emptying time with increased risk of vomiting and aspiration of feeds. Tube feeding may be wise for the first few days since there must be no fasting at night.

This diet can best be provided by dried skimmed milk and calcium caseinate (Casilan) for the protein, together with sucrose and cottonseed oil for the bulk of the calories. Dried skimmed milk alone is unsatisfactory since it provides insufficient calories to prevent the protein from being used for energy production instead of body building. Moreover, there is a large amount of lactose in skimmed milk which by itself would lead to diarrhoea because of lactase deficiency.

Hypothermia is the great danger so that the children must be nursed away from draughts and not be bathed in the early days. Regular rectal temperatures must be taken throughout the night as well as the day using a low-reading thermometer. A careful watch must be kept on blood sugar levels using a 'Dextrostix'.

All children in endemic malarial areas should be given a course of chloroquine. Hookworm should be treated if present. Tuberculosis is difficult to diagnose in malnourished children because the tuberculin test may be negative. If the chest X-ray is suggestive even in the absence of confirmatory bacteriological evidence, antituberculous treatment must be started. Routine antibiotic therapy is unwise since it may produce side effects as well as a false sense of security. The essential is a diligent and continuous hunt for infecting organisms followed by appropriate therapy.

Rickets may exist in the presence of a normal alkaline phosphatase since this does not rise if serum proteins are low. It can only be excluded by an X-ray of the wrist.

Progress in malnutrition is assessed by height and weight increments together with the measurement of skin-folds whose increase in size is particularly useful in the assessment of improvement. The mother's attitude is decisive in the outcome for her child; if she is not interested little can be done, but if she shows affection towards her child there is hope even for the worst cases.

In the long term prognosis the main hazard is intellectual stunting (Cravioto et al., 1966; Winick, 1969; Dobbing, 1974). Carefully controlled studies have shown that children malnourished during the first two years of life become intellectually retarded (Hertzig et al., 1972). No difference in the ultimate deficit could be detected for children malnourished at different age periods during the first two years. This corresponds to the finding that the human brain growth spurt during postnatal life lasts for two years.

## VITAMIN-DEFICIENCY DISEASES

These result either from a deficiency of vitamins in the diet or from failure of absorption owing to an intestinal disorder such as coeliac disease. Special precautions to prevent them must be taken when using synthetic diets in the management of metabolic disorders such as phenylketonuria (Mann et al., 1965). A deficiency of one vitamin alone seldom occurs, except under experimental conditions. The diseases which are recognized as being due to vitamin deficiency indicate a severe lack, it being probable that unrecognized subclinical states of vitamin insufficiency exist. In children the commonest conditions seen are rickets from lack of vitamin D, and scurvy from lack of vitamin C.

## VITAMIN A

Vitamin A is fat soluble and is present in milk, butter, cheese, eggs, liver and fish-liver oils. Carotene is a precursor of vitamin A and is present particularly in carrots and tomatoes. The first clinical sign of vitamin A deficiency is night blindness, though this is often overlooked. It results from a failure of regeneration of visual purple in the outer end of the rods.

Vitamin A is required for normal epithelial growth, its lack resulting in keratinization. The skin becomes dry and scaly, it develops follicular hyper-keratosis and is more liable to infection. Keratinization of the epithelium of the eyes causes xerophthalmia. The conjunctiva becomes dry, wrinkled and shrunken, pearly spots (Bitot's spots) appearing on the scleral conjunctiva. In advanced cases keratomalacia occurs in which the cornea is softened and hazy and finally ulcerates.

Lack of vitamin A may cause failure of growth but this is probably secondary to infection rather than to any specific action on growth.

The daily requirements are 2000 units. For therapy 20,000–50,000 units should be given daily for 2 weeks in addition to a diet rich in the vitamin.

## VITAMIN B

This is a complex containing several components so that a number of different deficiency states can be recognized, although they are often associated.

### Vitamin B₁ (thiamine)

This is contained in meat, especially pork, liver, fish, eggs, milk, cheese, yeast, marmite, green vegetables and fruit.

BERI-BERI

This disease results from lack of thiamine. The onset, which may be acute in infants, is shown by anorexia, listlessness, irritability, vomiting and constipation, followed by oedema. The heart enlarges and signs of cardiac failure may develop rapidly. Neurological involvement is shown by aching muscles, paraesthesiae and peripheral neuritis.

Daily requirements are 0·4–1 mg. In treatment 10–50 mg daily should be given with a high-thiamine diet. In view of the risk of cardiac failure, the treatment of beri-beri should be regarded as an emergency.

### Vitamin B₂ (riboflavin)

This is contained in milk, meat, fish, eggs and wholemeal bread. Lack of the vitamin causes cheilosis whereby the epithelium at the angle of the mouth becomes thinned and macerated leading to superficial fissures. Fissures may also appear on the red margin of the lips and on the nasolabial folds. Characteristically, the tongue becomes magenta-coloured and there is flattening of the papillae. Vascularization of the cornea and interstitial keratitis occur causing photophobia and excessive lacrimation.

Daily requirements are 0·2–2 mg. For therapy 3–10 mg daily are required and the diet corrected.

### Nicotinic acid (niacin, pellagra-preventive factor)

The best sources are liver and meat, but it is also present in milk and whole wheat. Lack causes pellagra.

PELLAGRA

The early signs are anorexia, headache and weakness. A photosensitive dermatitis develops causing symmetrical skin lesions to appear on the exposed areas; these consist of a well-demarcated erythema which is orange-red at first and brown later. On the face this has a characteristic butterfly distribution over the cheeks and bridge of the nose; on the neck the lower margin takes the form of a necklace. The tongue is bright red and swollen; at first the papillae are hypertrophic, later becoming flat from atrophy. Vomiting and diarrhoea occur. Although mental symptoms, such as apathy, sleeplessness and delirium may develop, they are less common in children than in adults.

Daily requirements are 4–16 mg. Therapy requires 50–300 mg orally and an appropriate diet.

### Vitamin $B_6$ (pyridoxine)

Lack of pyridoxine is occasionally responsible for convulsions in infancy. In such cases the electroencephalogram can be seen to improve during intravenous administration of the vitamin (see p. 414).

### Vitamin $B_{12}$ (cyanocobalamine)

Deficiency causes a megaloblastic anaemia (see p. 590).

## VITAMIN C (ASCORBIC ACID)

This is contained in fruit juices and fresh green vegetables; its lack causes scurvy. Breast milk has a high content of vitamin C so that scurvy is extremely uncommon in breast-fed infants. On the other hand, even fresh cow's milk has only about one-quarter the amount of vitamin C that breast milk has, presumably because the calf is able to synthesize the vitamin; the amount in bottled cow's milk is very low.

### Scurvy

Deficiency of ascorbic acid causes increased capillary permeability with consequent haemorrhage. Bone formation ceases, but calcification of cartilage continues so that a dense line of calcification appears at the growing ends of the long bones. Delayed healing occurs since ascorbic acid is necessary for the repair of tissues.

Scurvy may occur at any age but is seen mainly in infants of 7–12 months of age. The limbs become acutely painful and tender from the haemorrhages under the tight periosteum, this being the chief feature of the disease. The child is irritable and very apprehensive when approached, from fear of pain on handling. He lies quite still ('pseudo-paralysis') since the slightest movement or even jogging of the bed causes pain. The limbs adopt the characteristic 'frog position' with the thighs abducted and the knees slightly flexed. Subperiosteal haemorrhages may be large enough to be palpable or even visible as swellings in the limb. The costochondral junctions become prominent, forming a 'rosary' from subluxation of the sternum at these joints. The rosary in scurvy differs from that in rickets. In scurvy it is angular and sharp because it is due to epiphysial separation of the upper ribs with backward displacement of the costosternal plate. In rickets it is dome-shaped and semicircular because it is due to expansion of the rib end.

Haemorrhages may be present in the skin or orbit and haematuria or melaena may occur. The gums become spongy and swollen, though bleeding occurs only if the teeth have erupted. Anaemia results from loss of blood but possibly also from a specific effect of vitamin C lack on the bone marrow (see p. 591). The anaemia may be megaloblastic and, although this is sometimes corrected by vitamin C, folic acid also may be required.

X-rays of the long bones show generalized osteoporosis. There is a characteristic dense line of calcification at the epiphysis, with a thin subepiphysial line of rarefaction; this represents a break in the continuity of bone and may be the site of epiphysial separation. The dense line of calcification is sometimes continued beyond the edge of the shaft to form a spur (Fig. 124). When healing occurs the subperiosteal haemorrhage calcifies, causing a very striking picture as it may involve the whole length of the shaft. Absorption of this calcified mass eventually occurs, leaving no deformity.

Red cells are almost always found on microscopic examination of the urine so that a normal urine is strong evidence against the diagnosis. Further confirmation of the diagnosis is provided by a saturation test in which a known quantity of ascorbic acid is given. The amount of ascorbic acid excreted in the urine is then determined; this is less in scurvy than in a normal individual because of the amount taken up by the body.

*Prophylaxis.* Infants require 30–50 mg of ascorbic acid daily and this must be supplied to all artificially fed babies, being most conveniently given as orange or rose-hip juice. It is a wise precaution to give the same supplement to breast-fed babies. Mothers should be specifically told not to boil the

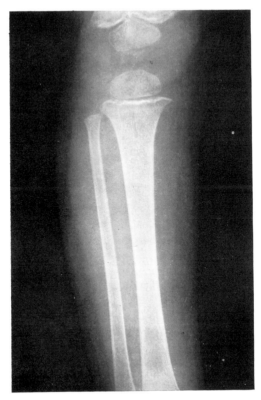

FIG. 124. Radiographic appearances in scurvy. There is a characteristic dense
line of calcification at the upper end of the tibia, extending medially to form
a short spur. A thin subepiphysial line of rarefaction lies just below this.

fruit juice since, having been so fully instructed about boiling the baby's milk,
it is understandable that some fall into the error of boiling the fruit juice as
well.

*Treatment.* 100–500 mg ascorbic acid daily or an equivalent amount from
fruit juice concentrates should be given. Nursing must be extremely gentle;
the child should not be taken out of the cot and a cradle should be provided
to keep the weight of the bed clothes off the legs. Wrapping the limbs in cotton
wool reduces some of the pain and analgesics may be required at first. Pain
is dramatically relieved within 1–2 days of starting ascorbic acid.


## VITAMIN D

This is fat soluble like vitamin A and its distribution in foods is similar, the chief source being fish-liver oils. It is also formed in the skin by the irradiation with ultra-violet light of sterols such as ergosterol. Vitamin D is present in milk but its content is very variable. The amount in milk is increased by the action of ultra-violet light, being at its lowest in the late winter.

Vitamin D is required for normal calcium and phosphorus metabolism. It aids their absorption from the bowel and is required for normal bone formation. Lack of vitamin D leads to rickets.

## Rickets

Lack of vitamin D causes a fall in blood phosphorus. In the early stages the calcium level does not fall since, although its absorption is affected, increased parathyroid activity maintains the normal serum calcium level. This is achieved at the expense of the bones from which calcium is withdrawn, with consequent osteoporosis. If this mechanism breaks down, the serum calcium level falls and tetany may result.

A knowledge of normal bone growth is necessary if the mechanism of vitamin D lack on bone development is to be understood. At the growing end of the bone there are four zones. In the first are resting cartilage cells. In the second these have arranged themselves in orderly columns. The third is the zone of preparatory calcification in which the cartilage cells have become swollen and degenerate; here the matrix is impregnated with calcium salts. In the fourth zone the spaces left by the degenerated cartilage cells are invaded by capillaries accompanied by osteoblasts which deposit a layer of osteoid on the calcified cartilaginous trabeculae. This osteoid is converted into bone by the deposition of calcium and phosphorus, the calcified cartilage being reabsorbed. As a result of these processes the zone of preparatory calcification lies between the layers of cartilage and osteoid, being seen as a straight line on the X-ray.

In rickets the cartilage cells fail to arrange themselves in columns, also they fail to undergo normal degeneration. Consequently, the invasion of capillaries occurs in an irregular manner. The matrix is not impregnated with calcium, and the osteoid, which remains uncalcified, is deposited irregularly. The result is a wide irregular zone of non-calcified cartilage and osteoid which has none of the rigidity of normal bone. Under normal circumstances bone is also formed under the periosteum, but in rickets a shell of osteoid is formed which surrounds the whole length of the shaft.

*Clinical features.* Rickets is more liable to occur in temperate climates than in the tropics since there is less ultra-violet light for the production of vitamin D in the skin. However, with improving diets rickets is now rare in England, except among the immigrant population. Presumably more cases are seen in developing countries because the effect of sunlight has been insufficient to compensate for the lack of vitamin D in the diet. The risk of rickets is particularly great if children in the tropics are brought up in a purdah household.

Rickets is a disorder of growing bones and therefore the bones affected in any patient are those which are growing fastest at the time of deficiency. On the other hand, if the child is not growing, rickets will not occur despite a lack of vitamin D. This situation is found in coeliac disease; these patients may develop rickets while being successfully treated, if they are not given extra vitamin D. Rickets is seldom seen during the first 3 months of life and mainly occurs between 6 months and 2 years of age. If it occurs in the first year, the skull is principally involved since it is growing the fastest. The excess of osteoid and non-calcified cartilage is heaped up, forming bosses over the frontal bones. Craniotabes indicates an abnormal softening of the skull bones which can often be indented; it is a common feature of rickets. There is also delay in closure of the anterior fontanelle.

The long bones are particularly affected from the second year onwards when they grow the fastest. Widening of the epiphyses at the wrists and ankles is visible and palpable (Fig. 125). The wrist deformity is increased by the pressure from crawling on the soft radius and ulna. Similarly, walking causes bowing of the long bones of the legs and a green-stick fracture may occur.

Prominence of the costochondral junctions results in the 'rickety rosary' and a wide Harrison's sulcus may develop with flaring of the costal margins (Fig. 126). The sternum may be depressed or excessively prominent (pigeon-chest). The spine may be deformed by kyphosis or scoliosis and deformities of the pelvis also result. Eruption of the teeth is delayed and dental caries is likely.

In addition to having bony deformities, children with rickets are fretful, hypotonic, pot-belled and have a tendency to head-sweating. They are often fat from excessive carbohydrates, since the vitamin D requirement of such babies is increased; consequently, their risk of a deficiency is greater. Sitting up and walking may be delayed; a child who develops rickets when he has already started to walk may go off his legs. Nasal catarrh and an iron-deficiency anaemia are common and the child is subject to attacks of bronchitis.

*Diagnosis.* Confirmation of rickets is obtained from X-rays, the changes being seen best at the wrist (Fig. 125). The lower ends of the radius and ulna are widened, cupped and indistinct. The appearance has been aptly likened to a frothing champagne glass. The distance between the epiphyses and the calcified portion of the shaft is greater than normal and, when healing takes place, irregular calcification occurs in the area. There is generalized osteo-porosis of bone and subperiosteal osteoid may produce a double contour along the shaft. The bone age is delayed.

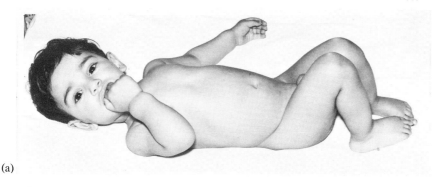

(a)

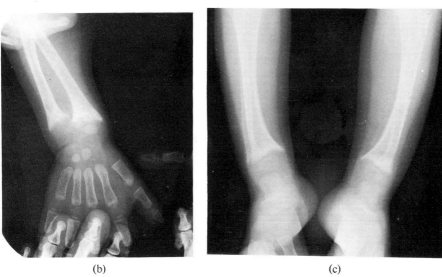

(b)                                    (c)

FIG. 125.
(a) Child aged 18 months with rickets. Widening of the wrists and ankles is apparent.
(b) The lower ends of the radius and ulna are widened, cupped and indistinct, causing the characteristic frothy champagne glass appearance. The bones are osteoporotic.
(c) Widening of the lower ends of the tibia and fibula is present.

The serum calcium is usually normal but the phosphorus is decreased and there is a considerable rise in the alkaline phosphatase, provided the child is not malnourished and therefore has low serum proteins (see p. 552). An increased urinary output of aminoacids occurs.

The mistake is sometimes made of diagnosing rickets in a child with simple

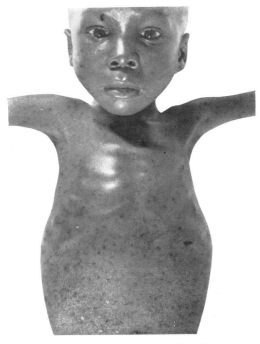

Fig. 126. Rickets. The prominent costochondral junctions have produced the 'rickety rosary'. (Note that the lower junctions are in the flanks; it is a common error to search for them too close to the midline.) The costal margins are flared.

bowing of the legs. A small degree of bowing is normal in toddlers, though this may be increased by the presence of bulky layers of napkin between the legs. Such children have none of the other manifestations of rickets, an X-ray showing normal bone growth.

*Prophylaxis.* Infants require 400 international units of vitamin D daily. Larger doses should not be given owing to the risk of hypercalcaemia (see p. 564). It should be given to artificially and breast-fed infants, being particularly important during the winter months when the vitamin D content of the milk is low and irradiation of the skin is less. All children should be exposed to sunlight whenever possible.

A new cause of rickets has now come to light—the disorder can be produced by prolonged administration of phenobarbitone or phenytoin in children with epilepsy. The anticonvulsant induces increased hepatic hydroxylase activity leading to inactivation of the vitamin D metabolites. Such children should therefore have regular estimations of calcium, phosphorus and alkaline phosphatase in order to detect the earliest evidence of this metabolic disorder.

*Treatment*. 10,000 units of vitamin D daily is sufficient for cure and at least 1 pint of milk a day should be given to cover calcium requirements. No weight bearing should be permitted until there is satisfactory radiological evidence of healing.

INFANTILE TETANY

This occurs as a complication of severe rickets when the calcium level falls below 7 mg per cent. In the latent stage the increased neuromuscular activity can be elicited only by mechanical means. In Chvostek's sign, tapping the facial nerve in front of the ear causes contraction of the side of the mouth. In Trousseau's sign, carpal spasm is elicited by constriction of the arm for 2–3 minutes.

In manifest tetany there are spontaneous muscle twitchings and carpopedal spasm. The hand assumes the position of *main d'accoucheur* in which the fingers are flexed at the metacarpo-phalangeal joints but extended at the interphalangeal joints. The feet are extended and the toes flexed. Laryngeal spasm and convulsions may occur together with tetany; they comprise the condition called spasmophilia.

*Treatment*. Immediate treatment in severe cases consists of the intravenous administration of 5–10 ml of 10 per cent calcium gluconate which must be given very slowly (see p. 134). If there is time for oral calcium therapy, calcium chloride is the most efficient form and can be given in 1 g doses up to a total of 4–6 g daily.

## Rickets of renal origin

Cases of rickets occur, due to renal disorders, which do not respond to the ordinary curative doses of vitamin D. This disorder may be glomerular or tubular in origin and, to prevent confusion, it is preferable to speak of 'glomerular rickets' and 'tubular rickets' rather than 'renal rickets'.

GLOMERULAR RICKETS

This form is often referred to as 'renal rickets' or renal osteodystrophy and results from chronic glomerular insufficiency. It may be due to congenital malformations such as bilateral renal hypoplasia, severe renal infections or chronic glomerulonephritis. The impaired glomerular function causes retention of urea, phosphate and creatinine. Lowering of the blood calcium occurs secondarily to the raised phosphate, an important diagnostic difference from tubular rickets.

*Treatment*. The rickets can be cured only if successful treatment of the primary renal condition is possible. If this is impossible high doses of vitamin D may effect an improvement.

## TUBULAR RICKETS

In these cases there is only slight or no retention of urea and creatinine; phosphate is low. The prognosis and response to treatment is quite different from glomerular rickets. Defective tubular reabsorption of phosphate is common to all types of 'tubular rickets', these being differentiated on the basis of the additional defects of reabsorption. Rickets result from the low serum phosphate.

*Defective phosphate reabsorption ± defective glucose reabsorption.* In this type renal glycosuria may or may not be present but there is never proteinuria. The condition may be genetically determined. It is often described as 'vitamin D resistant rickets' since the condition is resistant to ordinary doses of vitamin D. This is an unsatisfactory term since, on this basis, rickets in association with coeliac disease or 'glomerular rickets' might equally be described as 'resistant'. A preferable term is 'vitamin D refractory rickets'. The condition responds to massive doses of vitamin D since this is able to increase the reabsorption of phosphate by the tubules. As much as 500,000 units daily, or even more may be required. The dose should be gradually increased from a starting dose of 15,000 units daily. A careful watch must be kept for toxic symptoms as the difference between a curative and toxic dose is far less than in simple rickets.

*Defective reabsorption of phosphate, glucose and aminoacids (De Toni-Debré-Fanconi syndrome).* This group differs from the previous one by the additional feature of aminoaciduria and often of proteinuria. It also may be genetically determined. The children usually present at the age of 1–2 years with anorexia and failure to gain weight. The clinical features are very similar to mild hypercalcaemia (p. 564) and to infantile renal acidosis (p. 565). The child is irritable and develops vomiting, thirst and constipation followed by the appearance of rickets. Polyuria may be found and is due to an associated failure of reabsorption of water. There may be bouts of fever for which no infective cause can be found and which are probably due to dehydration. Episodes of weakness, lethargy and even coma may occur. These are due to electrolyte disturbances and to a low serum potassium which eventually appears if there is an associated defect of potassium absorption.

Some cases are associated with acidosis from a tubular defect which prevents the formation of an acid urine. The clinical features of such cases are more severe and the prognosis worse.

Microdissection of the individual nephron in the De Toni-Debré-Fanconi syndrome has shown a narrow elongated neck at the junction of the glomerulus with the proximal convoluted tubule (Darmady & Stranack, 1955).

Cystinosis (see below) is the cause of a few cases in this group where deposition of cystine crystals in the tubules causes dysfunction.

*Renal tubular acidosis* (*Butler-Albright syndrome*). In these cases, the primary defect is an inability of the tubules to form an acid urine, thus causing an inadequate elimination of metabolic acids with consequent acidosis. Ammonia formation by the tubules may also be defective, thus increasing the degree of acidosis. The acidosis leads to an increased excretion of phosphate and lowering of the plasma phosphate. Acidosis also causes an increased excretion of fixed bases, of which the most important are calcium, sodium and potassium. In the late stages calcification occurs in the renal tubules (nephrocalcinosis).

Renal acidosis of infancy (see p. 565) differs from renal tubular acidosis in that bone disease is not seen and nephrocalcinosis is less common and less severe. The disease is self-limiting, this probably accounting for the differences since the biochemical findings may be identical.

*Treatment of tubular rickets.* The same principles of treatment apply to all three types. A high dose of vitamin D should be given to all and, in addition, alkali therapy to those with acidosis. Vitamin D should be started in a dose of 50,000 units daily and gradually increased until the serum phosphate has risen to about 3 mg per cent. The lowest maintenance dose should then be determined which will keep the phosphate at this level and achieve radiological healing. Doses as high as 500,000 units daily may be required, but the risks of toxicity are great and the mother must be warned to stop the drug if the child develops anorexia, nausea, polyuria and dysuria from excessive urinary calcium. The blood calcium must be estimated regularly and vitamin D stopped if this rises above 11 mg per cent.

If acidosis is present, sodium bicarbonate or sodium citrate should be given, Albright's solution (p. 566) being a suitable preparation. In these cases the dose of vitamin D should be left at 50,000 units daily until the acidosis has been corrected and the effects observed.

### Cystinosis (Lignac's disease)

This is a rare metabolic disorder which is usually inherited as a recessive characteristic. Cystine is deposited in the reticulo-endothelial system, especially in the liver, spleen, lymph glands and bone marrow. It is deposited also in the renal tubules; when this occurs the tubular damage causes the identical features of the De Toni-Debré-Fanconi syndrome. Cystine crystals can be demonstrated in the cornea by slit lamp and in the bone-marrow samples. Most patients die before the age of 10 years.

**Cystinuria**

This must be differentiated from cystinosis. The only abnormality is the presence of cystine and other characteristic aminoacids in the urine, with the consequent chance of forming cystine stones in the urinary tract. Cystine is not deposited in other tissues so that, apart from the problem of stones, there is no risk to life.

**Idiopathic hypercalcaemia**

Two varieties of hypercalcaemia are described in infancy: the 'mild' and the 'severe' (Schlesinger *et al.*, 1956). It is probable that these represent different degrees of severity of the same condition since intermediate examples have now been reported. However, there are advantages in keeping at present to the two descriptions since, in clear-cut cases, the features are quite different. The aetiology is not yet understood; possibly the same factors work differently in the two types.

*Aetiology.* There is no doubt that vitamin D is involved and it is suggested that the disorder results either from an excess in the diet or from hypersensitivity to the vitamin, though probably both these mechanisms occur. In England, during the 1950's, doses of up to 4000 units daily were being given to normal babies as a result of fortification of milks and cereals (*Brit. med. J.*, 1960). Since this extra vitamin D has been removed and the amount in government cod liver oil reduced, the number of cases has fallen considerably. Hypersensitivity, as an additional factor, is suggested by the fact that only a small proportion of the babies who received these large doses developed any symptoms. Moreover, cases have been reported where, on a calcium-free diet, improvement occurred and the plasma calcium became normal but, whenever even a small dose of vitamin D was given, an exacerbation occurred.

However, neither excessive ingestion nor specific hypersensitivity explain all the features. It appears probable that small doses of vitamin D can produce hypercalcaemia only in those babies who have an inborn defect in the metabolism of the vitamin.

'MILD' IDIOPATHIC HYPERCALCAEMIA

The onset of symptoms occurs between the ages of 3 and 9 months when the infants are fed on cow's milk; this has a considerably higher calcium content than breast milk. Anorexia and irritability are the first symptoms, the child going off solids but at first continuing to accept milk. Soon he begins to refuse milk also but remains thirsty for clear fluids. This is followed by vomiting, constipation and often polyuria, so that the babies become wasted and sometimes dehydrated. The serum calcium and blood urea are raised but normal levels of phosphorus, phosphatase, chloride and bicarbonate are found. The plasma protein is raised, the increase being in the alpha 2 and gammaglobulin fractions. Nephrocalcinosis may be visible on X-ray. The urine may contain a trace of protein and a few white cells but the culture is sterile.

*Diagnosis*. The condition is most likely to be mistaken for a simple feeding difficulty, but the early history that solids were refused before milk and that thirst developed is very characteristic. Biochemical investigations will always settle the diagnosis. An erroneous diagnosis of pyelonephritis may be made on the urinary findings of protein and white cells, but the sterile culture and the other features of hypercalcaemia should prevent this mistake.

*Treatment*. The infants should be given a low-calcium diet; special low-calcium milk and cereal preparations are available. These should be made up with distilled water, as tap water may contain a considerable amount of calcium. No vitamin D should be given and the child should return to a normal diet only when the serum calcium and blood urea have fallen to normal, the alkaline phosphatase has risen above normal and there is a steady gain in weight. When a return has been made to a normal diet, not more than 400 units of vitamin D daily should be given, a careful check being kept on the serum calcium levels.

'SEVERE' IDIOPATHIC HYPERCALCAEMIA

In the severe cases there are additional features to those seen in the mild form. The children are both physically and mentally retarded and very irritable. They have characteristic facies described as 'elfin', in which the epicanthic folds are exaggerated and the nose retroussé. A squint is common and the lower lip hangs loosely. Hypertension occurs and a systolic murmur, which may be loud, is often present. Osteosclerosis occurs, causing an increase of density at the base of the skull and the ends of the long bones.

Investigations show a variable degree of renal impairment, the blood urea is raised, while protein and white cells are present in the urine. The serum calcium is always raised and the blood cholesterol frequently so.

*Treatment*. In the severe cases it is wise to give cortisone in addition to a low-calcium diet. Cortisone is a direct antagonist to vitamin D; it decreases the absorption of calcium so that a much more rapid fall in calcium is achieved. The prognosis for mental retardation and renal impairment is bad and the only hope is that cortisone used early may improve the children's future.

## Infantile renal acidosis

In this condition the tubules are unable to conserve bicarbonate, probably due to a deficiency of carbonic anhydrase. The condition is almost certainly due to mercury intolerance (MacGregor & Rayner, 1964; Husband &

McKellar, 1970). This would explain the declining incidence of the disease now that mercury has been eliminated from teething powders, but care must still be taken to avoid skin preparations containing mercury, especially in the treatment of napkin rashes. The age incidence and symptoms are identical with those of mild idiopathic hypercalcaemia (see p. 564).

Diagnosis is made by finding a persistently alkaline urine in the presence of a low plasma bicarbonate. The plasma chloride is high and the blood urea may be slightly raised. In a few cases the serum calcium is raised. Nephrocalcinosis may occur and, occasionally, the deposits of calcium may be sufficiently dense to show on a plain film of the abdomen. White cells may be present in the urine; the condition must be differentiated from pyelonephritis.

*Treatment.* Alkali therapy should be given to all patients, although mild cases may undergo spontaneous recovery. Albright's solution (sodium citrate 100 g, citric acid 60 g, water 1000 ml) is the most satisfactory form of alkali, starting with 15 ml three times daily and increasing gradually to as high as 60 ml three times daily if necessary. The dose is estimated from the serum bicarbonate level. When this and the clinical state have been normal for a month, the amount of alkali is slowly reduced while repeated checks on the bicarbonate level are made.

Tubular dysfunction is temporary only, since recovery continues after withdrawal of the alkali. No significant renal damage occurs even if nephrocalcinosis is present.

### Hypophosphatasia

This is a rare disease due to an inborn error of metabolism which is inherited as a recessive characteristic. The essential biochemical abnormality is a low or even absent alkaline phosphatase. All the tissues which normally produce phosphatase are involved but, from a clinical point of view, it is the skeletal tissues which are the problem since the osteoblasts and the hypertrophic chondrocytes are the principal source of phosphatase. An increased urinary excretion of phosphoethanolamine occurs and this finding, as well as a lowered alkaline phosphatase, has been shown in some of the parents, indicating the existence of a carrier state.

*Clinical features.* The majority of patients present in infancy and the bone lesions may be present at birth. Failure to thrive is the essential feature. There is anorexia, vomiting, irritability and intermittent fever. These symptoms are probably due to the associated hypercalcaemia. The fontanelle is often tense and bulging at first; this may be followed by premature fusion of the sutures (craniosynostosis). Congenital bowing of the long bones is sometimes associated as are congenital skin dimples on the limbs. The skeletal lesions resemble rickets and X-rays show grossly defective calcification so that the zone of provisional calcification disappears, irregular calcification only occurring in the metaphysis. Irregular formation of new bone may occur under the periosteum. The teeth are hypoplastic, often being lost early. Renal impairment may result from hypercalcaemia.

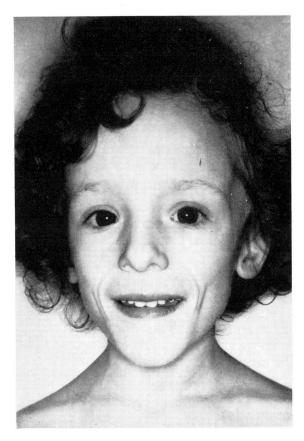

FIG. 127. Lipodystrophia progressiva in a girl aged 4 years. Loss of subcutaneous fat has led to hollow cheeks and an emaciated appearance.

*Treatment and prognosis.* A low-calcium diet should be given and although high doses of vitamin D have been used, the risks from hypercalcaemia make this a dangerous form of therapy, cortisone being safer. Craniectomy is required for craniosynostosis.

The prognosis is poor in cases presenting early, owing to hypercalcaemia and renal damage. In less severe cases, there is a tendency to improve during the first and second years of life; considerable healing of bone occurs although the low level of phosphatase persists.

## Lipodystrophia progressiva (Fig. 127)

In this disorder, which is of unknown aetiology, there is a progressive loss of subcutaneous fat from the face and upper part of the body, leading to an appearance of extreme emaciation. The diagnosis is easily made by the fact that the lower limbs remain normal and that, despite the facial appearance of ill health, the child continues to be well. The condition is more common in girls than boys, usually commencing in middle childhood.

# DISORDERS OF AMINOACID METABOLISM

## Phenylketonuria

In these patients the enzyme defect prevents the conversion of phenylalanine to tyrosine. A rise of phenylalanine occurs in the blood, its breakdown products, phenylpyruvic, phenyllactic and phenylacetic acids appearing in the urine. Mental defect results, either from the toxic effect of the excess phenylalanine or, more probably, from the accumulation of some phenylalanine metabolite. The incidence in the United States is 1 in 10,000 births (Hsia, 1966); the disease is transmitted by a recessive gene.

The babies seem normal at birth, but progressive mental deterioration occurs from the age of a few weeks. Vomiting, irritability and convulsions result from the accumulation of toxic metabolites. The children usually have fair hair, since tyrosine is required for melanin production, and blue eyes. Eczema is common. The incisors are widely spaced and the urine gives a musty smell from phenylacetic acid.

*Diagnosis.* Early diagnosis is essential in order to prevent mental retardation. All newborn babies should be screened on the 6th day of life using the Guthrie inhibition test (Guthrie & Susi, 1963) which detects a rise in serum phenylalanine. In this method, blood from a heel puncture is cultured with *B. subtilis* in media containing a growth inhibitor which is suppressed by phenylalanine; a positive test is therefore indicated by growth of the organism. The level of phenylalanine must be estimated quantitatively on all suspected cases and on the siblings of known cases.

*Treatment.* The child is given a low phenylalanine diet, the exact amount being determined by serial phenylalanine blood levels. Since this aminoacid is essential for growth it cannot be excluded completely but its level should be kept at 1·5–5 mg per cent. Escape from dietary control may occur during bouts of infection when a particular check on blood levels must be kept.

The duration of dietary control is still under investigation. It is probably safe to stop the diet when brain growth has been completed but pregnant women must return to a strict diet in order to avoid damage to the fetal brain.

### Maple syrup disease

The characteristic smell of the urine accounts for the name of this form of mental deficiency. The children become severely mentally handicapped and spastic, dying young. There is a multiple but patterned aminoaciduria involving valine, leucine and isoleucine. A special diet comprising synthetic aminoacids is required. This is more complicated than in phenylketonuria because each patient requires individual adjustment of the diet according to his metabolic pattern.

### Hartnup disease

This form of mental defect is named after the first family with the condition to be described. The defect is in tryptophan metabolism, appearing to be due to a specific defect in the transport of aminoacids in the cells of the jejunum and proximal renal tubules. The aminoaciduria is multiple but patterned. The mental defect comes on slowly and is not severe. In addition, there is photosensitivity which results in a pellagra-like rash, and cerebellar ataxia. Treatment with nicotinamide and a diet low in tryptophan may cause symptomatic improvement, although it does not alter the aminoaciduria.

### Homocystinuria

This is a more recently discovered inborn error of metabolism which, like the others, is also inherited on an autosomal recessive basis. The defect involves the metabolism of the essential aminoacid methionine leading to the urinary excretion of homocystine.

Children with this disorder are usually mentally handicapped and often suffer from convulsions. They are fair skinned with a malar flush. Many of the features of Marfan's syndrome (p. 235) are present: ocular defects, especially dislocation of the lens associated with iridodonesis; skeletal defects, especially arachnodactyly, chest deformities and a high arched palate. Thrombotic episodes, which do not occur in Marfan's syndrome, are a particular feature resulting from greatly increased platelet stickiness.

Since homocystinuria is a steadily progressive disease with the constant threat of thrombosis, treatment is worthwhile at any age. Pyridoxine may be sufficient to correct the metabolic defect; failing this the child should be given a low methionine diet with added cystine.

## DISORDERS OF CARBOHYDRATE METABOLISM

### Normal carbohydrate metabolism

All forms of carbohydrate must be reduced to monosaccharides since it is only in this form that they can be absorbed from the small intestine. The polysaccharides—starch and glycogen—are hydrolysed by salivary and pancreatic amylase to maltose and small quantities of isomaltose and glucose. Maltose and the other ingested disaccharides—lactose and sucrose—are hydrolysed to their component monosaccharides by a series of disaccharidase enzymes which are found in the brush border of the epithelial cells of the small intestine. The monosaccharides are then absorbed from the brush border into the mucosal cell by one of two methods. Glucose and galactose require active transport, the energy being supplied by the sodium pump. Fructose is passively absorbed by a diffusion process.

### Disaccharidase deficiencies

These may be primary or secondary. Primary deficiency involves either a combination of sucrase and isomaltase or a deficiency of lactase alone. Both are rare whereas secondary disaccharidase deficiencies are very common. This is understandable in view of their superficial location, the brush border, which is very liable to be damaged in diseases involving the intestine. This occurs in gastroenteritis, coeliac disease, kwashiorkor and lambliasis. It is also understandable that more than one enzyme is likely to be involved, although in practice lactase is the most severely reduced. This is particularly serious to a baby since lactose is the only disaccharide contained in human or cow's milk.

*Clinical features.* The established clinical picture is common to all types of disaccharidase deficiency though the onset will differ. Primary lactase deficiency causes symptoms from birth whereas sucrose–isomaltase deficiency will not show itself until sucrase is added to the diet. Secondary deficiencies cause a prolongation of symptoms, particularly diarrhoea, which begin with the onset of the causal disease. 'Chronic gastroenteritis' is almost always due to disaccharidase deficiency secondary to acute infection. The diarrhoea of kwashiorkor may have an infective element but a secondary disaccharidase deficiency is a far more important cause of the symptom; this knowledge is vital to the successful treatment of the disorder (pp. 549, 551).

Normally the absorption of the disaccharidases is completed in the upper jejunum. Since this is impossible the sugars pass along the small intestine acting as an osmotic agent and drawing fluid into the lumen of the bowel. This causes abdominal distension and an increase of peristalsis. In the lower ileum some of the sugar is fermented by intestinal bacteria to form lactic acid, carbon dioxide and water. This causes the stools to be gaseous and acid so that they severely excoriate the buttocks, increasing the infant's distress. The baby therefore fails to thrive, has abdominal distension, frothy diarrhoea and sore buttocks. Vomiting is not often a feature.

*Investigations.* The proof that the diarrhoea is due to malabsorption of sugar is made by demonstrating the acidity of the stool with pH papers. The pH is abnormally low if it is below 6. The presence of reducing substances is shown by a modification of the Clinitest method for urine. For these tests it is important that the stool is complete since the lactic acid and sugars are in the fluid part of the stool and this may have seeped into the napkin. This can be prevented by the use of a plastic liner. Since sucrose is not a reducing substance the stool must first be acidified with hydrochloric acid for its detection; any sucrose present is then hydrolysed.

An oral load of the appropriate disaccharide leads to a flat blood sugar curve. A normal response will be obtained when its component monosaccharides are given. Estimation of enzyme activity in an intestinal biopsy specimen may be required to prove a primary deficiency, but in a child with a secondary deficiency the clinical improvement after therapeutic exclusion of the appropriate disaccharidase is sufficient proof.

PRIMARY DISACCHARIDASE DEFICIENCY

*Sucrase–isomaltase deficiency*

This is the commoner variety, there being a combined defect of the two enzymes. An isolated defect of either of these has not been found. The clinical features described above commence when sucrose is introduced to the diet. Treatment requires a sucrose-free and low-starch diet.

*Hereditary alactasia and hypolactasia*

If there is total lack of lactase the symptoms are as already described but they start as soon as milk feeds are given. Hypolactasia has a racial incidence being particularly common in some negro tribes. It is much more common in the adults owing to a fall in lactase activity (Cook, 1967).

*Infantile lactase intolerance*

This is not due to a primary lactase deficiency and its cause is unknown. The infant becomes seriously ill in the first month of life with diarrhoea causing dehydration. There is evidence of renal tubular damage shown by aminoaciduria, lactosuria, glucosuria and sucrosuria.

A lactose-free diet is followed by recovery but the condition is not due to lactase deficiency since lactase activity returns when lactose is removed from the diet.

### Galactosaemia

This condition results from a deficiency of the enzyme galactose-1-phosphate uridyl transferase which is required for the conversion of galactose-1-phosphate into glucose-1-phosphate. An accumulation of glactose-1-phosphate

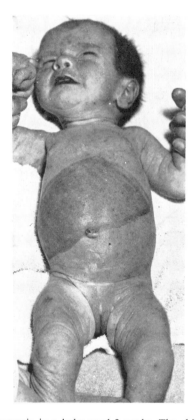

Fig. 128. Galactosaemia in a baby aged 2 weeks. The child was jaundiced and the liver, whose outline has been drawn in, much enlarged.

occurs which has a toxic action on the brain, lens, liver and kidney by inhibiting cell metabolism in these organs. The inhibition of carbohydrate metabolism in the liver leads to hypoglycaemia. The clinical features result from the damage to these organs and from hypoglycaemia. Galactose is formed in the body by the action of lactase on the lactose in milk, which for these patients, no matter what its source, acts as a poison.

*Clinical features.* The baby is normal at birth but within a few days of starting milk begins to vomit and to have diarrhoea, leading to progressive wasting. Jaundice develops at the end of the first or during the second week; this should not be confused with the more common causes of neonatal jaundice (p. 117) which occur sooner after birth. There is progressive enlargement of the liver, this being the most striking physical sign (Fig. 128). Hypoglycaemia causes lethargy, refusal to suck and may lead to convulsions.

Death may occur early. If the baby survives and is untreated, cataracts develop within a few weeks. There is also progressive mental retardation associated with retardation of growth.

Proteinuria and generalized aminoaciduria result from renal tubular damage. A reducing substance is present in the urine, shown by chromatography to be galactose.

The condition appears to be inherited as an autosomal recessive characteristic. The homozygous state is manifest clinically as galactosaemia, while the heterozygous state can be detected by an abnormal galactose tolerance curve. The enzyme defect can be demonstrated at birth in families at risk by making use of cord blood; if cord red cells are incubated in a medium containing galactose, there is an accumulation of galactose-1-phosphate.

*Treatment.* The child must immediately be placed on a diet from which lactose and galactose are excluded. Special milk substitutes are available.

*Prognosis.* With treatment, the acute symptoms from hypoglycaemia and the accumulation of galactose-1-phosphate, such as vomiting, diarrhoea, anorexia and lethargy disappear. Proteinuria and aminoaciduria also disappear at once. But mental retardation and cataract are irreversible and, for this reason, immediate diagnosis and treatment are essential if these complications are to be prevented.

### Fructosaemia

In many ways this condition resembles galactosaemia. It is due to a deficiency of hepatic fructose-1-phosphate splitting aldolase. When such patients are fed foods containing fructose or sucrose (which is converted to fructose) they develop severe hypoglycaemic attacks due to a secondary block in the release of hepatic glucose. The disorder is inherited as an autosomal, recessive characteristic.

The newborn baby remains perfectly well so long as he is fed only breast milk and is therefore not receiving fructose. When fed fructose or sucrose acute symptoms of hypoglycaemia (see p. 641) develop; these may be severe enough to lead to loss of consciousness and convulsions. The child fails to thrive and has a poor appetite associated with vomiting, hypotonia and hepatomegaly. If the child survives he is liable to become mentally retarded if hypoglycaemia has been prolonged. Older patients, who are usually found among the relatives of affected infants, have a strong aversion to sweet foods. By avoiding these they are able to remain perfectly well.

When estimating the blood sugar, the method used must be one which measures the true glucose level and not the total blood sugar which may not be much reduced. Due to an excessive accumulation of fructose-1-phosphate a proximal tubular defect occurs, causing proteinuria and aminoaciduria. These disappear as soon as fructose is omitted from the diet.

*Diagnosis.* This is made by an intravenous or oral fructose tolerance test which causes a fall in the blood glucose and serum inorganic phosphorus. Care should therefore be exercised and intravenous glucose may be required if hypoglycaemic symptoms develop.

Galactosaemia can be differentiated biochemically but, on clinical grounds, the major difference is that the baby with galactosaemia becomes acutely ill as soon as any milk is fed, whereas the baby with fructosaemia is normal while on breast milk.

*Essential fructosuria* is an entirely different condition, although it also causes fructosaemia and fructosuria. It is due to a deficiency of hepatic fructokinase but this does not result in hypoglycaemia. The condition causes no symptoms and is harmless.

*Treatment.* All foods containing fructose or sucrose must be excluded from the diet.

## Glycogen storage disease

In this disorder the body is unable to convert glycogen into glucose. It can be subdivided into a number of distinct groups, each characterized by a deficiency of a different enzyme along the pathway for the conversion of glycogen to glucose. Clinically, there are two main syndromes: hepatic glycogen disease, accounting for about 80 per cent of the cases, and the much more rare muscle glycogen disease.

HEPATIC GLYCOGEN STORAGE DISEASE (VON GIERKE'S DISEASE)

This is due to a deficiency of glucose-6-phosphatase. It is familial and probably inherited as a recessive characteristic. Hepatomegaly is present at birth but is not usually noticed since the child is otherwise well and is not jaundiced (in contradistinction to galactosaemia). The child presents during the first 2 years of life with failure to thrive, abdominal pain and progressive enlargement of the abdomen. Episodes of hypoglycaemia occur during periods of stress, causing vomiting, convulsions and sometimes loss of consciousness. Hyperglycaemia may also occur after meals because the liver cells are so filled with glycogen that they cannot absorb a sudden intake of glucose. Some of this unused glucose is converted to fat, accounting for the obesity shown by the patients. Owing to the overall lack of glucose there is excessive utilization of fat and protein, resulting in retardation of growth. The excessive metabolism of fat also causes acidosis from an accumulation of ketone bodies. Prothrombin deficiency may account for a bleeding tendency.

*Investigations.* The fasting blood sugar is low and there is no response to an injection of adrenaline or glucagon. The glucose tolerance curve is persistently high. Liver biopsy shows an increase in the amount of glycogen and is also used to demonstrate the specific enzyme defect.

*Treatment.* Symptomatic improvement can be achieved by adjusting the diet in order to maintain a reasonably constant flow of glucose into the blood and liver, so preventing hypoglycaemia and ketosis. Meals should be frequent and high in protein, the last being as late as possible or taken in the early hours of the morning. Steroid therapy may be of value since it increases the production of glucose from protein and fat.

## MUSCLE GLYCOGEN STORAGE DISEASE

The commonest form of this rare disorder is Pompe's disease due to a lack of acid maltase and affecting the heart and muscle. The patients present with heart failure in the early weeks of life. The condition should be suspected when this occurs in association with gross cardiac enlargement but no murmurs. Severe muscle weakness and hypotonia result from deposition of glycogen in skeletal muscles. The tongue also may be affected causing it to be thickened and protrude.

Mobilization of glycogen can be achieved so that hypoglycaemia does not occur. The prognosis is hopeless, the infants usually dying at about the age of 6 months.

# DISORDERS OF MUCOPOLYSACCHARIDES

## Gargoylism (Type 1 mucopolysaccharidosis, Hurler's syndrome)

This is due to an overproduction of certain acid mucopolysaccharides which are then stored in the body, causing the disorder. No physical abnormalities are present at birth, the diagnosis seldom being made before the age of 6 months. A grotesque facial appearance, associated with mental defect and dwarfism, gradually develops. The corneae are clouded (Fig. 130), the liver and spleen enlarged and an umbilical hernia is common. The umbilical hernia has not usually been present from birth and may be the reason for which the child is brought to the doctor. In the lateral X-ray of the spine is seen a beak-shaped deformity of one or two vertebrae, causing an angular kyphosis. Large quantities of chondroitin sulphate are found in the urine.

### Hunter's syndrome (Type 2 mucopolysaccharidosis)

Whereas in Hurler's type of gargoylism the disorder is inherited as an autosomal recessive trait, in this less frequent and separate type the condition is inherited as a sex-linked recessive trait so that boys only are affected. This type differs from the other in that the boys do not have clouded corneae (Fig. 129) and about half are deaf, whereas deafness seldom occurs in the other group.

There is no known treatment for the condition. Genetic counselling must be given (McKusick *et al.*, 1965).

### Morquio's syndrome (Type 4 mucopolysaccharidosis)

This type differs from the others in that skeletal deformities predominate and intelligence is normal. It is inherited as an autosomal recessive trait and is associated with the urinary excretion of keratosulphate.

The skeletal changes do not appear until after the first year. The neck becomes short, the chest barrel-shaped, the spine kyphotic and there is flattening of the lumbar vertebrae. This causes a semi-crouching stance and a waddling gait. The facial appearance is characteristic, the mouth being broad and the teeth widely spaced; the nose is short and the maxilla prominent. The wrists are enlarged and the fingers misshapen.

## DISORDERS OF LIPID METABOLISM

There are 4 major classes of serum lipids: cholesterol, phospholipids, triglycerides and non-esterified fatty acids. All are insoluble in water and therefore in order to be transported they are combined with proteins to form lipoproteins which are unloaded in the tissues. A number of hyperliproteinaemic and hypolipoproteinaemic states exist (Lloyd, 1968a, b). All are rare, but the most important disorder as far as children are concerned is familial hypercholesterolaemia, since in its heterozygous form, particularly, early diagnosis can prevent early death.

### Familial hypercholesterolaemia (Hyper-$\beta$-lipoproteinaemia)

This disorder is characterized by raised levels of $\beta$-lipoprotein, the form in which cholesterol is transported, and therefore by hypercholesterolaemia. It is inherited as an autosomal dominant with incomplete penetrance. The homozygous form of the disease is rare. It usually presents at the age of 2–3 years with the appearance of xanthomata over areas of friction such as the elbows, backs of knees and heels. Symptoms of coronary insufficiency may

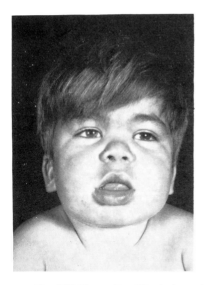 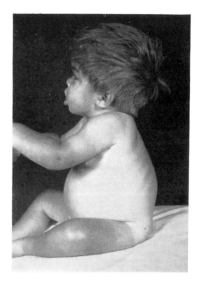

FIG. 129. Gargoylism (Hunter's syndrome). The facial features are coarse and an angular kyphosis is present in the lower thoracic spine. The patient is a boy and there is no clouding of the corneae.

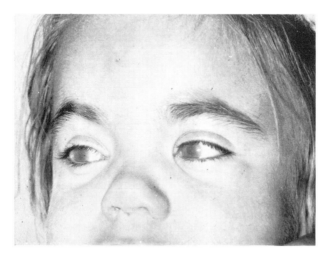

FIG. 130. Gargoylism (Hurler's syndrome). Clouding of the corneae in a girl with gargoylism.

occur as early as 7 years, becoming increasingly frequent as adolescence approaches. Death commonly occurs during teenage.

The heterozygous form usually shows no signs in childhood, though occasionally an arcus senilis appears from deposition of lipid in the cornea. In adult life xanthomata and coronary artery disease develop, leading to an early death if cholesterol levels are not reduced. This is achieved by replacing the saturated fats in the diet with poly-unsaturated fats such as corn oil. The intake of cholesterol from milk, eggs, lard and meat must be reduced. A number of drugs such as cholestyramine and clofibrate can also be used to reduce the cholesterol levels but diet is essential.

## LIPID STORAGE DISEASES (LIPIDOSES)

A number of disorders result from abnormal storage of phospholipids, mainly sphingolipids. They are genetically determined, occasionally with a racial predilection as in Tay-Sachs's disease which predominantly affects Jews. The cause is probably a lack of enzyme activity in the catabolic pathway of the respective lipid. The basic lesion is dysmyelination whereby abnormal myelin is formed. This differs from demyelination in which normally constituted myelin is later destroyed.

### Gaucher's disease

This condition results from a disturbance of cerebroside metabolism, whereby a large proportion of cerebrosides contains glucose rather than galactose, which is normally the only sugar component. This abnormal cerebroside is deposited in the reticulo-endothelial system of the liver, spleen, lymphatic system and bone marrow.

*Clinical features.* Two forms of the disease occur:

ACUTE INFANTILE GAUCHER'S DISEASE

Deposition of the cerebroside occurs in the brain as well as in the reticulo-endothial system. The infant appears normal at birth but soon becomes apathetic and there is progressive physical and mental retardation. Death occurs within the first year of life.

CHRONIC GAUCHER'S DISEASE

About half the cases present in older children, the rest during adult life. The child becomes wasted but there is no mental retardation as the brain is not involved. The abdomen enlarges from hepatomegaly and splenomegaly.

In both types there is anaemia from marrow involvement (leuco-erythroblastic anaemia), the bones fracturing easily. Thrombocytopenia may occur early, causing haemorrhagic manifestations. The typical Gaucher cells are striped, being found in the bone marrow or on rectal biopsy.

### Niemann-Pick's disease
In this condition there is an accumulation of sphingomyelin in the nervous system and elsewhere. The child, who is often Jewish, is normal at birth but during the first year of life there is a steady mental and physical deterioration; death, from progressive anaemia and wasting, occurs within the first 3 years of life. The liver and spleen enlarge, the skin becomes discoloured and lymph nodes palpable. A cherry-red spot at the macula may appear as in Tay-Sachs's disease. The abnormal cells can be seen on marrow or rectal biopsy; these are foamy as opposed to the striped cells seen in Gaucher's disease.

### Tay-Sachs's disease (amaurotic familial idiocy)
This disease is due to an accumulation of ganglioside in the nervous system. It results from a deficiency of hexosaminidase A which can be detected in the serum of carriers as well as cases and is therefore a vital aspect of genetic counselling. The patients are usually Jewish. The infant is normal for the first 3–6 months of life, then there is progressive mental retardation followed by spasticity, convulsions and blindness. A cherry-red spot at the macula is the characteristic feature. Hyperacusis is an early feature, causing an increased startle reflex; this sign precedes the development of the cherry-red spot. The degree of disturbance of the white matter is sufficient to cause the brain to increase in size so that enlargement of the head is detectable in the majority of cases.

### Metachromatic leucodystrophy
This is distinguished by the accumulation of metachromatically staining material in the areas of dysmyelination. The content of this material is cerebroside sulphate resulting from a deficiency of the enzyme cerebroside sulphatase. Normally about 15–20 per cent of cerebrosides exist as sulphate esters or sulphatides, but in metachromatic leucodystrophy as much as 80 per cent of the cerebroside exists in this form. Similar staining material is also found in the liver and kidney.

*Clinical features.* The disease may present at any time during childhood with the slow development of weakness and ataxia, and loss of tendon reflexes. Speech becomes impaired, vision lost and eventually there is complete dementia followed by death. Cranial nerve palsies often occur. The fundus usually shows optic atrophy, but a cherry-red spot as seen in Tay-Sachs's disease (see above) has been reported. The protein in the cerebrospinal fluid is raised. The wall of the gall bladder may be papillomatous, this involvement leading to absence of dye in a cholecystogram.

Diagnosis can be made by an examination of the urinary deposit which may show desquamated renal cells containing metachromatic material. Renal and rectal biopsy may show the same material. The nerve cells remain normal but the metachromatic material in the nerve fibres may extend right down the peripheral nerves, so that a skin biopsy can be used to show the material in myelinated nerves in the skin. Involvement of the peripheral nerves causes prolonged conduction time on the electromyogram.

### Krabbe's disease

This form of leucodystrophy is a disease of infants resulting from a reduction in cerebroside sulphotransferase. It is characterized by the presence of 'globoid' cells in the white matter, these being large multinucleated phagocytic cells surrounding the small blood vessels. The infant is normal at birth, but at about 3 months of age becomes irritable and vomits. This is followed by increasing rigidity associated with convulsions, blindness and deafness. Death usually occurs within 1 year of the onset. There is a rise of protein in the cerebrospinal fluid and nerve conduction velocity is decreased.

### Pelizaeus-Merzbacher disease

This variety of leucodystrophy is almost confined to males and is associated with a low level of cerebrosides. The onset is in infancy, often within a few days of birth, the course being one of slow progression with remissions, ending in death in young adult life. The characteristic presenting features are those of cerebellar dysfunction, particularly nystagmus. The cerebrospinal fluid shows no definite abnormalities.

There is no known treatment for these lipid storage diseases.


## DISORDERS OF MINERAL METABOLISM

### Wilson's disease

This disease follows from an abnormality of copper metabolism, resulting in damage from the excessive storage of copper, particularly in the brain, liver and kidneys. Brain damage occurs principally in the basal ganglia causing rigidity and tremor; liver damage leads to cirrhosis; renal tubular damage to aminoaciduria and glycosuria. The deposition of copper in Descemet's membrane of the cornea is responsible for the characteristic greenish-brown Kayser-Fleischer ring.

It is almost unknown for Wilson's disease to manifest itself as a neurological disorder before the age of 10 years, though it may present earlier as a haemolytic–hepatic episode (Wilson, 1972).

*Treatment.* There were strong hopes that dimercaprol (BAL) would be an effective mode of treatment but, unfortunately, these have not been realized as the drug produces unpleasant side effects and many of the patients become rapidly resistant to its cupruretic action. The chelating agent calcium disodium edathamil (EDTA) has also been disappointing, but penicillamine is a valuable form of treatment.

## BIBLIOGRAPHY

ANDERSON C.M. (1967) Intestinal malabsorption in childhood. *Arch. Dis. Childh.*, **41**, 571.

ANDERSON C.M. (1970) Malabsorption in childhood. In *Modern trends in paediatrics.* Ed. Apley, J. Butterworths, London.

*Brit. med. J.* (1960) Aetiology of idiopathic hypercalcaemia, **1**, 335.

CADELL J.L. (1965) Magnesium in the therapy of protein–calorie malnutrition of childhood. *J. Ped.*, **66**, 392.

CADELL J.L. (1967) Magnesium therapy in a Nigerian malnutrition clinic. *W. Afric. Med. J. and Nigerian Pract.*, **16**, 100.

COOK, G.C. (1967) Lactase activity in newborn and infant Baganda. *Brit. med. J.* **1**, 527.

CRAVIOTO J., DELICARDIE E.R. & BIRCH H.G. (1966) Nutrition, growth and neurointegrative development: an experimental and ecologic study. *Pediatrics*, **38**, 319.

DARMADY E.M. & STRANACK F. (1955) Microdissection of renal tubules. *Proc. roy. Soc. Med.*, **48**, 781.

DOBBING J. (1974) Later development of the brain and its vulnerability. In *Scientific Foundations of Paediatrics.* Ed. Davis, J.A. & Dobbing, J. Heinemann Medical, London.

GUTHRIE R. & SUSI A. (1963) A simple phenylalanine method for detecting phenylketonuria in large populations of newborn infants. *Pediatrics*, **32**, 338.

HERTZIG M.E., BIRCH H.G., RICHARDSON S.A. and TIZAND J. (1972) *Pediatrics*, **49**, 814.

HOLZEL A. (1967) Sugar malabsorption due to deficiencies of disaccharidase activities and of monosaccharide transport. *Arch. Dis. Childh.*, **42**, 341.

HSIA D.Y. (1966) *Inborn Errors of Metabolism.* Part 1. *Clinical Aspects.* Year Book Publishers, Chicago.

HUSBAND P. & MCKELLAR W.J.D. (1970) Infantile renal tubular acidosis due to mercury poisoning. *Arch. Dis. Childh.*, **45**, 264.

KING M. (1966) Ed. *Medical Care in Developing Countries.* Oxford University Press, Nairobi.

*Lancet* (1970) Classification of infantile malnutrition. *Lancet*, **2**, 302.

LLOYD J.K. (1968a) Disorders of the serum lipoproteins. I. Lipoprotein deficiency states. *Arch. Dis. Childh.*, **43**, 393.

LLOYD J.K. (1968b) Disorders of the serum lipoproteins. II. Hyperlipoproteinaemic states. *Arch. Dis. Childh.*, **43**, 505.

MCCANCE R.A. & WIDDOWSON E.M. (1966) Protein deficiencies and calorie deficiencies. *Lancet*, **2**, 158.

MCLAREN D.S. (1966) A fresh look at protein–calorie malnutrition. *Lancet*, **2**, 485.

MCKUSICK V.A., KAPLAN D., WISE D., HANLEY W.B., SUDDARTH S.B., SEVICK M.E. & MAUMANEE A.E. (1965) The genetic mucopolysaccharidoses. *Medicine*, **44**, 445.

MacGregor M.E. & Rayner P.H.W. (1964) Pink disease and primary renal tubular acidosis. *Lancet*, **2**, 1083.

Mann T.P., Wilson M. & Clayton B.E. (1965) A deficiency state arising in infants on synthetic foods. *Arch. Dis. Childh.*, **40**, 364.

Morley D. (1973) *Paediatric priorities in the developing world.* Butterworths, London.

Schlesinger B.E., Butler N.R. & Black J.A. (1956) Severe type of infantile hyper-calcaemia. *Brit. med. J.*, **1**, 127.

Stanfield J.P., Hutt M.S.R. & Tunnicliffe R. (1965) Intestinal biopsy in kwashiorkor. *Lancet*, **2**, 519.

Stewart W.K., Mitchell R.G., Morgan H.G., Lowe K.G. & Thomson J. (1964) The changing incidence of rickets and hypercalcaemia as seen in Dundee. *Lancet*, **1**, 679.

Wharton B. (1970) Hypoglycaemia in children with kwashiorkor. *Lancet*, **1**, 1970.

Whitehead R.G., Coward W.A. & Lunn P.G. (1973) Serum-albumin concentration and the onset of kwashiorkor. *Lancet*, **1**, 63.

Williams C.D. (1931–32) *Gold Coast Annual Report Med. Dept. for 1931–32*, Appendix E. Government Printing Office, Accra.

Williams C.D. (1933) A nutritional disease of childhood assiciated with a maize diet. *Arch. Dis. Childh.*, **8**, 423.

Wilson J. (1972) Investigation of degenerative disease of the central nervous system. *Arch. Dis. Child.* **47**, 163.

Winick M. (1969) Malnutrition and brain development. *J. Pediat.*, **74**, 667.

# CHAPTER 21

# DISORDERS OF THE BLOOD AND THE LYMPHATIC AND RETICULO-ENDOTHELIAL SYSTEMS

## DISORDERS OF THE BLOOD

### NORMAL HAEMOPOIESIS

The haemoglobin at birth is extremely variable and, even when the cord has been clamped as soon as possible after birth, it has been found to vary from 12–22 g per cent. With delayed clamping the variation may be still greater. No relationship has been found between the level of cord-blood haemoglobin and fetal maturity; by 2 months of age the level in all babies has reached a similar figure of about 11 g per cent.

After birth the haemoglobin and red-cell count rise during the first day and then remain approximately level until about the fourth day. They then start to fall, returning to the original cord level by about the ninth day. From then until the end of the second month, the haemoglobin falls to the level of 11 g per cent. This is the lowest point reached and, thereafter, there is a slow rise till the adult level is attained about the time of puberty. Consequently, the haemoglobin is lower throughout childhood than in adult life and a level of 11–13·5 g per cent (70–90 per cent Hb) may be regarded as normal for a child. When comparing haemoglobin and red-cell counts in infants, it must be remembered that capillary samples give somewhat higher readings than venous specimens for the first week of life. For accuracy, venous samples only should be used since the sample obtained from a finger-prick varies according to the depth to which the needle is inserted.

It is commonly stated that the fall in haemoglobin occurring after birth is due to excessive haemolysis, but it is now realized that this is not a significant factor. The principal factors which govern the level are the amount of erythropoietic activity of the marrow and the effect of body growth. Marrow activity is governed by the need to maintain the oxygen content of the blood at a constant level, the arterial oxyhaemoglobin being kept at about 11 g per cent, both in the fetus and in the newborn infant. After birth more oxygen is available so that there is no longer the need for the extra marrow activity of intrauterine life; consequently, the haemoglobin falls. The average total marrow-cell count in normal babies is 136,000 at birth. This drops to 35,000 by the ninth day, subsequently rising steadily to 201,000 by the age of 3 months. Confirmation of this mechanism is given by the fact that in babies with cyanotic congenital heart disease, the increased marrow activity of fetal life continues after birth.

In preterm babies the fall in haemoglobin tends to be exaggerated so that, although they start with a similar cord blood level, they fall lower than full-term babies by the end of the second month. This is due to the slow response of their marrow to the stimulus of anaemia and is exaggerated by their rapid growth. The administration of iron to full-term or preterm babies does not prevent the normal fall of haemoglobin, but it does reduce the extra fall in preterm babies since their iron stores are deficient. Even after the most premature birth these stores are sufficient for the first month of life, provided pathological haemorrhage or haemolysis has not occurred; it is satisfactory, therefore, to delay iron supplements until the age of 1 month. Absorption of iron has been shown to occur in full-term and preterm infants within the first week of life, though whether this causes any significant addition to the iron stores at that age is not yet clear. Additional iron should be continued for preterm babies until mixed feeding is established.

The red cells are 20 per cent larger at birth than in the adult, containing correspondingly more haemoglobin. The size of cell produced by the marrow gradually decreases, so that from 3–6 months of age they are actually smaller than in the adult. At birth nucleated red cells and reticulocytes in the peripheral blood film are more numerous than later on. There are about 5 per cent reticulocytes at birth, this figure falling to the normal level of less than 1 per cent by the end of the first week.

The total white-cell count at birth is extremely variable, but is greater than the average adult level due largely to an increase in polymorphs, a high proportion of which are young forms. During the first week there is a fall in the number of polymorphs and a rise in lymphocytes which then exceed the polymorphs by the end of the first week. The lymphocytes continue to exceed the polymorphs until about the age of 4 years when the two are equal; thereafter the adult proportions are slowly achieved. The higher lymphocyte count during the first 4 years is reflected in the response of the marrow to infection, since an increase in lymphocytes rather than polymorphs may take place. The formation of the white cells appears to be under relatively loose control at this time, so that diagnostic implications of the total and differential counts must be cautiously applied. Similarly, enlargement of the lymphoid tissue, such as the spleen and lymph glands, occurs readily with infection at this time. The sedimentation rate of the normal newborn baby is characteristically slow, though the reason for this is not clear.

During fetal life the bulk of the haemoglobin is of the fetal type (haemoglobin F). This is differentiated from adult haemoglobin (haemoglobin A) by the fact that cells containing fetal haemoglobin survive in alkali, whereas those containing adult haemoglobin succumb. Fetal haemoglobin shows a greater affinity for oxygen as shown by a shift of the oxygen dissociation curve to the left. This is advantageous to the fetus since oxygen can therefore be more readily transferred from the mother. Adult haemoglobin first appears about the thirteenth week, rising steadily to about 20 per cent at term. By 4 months, 90 per cent is of adult type and, in the normal adult, there are only traces of fetal haemoglobin. The two types of haemoglobin are contained mainly in different corpuscles but, during the period of changeover, intermediate cells containing both types are produced.

## ANAEMIA

### Classification

The types of anaemia in childhood fall into three groups:

1. Diminished production
2. Blood loss
3. Excessive breakdown (haemolysis)

1. DIMINISHED PRODUCTION

(a) *Lack of haemopoietic factors:*

(i) Iron
(ii) Protein
(iii) Folic acid
(iv) $B_{12}$
(v) Thyroid
(vi) Vitamin C

(b) *Lack of haemopoietic tissue:*

(i) Primary—aplasia or hypoplasia of marrow
(ii) Secondary
Interference with marrow function (leuco-erythroblastic or myelophthisic anaemia), e.g. leukaemia, secondary neoplastic deposits, lipidoses, osteopetrosis (Albers-Schönberg's disease)
Poisoning
Exogenous
Chemical—e.g. lead and certain drugs, such as sulphonamides, chloramphenicol

Physical—radiation
Endogenous
 Chronic infection
 Chronic illness, e.g. nephritis

2. BLOOD LOSS

(a) *Without blood disease:*

 (i) Acute
   Trauma, epistaxis, fetal from placenta, gastrointestinal—bleeding more
   often chronic (see below)
 (ii) Chronic
   Particularly gastrointestinal, e.g. oesophagitis, oesophageal varices, peptic
   ulcer, hookworm disease, Meckel's diverticulum, ulcerative colitis,
   chronic dysentery, polyps or haemorrhoids
   Idiopathic pulmonary haemosiderosis

(b) *With blood disease:*

   Haemorrhagic disease of newborn, haemophilia, purpura, leukaemia,
   scurvy

3. EXCESSIVE BREAKDOWN (HAEMOLYSIS)

(a) *Congenital abnormality of red cells:*

 (i) Hereditary spherocytosis
 (ii) Sickle-cell disease
 (iii) Thalassaemia
 (iv) Deficiency of glucose-6-phosphate dehydrogenase

(b) *Circulating antibodies:*

 (i) Haemolytic disease of the newborn
 (ii) Auto-immune haemolytic anaemia

(c) *Due to extracorpuscular agents unassociated with antibodies*

 (i) Infection
 (ii) Drugs
 (iii) Chemical poisons
 (iv) Haemolytic–uraemic syndrome
 (v) Hypersplenism

**Clinical features**

Although tiredness is a feature of anaemia in adults, children can be remarkably unaffected by anaemia. Breathlessness and oedema are seen only
in the most extreme cases. The symptoms are most obvious if anaemia has
developed rapidly (as from blood loss) so that the body has had no time to

adjust. In chronic anaemia, haemoglobin levels of 2·8 g per cent (20 per cent Hb) are tolerated with surprisingly little trouble and, particularly in tropical countries, patients may even walk up to hospital with a haemoglobin of less than 1·4 g per cent (10 per cent Hb).

Pallor is often the only sign. Its assessment must be made from the mucous membranes not the cheeks whose pallor is often unrelated to the level of haemoglobin. The colour of the lobes of the ears and the palms is often useful, especially in babies; the palms are also valuable in the assessment of anaemia in coloured children.

## ANAEMIA FROM LACK OF HAEMOPOIETIC FACTORS

### Iron deficiency anaemia

Lack of iron causes microcytic hypochromic anaemia. This is due to many factors, the most important being insufficient intake. Lack of iron in the diet occurs with prolonged milk feeding in infancy, since the antenatal stores of iron are exhausted after 6 months of age and milk alone does not provide sufficient iron. Even in children who have started mixed feeding the amount of iron-containing foods, such as green vegetables, meat and eggs, may be insufficient.

Prematurity is often a factor in the production of an iron deficiency anaemia (see p. 584). Multiple pregnancy may result in lack of iron since the amount available for storage must be divided. Maternal iron deficiency anaemia does not cause anaemia in the early weeks of life because the fetus lives as a parasite, extracting all it requires at the expense of the mother's own needs. Maternal anaemia is only a causative factor if breast feeding is prolonged; the milk from an anaemic mother contains little or no iron.

Infection is important and acts in several ways: it interferes with the ingestion and absorption of iron by causing loss of appetite, vomiting or diarrhoea and it causes bone-marrow depression. In the presence of infection iron is diverted from the marrow and immobilized in the tissues. Since anaemia predisposes to infection, a vicious circle is set up. Failure of absorption of iron also occurs in association with steatorrhoea, as in coeliac disease.

*Clinical features.* Iron deficiency anaemia often produces no symptoms apart from pallor. Loss of appetite may occur, due presumably to a deficiency of iron-dependent enzymes in the body and to diminished efficiency of cell function throughout the body (Clement, 1964). Pica (p. 465) is another symptom of iron deficiency anaemia; with iron therapy an improvement in the habit often precedes the rise in haemoglobin.

*Prophylaxis.* Prevention of prematurity and infection reduces the incidence of iron deficiency anaemia. All preterm babies require iron supplements from the age of 4 weeks until mixed feeding is established. Iron-containing foods should be given to all babies from the age of 6 months.

*Treatment.* The first step is to treat any infection and to correct the diet. Iron supplements are available in many forms, but since the iron is absorbed in the ferrous state, ferrous salts are preferable to ferric. The dose of an iron preparation should be calculated in terms of elemental iron; 6 mg/kg/day is effective, being given in three divided doses. Iron salts differ appreciably in their content of elemental iron. Ferrous sulphate contains 20 per cent iron whereas ferrous gluconate contains only 10 per cent. Ferrous sulphate, in a dose of 20 mg/kg/day in divided doses, is satisfactory. Mixtures of iron salts with other metals, vitamins or extracts of stomach or liver are deplorable. Such preparations are very expensive and less effective.

The iron supplement should be given between meals to be most effective since absorption is greatest when the stomach is empty. It is also less likely to cause a gastrointestinal upset when given in this way. Mothers should be warned that the stools will turn black.

If vomiting occurs, a different preparation, such as colloidal iron can be tried. Intramuscular iron should be given to patients who develop gastro-intestinal symptoms from more than one preparation of oral iron or have a defect of adsorption; it is also indicated if it is thought that the child will not receive the therapy prescribed. Parenteral iron replenishes the iron stores much more rapidly than oral iron. Traces of copper are required for normal haemopoiesis, but this is present as a contaminant in iron preparations so that additional copper is unnecessary.

Administration of iron causes a reticulocyte response and a daily haemo-globin rise of 0·1–0·3 g per cent, the more rapid rates occurring in the more anaemic. Iron therapy should be continued for 2–3 months after the haemo-globin has returned to normal in order to replenish the iron stores in the body.

Failure to respond may be due to several causes: the drug may be ineffective or it may not have been given. Alternatively, the dose may be insufficient. The possibility that blood is being lost from the body should be checked as well as the possibility of haemolysis. Chronic infections should always be borne in mind as well as collagen diseases. Malabsorption is a rare cause for failure of therapy.

A blood transfusion is required only if the symptoms are very severe, particularly cardiac failure or associated infection, or a rapid rise in haemo-globin required—such as before an operation. Otherwise, even levels of haemoglobin as low as 2·8 g per cent (20 per cent Hb) can be treated with oral iron. Blood transfusions must be given slowly because of the risk of cardiac failure, particularly in severe chronic anaemia when the danger that cardiac failure will be precipitated is great. An intraperitoneal transfusion of blood is an effective alternative when intravenous administration of blood is impractical from lack of skill or lack of veins. It has the advantage that there is little risk of inducing cardiac failure, especially if given by drip.

## Protein lack

Adequate protein is necessary for the formation of globin, the protein portion of haemoglobin. However, anaemia from lack of protein is rare since the formation of haemoglobin takes precedence over the formation of plasma proteins, so that the protein stores must be seriously depleted before anaemia from this cause develops. Moreover, any patient with such a serious deficiency of protein would be likely to have a deficiency of some other haemopoietic factor as well.

However, under experimental conditions it has been possible to produce anaemia from lack of protein alone. Protein lack must therefore be considered to be a possible additional factor in the anaemia of malnutrition; it could also be a factor in disorders causing an excessive loss of protein, such as nephrosis or protein-losing enteropathy (p. 311).

## Folic acid deficiency anaemia

All cells require folic acid for growth, the need being greatest where the cells are most active, as in the bone marrow. Lack of folic acid results in a megaloblastic anaemia and, since it cannot be stored in significant quantities, the balance is always precarious, particularly in infants, because of the requirements of rapid growth. Folic acid is necessary for skeletal growth. In children with sickle-cell disease there is a failure of growth including sexual maturation which responds to folic acid alone. Lack of folic acid occurs in a number of different ways:

### 1. DEFICIENT FOLIC ACID IN THE DIET

Folic acid is contained in green vegetables, liver, meat and milk. Folic acid content is similar in cow's milk and breast milk but the level in cow's milk is reduced by boiling. Dietary deficiency of folic acid is most often seen in infancy. It is particularly likely to occur in association with scurvy and may also be seen in children with kwashiorkor.

### 2. MALABSORPTION OF FOLIC ACID

This frequently occurs in coeliac disease and, occasionally, in gastroenteritis or ulcerative colitis if the lesions are very extensive. Any severe infection may diminish the absorption of folic acid.

### 3. INCREASED REQUIREMENTS OF FOLIC ACID

This is the main factor in the lack of folic acid in sickle-cell disease owing to the rapid destruction and formation of red cells. The same mechanism may also operate in spherocytosis, thalassaemia and chronic malaria. Folic acid deficiency may occur in leukaemia, presumably because the leukaemic cells take up much of the available folic acid.

### 4. DRUGS

Methotrexate and aminopterin are primary folic acid antagonists which are used in the treatment of leukaemia. A similar action may occur as a side effect with some of the anticonvulsant and antimalarial drugs, notably phenytoin.

### Megaloblastic anaemia of infancy

This condition is more common than is often realized; it usually occurs in the second half of the first year. The patients may be obviously malnourished but this is not necessarily so. The striking symptom is anorexia associated with pallor, the child being more ill than would be anticipated from the degree of anaemia. Infection is often present and is a factor in producing the deficiency of folic acid. The liver is invariably enlarged and extramedullary erythro-poiesis has been found in the liver at autopsy. There may be evidence of scurvy. The bone marrow is megaloblastic and the granulocyte precursors show characteristic changes; the myelocytes are large and, though the cells are obviously immature, the nuclei have undergone lobulation. Since the megaloblasts are not always found in the peripheral film, a bone-marrow examination should be carried out in all cases of normochromic anaemia in infancy. Leucopenia, neutropenia and thrombocytopenia are also present.

If the condition is not recognized, the child may succumb early to an associated infection. It responds dramatically to the administration of folic acid in a dose of 15–20 mg daily; this produces a lasting cure so that the condition clearly differs from pernicious anaemia. The frequent association with scurvy has suggested the possibility that a deficiency of ascorbic acid might inhibit the utilization of folic acid, but it is now thought more likely that the changes in scurvy cause a greater demand for folic acid which cannot be met.

### $B_{12}$ deficiency anaemia

This is a rare form of megaloblastic anaemia in children, which may occur in more than one member of a family, is associated with lack of intrinsic factor and which responds to intramuscular vitamin $B_{12}$. Maintenance therapy is required for life to prevent a relapse. The condition is comparable to pernicious anaemia of adults except that almost all the cases have had normal gastric acidity whereas, in adults, gastric achlorhydria and an atrophic gastric mucosa on biopsy are regarded as essential features.

Pernicious anaemia results from a deficiency of intrinsic factor which is secreted by the stomach and enables vitamin $B_{12}$ to be absorbed, mainly in the ileum. In adults the deficiency of intrinsic factor is associated with gastric atrophy, whereas in these children the loss of intrinsic factor is an isolated defect. Whether these are the same condition is debatable, but possibly the deficiency of intrinsic factor is the primary defect in pernicious anaemia and predisposes to gastric atrophy. The fact that juvenile pernicious anaemia and the classical form have been described in different members of the same family is strong evidence that they represent different stages of the same disorder.

### Vitamin C deficiency anaemia

Whether vitamin C has a primary or only a secondary role in haemopoiesis is still uncertain. Its relationship with folic acid and the occurrence of megaloblastic anaemia in scurvy have already been discussed (p. 555). The hypochromic anaemia which develops in scurvy responds to vitamin C. However, this could be due to a return of normal capillary function, since haemorrhage resulting from increased capillary permeability is the main cause of the anaemia.

### Thyroid deficiency anaemia

Some children with thyroid deficiency develop a hypochromic anaemia. Treatment with thyroid alone causes a reticulocyte response and a return to a normal blood picture.


## ANAEMIA FROM LACK OF HAEMOPOIETIC TISSUE

### Congenital aplastic anaemia

This is a rare condition resulting from aplasia of the bone marrow; it is sometimes genetically determined. The white cells and platelets are affected as well as the red cells, causing an increased liability to infection and bleeding. Associated multiple congenital anomalies may be present, the condition then being termed 'Fanconi's anaemia'. The most frequent anomaly is hyperpigmentation. Skeletal defects are common, especially those involving the radius. The heart and genito-urinary tract may be malformed and mental retardation may occur. In some of these cases the anaemia does not become apparent until the age of 2–3 years. The prognosis is very serious but some cases have responded to steroid therapy.

### Congenital hypoplastic anaemia (erythrogenesis imperfecta)

In this condition the depression of the bone marrow involves the red-cell series only; it is regarded as a congenital anomaly of the erythron. Anaemia is not present at birth but is usually apparent by the age of 3 months. Some of the children resemble each other, being fair-haired with a low nasal bridge and snub nose. Reticulocytes are few or absent. Bone-marrow examination shows the failure of red-cell development to be at the late normoblast stage in most cases.

Some patients have responded to steroid therapy, others to testosterone. If there is no response to therapy, repeated transfusions are the only form of treatment, but there is considerable risk of secondary haemosiderosis from deposition of the iron present in the transfused red cells (see p. 612).

### Leuco-erythroblastic anaemia (myelophthisic anaemia)

Interference with marrow function occurs in osteopetrosis (Albers-Schönberg's disease), secondary neoplastic deposits such as neuroblastoma and in the lipid storage diseases (p. 578). This same mechanism is also a factor in the anaemia which develops in patients with leukaemia.

The nutrition of the erythropoietic tissue is disturbed, causing disordered erythropoiesis so that anaemia develops, immature red cells appearing in the peripheral blood. Maturation of platelets is also disturbed so that thrombocytopenic purpura may develop.

### Leukaemia

Leukaemia in children is almost always acute. It is by far the commonest form of malignant disease in childhood. The predominant cell is so primitive that it may be impossible to determine whether it is a lymphoblast or a myeloblast and it can be described only as a stem or 'blast' cell. In childhood all cases of undifferentiated leukaemia are treated as acute lymphatic. Using this definition approximately 75 per cent of the cases are acute lymphatic and about 15 per cent are acute myeloid. Acute monocytic leukaemia is very uncommon. Chronic leukaemia accounts for only about 2 per cent of leukaemias in childhood; this is almost always myeloid, and usually starts after the age of 8 years.

An association exists between leukaemia and chromosomal abnormalities. Children with Down's syndrome show a ten times higher frequency of leukaemia than normal children (Hug, 1965). Adults with chronic myeloid leukaemia possess an abnormal chromosome, termed 'Philadelphia' (Ph); this is a small remnant resulting from partial deletion of chromosome 21. Tough *et al.* (1961) put forward the suggestion that this chromosome might carry a locus concerned with leucopoiesis. Triplication of this locus would increase the liability to acute leukaemia whereas its deletion could cause myeloid leukaemia. Maternal irradiation during pregnancy increases the risk of later leukaemia for the child (Stewart *et al.*, 1958); this could be due to chromosomal damage.

## ACUTE LEUKAEMIA

This is almost entirely a disease of young children, the peak incidence occurring between 2 and 4 years of age. The onset is relatively sudden, the child being brought usually because of pallor from the severe anaemia due to interference with marrow function by the leukaemic tissue. Limb pains from bone deposits are common and haemorrhages occur from thrombocytopenia. The haemorrhages are usually seen in the skin or mucous membranes as petechiae or bruises, but may occur into any organ. Haematuria is occasionally a presenting symptom. Fever is usual and some degree of lymphadenopathy is often present. The spleen and liver are often enlarged but splenomegaly is not constant. The kidneys, though seldom enlarged clinically, are often found at autopsy to be completely infiltrated with leukaemic tissue. Renal failure is uncommon, although an intravenous pyelogram may show distortion of the renal outline.

Intracranial manifestations are now seen often since treatment prolongs life but the antimetabolites used do not cross the blood–brain barrier. They occur in about half the children with acute lymphatic leukaemia but are rare in the other forms. These manifestations result from leukaemic infiltration of the brain, meninges or cranial nerves, the most common being raised intracranial pressure, causing headache, vomiting and papilloedema. In such cases leukaemic cells may be found in the cerebro-spinal fluid. Intracranial manifestations occur as often in remissions as in relapses because the drugs do not cross the blood–brain barrier.

Radiological signs are present in more than half of the patients; these most often involve the femur and tibia, but may affect the skull and spine. Rarefaction causing translucent bands at the metaphysis is the commonest finding in the long bones; more extensive areas of rarefaction may occur in the diaphysis, causing spontaneous fractures. Sclerosis occurs only occasionally. Periosteal involvement results in a double outline from new bone formation.

The white-cell count is usually lowered but it may be normal or raised, though the high white-cell count to be found in chronic cases is not a feature of acute leukaemia. There is nothing to gain from the use of the term *aleukaemic leukaemia* since the pattern in the peripheral blood is not constant. Immature white cells may be present in the peripheral blood or only in the bone marrow which should be examined for confirmation of the diagnosis.

In young children, the iliac crest is the most suitable site for puncture since a sternal marrow puncture is more frightening for them.

The red-cell count and haemoglobin are always lowered; the anaemia is usually normochromic. Some degree of thrombocytopenia is usual and the bleeding time is prolonged.

*Diagnosis.* The condition must be differentiated from other causes of anaemia; this is not difficult once the increase in 'blast' cells has been seen in the peripheral blood or marrow. The real difficulty is differentiation from aplastic anaemia, particularly since the picture of aplastic anaemia with suppression of all marrow elements may be an early manifestation of leukaemia. In such cases the correct diagnosis can be made only by repeated marrow examinations until the immature cells of acute leukaemia appear. The limb pains may resemble those in rheumatic fever and rheumatoid arthritis, but the pain is in the bones rather than in the joints.

A *leukaemoid reaction* indicates a high white-cell count, with or without immature white cells in the peripheral blood; this occurs in conditions other than leukaemia. It may occur in any severe infection, especially in young children, in pertussis, varicella, measles, miliary tuberculosis, rheumatoid arthritis and Hodgkin's disease. It may also occur when there is sudden erythropoietic activity from acute haemolysis or haemorrhage. Invasion of the bone marrow by tumour cells may cause a leukaemoid reaction and occurs particularly with a lymphoma or neuroblastoma because these frequently involve the bone marrow.

It may be difficult to decide on clinical grounds whether the child has thrombocytopenic purpura or acute leukaemia when haemorrhagic manifestations are widespread, but bone marrow examination will differentiate the conditions.

*Prognosis and treatment.* The outlook for acute leukaemia has been radically altered by modern treatment. Without treatment the majority of children died within 4 months. With treatment, remissions can be induced in about 90 per cent of patients in whom the average survival is likely to be about 4 years provided the child is managed in an experienced centre. A very small proportion of children with acute leukaemia survive for many years and probably outlive their disease.

Before starting treatment, once the diagnosis has been established, the condition must be discussed fully and frankly with the parents. The aim of treatment is not only to prolong the child's life but also to reduce the suffering of the parents; this cannot be achieved if the parents are not fully informed. It might be argued that the parents' suffering is increased by prolonging the child's life but this is not the case. By giving treatment the parents feel that something is being done, quite apart from the fact that their child's life is being prolonged. Moreover, without giving any false claims for existing method of treatment it is not unreasonable to give the parents the hope that the continued search for drugs may, during their child's lifetime, produce a more effective mode of treatment. It is essential that in prolonging life no increased suffering is caused to the child; correct treatment reduces bone pains.

Treatment is complex and it is for this reason that it should be undertaken in a special centre. It is divided into two parts: induction of remission and maintenance of remission. The remission is induced by drugs which, while destroying the blast cells, are not so toxic as to suppress marrow regeneration; they must also act fast. For this purpose a combination of prednisone and vincristine is commonly used. Remission is achieved in about 90 per cent of cases but this would only last 6–12 weeks without maintenance therapy. An early sign of remission is the return of the temperature to normal.

Maintenance therapy usually involves continuous treatment with 6-mercaptopurine, methotrexate or cyclophosphamide which are slower acting drugs. The drugs may be given sequentially, the change being made at the earliest sign of relapse. The bone marrow is checked every 6–8 weeks, and if maintenance therapy fails to control the disease an induction course with prednisone and vincristine is repeated, followed by a return to maintenance therapy. This is discontinued after 3 years if no relapse has occurred.

New drugs continue to appear. Thus daunorubicin (rubidomycin), cytosine arabinoside and colaspase (asparaginase) are additionally in use for the induction of remission. New and more intensive cycles of treatment are being evolved with the aim of such radical therapy as to achieve total leukaemic cell kill.

The progress of treatment has required an intensive drive to overcome the complications which were not previously seen or not to the same extent. Of these the most serious is meningeal leukaemia which should be treated prophylactically by irradiation of the skull and intrathecal methotrexate.

Infection is the usual cause of death, due partly to the depression of circulating granulocytes and partly to ulceration of the buccal and pharyngeal mucosa leading to secondary monilial infection. Prophylactic mouth washes and amphotericin lozenges may reduce the liability to monilial infection.

Haemorrhage usually results from thrombocytopenia and can be prevented by a platelet transfusion. Anaemia requires blood transfusion. Hyperuricaemia occurs and is secondary to extensive white cell destruction; it may lead to renal damage and secondary gout. If this is anticipated because of a high blast cell count the risk can be reduced by ensuring good hydration and alkalinization of the urine together with the administration of allopurinal. Vincristine and cyclophosphamide cause loss of hair of which prior warning should be given to the child and his parents. Regeneration of hair always occurs when the drugs are stopped, meanwhile a wig can be worn if necessary.

Acute lymphatic leukaemia is more responsive to treatment than acute myeloid. Good prognostic signs are a low total leukaemic-cell mass at the onset as shown by minimal organ involvement and a relatively low blast cell count in the peripheral blood. A normal platelet count at the time of diagnosis is also a favourable sign (Till *et al.*, 1973).

As soon as possible once treatment has been started, the child should be discharged home and encouraged to attend school and lead a normal life. When readmission to hospital is necessary, it should be for not more than 1–2 days.

## ANAEMIA FROM BLOOD LOSS

### Fetal haemorrhage

The route for blood loss occurring earliest in the child's life is across the placenta into the maternal circulation during intrauterine life. This subject is discussed on p. 131.

### Bleeding diatheses

The term 'haemophilia', as originally understood, is now known to be a group of disorders comprising haemophilia A and B and pseudo-haemophilia A and B.

#### HAEMOPHILIA A

This is a sex-linked, recessively inherited, bleeding disorder which is transmitted by females but apparent only in males. A male develops haemophilia when heterozygous for the gene causing the condition, whereas a female must be homozygous if haemophilia is to occur. Very occasionally a female with haemophilia has occurred when a female carrier has married an affected male. The severity of haemophilia tends to decrease with succeeding generations. Sporadic cases occur, these being usually more serious than the hereditary form.

The defect in haemophilia is an absence of antihaemophilic globulin (factor 8), one of the factors in plasma required for the formation of thromboplastin. In normal clotting, prothrombin is converted to thrombin by thromboplastin acting in the presence of calcium; the thrombin then interacts with fibrinogen to form fibrin. The deficiency in haemophilia results in defective clotting.

It has been estimated that there are one to two haemophiliacs for every

100,000 of the population of the British Isles. The Japanese are the only non-white race in which haemophilia has been observed.

The condition manifests itself in early childhood and may come to light when prolonged bleeding follows circumcision or other minor operation. There is a tendency for the condition to improve once adult life is reached, but it is probable that this is largely due to a greater avoidance of trauma. Bleeding occurs as a result of trauma, which is usually minimal, but there is no tendency to spontaneous haemorrhage. The joints are particularly affected, haemorrhage occurring mainly into those that are weight-bearing, especially the knees; as a result of repeated haemarthroses the joints become damaged. Prolonged hyperaemia results in overgrowth of the ends of the bones, causing further diability. Apart from the joint changes, X-rays commonly show Harris's lines of arrested growth which have developed during the frequent periods of ill-health and confinement to bed.

Bleeding may also occur from the skin or mucous membranes, or into the tissues as a result of mild trauma; massive haemorrhages may occur into the lips, periorbital tissues, muscles and retroperitoneal tissue. Bleeding tends to occur about 2 hours after a blow since there is initial platelet blockage of the injured blood vessel but the impaired clotting mechanism is unable to complete the repair. It is interesting that affected members of the same family have a strong tendency to produce the same manifestations.

*Management.* Every possible step must be taken to prevent trauma, particularly in the early years of life. Young children should wear a protective helmet to guard the face and head. Long trousers should be worn, a rubber pad being sewn into them in front of the knees. A high standard of conservative dental care should be maintained in order to avoid dental extractions which are likely to lead to prolonged bleeding. If dental extractions are required, a splint to cover the socket should be prepared beforehand. The aim of this splint is not to provide pressure but to stop the patient traumatizing the site with the tongue.

Special attention must be paid to schooling since these patients will have to earn their living by their brains rather than by their muscles. Teaching must always be continued when in hospital. Many sports have to be denied to these children but swimming is ideal. If they are taught to swim early, they have a chance of outshining their compatriots in a sporting activity.

The specific treatment to stop bleeding is the intravenous administration of factor 8 which is available as a cryoprecipate preparation and as factor 8 concentrate. This concentrate is very expensive and in short supply. However, since it can be given as a single intravenous injection instead of by drip, it is ideal for immediate home treatment by parents as soon as bleeding is suspected. If factor 8 is not available, a preparation of fresh frozen plasma is preferable to blood since it is less likely to be antigenic. If blood has to be used it must be fresh since AHG, being unstable, is not present in stored blood.

Bleeding should be stopped by pressure rather than by suture which may cause additional bleeding. Haematomata should not be aspirated owing to the risk of further bleeding and infection. If a haemarthrosis occurs the child should immediately be admitted to a special centre where the coagulation defect can be corrected. Under cover of this correction the joint is aspirated and a compression bandage applied. Immobilization by means of a plaster slab over the bandage is maintained for 48 hours. After this, rehabilitation of joint movement is encouraged through physiotherapy.

Prior to major surgery, administration of factor 8 to raise its level to at least 30 per cent of normal is required. Blood samples must never be taken from the femoral vein since the site prevents total control of bleeding into the tissues as is possible in the arm.

### HAEMOPHILIA B (CHRISTMAS DISEASE)

This disease has been named after the first patient to be recorded. It is due to an absence of a different plasma factor required in the formation of thromboplastin; this is the Christmas factor or plasma thromboplastin component (factor 9). The disease is inherited as a sex-linked recessive trait; it has been recorded only in males. The clinical symptoms tend to be milder than in the classical form of haemophilia but are otherwise identical. Christmas factor is stable so that frozen plasma or stored blood can be used in treatment. Concentrates of factor 9 are in short supply.

### VON WILLEBRAND'S DISEASE

This resembles haemophilia superficially in that minor injuries cause disproportionate bleeding, but the bleeding time is prolonged and the clotting time normal. The disease is transmitted as an autosomal dominant trait, the sexes being equally affected.

There is reduced synthesis of factor 8 and reduced platelet adhesiveness though all other measures of platelet activity are normal. These disorders are thought to be due to an unidentified plasma factor. The previous concept of an underlying vascular defect causing the capillaries to be distorted is no longer held now that it is realized that normal capillaries vary widely in tortuosity.

Haemarthroses occur but the bleeding tendency is not so serious as in haemophilia; only rarely do the patients die from haemorrhage. Since the patient can synthesize factor 8 to some extent an infusion of fresh or fresh-frozen plasma is usually adequate to stop the bleeding.

## PURPURA

The different varieties of purpura can be separated into those which are associated with a low platelet count in which there may also be a vascular defect, and those in which the platelets are normal, purpura being due to a vascular defect alone.

### Thrombocytopenic purpura

1. Primary (Werlhof's disease)
2. Secondary to:

(a) Marrow defect

(i) Infections
(ii) Blood disorders—leukaemia, aplastic anaemia
(iii) Toxic factors, e.g. poisons such as benzol, and irradiation

(b) Hypersplenism. In association with Gaucher's disease, sickle-cell disease, thalassaemia and the splenomegaly of some parasitic infections, the spleen may destroy the platelets at an excessive rate.

### Purpura due to vascular defect

1. Anaphylactoid purpura (p. 659)
2. Scurvy (p. 554)
3. Infections

### IDIOPATHIC THROMBOCYTOPENIC PURPURA (ITP)

This disorder is believed to be due to an auto-immune process although platelet antibodies can often not be detected, possibly because they adhere to the platelets. Support for this comes from the occasional association of auto-immune haemolytic anaemia in the same patient. Moreover, mothers who have had the disease but have been cured by splenectomy have caused thrombocytopenia in their newborn infants, presumably from placental transfer of platelet antibodies. The response of the disease to steroids is additional evidence.

The majority of cases in children occur under the age of 6 years. They present with bruising and petechiae; they may also bleed from any mucosal surface, especially the nose, gums and urinary tract. Splenomegaly is so seldom present that a palpable spleen raises the strong possibility of an alternative diagnosis. The platelet count is reduced, being usually less than 50,000. There is increased capillary fragility, the bleeding time is prolonged and the clotting time normal. Hess's tourniquet test is positive.

The condition tends to be milder in children than in adults but more cases are acute. The patients usually fall without difficulty into an acute or a chronic group.

*Acute cases.* These patients give no previous history of any bleeding tendency but a history of a recent infection, especially of the upper respiratory tract, is obtained in about half the cases. The onset of bleeding is sudden and the increased capillary fragility, in addition to the low platelet count, results in severe bleeding for the first few days. Bleeding then becomes reduced as the capillary involvement declines, although the thrombocytopenia remains unchanged for some time. The patients either recover completely within 6 months or die in the acute stage from uncontrollable bleeding or intracranial haemorrhage. Very few acute cases pass into the chronic stage.

*Chronic cases.* These patients may have a long history of bleeding or bruising tendency, the course of the illness being marked by relapses and remissions. Bleeding is usually less severe than in acute cases, probably because there is less capillary involvement. A history of antecedent infection is seldom obtained, although the length of the disease and its less dramatic onset would in any case make this less likely to be obtained. Chronic cases seldom die from the condition but it may persist for years.

The platelet count is extremely variable in both groups; in some fulminating cases it may still be high, so that it is of no prognostic value. The bone marrow shows a normal or increased number of megakaryocytes.

*Diagnosis.* The disorder must be differentiated from cases in which thrombocytopenia is part of another blood disease, particularly aplastic anaemia or leukaemia. In these conditions there is a severe degree of anaemia, whereas the anaemia in primary thrombocytopenic purpura is related to the actual blood loss. In doubtful cases an examination of the bone marrow will soon decide the diagnosis. An investigation must be made into the possibility that the low platelet count has resulted from the toxic action of drugs or poisons or from infection.

*Treatment.* Acute cases must always be given steroid therapy in view of the risk of a major bleed, especially intracranial haemorrhage. Steroids reduce the increased vascular fragility as well as increasing the platelet count. Blood transfusion may be necessary. Splenectomy should not be advised unless the condition persists for over 12 months. For chronic cases a period of 12 months' watchful waiting is recommended and steroids can be used during this time. Steroid therapy is less effective in chronic than in acute cases, since its principal action is to control the vascular component of the disease rather than to affect the platelet count. If symptoms persist for longer than 12 months, splenectomy is advisable; at least half of the cases can then be expected to respond.

CONGENITAL THROMBOCYTOPENIC PURPURA

Three groups can be separated. In the first the mother has primary thrombocytopenic purpura, platelet antibodies having been detected in some of the affected infants. In the second the mother is normal, while in the third there is congenital hypoplasia of the megakaryocytes and the child may show other congenital malformations.

PURPURA DUE TO INFECTION

*Acute thrombocytopenic purpura*

Some 50 per cent of cases of acute thrombocytopenic purpura are preceded by a history of infection within the previous 3 weeks, particularly an upper respiratory infection. The condition may also follow one of the infectious fevers, especially rubella, measles, chicken pox and scarlet fever. This complication bears no relationship to the severity of the primary infection which may have been mild or severe.

The cause of the thrombocytopenia is unknown, but possibly the virus alters the antigenicity of the platelets so that they become foreign and are destroyed by antibody.

Clinical differentiation from ITP is not possible, but this disease is essentially a benign self-limiting condition in which the platelet count usually recovers in about 6 weeks, though it may take up to one year. The indications for steroid therapy depend on the severity of the illness and the considered risk of haemorrhage.

## Disseminated intravascular coagulation (DIC)

This is not a primary disease process but is a response to certain stimuli, especially septicaemia, hypothermia, hypoxia and acidosis. Intravascular coagulation is triggered either directly by the entry of foreign material into the blood or indirectly as a result of endothelial injury. A massive consumption of platelets and coagulation factors then takes place leading to thrombosis from fibrin micro-emboli, and haemorrhage.

Clinically the patient is in a state of shock associated with purpura. Multiple organ involvement with thrombosis or emboli may occur.

Fragmentation of red cells is seen in the blood film and the platelet count falls. There is also a fall in the levels of factors 2, 5, 8, and of fibrinogen and prothrombin. Fibrin degradation products rise.

Treatment is directed at the underlying disease and at the coagulation abnormality. Heparin is required to inhibit coagulation and break the vicious circle.

# ANAEMIA FROM EXCESSIVE BREAKDOWN
# OF RED CELLS (HAEMOLYSIS)

Normal red cells survive 120 days. Haemolysis is taking place whenever premature destruction of red cells occurs. The disorders causing this are either the result of a defect in the cell or of something abnormal in the circulation—an antibody or some other agent.

## 1. Haemolysis due to congenital abnormality of red cells

### (A) HEREDITARY SPHEROCYTOSIS (ACHOLURIC JAUNDICE)

The primary disorder in this condition is the abnormal shape of the red cells. They are spherocytic, causing them to be more fragile than normal and so more liable to haemolysis. The condition is inherited as a dominant characteristic and may be transmitted through either sex.

The disease may become apparent at any age but it is only rarely a cause of neonatal jaundice. In childhood the disorder is usually one of a mild chronic haemolytic anaemia. At times the haemolytic process may be intensified, causing a haemolytic crisis. In the chronic phase there is a mild anaemia associated with splenomegaly and reticulocytosis. The bilirubin is slightly raised and may be sufficient to show as clinical jaundice, but none appears in the urine. During the crisis the level of red cells falls acutely, jaundice becomes marked and fever is common. In these crises there is usually a rise in reticulocytes, but occasionally an aplastic crisis may occur when a lowered reticulocyte level occurs for a few days. Gall-stones may develop as a result of prolonged hyperbilirubinaemia but these are uncommon in children.

Examination of the blood shows a normochromic and normocytic anaemia; the reticulocyte count may be as high as 30 per cent. The red cells are spherocytic and show increased fragility. Incubation of the red cells increases their fragility, thereby rendering the test more sensitive. The Coombs' test is negative.

*Prognosis and treatment.* Some patients are very little disturbed by the disorder, while others have repeated crises. If the symptoms in childhood are severe, growth is retarded and there is an increased risk of infection. It is probably wise that all children showing clinical or even only laboratory evidence of the disease should have splenectomy performed in order to reduce the risk of these complications. The only disadvantage of splenectomy in any individual is the increased possibility of infection and its greater severity. This question is still unanswered in hereditary spherocytosis since it is a disease in which there is already a greater liability to sepsis. Splenectomy does not affect the abnormal shape of the red cells which persists throughout life, but it does reduce their liability to haemolysis.

## (B) HEREDITARY HAEMOGLOBINOPATHIES

Haemoglobin consists of haem, which is an iron-porphyrin, and globin, which is a protein. Variations can occur in both portions of the molecule. Alterations in the haem portion cause impairment of the oxygen-carrying capacity, as in methaemoglobinaemia and sulphaemoglobinaemia. Alterations in the globin fraction produce abnormal haemoglobins whose oxygen-carrying capacity is unimpaired but which render the red cell more liable to haemolysis. About thirty varieties of abnormal haemoglobin have now been identified, though most of these are very rare. The two most important diseases caused by abnormal haemoglobin are sickle-cell disease and thalassaemia; these are confined to specific races.

### SICKLE-CELL DISEASE (DREPANOCYTOSIS)

In this condition haemoglobin S is present in the red cells instead of haemoglobin A, the adult form. Haemoglobin S, when deprived of its oxygen by tissue respiration, undergoes molecular rearrangement to form long rod-like particles which alter the contour of the red cells to a sickle shape rendering them more liable to haemolysis. These cells are therefore destroyed prematurely by the reticulo-endothelial system, the red-cell survival being only 15–60 days as compared with the normal 120 days. The reserves of the marrow are enormous and they can increase its capacity so as to compensate for a red-cell survival time as low as 20 days, but in sickle-cell disease the compensation is never quite complete, hence the moderately severe anaemia which is usually present. The abnormally shaped red cells are liable to adhere to each other, causing intravascular thrombi. Consequently, the clinical effects of the disease result from anaemia and thrombosis.

In addition to the presence of haemoglobin S there is also persistence of haemoglobin F, the fetal form. Up to 20 per cent of the haemoglobin may be of the fetal form; there is evidence that fetal haemoglobin can exercise a protective effect against sickling.

Identification of the different varieties of haemoglobin is determined by filter-paper electrophoresis since the rate of movement of each type of haemoglobin is different. Eighty per cent of the haemoglobin in all babies at birth is fetal; this obscures the adult pattern so that it is not usually possible to diagnose sickle-cell disease before the age of 3 months. By this time the level of fetal haemoglobin has fallen so that the presence of haemoglobin S, instead of haemoglobin A, can more easily be detected.

Since sickling occurs in a low oxygen tension, this can be induced by tests if such cells are present in the circulation. The quickest method is to mix a drop of blood with a drop of 2 per cent sodium metabisulphite on a glass slide; a positive result is shown by the presence of any sickled cells after 30 minutes. Sickling is not usually present at birth, this being probably due to the small percentage of haemoglobin S present. If it is present, or can be induced at birth, sickle-cell disease can be diagnosed with confidence.

Patients with sickle-cell disease are homozygous for the abnormal haemoglobin so that their genotype is SS. Carriers have the genotype AS and are described as showing the sickle-cell trait. Haemoglobin S occurs exclusively in the Negro race; in Central Africa up to 45 per cent of the population may carry the gene. Approximately 9 per cent of American Negroes are carriers.

*Clinical features.* Sickle-cell disease begins as a mild disease about the third month of life. From the sixth month its evolution becomes rapid so that many of the children die before the age of 2 years. The child is most likely to present in a crisis, though before this the picture of chronic haemolytic anaemia with pallor and faint jaundice, associated with tiredness, may have been apparent. Sickle-cell disease has many manifestations; it has been called 'a great masquerader' (Winsor & Burch, 1945).

Two forms of crisis occur: the *aplastic* and the *painful*. The *aplastic crisis* is often precipitated by an infection; it may also be brought on by a deficiency of folic acid. Pain is not a feature but the mother may notice a sudden increase in pallor. The sudden fall in red-cell count is due to a temporary failure of erythrocyte production in the bone marrow. It is not due to increased haemolysis as is often stated. The mechanism is comparable to that which causes the fall in red-cell count in normal babies after birth where the same mistake regarding a haemolytic mechanism has been made (see p. 583).

The *painful crisis* results from intravascular thrombosis and there is little effect on the blood picture, though fever is common. Pain is felt particularly in the bones but also occurs in the abdomen and in the joints. An 'acute abdomen' presenting in a Negro child should always be investigated for sickle-cell disease. The joint pains may resemble rheumatic fever. Pulmonary infarction, bone infarction, cerebral vascular accidents and renal infarction causing haematuria, may also occur.

Physical examination shows general underdevelopment with long and spindly extremities. The abdomen protrudes and the chest is barrel-shaped (Fig. 131). Chronic jaundice is common since the sickle-cells are consistently haemolysed more rapidly than normal cells; the liver may be enlarged. The spleen is usually enlarged in children and may then exert a hypersplenic action, thereby causing an even more rapid destruction of red cells than is usual in the disease. As the child gets older the spleen becomes smaller as a result of fibrosis caused by repeated infarcts; on the other hand, the liver gets larger and may induce liver failure.

Infarction of bone causes its destruction with consequent new bone formation. This osteopathy occurs especially in young children, seldom being seen

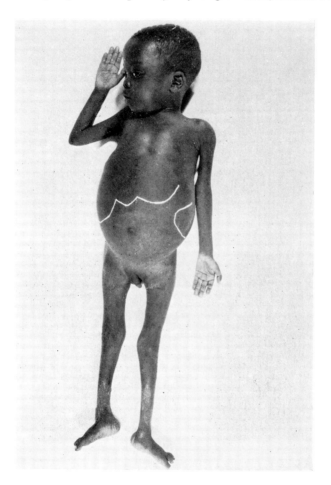

Fig. 131. Sickle-cell disease. Child aged 5½ years showing under-development, associated with a barrel-shaped chest, distended abdomen and long spindly legs. The edges of the enlarged liver and spleen have been marked on the skin.

over the age of 6 years. During the first 2 years of life the bones of the hands (Fig. 132) and feet are those most often affected. The lesion may show as a painful swelling of the dorsum of the hand or foot which does not pit on pressure and is often symmetrical; this is termed the 'hand and foot syndrome' (Fig. 133a). Sometimes, painful spindle-shaped swellings of the digits occur, these also often being symmetrical (Fig. 133b). In children between the ages of 2 and 6 years the long bones are more often involved. In an acute stage

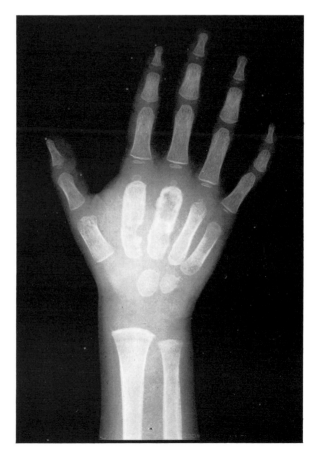

FIG. 132. Sickle-cell disease affecting the second and third metacarpals. Multiple small infarcts have led to loss of bone and periosteal new bone formation.

it may be difficult to differentiate from osteitis, a problem which may easily arise since these children are particularly liable to salmonella osteitis but, if the distribution of the lesions is symmetrical, a diagnosis of sickle-cell osteopathy can be made with confidence. Bossing of the skull from bone changes causes a characteristic head shape and there is generalized osteo-porosis.

Older children may develop the leg ulcers which are characteristic of the adult with sickle-cell disease. Puberty may be delayed. Gall-stones may develop but in children these are rare.

The blood picture shows a normochromic, normocytic anaemia with a variable reticulocyte response and haemoglobin level depending on the degree of marrow activity. Polychromasia, target cells, occasional sickle cells and nucleated red cells are regularly seen. The Coombs' test is negative. An associated megaloblastic anaemia is not uncommon owing to the increased

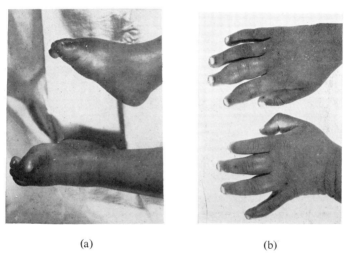

(a)                                      (b)

FIG. 133. (a) Symmetrical oedema of the dorsum of the feet in an infant with
sickle-cell disease.
(b) Symmetrical spindle-shaped swellings of the fingers in an infant
with sickle-cell disease.

need of the bone marrow for folic acid, aggravated by its frequent shortage in the diet.

There is a threefold increase in the incidence of glucose-6-phosphate dehydrogenase (G-6-PD) deficiency in Africans with sickle-cell disease (Lewis et al., 1966). This may be masked by the high reticulocyte count since these cells are not deficient in the enzyme (p. 112).

*Prognosis and treatment.* The number of patients who survive to adult life is small and, therefore, the number who will bear children is very limited. Despite this, the frequency of the disease in tropical Africa is very high due to the large number of carriers. A further factor which tends to increase the proportion of carriers in the population is the fact that AS individuals are more resistant to malaria than normal adults. Malaria increases the sickling rate but since these cells are more rapidly phagocytosed than normal cells the malarial parasite is destroyed in the process.

Treatment is essentially prophylactic to reduce the liability to crises, and symptomatic; there is no cure for the condition. Early treatment of infection by antibiotics and fluids may prevent a crisis. Hypoxia must be avoided during anaesthesia; for this reason a local or spinal anaesthetic is preferable to a general anaesthetic. Blood transfusions should be used as little as possible since a higher haemaglobin increases the liability to thrombosis. Moreover, a transfusion of blood causes temporary inhibition of erythropoiesis. A low haemoglobin is less serious than in a normal child since Hb S releases its oxygen more easily than Hb A, its oxygen dissociation curve being to the right of normal.

All patients should be checked for G-6-PD deficiency since aspirin and many other analgesics will precipitate haemolysis in such individuals.

Folic acid should be given to all patients in view of their increased requirements. The administration of folic acid alone to untreated dwarfed and immature young adults with the disease has caused growth and sexual maturity to take place. In cases where the spleen is enlarged and overactive in destroying red cells, splenectomy may be required to eliminate this hypersplenic action.

Intravenous bicarbonate solutions have been recommended for crises but their value is questionable. Acetazolamide, which inhibits the occurrence of sickling *in vitro*, has been tried in treatment but unfortunately has little influence on the disease.

### SICKLE-CELL TRAIT (AS)

These individuals usually have no symptoms, since less than 1 per cent of their red cells are sickled in comparison with 30–60 per cent of those with the disease. Haematuria may occasionally occur and more serious symptoms can result if they are subjected to low oxygen tension as might occur when flying. The risks are less in a pressurized aeroplane but it is safer if air travel is avoided.

### SICKLE-CELL HAEMOGLOBIN C DISEASE (SC)

Haemoglobin C is another abnormal haemoglobin. Patients with SC genotype present as a mild form of sickle-cell disease with later onset and a longer expectation of life. The characteristic finding is the number of target cells in the peripheral blood which may be as high as 80 per cent.

THALASSAEMIA

This condition occurs particularly in those of Mediterranean parentage but is sometimes seen in other races. No specific abnormal haemoglobin has been detected, but there is a defect in the synthesis of haemoglobin A leading to the production of abnormally shaped cells which are deficient in haemoglobin and more liable to haemolysis. Large quantities of fetal haemoglobin are produced, presumably as a compensation for a defect in the ability to produce haemoglobin A.

The condition exists in two forms: thalassaemia minor, which is the heterozygous trait; and thalassaemia major or Cooley's anaemia, which is the homozygous form.

THALASSAEMIA MINOR

Affected individuals may be asymptomatic or may show symptoms which simulate mild Cooley's anaemia. The level of fetal haemoglobin may be up to 20 per cent and there is a characteristic increase in the level of haemoglobin $A_2$ in most cases. In normal adults 97 per cent of the adult haemoglobin is in the $A_1$ form, and only 3 per cent as $A_2$, which has different polypeptide chains. Proving that a parent has the thalassaemia trait helps in the diagnosis of thalasaemia major in the child.

THALASSAEMIA MAJOR (COOLEY'S ANAEMIA, MEDITERRANEAN ANAEMIA)

This is an extremely severe clinical syndrome with profound haemolysis and anaemia so that few patients survive to adult life. The condition manifests itself from the age of 3 months. Hyperplasia of the bone marrow leads to thickening of the skull and face bones and a somewhat mongoloid appearance. The skin is a muddy yellow colour. The liver and spleen are much enlarged.

The blood picture shows all the changes of a severe haemolytic anaemia. The red cells are irregular and fragmented and target cells are numerous. Up to 90 per cent of the haemoglobin is fetal. Jaundice is not a feature since the red cells are so poorly haemoglobinized that a sufficient rise in bilirubin to produce clinical jaundice seldom occurs.

X-rays of the skull show radiating spicules in the widened diploe resulting from hyperplasia, giving a characteristic picture like hair standing on end.

*Treatment.* There is no cure for the disease, but transfusions should be given frequently in order to maintain the haemoglobin at a high level. The reason for this is that Hb F does not release its oxygen as freely as Hb A, its oxygen dissociation curve being to the left of normal. This high transfusion regime also reduces the expanded blood volume which occurs in thalassaemia. Iron is contraindicated since the frequent transfusions of blood cause the tissues to contain an excess of iron, so that secondary haemosiderosis becomes a problem (see below). Splenectomy is of value if the spleen is so much enlarged as to produce symptoms from its size or if it is exerting a hyper-splenic action, thereby causing an even more rapid destruction of red cells and sometimes of platelets also.

SICKLE-CELL THALASSAEMIA

This condition shows the features of both diseases, though usually it is less severe than either sickle-cell anaemia or Cooley's anaemia. It cannot be definitely distinguished from sickle-cell anaemia by electrophoresis since the two disorders can produce identical patterns. Family studies are therefore necessary to confirm the diagnosis.

## Glucose-6-phosphate dehydrogenase (G-6-PD) deficiency

Glucose-6-phosphate dehydrogenase is required for the pentose–phosphate pathway involving glutathione metabolism. Glutathione is necessary for the maintenance of the normal architecture of the red cell; a deficiency of G-6-PD therefore leads to weakening of the structure of the cell and consequent greater liability to haemolysis.

The deficiency occurs on the X chromosome. Full expression occurs in heterozygote males and in the rare females in whom both X chromosomes carry the mutant gene. Intermediate expression occurs in heterozygous females who have two red cell populations, one normal and one indistinguishable from deficient males. The proportion of abnormal cells varies from about normal to that found in heterozygote males and it is this proportion which governs the severity of the disorder.

Over 50 variants of this deficiency have now been described but 3 only are particularly important to children.

TYPE 1

Occurs in Negroes and is the mildest form. Haemolysis is provoked by high doses of haemolytic drugs such as sulphonamides, sulphones, primaquine, pamaquin, mepacrine, acetylsalicylic acid, phenacetin, synthetic vitamin K analogues, nalidixic acid, naphthalene and aniline dyes. Haemolysis does not occur spontaneously, nor is it provoked by fava beans.

In this type (unlike type 2) the reticulocytes have a relatively high level of G-6-PD. In affected full-term Negro babies there is no significantly increased incidence of jaundice nor is there a danger of this from giving 1 mg vitamin K routinely to newborn babies (Capps et al., 1963).

TYPE 2

This type is called *favism* and affects Caucasians, especially the Mediterranean races. Oriental individuals may be similarly affected. There is a greater susceptibility to all the haemolytic drugs and especially to fava beans. The reticulocytes carry a low level of G-6-PD, therefore the risk of hyperbilirubinaemia leading to kernicterus is great. Spontaneous haemolysis occurs in this type.

TYPE 3

This occurs mainly in N. Europeans. The deficiency causes a congenital chronic non-spherocytic anaemia even in the absence of drugs. Hyperbilirubinaemia always occurs in the neonate. The reticulocytes in this type show no difference in enzyme activity from adult red cells. In newborn babies great care must be taken to ensure there is no risk of haemolytic drugs reaching the baby through the breast milk.

## 2. Haemolysis from circulating antibodies

(a) *Haemolytic disease of the newborn* (*Erythroblastosis fetalis*), see p. 120.

(b) *Auto-immune haemolytic anaemia.* In these patients haemolysis results from circulating autoagglutinins; the direct Coombs' test is usually positive. The process may involve the circulating blood only so that immune antibodies destroy the erythrocytes and reticulocytes but leave the erythropoietic elements of the marrow intact. In such cases the peripheral blood suggests an aplastic anaemia but the marrow shows erythroid hyperplasia. Alternatively, the marrow may also be involved, so that the condition of immune aplastic haemolytic anaemia results. These processes may take place in the same patient at different stages of the disease. Thrombocytopenia may also be present (see p. 599).

This condition may be precipitated by infection. It is usually acute and tends to be self-limiting so that there is a good chance of recovery. Steroid therapy should be used in all cases. Splenectomy may be of value by reducing the amount of destruction of red cells and platelets.

## 3. Haemolysis due to extra corpuscular agents unassociated with antibodies

This may result from infection, drugs or chemical poisons.

*Infection.* This may be due to a bacterial toxin such as that derived from *E. coli*, haemolytic streptococcus or *C. welchii*, or it may be due to an organism such as malaria which directly attacks the red cell.

*Drugs.* The most frequent reason for haemolysis following the ingestion of drugs is that the patient is deficient of glucose-6-phosphate dehydrogenase (see above). Drugs can also cause haemolysis in individuals who are not enzyme deficient; for example, large doses of vitamin K analogues can cause severe haemolysis in newborn babies, especially if preterm.

*Chemical poisons.* Those which cause haemolysis include lead, benzol and its derivatives, and nitro-derivatives of toluol and phenol.

The onset of this form of haemolytic anaemia is usually acute; haemoglobinuria may occur early in the disease. The blood shows a normochromic and normocytic anaemia which may be profound; a high reticulocyte count is present, indicating the intense regenerative activity taking place. Nucleated red cells may be present in the peripheral blood, the toxic action being shown by fragmentation of the red cells and Heinz bodies. Erythrophagocytosis is often found in the peripheral blood and bone marrow. The red cells may become spherocytic, in which case tests show increased fragility.

### Haemolytic–uraemic syndrome

This disorder mainly affects toddlers. It is of unknown cause but occasionally there is evidence of a preceding viral or bacterial infection; sometimes small epidemics have occurred. There is an acute onset of severe anaemia, thrombocytopenia and uraemia.

Disseminated intravascular coagulation (p. 601) occurs, leading to the characteristic blood picture of burred and fragmented red cells, due to their damage by fibrin strands.

Treatment comprises repeated transfusions with packed cells and the management of acute renal failure by restricting the intake of fluid, protein and potassium. Peritoneal dialysis may be required. Heparin is necessary for the management of the coagulation defect.

### Hypersplenism

This is a syndrome in which a spleen enlarged from any disorder causes a reduction in the circulating level of red cells, white cells or platelets. Marrow activity must be normal or increased, especially in regard to the cell line(s) affected. There should be no immature cells in the peripheral blood.

In deciding whether splenectomy is required an estimation of red cell survival is helpful. Retrospective confirmation of the diagnosis is shown by correction of the defects following removal of the spleen.

### Secondary haemosiderosis

With all chronic haemolytic anaemias the problem of secondary haemosiderosis must be considered in relation to therapy. Haemolysis results in an excess of iron in the tissues which is stored in the reticulo-endothelial system. This causes enlargement of the liver, spleen and sometimes of the lymph glands, as well as producing a grey colour in the skin; in severe cases there is impaired liver function.

Iron therapy is therefore contraindicated and, since blood transfusions increase the degree of haemosiderosis, this aspect must always be considered before giving a transfusion, in order to achieve a balance between the problems of anaemia and those of haemosiderosis. Chelating agents, such as desferrioxamine, which have an affinity for iron should be considered for those who are liable to secondary haemolysis, especially patients with thalassaemia in which this is such a serious problem because of the frequent transfusions required. It is given by daily intramuscular injection, which unfortunately is painful, and it should be added to the blood before transfusion (Sephton Smith, 1964).

## Methaemoglobinaemia

This exists both as a congenital disease due to an inborn error of metabolism and as an acquired condition from poisoning.

### CONGENITAL METHAEMOGLOBINAEMIA

This is a rare inborn error of metabolism which is usually familial; transmission may depend on either dominant or recessive genes. It is due to a deficiency of the methaemoglobin reductase system in the red cells. The infants are cyanosed and are often thought first to have congenital heart disease, but the absence of distress, the normal heart size and the peculiar lavender-blue colour should suggest the correct diagnosis. The diagnosis is made by spectroscopic examination of the blood.

Many of the children with the disease become mentally retarded. It has been suggested that this is due to the effect of the methaemoglobin, but the occurrence of normal mentality in some individuals with a high level of methaemoglobin makes it more likely that the mental defect and the methaemoglobinaemia are inherited separately.

*Treatment.* Methylene blue or ascorbic acid result in reduction of the methaemoglobin. Methylene blue is more effective and is therefore the drug of choice. It is given in a dose of 4 mg per kg daily by mouth in three divided doses. If intolerance to methylene blue develops, ascorbic acid should be used alone or in combination with a smaller dose of methylene blue. Large doses (300–500 mg daily) of ascorbic acid are required.

### ACQUIRED METHAEMOGLOBINAEMIA

Drugs such as sulphonamides, and poisons such as nitrites or aniline derivatives may cause this condition. Poisoning has occurred from the accidental ingestion of nitrites or the contamination of drinking water with nitrates which are converted to nitrites in the intestine. Aniline derivatives may be ingested in the form of wax crayons or disinfectants, or they may be absorbed through the skin when aniline dye has been used to mark napkins.

## Hypogammaglobulinaemia

When first described, this condition was termed agammaglobulinaemia; since then more sensitive techniques have shown that gammaglobulin is probably never completely absent and it is, therefore, preferable to speak of hypo-gammaglobulinaemia. The condition is probably not rare and manifests itself in a number of ways.

*Congenital hypogammaglobulinaemia.* This is inherited as a sex-linked recessive characteristic, being virtually confined to boys. The lymph nodes are.almost totally devoid of normal follicles and plasma cells. Since these are responsible for the synthesis of gammaglobulin (see p. 481) there is a severe lack of it.

*Primary acquired hypogammaglobulinaemia.* This is equally common in both sexes and is not a hereditary disease. In this form the lymph glands are enlarged and show either follicular hyperplasia or reticulum-cell hyperplasia.

*Secondary acquired hypogammaglobulinaemia.* This is found in some cases of multiple myeloma, lymphoma, and chronic lymphatic leukaemia and nephrosis.

Individuals with hypogammaglobulinaemia are particularly susceptible to recurrent bacterial infections, especially with Gram-positive organisms and *Pneumocystis carinii*. Some children have presented with chronic bronchiec-tasis which has progressed despite all forms of therapy. Somewhat surprisingly, they appear to respond normally to most virus diseases except hepatitis, although they cannot produce antibodies against virus antigens. The level of gammaglobulin should be below 200 mg per cent before the diagnosis is made. Treatment should be by the weekly intramuscular injection of pooled gammaglobulin in a dose of 0·025 g per kg. Diarrhoea and steatorrhoea are common in these patients and rheumatoid arthritis sometimes occurs.

*Transient hypogammaglobulinaemia of infancy.* A fall in gammaglobulin is normal shortly after birth when the maternal gammaglobulin is gradually disappearing and the infant's own synthesis has not yet got under way. In some this natural fall may be excessive. These patients differ from those already described in that the condition is transient. They show a specific sensitivity to viruses so that generalized vaccinia has occurred following vaccination.

# DISORDERS OF THE LYMPHATIC SYSTEM

## Lymphosarcoma

This condition is closely related to lymphatic leukaemia. It is probable that both represent different manifestations of the same condition, the difference being the presence of malignant cells in the peripheral blood in leukaemia, and their absence in lymphosarcoma. Some cases of lymphosarcoma develop the typical blood picture of lymphatic leukaemia in the late stages.

The disease may affect any of the lymph gland groups, the cervical, mediastinal and abdominal being the most frequently affected. Symptoms depend on the area affected; if the cervical glands are involved, a mass is visible in the neck which is hard and fixed; pain is not a feature and pressure symptoms occur late. Mediastinal involvement causes early pressure symptoms from tracheal or bronchial obstruction and a pleural effusion commonly develops. Abdominal disease may affect the retroperitoneal or mesenteric glands, causing abdominal pain and disturbance of bowel function.

As the disease spreads there may be widespread involvement of lymphatic tissue throughout the body, the child becoming increasingly wasted. The condition is confirmed by biopsy and is always fatal.

*Treatment.* Chemotherapy by means of cytotoxic drugs still has little to offer in this disease but may afford temporary relief. Surgery can do little except to relieve obstruction of the respiratory passages or intestinal tract.

### Malignant lymphoma (Burkitt tumour)

This is a common condition affecting children in Africa. It has a remarkable geographical distribution and, in the countries involved, is the commonest cause of cancer in children. The tumour lymphocytes are larger than normal lymphocytes and dispersed among them are non-malignant histiocytes, thus giving a different picture from the ordinary form of lymphosarcoma in which there are sheets of neoplastic lymphocytes only. It is characteristic that the lymph glands and spleen are seldom involved. The tumour deposits appear in many widely separated organs simultaneously and, in the early stage of development in one organ, the lesions are often multiple before they coalesce to form a single mass. The possibility of blood-stream spread is made unlikely by the fact that the lungs are seldom involved; it is probable that multiple primary tumours occur simultaneously in different sites.

*Aetiology.* The tumour has a geographical distribution from the west to the east coast of Africa—in the equatorial belt across the middle of the continent. It rarely occurs in high altitudes or in hot dry areas (Burkitt & Wright, 1966). The disease is almost certainly due to EB virus infection of lymphoid tissue which has been damaged previously by chronic malarial infection.

*Clinical features.* The condition seldom occurs before 2 years or after 14 years of age, the majority of patients being between 4 and 7 years old. The commonest modes of presentation are as a tumour of the jaw, orbit or abdomen, or as paraplegia from extradural involvement of the spinal cord.

The jaw tumour (Fig. 134a) is the most characteristic form of presentation; the teeth soon become displaced and then drop out. In many cases more than one quadrant of the jaw is affected and it is not unusual for all four quadrants to be involved simultaneously. The orbital tumour (Fig. 134b) causes the rapid development of chemosis and proptosis of the eye. The abdominal tumour most often presents in one or both loins from renal

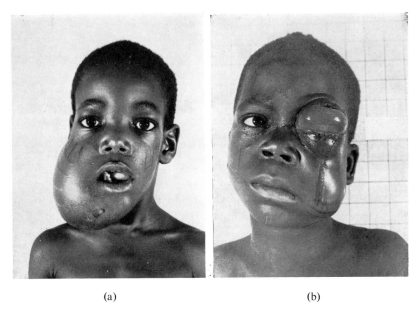

(a)                                                    (b)

FIG. 134. Malignant lymphoma.
(a) Involving the right maxilla and mandible. The displaced teeth are visible inside the mouth.
(b) Arising from the left maxilla to involve the orbit. There is gross chemosis, with upward displacement of the eye.

involvement; the liver may be affected also. Bilateral ovarian tumours are characteristic, being detected as freely mobile masses in each iliac fossa. Paraplegia is caused by neoplastic deposits in the extradural space in the lumbar and lower thoracic spine which compress the spinal cord. It is distinguished from that of tuberculous origin by the absence both of kyphosis and radiological changes in the vertebrae.

The tumours may also be found in the long bones, salivary glands, thyroid, testicle and breast. In every patient it is usual to find more than one site involved. Growth of the tumours in all sites is very fast so that the condition is rapidly fatal, but hideous facial deformities occur in the course of the disease.

*Treatment.* Chemotherapy with cytotoxic drugs such as cyclophosphamide offers some hope, the tumours usually melting away for a time when treatment is begun. BCG enhances the degree of cell mediated immunity although it does not affect the relapse rate.

### Hodgkin's disease

This condition is uncommon in children, rarely occurring before the age of 5 years; it is more frequent in boys than girls. There is a slowly progressive painless enlargement of the lymph glands, most often in the cervical region. The glands characteristically remain discrete and rubbery even when much enlarged. Pressure symptoms result from mediastinal and abdominal gland involvement. The spleen is usually enlarged and spread to the liver and bone marrow may occur.

In most cases the appearance of enlarged cervical glands is the first sign; there is little constitutional disturbance. However, in some patients there are general symptoms of anorexia and loss of weight associated with periods of high fever lasting 1–2 weeks, followed by a remission (Pel-Ebstein fever).

The blood may be normal but a hypoplastic anaemia develops as the bone marrow is invaded. The white-cell findings are variable; eosinophilia sometimes occurs. Confirmation of the diagnosis is made by lymph-gland biopsy.

*Treatment.* There is no cure but life can be prolonged by therapy. Localized disease should be treated by radiation; cytotoxic drugs should be given if the disease is generalized.

## DISEASES OF THE RETICULO-ENDOTHELIAL SYSTEM

### HISTIOCYTOSIS-X

#### Eosinophilic granuloma, Hand-Schüller-Christian disease, Letterer-Siwe disease

These three conditions, once regarded as distinct, are now accepted as clinical variations of one pathological disorder. The basic lesion is a proliferation of histiocytes which is probably neoplastic in origin. The main sites of the reticulo-endothelial system are the bone marrow, lymphoid tissue, liver, spleen, lungs and skin; therefore it is these organs which are involved singly or together in the disease process. The bone-marrow lesions usually cause clear-cut areas of bone destruction and this may stimulate the formation of new bone. It is possible for the bone marrow to be extensively infiltrated without any absorption of bone taking place.

Involvement of lymphoid tissue causes medullary proliferation with loss of normal architecture, thereby causing enlargement of the liver, spleen, lymph glands and thymus. In the liver the histiocytic proliferation is largely confined to the portal zones and may lead to biliary obstruction and cirrhosis.

Multifocal lung lesions occur, consisting of interstitial and peribronchial cellular infiltration which produce miliary shadows radiographically. Bronchial damage and necrosis of the abnormal tissue leads to cavitation and an X-ray appearance of a honeycomb lung.

*Clinical features.* Reference to the earlier clinical categories has some value from a descriptive angle, provided it is understood that intermediate forms are seen and that one pattern may undergo transition into another.

### Eosinophilic granuloma

This is a slow-growing lesion of bone seen in older children, occurring especially in the skull, pelvis or long bones. The lesions are focal, either single or multiple. The disease may present as a visible tumour of bone, usually with some pain, or be discovered on routine radiography.

### Hand-Schüller-Christian disease

In this form of the disease the bone lesions are multiple, occurring in the same sites as those where the eosinophilic granuloma may be found. Soft-tissue swellings may be palpable over the bone lesions. The classical description comprised a triad: bony defects in the skull, exophthalmos and diabetes insipidus, but all of these are seldom seen together. The disease occurs during the first 6 years of life. The condition progresses more rapidly than the eosinophilic granuloma.

Jaw involvement leads to extrusion of the teeth, and mastoid involvement to an aural discharge. Skin rashes and nodules may develop as in Letterer-Siwe disease. Exophthalmos is caused by retro-orbital infiltration, and compression of the pituitary gland may lead to retardation of growth or sexual development, or to diabetes insipidus from pituitary insufficiency.

The skull lesions show on X-ray as clear-cut, oval or circular areas of bone destruction which may be very numerous, with slight surrounding increase in bone density. The appearance in the long bones may be more variable and less distinctive. Any part of the shaft may be affected, though the region near the metaphysis is the most commonly involved. The shaft may be expanded, surrounding sclerosis may occur and, if the cortex is involved, periosteal new bone formation takes place. A pathological fracture results occasionally only.

## Letterer-Siwe disease

This is an acute illness, principally affecting infants in the first 2 years of life. There is enlargement of the liver, spleen and lymph glands. Skin changes are always present, a pink macular rash being characteristic in the early stages, infiltrative papules appearing later; these may become so extensive as to give an appearance similar to seborrhoeic eczema. Such lesions are most marked in the scalp and flexures and may be intensely irritating. Thrombocytopenia from marrow involvement causes petechial and purpuric eruptions. The nail beds may be affected so that the nails are loosened and eventually drop off. Pulmonary involvement causes miliary mottling or a honeycomb appearance in the chest X-ray. Skeletal lesions, though present, do not dominate the condition as in the other two forms of the disease.

*Diagnosis.* This is confirmed by skin or lymph-gland biopsy. The miliary mottling in the chest film must be distinguished from miliary tuberculosis and the honeycomb lung from the changes seen in cystic fibrosis.

*Prognosis.* Letterer-Siwe disease is the most fulminating form of the disease; without treatment the condition is usually fatal within a few months, although spontaneous recovery has occurred. Eosinophilic granuloma is the most chronic form, especially in the older patient. It may cause little clinical disturbance and has a strong tendency to heal spontaneously, though it may progress to the multiple bone involvement seen in the Hand-Schüller-Christian form.

Hand-Schüller-Christian disease lies between these two forms. It causes a chronic disease lasting for years; death may occur from intercurrent infection.

*Treatment.* The eosinophilic granuloma can be rapidly cured by surgical excision or radiotherapy. For the other two forms of the disease treatment as for acute leukaemia should be given. Since the individual lesions are radiosensitive, X-ray therapy may also be used in Hand-Schüller-Christian disease.

## BIBLIOGRAPHY

BRITTEN M.I., SPOONER R.J.D., DORMANDY K.M. & BIGGS R. (1966) The haemophilic boy in school. *Brit. med. J.*, **2**, 224.

BURKITT D. (1962) A tumour syndrome affecting children in tropical Africa. *Postgrad. med. J.*, **38**, 71.

BURKITT D. & WRIGHT D. (1966) Geographical and tribal distribution of the African lymphoma in Uganda. *Brit. med. J.*, **1**, 569.

CAPPS F.P.A., GILLES H.M., JOLLY H. & WORLLEDGE S.M. (1963) Glucose-6-phosphate dehydrogenase deficiency and neonatal jaundice in Nigeria. Their relation to the use of prophylactic vitamin K. *Lancet*, **2**, 379.

CLEMENT D.H. (1964) Pitfalls in the diagnosis and treatment of iron deficiency anaemia in pediatrics. *Pediatrics*, **34**, 117.

EVANS H.E. & NYHAN W.L. (1964) Hodgkin's disease in children. *Bull. Johns Hopk. Hosp.*, **114**, 237.

HUG I. (1965) Die leukämiefälle des kinderspitals Zürich 1954–63. *Helv. Paed. Acta*, **20**, 56.

KELLY F. (1965) Hodgkin's disease in children. *Amer. J. Roentgenol*, **95**, 48.

KONOTEY-AHULU F.I.D. (1965) Sicklaemic human hygrometers. *Lancet*, **1**, 1003.

LAMBERT H.P., PRANKERD T.A.J. & SMELLIE J.M. (1961) Pernicious anaemia in childhood. *Quart. J. Med. N.S.*, **30**, 71.

LEWIS R.A., KAY R.W. & HATHORN M. (1966) Sickle cell disease and glucose-6-phosphate dehydrogenase. *Acta haemat.* (Basel) **36**, 399.

MCINTYRE O.R., SULLIVAN L.W., JEFFRIES G.H. & SILVER R.H. (1965) Pernicious anaemia in childhood. *New Engl. J. Med.*, **272**, 981.

MIDDLEMISS J.H. (1960) Haemophilia and Christmas disease. *Clin. Radiol.*, **11**, 40.

PINKEL D. (1973) *Treatment of acute lymphocytic leukemia.* Leuk. Research Fund.

SEPHTON SMITH R. (1964) Chelating agents in the diagnosis and treatment of iron overload in thalassemia. *Ann. N.Y. Acad. Sci.*, **119**, 776.

STEWART A., WEBB J. & HEWITT D. (1958) A survey of childhood malignancies. *Brit. med. J.*, **1**, 1495.

TILL M.M., HARDISTY R.M. & PIKE M.C. (1973) Long term survivals in acute leukaemia. *Lancet*, **1**, 534.

TOUGH I.M., COURT BROWN W.M., BAIKIE A.G., BUCKTON K.E., HARNDEN D.G., JACOBS P.A., KING M.J. & MCBRIDE J.A. (1961) Cytogenetic studies in chronic myeloid leukaemia and acute leukaemia associated with mongolism, *Lancet*, **1**, 411.

WINSOR T. & BURCH G.E. (1945) Sickle cell anaemia, 'a great masquerader'. *J. Amer. med. Ass.*, **129**, 792.

CHAPTER 22

# DISEASES OF THE ENDOCRINE GLANDS

## PITUITARY

The influence of the pituitary gland on the other endocrine organs is such that clear-cut syndromes resulting from its over- or under-activity are less easily identified than those of the other organs. Thus hypopituitary causes of dwarfism may consist of an isolated deficiency of growth hormone or comprise panhypopituitarism in which case there is evidence of thyroid or adrenocortical failure due to insufficiency of thyrotrophic or adrenocorticotrophic hormone. Similarly, Cushing's disease (p. 632) which is due to excessive adrenocortical hormones, may be due to a pituitary or an adrenal lesion. A multiplicity of endocrine disorders increases the likelihood that the primary fault lies with pituitary.

Disorders caused by underactivity of the pituitary, since they lead to growth failure, have been discussed on p. 278. Overactivity of the pituitary gland is extremely rare, the only syndromes from this cause in children being gigantism, due to an eosinophil adenoma (p. 281), and Cushing's disease (p. 632), one cause of which is a basophil adenoma of the pituitary.

### Diabetes insipidus

There are three types of diabetes insipidus:

### 1. HORMONAL TYPE

In this type there is a lack of antidiuretic hormone from the posterior pituitary owing to an organic brain lesion. The lesion can involve either the posterior pituitary itself or the hypothalamus since a close functional relationship exists between them; it may be due to trauma, neoplasm or infection, especially encephalitis or tuberculous meningitis. There may be associated neurological abnormalities, such as ocular defects, anosmia or raised intracranial pressure. There may also be evidence of other endocrine disorders from more extensive involvement of the pituitary or hypothalamus.

This is the only disorder which results from diminished activity of the posterior pituitary gland.

## 2. RENAL TYPE (NEPHROGENIC DIABETES INSIPIDUS)

In this type, a defect of the distal renal tubule renders it insensitive to the action of antidiuretic hormone. The condition is confined to males and is inherited as a sex-linked recessive character. It is transmitted by females who can be discovered by their defective water concentration tests; these females may develop polydypsia and polyuria during pregnancy.

## 3. IDIOPATHIC TYPE

No organic lesion can be detected in this type. It may be inherited as a dominant characteristic.

*Clinical features.* The symptoms of diabetes insipidus are the same in all three types—polyuria and thirst. This may be so intense as to cause the child to drink water from flower vases if ordinary sources are denied to him. Enuresis may be the presenting feature. In infants, the lack of fluid causes severe irritability and restlessness, leading to dehydration, collapse and high fever. Mental retardation develops if the thirst is not satisfied.

## Treatment

### HORMONAL TYPE

The organic lesion should be treated directly if possible. However, such treatment is not always possible in which case the patient should be given vasopressin tannate. This is injected intramuscularly, on alternate days, starting with 0·2 ml and working up to 2 ml if a satisfactory response has not been produced earlier. Great care must be taken to locate the brown oil spot in the ampoule since it is this which contains the pitressin. If the ampoule has been stored upside down and not shaken before opening, the pitressin could easily be thrown away with the cut end of the ampoule. This risk is so great as to cause some clinicians to prefer the watery solution, even though this must be given intravenously.

### RENAL TYPE

Chlorothiazide and hydrochlorothiazide are effective in this form of the disorder. Their mode of action is probably by depletion of body sodium (Schotland *et al.*, 1963).

### IDIOPATHIC TYPE

Patients with this form of the disorder respond to pitressin tannate, given as above.

In all three forms of the disease the child must be encouraged to drink as much as he wants if mental retardation is to be prevented.

# THYROID

## HYPOTHYROIDISM

### DYSGENESIS OF THE THYROID GLAND

In childhood, hypothyroid states are much commoner than hyperthyroid. These most frequently result from dysgenesis of the gland which can cause its total absence or its maldevelopment, resulting in a correctly situated but inadequate remnant. More common than either of these causes of hypothyroidism is maldescent leading to an ectopic thyroid gland placed above the hyoid bone. Total lack of thyroid causes severe cretinism whereas maldescent or maldevelopment result in mild cretinism or juvenile hypothyroidism.

### DYSHORMONOGENESIS

Hypothyroidism can also be due to metabolic blocks in the synthesis of the two thyroid hormones: tri-iodothyronine (T3) and thyroxine (T4). These are genetically determined on an autosomal recessive basis and are less frequent than dysgenesis of the gland. Five enzyme defects are recognized at present: failure of the thyroid trapping mechanism of iodine; failure of organic binding of iodide; failure of coupling of iodotyrosine; failure of deiodination of iodotyrosines; production of abnormal thyroproteins. The diminished production of thyroid hormones results in an increased secretion of TSH by the pituitary causing thyroid hyperplasia and the formation of a goitre—hence *familial goitrous hypothyroidism*.

Synthesis of thyroxine in the fetus can also be interrupted by the ingestion of antithyroid drugs in pregnancy, such as thiouracil or carbimazole given to the mother for the treatment of thyrotoxicosis. A similar situation occurs if the pregnant mother takes excessive iodide, commonly in the form of cough mixtures or 'asthma cures'. Fetal thyroid lack due to the maternal ingestion of drugs is temporary only but the baby may be born with a goitre and can suffer permanent brain damage.

### ENDEMIC CRETINISM

This condition is due to iodine deficiency. It occurs in some but not all areas of endemic goitre. It does not occur in the United Kingdom.

### Cretinism

These children commonly appear normal at birth because they have been receiving some thyroid hormone from the mother. However, the placental transfer of tri-iodothyronine and thyroxine is slow, probably because it is bound to protein. Severe cretinism can therefore be diagnosed within a few days of birth although mild cretinism will not be obvious until 6–12 months of age.

The baby becomes increasingly sluggish so that feeding is difficult. Severe constipation develops and there are often respiratory difficulties due to nasal obstruction. It is essential to be aware that these symptoms occur before the physical signs appear. The physical features, which make all cretins look alike, appear slowly (Fig. 135a). The face becomes coarse and somewhat pig-like, with heavy eyelids, a squat nose and thick lips. The hair is scanty, dry and brittle and the eyebrows become thinned. The complexion is sallow and the skin is cold and thick from myxoedematous tissue which produces supra-clavicular pads and, by thickening the vocal cords, causes the voice to become deep and hoarse. Prior to the development of the deep cry it may be noticed that facial contortion occurs some seconds before the actual cry is heard. The tongue is large so that it protrudes through the open mouth, the pulse is slow and the temperature subnormal. The abdomen is pot-bellied and an umbilical hernia is common. Growth becomes retarded, there is delay in the eruption of teeth and closure of the fontanelle and, most important of all, there is progressive mental retardation. Prolonged physiological jaundice (p. 119) sometimes occurs.

Some degree of hypochromic anaemia is always present, due to a specific effect of thyroid lack. The bone age is retarded so that in a cretin diagnosed in the early weeks of life there is absence of the lower femoral and upper tibial epiphyses which should be present at birth. The bone age in hypothyroidism is even more retarded than the height age, whereas a deficiency of growth hormone causes the bone age and height age to be equally retarded.

The rise in serum cholesterol is a crude test of hypothyroidism, there often being no change during the first 2 years of life. A more sensitive test is the level of protein-bound iodine (PBI) which is lower than normal. However, in the newborn the normal levels of PBI are high so that estimation of red blood cell uptake of tri-iodothyronine or the level of thyroxine should be undertaken.

*Diagnosis.* The younger the infant the more difficult the diagnosis, but successful treatment requires early diagnosis and this is often unnecessarily late. Constipation is the most useful early sign. Severe constipation in a young baby is unusual; no baby should be treated for constipation without the possibility of cretinism being first considered. The hoarse cry of the cretin is also very typical and may become apparent in the maternity hospital. (One such baby received the nickname of 'basso' before the correct diagnosis was considered.)

Much has been written of the similarities between cretins and mongols but the differences are far greater. The essential difference is that the mongol is an active baby who is not constipated and has a high colour, whereas the cretin is sluggish, pasty-faced and always constipated. These striking differences should prevent the tragic mistake of diagnosing a cretin as a mongol, thereby failing to give thyroid.

*Treatment.* Without treatment all cretins become grossly mentally defective, their growth remaining very stunted. The earlier treatment is started the better the chance for future mental development. Thyroxine should always be used in preference to thyroid extract whose biological potency is variable.

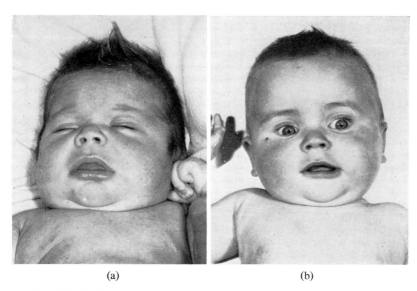

(a)                                             (b)

Fig. 135. Cretin.
(a) Before treatment, aged 4 months. The appearance is sluggish, the features coarse and thick. The eyebrows are thinned and the tongue protrudes.
(b) Under treatment, aged 8 months. The child is now alert and looks normal.

0·1 mg 1-thyroxine sodium is equivalent to 60 mg of thyroid, a starting dose of 0·05 mg daily being given. This is gradually increased until there is evidence of excess, shown by restlessness, tachycardia or diarrhoea; the dose should then be reduced a little. The amount required by individual cretins is very variable and it is, therefore, essential to push the dose to the limit of tolerance rather than plan a fixed dose according to age; many cretins are undertreated because of failure to appreciate this fact. The maintenance dose will need to be increased a little as the child grows older and must be continued for life. In determining the dose for long-term control, the rate of skeletal maturation is valuable, this being assessed by the height and the radiological bone age. The parents must understand that the drug is required for life since they often fail to continue it unless supervision is close. Under treatment the child's physical appearance returns to normal (Fig. 135b). This sometimes causes a new doctor at a later date to doubt the diagnosis and stop the thyroid. To prevent this, the parents should be given a clinical photograph of the patient before treatment which they can show to any doctor.

The administration of thyroxine corrects the anaemia, its specific action being shown by a rise in reticulocytes. The final mental state depends largely on the age at which treatment is initiated but, unfortunately, mental progress in some patients is less satisfactory than might have been anticipated, presumably because intrauterine thyroid lack has produced irreversible changes.

### Juvenile hypothyroidism

These children have some thyroid gland but its function is insufficient for their growing needs. The commonest cause is failure of descent from the back of the tongue to the cricoid cartilage which normally occurs during intrauterine life. The thyroid gland is therefore ectopic, consequently it functions poorly.

The child is normal for the first few years, then signs of hypothyroidism slowly appear. Growth becomes retarded and the child less mentally alert but, because this change is slow, it may not be obvious. Constipation develops, the build becomes stocky and the hands proportionately short and stubby. Myxoedematous deposits, as in cretinism, may be present. Epiphysial dysgenesis occurs so that the epiphyses become irregular and stippled. This change is usually best seen in the upper femoral epiphyses; it may first bring the patient to the orthopaedic surgeon, who must differentiate the condition from Perthes's disease (see p. 693).

Treatment is the same as for cretins, thyroxine being required for life.

### Thyrotoxicosis

This is due to long-acting thyroid stimulator (LATS), an immunoglobulin of the IgG type. This has a TSH-like action but is more powerful and its action more prolonged. It differs from TSH in that its serum levels are not reduced by the administration of thyroxine. Thyrotoxicosis is therefore one of the auto-immune thyroid diseases. It is rare in childhood but the clinical features are the same as in adults though, in addition, the children become taller than normal and have an advanced bone age. It is commoner in girls than in boys and emotional instability is a prominent feature; sometimes the onset seems to be precipitated by an emotional upset. Weight falls despite a good appetite.

The thyroid gland is enlarged and there is tachycardia, excessive sweating and exophthalmos. The level of protein bound iodine is raised. Thyrotoxicosis is sometimes mistaken for chorea.

*Treatment.* The question whether thyrotoxicosis in children should be treated by subtotal thyroidectomy or anti-thyroid drugs, such as carbimazole or methylthiouracil, remains unresolved. About 50 per cent of the patients can be expected to do well on medical treatment, but relapses and toxic reactions are frequent (Saxena *et al.*, 1964). The problem with surgery is the assessment of the future thyroid needs of the child once she has passed through puberty. Consequently, post-operative hypothyroidism is liable to occur.

Rigid adherence to one method of treatment is wrong; each child should be treated as an individual. The problem is eased if, by medical treatment, the child can be brought successfully through puberty. Surgery may still be found necessary later but the liability to post-operative hypothyroidism is reduced. Relapse on medical treatment is an indication for surgery.

Radioactive iodine therapy is simpler and more efficient than either of the other methods, but the increased risk in children of inducing malignancy has largely prevented its use.

*Congenital thyrotoxicosis.* Occasionally, babies are born with the condition if their mothers have been thyrotoxic during pregnancy or treated recently for it. The condition is temporary, resulting from the transplacental passage of LATS. The disorder is usually rapidly controlled by the administration of potassium iodide but carbimazole is occasionally required.

NON-TOXIC GOITRE

The commonest cause is an increased secretion of thyrotrophic hormone in response to inadequate circulating levels of thyroid hormone, the thyroid gland enlarging to compensate for this partial deficiency. The thyroid lack can occur during intrauterine life if the mother is receiving anti-thyroid drugs, the baby being born with a goitre. Such babies should not be breast fed if the mother is still on the drugs, since these are excreted in breast milk. Lack of thyroid, causing a goitre, may also result from inherited defects of the enzymes necessary for the synthesis of thyroid hormone (p. 623).

Lack of iodine in the diet is another cause of goitre. This may occur endemically in iodine deficient areas and can be prevented by the routine administration of iodine.

*Treatment.* Thyroxine should be given to all cases, including those due to iodine lack. The adminstration of iodine usually causes further enlargement of the gland.

## PARATHYROIDS

### Primary hyperparathyroidism

This is extremely rare in childhood, being usually due to a parathyroid adenoma. Calcium is withdrawn from the bones so that the blood calcium rises, the bones becoming decalcified and sometimes cystic. Bone deformities result and calcium may be deposited in the renal tract. Gastrointestinal symptoms, particularly constipation, and muscle weakness also occur.

*Secondary hyperparathyroidism* may occur in children with chronic renal failure. Phosphate retention causes a decrease in serum calcium which leads to overactivity and hyperplasia of the parathyroids.

### Hypoparathyroidism

This is less rare than hyperparathyroidism but is of unknown aetiology. The low serum calcium causes neuromuscular irritability leading to carpopedal spasm, laryngeal stridor, tetany and convulsions. Gastro-intestinal symptoms result from irritability of the intestine. Cataracts develop and photophobia may be a presenting symptom. Ectodermal structures are affected so that the enamel of the developing teeth is pitted, the skin thick and rough and the nails thin and short. Monilial infection of the nails, skin and tongue sometimes occurs, being probably secondary to the trophic changes. Fine granular calcification may occur symmetrically in the basal ganglia on both sides and show on an X-ray of the skull. The low level of parathyroid hormone can be measured.

*Treatment.* The condition responds to dihydrotachysterol or large doses of vitamin D, so that parathyroid hormone, which must be given by injection and is expensive, can be avoided. Moreover, patients become resistant to parathormone after a time.

*Pseudohypoparathyroidism.* This familial disorder is due to failure of the renal tubules to respond to parathyroid hormone, by which test the two conditions are differentiated. The clinical features are the same as in hypoparathyroidism but there are additional congenital abnormalities. The patients are short and stocky with round faces; the index finger is longer than the rest owing to shortening of all the other metacarpals. Subcutaneous calcification is common; mental retardation and obesity may be present.

*Treatment.* The condition responds to large doses of vitamin D or dihydrotachysterol.

## ADRENALS

There are three groups of adrenal corticosteroids:

## 1. Androgen S, e.g. testosterone

This has masculinizing and virilizing properties and encourages growth by protein anabolism. It is sometimes known as the nitrogen-retaining or 'N' hormone. 17-ketosteroids are the excretion product.

## 2. Glucocorticoids, e.g. hydrocortisone and cortisone

Their main function is the control of carbohydrate metabolism. This is largely effected by increasing the breakdown of protein to form glycogen, a process which inhibits growth. It is known as the sugar or 'S' hormone. 17-hydroxy-cortico-steroids are the excretion product.

## 3. Mineralocorticoids, e.g. aldosterone

This is concerned with the control of electrolyte balance. It causes retention of sodium and loss of potassium. It is sometimes known as the salt-retaining hormone.

The adrenogenital syndrome results from an excess of androgens; if the child also suffers from the salt-losing syndrome there is a lack of mineralo-corticoids. Cushing's disease results from an excess of all three groups, but most of the effects are due to an excess of glycogenetic hormone.

## DISORDERS OF THE CORTEX

### Adrenogenital syndrome

This occurs as a congenital or an acquired disorder. The congenital form is always due to adrenal hyperplasia whereas the acquired, which is less common, may be due to hyperplasia or tumour.

### Congenital adrenal hyperplasia

This is due to an inborn error of metabolism in the synthesis of cortisol (hydrocortisone) which is determined by an autosomal recessive gene. At least six different enzyme defects can cause the condition but the commonest is 21-hydroxylase deficiency. The resultant lack of hydrocortisone causes the pituitary to secrete excess ACTH, thereby producing hyperplasia of the fetal adrenal cortex. This causes excessive production of androgens and, if the fetus is female, a female pseudohermaphrodite results. This condition is described on p. 195 since the baby is physically abnormal at birth. The clitoris is enlarged and there is a persistence of the urogenital sinus so that in most cases a single external orifice serves both the vagina and the urethra. Without treatment there is progressive virilization so that the clitoris continues to enlarge and pubic hair appears. Rapid growth is associated with an advanced bone age, deepening of the voice and acne.

If the fetus is a male, the baby appears normal at birth but, during the next few months, the rate of growth and muscular development is greater than normal. Between the ages of 2 and 5 years the penis enlarges, pubic hair develops, the voice deepens and acne appears on the face and back. The testicles remain infantile. The bone age is advanced and the urinary excretion of 17-ketosteroids and pregnanetriol is increased from birth.

Confirmation of the diagnosis at birth is made by finding a raised level of pregnanetriol. The rise in 17-ketosteroids may not be evident until after the first 2 weeks of life. In girls the nuclear sex chromatin shows a normal female pattern.

*Diagnosis.* In girls the condition must be differentiated from other causes of intersex (p. 194). In boys the condition must be diagnosed from other causes of sexual precocity (see p. 282). That the testicles remain infantile is the most useful sign to differentiate it from precocious puberty of constitutional or organic cerebral origin (see Fig. 96). An interstitial cell tumour of the testis produces the same signs and, in the early stages, it is easy to overlook the increased size of one testicle unless special care is taken. The 17-ketosteroids in constitutional precocious puberty are raised to the normal adult level, whereas in adrenal hyperplasia they are very much higher; an interstitial cell tumour also causes a rise but it is seldom as high as in adrenal hyperplasia.

SALT-LOSING TYPE

Virilization is common to all patients with adrenal hyperplasia but about one-third of those with 21-hydroxylase deficiency develop a severe salt-losing syndrome soon after birth, within the first 3 weeks of life, which if untreated often causes death. These patients have a more severe degree of 21-hydroxylase deficiency and affected families breed true so that they either produce children with a defect causing virilization only or virilization and salt loss. The sexes are equally affected in both groups. These patients frequently show hyperpigmentation prior to treatment.

The onset of symptoms is acute. The infant goes off feeds, developing vomiting and diarrhoea which lead to severe dehydration and collapse. The serum sodium and chloride fall while the serum potassium rises; the bicarbonate may fall.

The vomiting sometimes causes the condition to be mistaken for pyloric stenosis (p. 157), especially in boys since they show no genital abnormality at this age. But collapse is not a feature of pyloric stenosis and a pyloric tumour would be felt. The serum chloride is likely to be low in pyloric stenosis, but the serum sodium is much lower in the babies with adrenal failure, whilst their serum potassium is raised.

HYPERTENSIVE TYPE

A very small group of patients develop hypertension after 2–3 years. This is due to a deficiency of 11-β-hydroxylase instead of the much more common 21-hydroxylase deficiency.

*Treatment of congenital adrenal hyperplasia.* Continuous steroid therapy for life is required in both sexes. Steroids suppress the pituitary by removing the exciting stimulus, namely the low level of circulating cortisol. Once the pituitary has been suppressed the excessive production of androgens ceases. Steroids are best given as hydrocortisone since this is the hormone secreted by the adrenals. Its dose is decided by the level of 17-ketosteroids or preg-nanetriol, being the smallest amount which will maintain these substances at a normal level. In view of the circadian rhythm of ACTH production with a peak at 8 a.m., a larger dose of hydrocortisone should be given at night, to deal with this extra ACTH, than in the morning.

Hydrocortisone therapy makes little difference to the size of the penis if it is already enlarged when treatment is begun, but it does cause some diminution in the size of the clitoris and stops the painful erections which sometimes occur. However, a large clitoris should be removed surgically within the first year, once treatment is stabilized. This is necessary because 'gender-aware-ness' becomes established at about the age of 18 months. Moreover, a large clitoris is distressing to the mother. If a plastic repair of the vagina is required, this is deferred until the pubertal period.

*Salt-losing type.* If this condition is first discovered during a crisis, im-mediate intravenous normal saline is required as an emergency. Intravenous hydrocortisone in a dose of 100 mg daily is also necessary, together with 2–5 mg deoxycortone intramuscularly daily.

Once over the acute crisis the infant should be maintained on oral salt and steroid therapy. The starting dose of salt is 4 g daily, this being adjusted as necessary. The most suitable form of steroid for maintenance therapy is 9-alpha-fluoro-hydrocortisone (fludrocortisone), since this has powerful salt-retaining properties; the dose is 0·05–0·2 mg daily. The alternative to this steroid is a combination of hydrocortisone and deoxycortone.

The tendency to salt loss in these patients disappears by the age of 4–5 years. However, it is still wise to keep them on fludrocortisone (Komrower & Bailey, 1974). The dose of salt and salt-retaining hormone should be increased during periods of stress, such as bouts of infection, or when surgery is required.

## Acquired adrenogenital syndrome

If the condition develops after birth it is due to hyperplasia or a tumour, either adenoma or carcinoma, of the adrenal cortex. In the male, the excess of androgen causes the same changes as are seen in congenital adrenal hyperplasia (see p. 629). In the female, virilization occurs as in the congenital form but the external genitalia are normal since fetal development was not affected. Hyperplasia and tumour are differentiated by giving cortisone; this reduces the level of 17-ketosteroids if hyperplasia is present, but there is no change in the case of an adrenal cortical tumour.

### Cushing's disease

This disease results from excessive secretion of adrenocortical hormones. Most of the symptoms result from excess of glucocorticoids, but the two other adrenal corticosteroid hormones, androgens and mineralocorticoids, are increased, being responsible for some of the features of the disease.

The condition is due either to a basophil adenoma of the anterior pituitary causing an excessive production of ACTH, or to a lesion in the adrenals themselves. In all cases there is a hyaline change in the basophil cells of the pituitary (Crooke's hyaline change). The adrenal lesion is either bilateral hyperplasia or a tumour of the cortex. In children, in contrast to adults, an adrenal cortical tumour is by far the commoner cause, the majority being in girls. The patients become 'moon-faced', their faces being round, flushed and bloated. They develop a characteristic obesity which produces a 'buffalo hump' on the upper part of the back, a fat abdomen and thick hips. The limbs remain thin. Purple striae appear on the trunk and limbs and osteoporosis occurs, causing pain in the back. Signs of virilization are less than in the adrenogenital syndrome so that, although excessive hair and acne appear, the penis or clitoris are not necessarily enlarged. Hypertension is usually present and glycosuria with diminished glucose tolerance is common. The circadian rhythm of ACTH production is lost and this has diagnostic value.

*Treatment.* If an adrenal tumour is present it should be removed, but for other cases radiotherapy to the pituitary is the most rational form of therapy. This may need to be combined with subtotal adrenalectomy.

### Adrenal cortical insufficiency

This is seen in its most fulminating form in the Waterhouse-Friderichsen syndrome (see p. 403) when haemorrhage occurs into the adrenals during the course of meningococcal septicaemia. The syndrome may occur also with other fulminating bacterial infections, especially *Pseudomonas pyocanea*. Adrenal insufficiency may also be seen in babies with the adrenogenital syndrome (p. 629) and in newborn babies whose mothers have been receiving steroid therapy. Whenever possible, steroid therapy should be discontinued during pregnancy. If this is impossible, the newborn baby must be closely observed for the earliest evidence of adrenal insufficiency. This is indicated by vomiting, tachycardia and a fall in temperature and blood pressure leading to collapse. Serum electrolyte studies show a low sodium, high potassium and often a low bicarbonate.

*Treatment.* Immediate hydrocortisone therapy and salt replacement is required as for treatment of the salt-losing type of congenital adrenal hyperplasia (p. 631).

### Addison's disease

This is rare in childhood; the majority of cases have been due to tuberculosis of the adrenal and the remainder to adrenal atrophy. The children develop a slowly progressive debility with loss of weight, loss of appetite, general weakness and low blood pressure. A generalized brown pigmentation of the skin develops, together with bluish pigmentation in the mouth. Bouts of vomiting, diarrhoea and abdominal discomfort are common, resulting from acute adrenal insufficiency.

*Treatment.* Continuous therapy with salt and 9-alpha-fluoro-hydrocortisone, or salt, hydrocortisone and deoxycortone is required, as discussed on p. 631.

## DISORDERS OF THE MEDULLA

### Neuroblastoma

This tumour may arise either from the adrenal medulla, or from anywhere in the sympathetic nervous system as both have a similar origin from neuroblasts, which are immature ganglion cells. The majority develop in the adrenal medulla or in the adjacent abdominal sympathetic chain, only a small proportion being cervical, thoracic or pelvic in origin.

The tumour usually occurs within the first 4 years of life. It has no endocrine function and commonly presents as an abdominal mass in an ill child. A large proportion of patients show evidence of metastases at the time they are first seen (Fig. 136), these being usually in the skeleton, lymph glands or liver. The tumour cells cause an increased urinary excretion of catecholamines and of their metabolite vanillyl mandelic acid (VMA).

Occasionally, the highly malignant neuroblast cells become differentiated into mature ganglion cells so that a benign ganglioneuroma (see below) is produced. Spontaneous disappearance of a neuroblastoma sometimes occurs, even after it has metastasized.

The principal problem is to differentiate this tumour from a nephroblastoma (this is discussed on p. 393). The outlook is extremely poor since the tumour is usually inoperable when first seen and has often undergone necrosis. Cytotoxic drugs, especially cyclophosphamide and vincristine, are of value. Radiotherapy can be palliative only, for the relief of pain. Vitamin $B_{12}$ has been tried for some time but has been shown to be ineffective (Sawitsky & Desposito, 1965).

## Ganglioneuroma

This tumour is composed of sympathetic ganglion cells and arises in the same sites as the neuroblastoma. The cells are usually completely differentiated so that the tumour is benign, but tumours with less differentiated cells may occur, merging in their most immature form into the neuroblastoma.

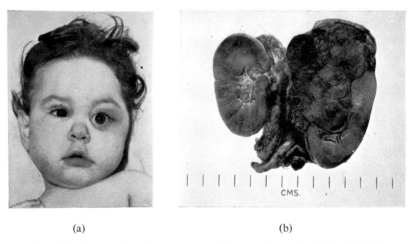

(a)             (b)

FIG. 136. (a) A patient who presented with a swelling in the left orbit. This was due to a metastasis from a neuroblastoma of the left adrenal (b).

## Phaeochromocytoma

These tumours are rare in childhood. They consist of chromaffin cells which produce large quantities of adrenalin and noradrenaline. This causes hypertension which is usually sustained but may be paroxysmal, the child having attacks of headache and vomiting, associated with pallor, sweating and palpitations. The increased urinary excretion of catecholamines and VMA is the most direct test.

## PANCREAS

### Diabetes mellitus

*Aetiology.* The clinical features result from a lack of available and effective insulin. The earlier explanation that this was due to a simple failure of the pancreatic beta islet cells is no longer completely satisfactory, even though the rare occurrence of diabetes after mumps shows that such a mechanism can exist. Probably there is no single cause, the disease being of multifactorial aetiology. Possible factors are: failure of insulin synthesis in the beta cells or of its release from the secretion granules which occurs separately; inhibition of insulin action in the blood by inhibitors such as synalbumin; abnormalities of tissue response to insulin.

Genetic factors are more important in young diabetics than in the elderly. The exact mode of inheritance is unknown and probably multifactorial; this includes a delayed or decreased insulin response to a glucose load. In view of this genetic predisposition some clinicians advise that the siblings of diabetic patients should have a monthly urine check for sugar by the mother and also when ill with infection. Such siblings should also be warned against obesity which can precipitate diabetes.

*Clinical features.* Childhood diabetes accounts for about 5 per cent of all diabetic patients and, although rare under the age of 2 years, its onset has been reported at the age of 9 days. Its onset in childhood is always acute, with thirst and polyuria as the presenting symptoms. A mother may not be able only to state the day of onset, but even the actual hour. For this reason many children present in pre-coma or coma; the discovery of diabetes by finding sugar on routine urine testing seldom occurs. The patients are usually irritable from thirst and dehydration, though polyuria may cause enuresis to be the presenting feature. Abdominal pain and vomiting may by prominent, hence the importance of testing the urine of all children suspected of appendicitis. Unlike adults who are commonly fat at the onset of diabetes, children are thin and may be wasted.

Infection and emotional stress are both precipitating factors in the onset of diabetes. The disorder is uncommon in developing countries, but in such countries it increases with urbanization and rising standards of living.

Diabetic coma presents with increasing drowsiness and dehydration. The breath smells of acetone and there is air-hunger, vomiting and constipation.

*Diagnosis.* Glucose is present in the urine and, in cases of coma or pre-coma, ketonuria is also found. The raised blood sugar is merely required to confirm the diagnosis. Renal glycosuria, which results from a lowered renal threshold, is differentiated by a glucose tolerance curve but this test is not required routinely for the diagnosis of diabetes.

Salicylate intoxication must be differentiated in young children since it produces similar clinical features with glycosuria and even hyperglycaemia. The urinary ferric chloride test will differentiate if precautions are taken (p. 713). A salicylate blood level should be estimated in any doubtful case.

*Treatment.* There is agreement that all children with diabetes require insulin. Management by diet alone would restrict normal growth and the oral preparations, such as the sulphonylureas and diguanides, are unsuitable by themselves for children but can be a useful adjunct to insulin in selected cases (p. 638).

The unanswered question is whether the diet should be 'restricted' or 'free'; there is now considerable support for an unrestricted diet. On a free diet the dose of insulin is adjusted to prevent ketonuria but some glucosuria is per-mited, whereas on a restricted diet rigid control to prevent glucosuria as well as ketonuria is practised. There are two possible reasons for advocating a strict regime: first, that this reduces the risk of diabetic coma; and secondly that it lessens the chances of future complications. Present evidence is that the precipitating cause of diabetic coma is not the sudden ingestion of excessive amounts of carbohydrate but lack of insulin, a situation which is clearly seen in a diabetic at the onset of infection when more insulin is required. If this increased requirement is not met, coma is likely to develop. There is no certain evidence that the complications of diabetes are due to hyperglycaemia, a long-term follow-up of the two regimes being necessary to determine this point. It is very possible that the vascular complications are due to elevation of the serum lipids, since it is known that lipaemia precedes the development of atheroma in older non-diabetic patients. It is also possible that the high level of insulin-antagonists is responsible for the complications, since these are so similar in the two age groups of diabetics, despite their clinical differences—on the one hand the patient whose diabetes starts in childhood and is particularly liable to ketosis and, on the other, the patient whose diabetes starts in adult life and is resistant to ketosis.

The advantage to a child of the unrestricted diet is that he is much less likely to develop the psychological complications seen in those on a strict diet. Such children feel different from others, constant parental supervision being required if the diet is to be strict. Those on an unrestricted diet are warned not to over-indulge themselves and, when first being stabilized on insulin, some measure of dietary control is wise, especially regarding the in-take of carbohydrates. This assists in stabilization and teaches the parents some of the rudiments of diet so that they may more easily understand the disease.

During this initial period the constituents of the diet are calculated from the infant's age. At birth a diet providing 1000 calories a day is required. Thereafter 100 calories is added for each year of life up to a maximum of 3500 calories for girls and 4000 calories for boys, at the age of 13 years. Ten per cent of the total calories is the number of grams of carbohydrate required. A 10-year-old child whose requirement is 2000 calories would receive 200 g of carbohydrate. The amount of protein and fat required is half the number of grams of carbohydrate, in this case 100 g of each (1 gram of protein and carbohydrate each provide 4 calories and 1 gram of fat provides 9 calories).

*Insulin.* When stabilizing a child on insulin he should be allowed to lead as normal a life as possible and not be kept in bed. Bed rest leads to increased insulin requirements, exercise to decreased requirements. The child should be allowed home as soon as possible since the requirements are then likely to change; a long period of hospital stabilization is a waste of time. The main reason for the period in hospital is to instruct the mother in the disease and teach her, and the child if old enough, how to inject insulin and test urine.

Soluble insulin is used at first, being given subcutaneously three times a day 20 minutes before meals. It reaches its maximum action 3–4 hours after injection. The dose required varies considerably in different children but is of the order of 1 unit/kg/day. Further doses are calculated from testing the urine with Benedict's reagent or Clinitest immediately before the insulin is to be given:

*If green or blue no insulin is given.*
*If yellow give 5–10 units.*
*If orange give 10–15 units.*
*If red give 15–20 units.*

It will be found that the amount of insulin required will gradually decrease until a maintenance level is achieved. At this point a change should be made to a long-acting preparation such as lente or a medium-acting preparation, such as isophan, combined with soluble insulin.

The insulin zinc suspensions—lente, semilente and ultralente are satisfactory since they contain no added protein and are therefore unlikely to provoke cutaneous reactions. Lente is most frequently used since its action commences 1–2 hours after administration and lasts about 24 hours. If given half an hour before breakfast its peak action will be reached between noon and 6 p.m.; the bulk of carbohydrate can then be eaten in the middle of the day and at bed-time. The dose is the same as the total soluble insulin previously being given. The action of semilente lasts about 12 hours and of ultralente 24–36 hours.

Isophane insulin has largely replaced globin insulin. It has its main action 8–16 hours after injection. Since it contains no excess of protamine, added soluble insulin retains its full effect.

Protamine zinc insulin should not be used for children since its action is too long and imprecise. It usually has to be combined with soluble insulin to achieve a sufficient hypoglycaemic effect early in the day, but the excess of protamine in the preparation results in a variable proportion of the soluble insulin being converted to the long acting form.

Oral hypoglycaemic drugs cannot replace insulin but may be useful to assist control in children with wide swings in blood sugar levels. They can also be used in mild cases at the start of treatment when the child is adjusting to dietary restrictions and before introducing the additional burden of daily insulin injections. One of the sulphonylurea group, such as tolbutamide, is the most suitable. These act by stimulating the beta cells to increased insulin secretion.

Treatment should aim at keeping the urine free of ketone bodies, but no attempt made to keep it free of sugar since this is bound to cause hypoglycaemic reactions in a child. After the child has been on insulin for a few weeks the requirements are likely to fall quite suddenly. Therefore, a careful watch must be kept for hypoglycaemic reactions which are the great hazard for children with diabetes. An explanation of hypoglycaemic symptoms should be given to the child and his parents; it is wise that he should deliberately be given a mild hypoglycaemic attack while in hospital, in order that he may experience the symptoms. He should always carry lumps of sugar in case this occurs. Insulin requirements are likely to increase with the onset of puberty, particularly in girls.

*Prognosis.* Providing the children receive close supervision, the outlook for life is good, though the risk of later complications is considerable. These consist of atheroma, cataract and retinitis, peripheral neuritis and renal lesions. There is an increased liability to tuberculosis and all patients should be given BCG if they are Mantoux negative.

Normal growth is an indication of good diabetic control. The presence of hyperlipidaemia almost always signifies inadequate control. Careful psychological management is essential so that as far as possible the child is helped not to feel different from his peers. Hospital care should be kept to a minimum but occasionally a residential hostel will be needed for the child who cannot be controlled adequately at home. Atrophy at the site of injection can lead to embarrassment, therefore the arms should never be used for injections in girls.

### DIABETIC COMA

This is particularly liable to occur at the onset of diabetes in children, or if infection occurs. The parents should be warned that increased insulin will be needed during an infection. When vomiting occurs with an infection parents often make the mistake of withholding insulin, causing the situation to be doubly serious.

Insulin must be given immediately the child is seen, without waiting for the blood sugar results. Speed is essential if the child is to survive; insulin resistance develops rapidly as acidosis advances. The initial amount required varies with the age of the child, the degree of acidosis and dehydration, and the severity of any infection; an average dose is 2 units/kg, half being given intravenously and half intramuscularly. If the general practitioner is certain of the diagnosis, the insulin and the penicillin should be given before the patient leaves home for the hospital.

After giving insulin and penicillin the next step is to provide parenteral fluids in order to correct the dehydration and acidosis. Blood is taken for biochemical estimations, but intravenous saline should be started without waiting for the results. At this stage the saline should not contain glucose which, by increasing the glycosuria, would cause an increased urinary loss of valuable electrolytes. Physiological saline (0·9 per cent) is used with added bicarbonate to correct the acidosis. Early correction of the acidosis hastens recovery. The rate of the infusion depends on the severity of the dehydration but in severe cases up to 5 ml/kg can be given in the first hour. After this the usual rate of not more than 2·5 ml/kg/hour should be kept.

Once the intravenous infusion has been started and provided the patient is not *in extremis*, gastric lavage should be performed to relieve abdominal distension and prevent the risk of vomiting with consequent aspiration of fluid. Five per cent sodium bicarbonate is used for the lavage but no fluid should be left in the stomach because of the risk of vomiting. Repeated blood pressure estimations must be made. If hypotension persists, intravenous noradrenaline should be given.

When the blood sugar level starts to fall it is safe to give intravenous solutions containing glucose, such as 5 per cent glucose in 1/5 normal saline. As the blood sugar falls so will the serum potassium, provided there is a satisfactory flow of urine. Potassium supplements now become an urgent necessity, since the already diluted plasma potassium tends to move into the cells under the influence of insulin. Potassium can always be given safely by mouth up to 1 or even 2 g per day, but if this is not yet possible it can be given intravenously to a total of not more than 3 mEq/kg/day. The fluid given must not contain more than 40 mEq of potassium per litre. Potassium must never be given intravenously until renal function is re-established since cardiac arrest might result from a dangerously high level of potassium.

Further dosage of insulin is decided by the blood sugar level and not by the amount of sugar in the urine which gives no indication of the level in the blood when this is high. The second blood sugar should be taken 90 minutes after the first so that a result is available 2 hours from the onset of treatment. If the level has risen, double the dose of insulin should be given; if it is unchanged the first dose should be repeated; if it has fallen no insulin should be given, a further estimation being made 90 minutes later. Two hourly blood sugars should be continued until the renal threshold is reached; the dose of insulin is then decided by the amount of sugar in the urine according to the scheme on p. 637.

Intensive carbohydrate metabolism follows treatment of diabetic coma. This increases the requirement of co-enzymes derived from vitamin B complex so that parenteral vitamin B supplements should be provided.

If the child is in a state of pre-coma rather than coma, that is, ketone bodies are present in the urine but the child, although drowsy is not unconscious, the intramuscular dose of insulin is 1 unit per kg. It should be possible to give fluids by mouth, but vomiting may make intravenous therapy necessary. In all cases of diabetic coma fluids should be given by mouth instead of intra-venously, once the condition permits.

Constipation may be very severe in these patients, adding to the abdominal discomfort. It should be relieved by an enema.

TRANSIENT DIABETES OF THE NEWBORN

In this disorder a neonate develops the clinical picture of severe diabetes with marked dehydration, loss of weight and polyuria. The condition differs from diabetes in that it is transient and the baby may become normal by the age of 6 months or earlier. Moreover, these patients are extremely sensitive to insulin so that, although the blood sugar may be in the region of 900 mg per cent, a dose of 2 units of insulin may produce hypoglycaemia and 0·5 unit may be the correct dose. The condition is believed to be due to delay in functional maturation of the fetal beta cell (Milner *et al.*, 1971). Early treat-ment is essential to prevent residual brain damage.

## Hypoglycaemia

Hypoglycaemia is usually regarded as being present when the blood glucose falls below 40 mg per cent. The level at which symptoms appear is variable, being usually lower than this, especially in babies. Whenever hypoglycaemia is suspected a rough estimate of the blood sugar should be made using the Dextrostix strip. If no colour develops on the strip the blood glucose is less than 40 mg per cent, indicating the need for immediate treatment and a laboratory estimation of blood glucose.

Apart from excessive administration of insulin, hypoglycaemia may develop in children from a number of causes; it is most common in the neonatal period.

INSULIN HYPOGLYCAEMIA

This results from an excessive dose of insulin and occurs shortly before a meal is due, when the blood sugar is likely to be at its lowest. It produces sweating, pallor, palpitations and tremor. Hunger and drowsiness are common; nausea and headache may occur. Ataxia and changes in mood are symptoms which in adults may be mistaken for drunkenness, so that police in the region of diabetic clinics are warned not to make this error; in young children naughtiness may be an early sign. In severe cases, convulsions and coma result. The urine contains no sugar unless the bladder contained urine secreted some time previously. The blood sugar is low.

*Treatment.* Patients must be taught to give themselves sugar at the earliest sign of hypoglycaemia. Every child should be given a mild hypoglycaemic attack while in hospital so that he can become acquainted with the symptoms. If oral glucose cannot be taken he can be given 5–20 ml of 50 per cent glucose intravenously. One mg of glucagon is an alternative to intravenous glucose and is easier to administer. It can be given by parents who must be told to use an intramuscular and not an insulin needle. This will bring him round sufficiently to permit glucose administration by mouth. Glucose may also be given by stomach tube.

NEONATAL HYPOGLYCAEMIA

Diagnosis is difficult because many babies have abnormally low blood sugar levels by adult standards, yet have no symptoms. Asymptomatic infants with demonstrable hypoglycaemia on repeat testing should be treated. The condition may occur in preterm infants and in babies of diabetic and toxaemic mothers. It particularly occurs in babies who are small for dates (p. 54), especially when associated with hypoxia, hypothermia or intracranial injury.

Toxaemia, an important cause of babies being small for dates, is associated with half the cases of neonatal hypoglycaemia. The cause is not known, but it may be due to an immaturity of the enzyme systems responsible for raising the blood sugar, or to an increased sensitivity to insulin. Liver glycogen is not laid down until late in pregnancy; it is probable that the level of liver glycogen is low in preterm babies and in those babies whose nutrition during pregnancy has been inadequate; insufficient reserves of liver glycogen could well be an important factor in the aetiology. In the babies of diabetic mothers the hypoglycaemia is due to fetal hyperinsulinism resulting from hyperplasia of the islets of Langerhans (p. 133).

There is no way of forecasting which baby with a low blood sugar will develop symptoms. The child is usually well for the first 24 hours, then becomes drowsy and refuses to suck. Unusual irritability may be a feature. This is followed by bouts of apnoea with cyanosis which are the most constant feature and lead to convulsions. Since these symptoms are the same as might be expected from intracranial injury, anoxia or infection, the blood sugar must be checked when these occur. The conditions may coexist. Convulsions usually occur after the first 48 hours; therefore, hypoglycaemia should be suspected if convulsions develop after this interval and birth was normal.

*Treatment.* Immediate treatment is essential to prevent permanent brain damage. Ten per cent glucose should be given intravenously for 24–48 hours by scalp vein infusion. There is a risk of portal vein thrombosis if the umbilical vein is used. Oral glucose alone is not effective, but if intravenous therapy is impractical, a combination of 5–10 per cent glucose through an indwelling gastric tube and 25 mg hydrocortisone intramuscularly may be satisfactory. The blood glucose must be kept above 20 mg per cent. This will require continuous therapy for several days owing to the remarkable ability of these babies to metabolize glucose.

Early feeding of newborn babies reduces the incidence of this disorder.

### SYMPTOMATIC HYPOGLYCAEMIA

In the neonatal period, hypoglycaemia may occur as a result of glycogen storage disease, galactosaemia, fructosaemia or adrenal hyperplasia. An insulinoma or hyperplasia of the islet cells, causing hypoglycaemia from excessive production of insulin, is extremely rare in childhood.

### REACTIVE HYPOGLYCAEMIA

These patients develop hypoglycaemia shortly after meals. This is thought to result from an excessive output of insulin in response to the intake of food. Such patients should be given a low carbohydrate diet so as to reduce the stimulus to the pancreas to produce insulin. The diet should be high in protein, since this produces a slow liberation of carbohydrate, causing less stimulation of the pancreas.

### IDIOPATHIC HYPOGLYCAEMIA

This condition occurs usually within the first 2 years of life, being often familial. It probably contains a heterogeneous group of unrelated entities; one of these has been separated with the discovery that some children with hypoglycaemia are sensitive to leucine in the diet (Cochrane *et al.*, 1956). The diet of such patients should not contain excessive protein, and extra carbohydrate should be given about half an hour after meals to counteract the effect of the protein in lowering the blood sugar. The hypoglycaemic attacks in 'idiopathic' cases can be largely prevented by daily ACTH. This will need to be continued for some months but the dose can then be reduced and, in some cases, can be discontinued without recurrence of symptoms.

The importance of all forms of hypoglycaemia is the risk of future mental impairment. In order not to overlook the possibility of hypoglycaemia as a cause of convulsions, it should be the rule for a blood glucose to be performed in every child presenting with convulsions. If the level of sugar in the cerebrospinal fluid is less than 20 mg per cent, hypoglycaemia is the probable cause of the convulsions.

# GONADS

## TESTIS

The mature testis is composed of seminiferous tubules, which make up the bulk of the organ, and the interstitial cells of Leydig. The seminiferous tubules are composed of the germinal cells and the Sertoli cells. The germinal cells develop into spermatozoa under the stimulus of follicle-stimulating hormone (FSH) from the pituitary. The Sertoli cells become differentiated only at puberty; their function is unknown.

At puberty the interstitial cell stimulating hormone of the pituitary causes the Leydig cells to secrete androgenic hormone which is almost entirely testosterone, and probably also oestrogen. During childhood it is likely that the testis has no endocrine function.

Testicular deficiency results from anterior pituitary insufficiency or from a primary abnormality of the testis due to an embryological defect, neoplasm, trauma or inflammation, such as mumps or tuberculosis. Patients with an embryological defect of the testis can be differentiated by their high FSH level from those in which the testicular deficiency is secondary to pituitary insufficiency.

### Testicular tumours

INTERSTITIAL CELL TUMOUR

This tumour is usually benign and causes sexual precocity (see p. 285).

TERATOMA

A rare tumour which presents as enlargement of one testicle. Despite the fact that the neoplastic cells are usually very primitive and therefore malignant, the prognosis is reasonably good, presumably because its situation permits early diagnosis.

### Klinefelter's syndrome

These patients are males with one extra chromosome. The chromosomal constitution is usually XXY (see p. 194) and they are therefore chromatin positive. The condition is seldom diagnosed before adolescence because the external genitalia are normal. Secondary sexual characteristics develop at puberty but the testicles remain small and are soft. Biopsy shows hyalinization of the seminiferous tubules and hyperplasia of the Leydig cells. There is increased FSH in the urine after the age of 10 years. Gynaecomastia is common; the patients may grow very tall, developing eunuchoid proportions. Some are mentally handicapped. Diagnosis in childhood is suggested by the presence of unusually long legs or mental handicap and can be confirmed by finding an apparent male to be chromatin positive.

A few cases of Klinefelter's syndrome are not due to a chromosomal anomaly; these are chromatin negative. The disorder may be congenital from an absence of germinal cells (del Castillo's disease) or acquired from postpubertal testicular atrophy without any history of orchitis or trauma.

### Undescended testicles

Failure to palpate the testicles in the scrotum is due to one of three causes: a 'retractile' testicle; a congenital malformation preventing normal descent; or, very rarely, an endocrine disorder causing hypogonadism. In the majority of cases the testicles are 'retractile' and have been pulled up by a strong cremasteric reflex. Examination with warm hands in a warm room and in an atmosphere which does not make the boy feel tense, will then demonstrate that they can be brought into the normal site. Obesity renders the palpation of retractile testicles less easy.

A 'retractile' testicle is found in the upper part of the scrotum or in the superficial inguinal pouch which is the abdominal extension of the scrotum, lying between the superficial abdominal fascia and the external oblique muscle, directly over the inguinal canal. The appearance of the scrotum is useful in deciding whether the testicles have ever been in the scrotum, since it is commonly hypoplastic if they have never descended. In cases of unilateral failure to descend, the affected half is smaller than the other. A testicle in the inguinal canal cannot be felt since it lies deep to the strong tendon of the external oblique muscle; the majority described as being felt in the inguinal canal are in the superficial inguinal pouch. Moreover, testicles do not slide up and down the inguinal canal unless an inguinal hernia is also present, since the canal is filled with connective tissue surrounding the cord.

Congenital malformations, such as a tight inguinal ring, are more likely to be unilateral than bilateral. An indirect inguinal hernia is sometimes associated. Ectopic testicles are included in this group.

When the cause is an endocrine disorder both testicles are involved. The condition is due either to hypopituitarism or to primary testicular deficiency. In all apparent males with bilateral cryptorchidism a buccal smear should be examined in order to exclude female pseudohermaphroditism due to adrenal hyperplasia (p. 195).

*Treatment.* 'Retractile' undescended testicles should be left alone since they will descend. The unilateral undescended testicle usually requires surgery; this is always necessary if the testicle is ectopically placed or associated with an inguinal hernia. Orchidopoxy should be carried out at the same time as the repair of the hernia.

The chief problem is the boy with bilateral undescended testicles, since if these are still within the abdomen after puberty, the tubules fail to mature and the testis may atrophy or, rarely, may undergo malignant change. (Bringing the testicle down does not reduce the risk of malignancy but it makes earlier diagnosis possible.) Very few descend spontaneously after the first year of life, therefore, surgery at the age of 4–5 years is a reasonable compromise. One side only should be dealt with at a time owing to the risk of vascular damage.

It is sometimes difficult to differentiate the high 'retractile' testicle from one which is ectopically placed. A therapeutic trial with human chorionic gonadotrophin will bring down the high 'retractile' testicle. This can be given when the child is 9 years old in a dose of 500 units twice weekly for 10 weeks. It will bring down only those testicles which would have descended normally at puberty. If it fails, surgery should be carried out without delay.

**Torsion of the testicle**

This condition is not uncommon and may occur at any age, including the neonatal period. It results from a congenital anomaly of the testis rendering it more liable to rotate. This anomaly is commonly an upward extension of the tunica vaginalis but, in addition, the mesorchium may be lengthened so that the testicle lies in a horizontal position when the patient is upright.

The scrotum on the affected side is red and oedematous while the testicle is swollen and acutely painful. These features, together with the fact that fever is often present and the onset not always dramatic, are the cause of the common and disastrous mistake of misdiagnosing the condition as epididymo-orchitis and giving medical treatment. The anomaly is often bilateral, so that a horizontal testicle on the other side is important confirmatory evidence.

*Treatment.* Immediate surgery is required in order to prevent atrophy of the testicle from loss of blood supply. The testicle should be anchored in the scrotum to reduce the possibility of a recurrence. Since the same predisposing anomaly often involves the opposite testicle it is a wise precaution that this also should be anchored. Treatment of the opposite side can be carried out at the same time as the emergency operation if the patient's condition is satisfactory.

**Orchitis**

Orchitis occurs as a complication of mumps but this is seldom before adolescence, when it becomes common. It occurs occasionally with a Coxsackie virus infection, but again largely only in adults. The condition may also result from trauma. *Epididymo-orchitis* may be due to infection with the streptococcus, staphylococcus, gonococcus, pneumococcus, *E. coli* and the tubercle bacillus; it must be differentiated from torsion of the testicle (see above).


# OVARY

## Ovarian tumours

GRANULOSA CELL TUMOUR

This tumour is very rare but its importance arises from the fact that it causes sexual precocity (see p. 285).


TERATOMA

This is usually benign, presenting as an abdominal mass or with pain following torsion of the tumour.

## Ovarian dysgenesis (Turner's syndrome)

The majority of these patients are chromatin negative and their chromosomal pattern is xo (see p. 194). They have forty-five chromosomes instead of the normal forty-six since there is only a single x chromosome. The gonads are absent or grossly hypoplastic. The patients are stunted, though for no clear reason; castration leads to eunuchoidism in which the height is increased, so that it cannot be due to the absence of gonads. After the age of 10 years the pituitary gland becomes more active than normal, this being shown by the increased urinary content of gonadotrophins (FSH).

Associated abnormalities are usually present, including webbing of the neck, a wide carrying angle at the elbow, a shield-shaped chest with widely spaced nipples and congenital heart defects, particularly coarctation of the aorta (Fig. 137a). Some of the patients are mentally handicapped. Pigmented naevi, widely distributed over the body are common. In infancy, oedema of the feet and, to a lesser extent, of the hands, may be found and should immediately suggest the correct diagnosis (Fig. 137b). This is lymphoedema resulting from hypoplasia of the superficial lymphatic channels.

There is failure of breast and genital development at the time of expected puberty owing to lack of oestrogen, but pubic and axillary hair appear since these result from adrenal androgen.

Diagnosis is made by finding a stunted girl with the characteristic congenital anomalies who is chromatin negative and, after the age of 10 years, has a high FSH. After puberty, differentiation from sexual infantilism due to hypopituitarism is made by the presence of sexual hair; this is absent in hypopituitarism since there is also a lack of adrenal androgen.

*Treatment.* No hormonal treatment is indicated in childhood, but at the usual age of puberty substitution therapy with oestrogen and progestogen should be started. These patients have a tendency to keloid formation which may prove troublesome after plastic surgery for webbing of the neck.

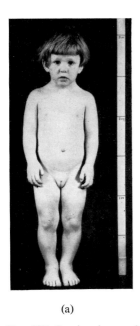
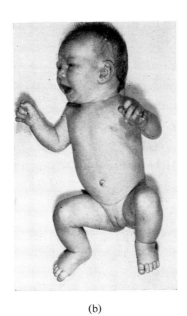

(a)                                                    (b)

FIG. 137. Ovarian dysgenesis.
(a) Illustrating webbing of the neck, widely separated nipples and a shield-shaped chest.
(b) The diagnosis was made in infancy as the child presented with oedema of the feet.

## BIBLIOGRAPHY

ADAMS D.D., LORD J.M. & STEVELY H.A.A. (1964) Congenital thyrotoxicosis. *Lancet*, **2**, 497.

BACON G.E. & LOWREY G.H. (1965) Experience with surgical treatment of thyrotoxicosis in children. *J. Pediat.*, **67**, 1.

BURLAND W.L. (1964) Diabetes mellitus syndrome in the newborn infant. *J. Pediat.*, **65**, 122.

COCHRANE W.A., PAYNE W.W., SIMPKISS M.J. & WOOLF, L.I. (1956) Familial hypoglycemia precipitated by amino acids. *J. clin. Invest.*, **35**, 411.

CORNBLATH M., WYBREGT S.H., BAENS G.S. & KLEIN R.I. (1964) Symptomatic neonatal hypoglycemia. *Pediatrics*, **33**, 388.

COUR-PALAIS I.J. (1966) Spontaneous descent of the testicle. *Lancet*, **1**, 1403.

CROMBIE, D.L. (1964) The diabetic syndrome. *Lancet*, **1**, 627.

GLASS S.D., TOWNSLEY J.T. & GEPPERT L.J. (1964) Neonatal hyperthyroidism. *J. Pediat.*, **64**, 906.

KOMROWER G.M. & BAILEY C.C. (1974) Congenital adrenal hyperplasia. *Arch. Dis. Childh.*, **49**, 830.

MILNER R.D.G., FERGUSON A.W. & NAIDU S.H. (1971) Aetiology of transient diabetes mellitus. *Arch. Dis. Childh.*, **46**, 724.

NEWNS G.H. (1974) Congenital adrenal hyperplasia. *Arch. Dis. Childh.*, **49**, 1.

RAITI S. & NEWNS G. (1971) Cretinism: early diagnosis and its relation to mental prognosis. *Arch. Dis. Childh.*, **46**, 692.

ROOT A.W., BONGIOVANNI A.M., HARVIE F.H. & EBERLEIN W.R. (1963) Treatment of juvenile thyrotoxicosis. *J. Pediat.*, **63**, 402.

SAWITSKY A. & DESPOSITO F. (1965) Survey of American experience with vitamin $B_{12}$ therapy of neuroblastoma. *J. Pediat.*, **67**, 99.

SAXENA K.M., CRAWFORD J.D. & TALBOT N.B. (1964) Childhood thyrotoxicosis: a long-term perspective. *Brit. med. J.*, **2**, 1153.

SCHOEN E.J. (1960) Renal diabetes insipidus. *Pediatrics*, **26**, 808.

SCHOTLAND M.G., GRUMBACH M.M. & STRAUSS J. (1963) The effects of chlorothiazide in nephrogenic diabetes insipidus. *Pediatrics*, **31**, 741.

SCORER C.G. (1964) The descent of the testis. *Arch. Dis. Childh.*, **39**, 605.

SHELLEY H.J. & NELIGAN G.A. (1966) Neonatal hypoglycaemia. *Brit. med. Bull.*, **22**, 34.

VALLANCE-OWEN J. & LILLEY M.D. (1961) An insulin antagonist associated with plasma albumin. *Lancet*, **1**, 804.

CHAPTER 23

# COLLAGEN DISORDERS

Those disorders which affect collagen, the main constituent of connective tissue, are conveniently grouped together since they have much in common, although our knowledge of their aetiology is limited. The disorders included are: rheumatic fever, rheumatoid arthritis, anaphylactoid purpura, dermatomyositis, scleroderma, disseminated lupus erythematosus and polyarteritis nodosa. Chorea will also be considered here since it is closely related to rheumatic fever, although perhaps not itself a collagen disorder.

**Rheumatic fever**

The exact aetiology is still unexplained, but it certainly represents a hypersensitivity reaction to infection with beta-haemolytic streptococci of Lancefield's group A. It occurs mainly between the ages of 5–15 years, being exceptional under the age of 3 years. Its incidence is closely related to poor environment, bad hygiene and damp; it is more common in towns, especially where there is overcrowding. It is associated with poverty, and a large factor in the reduced incidence which has occurred since the turn of the century is thought to be the rise in the standard of living. Its relation to damp renders it particularly a disease of temperate climates, but it is also surprisingly common in poor communities in tropical countries. Recently there has been an increased incidence in England though the disease is still much less severe than it was at the beginning of the century. The disease is no longer more common in winter than in summer as used to be the case.

The seriousness of rheumatic fever is entirely due to the carditis which often accompanies the condition. It is a disease which affects connective and other mesenchymal tissues. The changes are of two kinds: a degeneration of connective tissue which is best seen in the cardiac valves; and a focal inflammatory reaction which is the basis of the Aschoff nodule, seen in the pericardium, myocardium and elsewhere.

The preceding streptococcal infection is most often upper respiratory, particularly tonsillitis. The latent period before the onset of rheumatic fever is usually 10 days but may vary from 1–4 weeks. This streptococcal infection may pass unnoticed.

The onset of rheumatic fever may be insidious or acute, but in either case the joint pains are characteristic. The pain is in the joint rather than in the muscle; the large limb joints are affected, the pain moving from one joint to another. The joints commonly affected are the knees, ankles, elbows and wrists, in that order of frequency; the pain usually stays in one joint for 1–2 days before moving to the next. The child is feverish, pale, obviously unwell and may sweat excessively. The joint signs are variable; in severe cases the local signs of inflammation are acute so that the joint is red, hot and swollen, the slightest movement being extremely painful. In other cases the joint signs are minimal, especially in children under 5 years of age. The change in the pattern of the disease over the last years has been associated with a reduction in the number of cases with very acute joint signs. The severity of

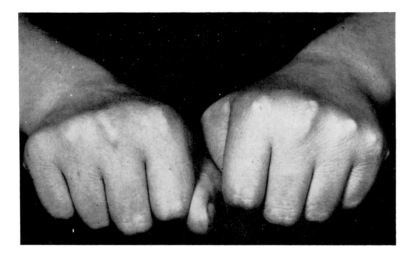

Fig. 138. Rheumatic nodules over the knuckles.

the cardiac signs bears no relation to the degree of joint involvement. Permanent cardiac damage may occur more easily in cases with mild joint involvement because the initial attack passes unnoticed and untreated.

*Rheumatic carditis.* The heart is frequently involved in rheumatic fever and there are some who believe that it never escapes. Tachycardia is the most significant sign and a systolic murmur is invariable. However, the mere presence of a systolic murmur is not diagnostic of carditis, most soft mid-systolic murmurs being innocent. A pansystolic murmur is almost certain evidence of carditis. The definite signs of carditis are a diastolic murmur, cardiac enlargement, pericarditis, rheumatic nodules and electrocardiographic changes. Rheumatic nodules (Fig. 138) are small subcutaneous lumps about the size of a small pea found over the occiput, behind the elbow, in front of the knee and on the dorsal aspects of the hands and feet. They are not tender and are more easily felt than seen. Histologically their appearance is similar to that of the Aschoff nodule. The most common change in the electrocardiogram is prolongation of the P–R interval, this being the earliest sign of a conduction defect.

In severe cases and especially those with pericarditis, signs of heart failure appear. Two symptoms are particularly significant in heralding its onset: vomiting and abdominal pain. The child becomes breathless, the neck veins distended and the liver enlarges. Oedema is less often a feature of heart failure in children than in adults. Heart failure in the acute attack is due to myocarditis and not to valvular disease.

Skin rashes often accompany the attack; these are varieties of erythema multiforme, especially erythema annulare (erythema marginatum). Erythema nodosum (p. 518) which may be due to the haemolytic streptococcus, is not a sign of rheumatic fever.

There is usually a moderate degree of hypochromic anaemia and leucocytosis. The erythrocyte sedimentation rate is raised; this indicates an inflammatory reaction only, not being a specific sign of rheumatic fever, although in rheumatic fever its rise is generally high and out of proportion to the other features of the disease. The anti-streptolysin O titre is high, unless the original streptococcal infection was treated with antibiotics which suppress the anti-streptolysin O response.

DIAGNOSIS

*Limb pains.* Perhaps the most frequent diagnostic error is to mistake the common condition of limb pains (see p. 472) or, as they used to be called, 'growing pains'. Particularly is the error likely to be made if the child happens to have a systolic murmur. But the pain, usually in the legs, is in the muscles and not in the joints, it does not prevent walking and there are no joint signs. The pain usually comes on in the evening when the child is tired; there is no pathological lesion. Carditis is absent and particularly is there no tachycardia, although if the child is nervous it may be necessary to determine the normal cardiac rate from the sleeping pulse.

*Congenital heart disease.* Limb pains in a child with congenital heart disease may make the diagnosis more difficult but, despite the cardiac signs, there will be no evidence of carditis. It is exceptional to have rheumatic fever before the age of 3 years.

*Single joint disease.* Osteomyelitis near a joint, acute pyogenic arthritis and tuberculous arthritis may all raise diagnostic difficulties. The fact that a single joint is involved should arouse suspicion, but occasionally rheumatic fever does involve one joint only. In such cases reliance must be placed on the other signs of rheumatic activity.

*Rheumatoid arthritis.* This condition affects the hands as well as the large joints, cardiac involvement seldom occurring. It is a relapsing illness with high fever and often with enlarged glands and spleen. There is no dramatic response to salicylates.

*Anaphylactoid purpura.* The typical rash usually makes diagnosis easy. Under the age of 5 years florid arthritis with visible external signs is more commonly due to anaphylactoid purpura than to rheumatic fever.

*Acute poliomyelitis.* Limb pains may be a prominent feature in the early stages of the disease but the pain is felt in the muscle rather than in the joint.

*Acute leukaemia.* Limb pains from bone deposits are often a feature but the pain occurs in the bone rather than in the joints. Other features of leukaemia are present, such as severe anaemia and haemorrhagic manifestations.

TREATMENT

All cases should be treated in hospital and confined to bed, but it is unnecessary to insist that the child remains lying flat all the time as was the practice in the past. Pillows should be permitted so that the child can obtain the position of greatest comfort. No harm results from allowing him to sit up and play if he so desires. Nursing between blankets is unnecessary and uncomfortable.

Salicylates are so specific that if they fail to relieve the pain the diagnosis is almost certainly wrong. Their mode of action in rheumatic fever is uncertain but it is unlikely that they prevent the onset of carditis or reduce the chance of permanent cardiac damage. It has been customary to give them in all cases, but there is a risk in those with cardiac enlargement that the drug may precipitate heart failure; they should not therefore be used in such cases. For the remaining cases soluble acetylsalicylic acid is a palatable form and should be given in a dose of 120 mg/kg/day up to a maximum of 8 g per day. This full dose should be continued for 2 weeks, followed by half the amount until rheumatic activity has ceased. The dose should be reduced if there is evidence of salicylism shown by vomiting, headache, hyperpnoea, tinnitus or deafness. Hyperpnoea is a common toxic sign in children, though skill is required for its early recognition.

The place of steroids is still undecided. They have been shown to be of definite benefit in those with carditis and should always be given in such cases. The debatable group consists of those patients without evidence of carditis. However, in view of the difficulty of being certain that carditis is not present, and the possibility that it exists in all cases, it is recommended that steroids be given to all cases. The type of steroid used should be one with minimal salt-retaining properties; prednisolone is a suitable preparation; it should be continued until there is no evidence of rheumatic activity.

An intensive intramuscular course of penicillin should be given to all cases at the outset in order to ensure eradication of the streptococcus, this being checked by throat swabs. Relief of pain in the joints can be achieved by wrapping them in cotton wool. A bed cradle should be used to relieve pressure on the feet.

There is at present no agreement with regard to the duration of bed rest. In the past it has been the practice for the child to be kept in bed until 4 weeks after signs of activity have disappeared, with 6 weeks as the minimum period of bed rest in all cases. Absence of activity is shown by a normal pulse, temperature and sedimentation rate; a systolic murmur does not indicate activity. Present opinion favours earlier ambulation; no harm has resulted from allowing children to be up for short periods after the first few days, if they feel like it, even in the presence of continued rheumatic activity. A suitable compromise is to keep all patients in bed for 3–4 weeks, but during this period to allow them the freedom of the bed and, if they feel well enough, they can get out of bed to use the lavatory.

Early ambulation reduces the incidence of neurosis and cardiac invalidism which often occurred in the past. During the convalescent stage it is important that the mother is not given an impression that the heart is weak, a situation which may arise if unnecessary limitations are placed on her child's activity. While convalescent, the only limitation on activity is that the child should not be permitted to exhaust himself.

PROPHYLAXIS

Rheumatic fever can be prevented by the early and efficient treatment of streptococcal infections. Such patients should be supervised for 4 weeks after the acute attack in case rheumatic fever develops.

Inherent in every attack of rheumatic fever is the threat of another. Anyone who has had one attack must receive prophylactic penicillin or sulphadiazine, the only difficulty being to decide how long this should be continued. Some authorities go so far as to recommend that it should be continued for life but since recurrences are more liable to occur in children, a useful compromise is to give penicillin until puberty, or for 5 years whichever is the longer. The penicillin may be given either daily by mouth in a dose of 125–250 mg phenoxymethyl penicillin or once a month as a depot injection of one million units of benzathine penicillin. The single injection is of advantage where there is doubt whether the child will receive the daily dose, but it has the disadvantage that it is painful. Sulphadiazine can be used as an alternative to penicillin in a dose of 0·25 g b.d. for children of 5 years and under, and

0·5 g b.d. for those over 5. Fortunately, the streptococcus does not develop resistance to penicillin and only seldom to sulphadiazine. Penicillin resistant staphylococci may, however, co-exist in the throat.

PROGNOSIS

The younger the patient the greater the chance that the heart will be affected, about half the patients being left with cardiac lesions. Permanent cardiac damage occurs in almost all of those who develop pericarditis or heart failure. Neither steroids nor salicylates can prevent residual heart disease. Residual cardiac damage is unrelated to the severity of the joint lesions and may be found in patients without any history of preceding rheumatic fever, presumably because the infection was mild. The pattern of the first attack is of great value in forecasting the liability to cardiac complications should there be a recurrence. If a patient has emerged from the first attack without cardiac damage, then the heart is unlikely to be affected by future attacks. On the other hand, if the first attack has affected the heart, recurrences are likely to make it worse.

*Established rheumatic carditis.* The assessment of sequelae must be left until the acute attack has completely subsided. The heart may return to normal even though a diastolic murmur has been heard during the acute attack. The mitral valve is most often involved, the most frequent valvular lesion being mitral stenosis, with aortic incompetence the next. The development of these lesions takes at least 2 years from the acute attack. The general management of these children is the same as for those with congenital heart disease (see p. 190), and they should be allowed to undertake such activity as they feel themselves capable. Wholesale restriction of activity is wrong and leads to cardiac invalidism. Any source of chronic sepsis should be dealt with, but the indications for tonsillectomy are no different from usual because a child has a cardiac lesion. Antibiotic cover should be prescribed for dental extractions and other operations which might cause bacterial endocarditis (see p. 373). Children with severe cardiac lesions should attend special schools so that they may receive adequate medical supervision. Their interests should be directed towards a future sedentary occupation.

## Chorea (Sydenham's chorea, St Vitus's dance)

The inclusion of chorea among the collagen disorders could be criticized on the grounds that remarkably little is known about its pathology. But since it is closely related to rheumatic fever there are good reasons for describing the two conditions together. About three-quarters of the patients give a previous history of rheumatic fever, or show evidence that such has occurred. The relationship to infection with the haemolytic streptococcus is not clear cut since this has occurred weeks or months before the onset of chorea. Evidence from streptococcal antibody levels studied during the course of the disease suggests a latent period of months between the streptococcal infection and the onset of chorea. The disease is exceptional amongst rheumatic manifestations in that there may be no accompanying evidence of inflammation; it is not therefore surprising that there is no response to steroid therapy.

The average age of the patients is older than those with rheumatic fever, being 10–15 years instead of 5–15 years; there is a striking predilection for girls. The onset is insidious, the child develops uncontrollable fidgets and drops things, for which, in the early stages, she is liable to be punished by her unsuspecting mother. Changes in her handwriting may have been noticed. Emotional factors play a part; the child is likely to have been described as a nervous individual before the attack and in the attack she is easily upset, showing rapid changes of mood. Sighing, an unusual occurrence in children, may be prominent.

When the child is examined, she is found to have involuntary, purposeless movements which are non-repetitive and are increased when she is watched or asked to perform an intricate manoeuvre such as undoing buttons. These movements may be so severe that the child has to be protected in bed. They may be confined to one-half of the body, a condition termed *hemichorea*. Facial grimacing is common and when asked to protrude the tongue she will suddenly have to withdraw it when involuntary closure of the jaws would otherwise cause it to be bitten. With the arms and hands extended 'piano-playing' movements of the fingers can be observed, and the hand adopts an unusual degree of hyperextension at the metacarpo-phalangeal joint so that the fingers are bent far back. Inconstancy of the grip, felt when the examiner's hand is held, is a most useful sign. Dysarthria may be caused by the facial movements and, in severe cases, speech may be lost entirely for a few weeks.

Muscle weakness is a cardinal feature of the disease, being associated with diminished tone. In some cases, this may be so severe that one or more limbs are flaccid instead of always moving, appearing to be paralysed, although complete paralysis never occurs; this condition is termed *chorea mollis*.

The sedimentation rate is often normal and there may be no rise in pulse or temperature. The incidence of carditis is lower than in rheumatic fever, but occurs more often than was previously believed (Aron *et al.*, 1965).

*Diagnosis.* The only diagnostic difficulty lies in the differentiation of habit spasm (p. 469) which is often mistaken for chorea, whereas chorea itself is so obvious that no such mistake is likely to be made. Children with habit spasm repeat the same movement, often one of head shaking, grimacing or shrugging of the shoulders. Although this is an involuntary movement they can repeat it on request, something a child with chorea cannot do. If the child's attention is held, the movements cease or become very much less. The hand grip is constant and there are no 'piano-playing' movements.

*Prognosis.* The condition may last for months, with relapses being common. Progress can be followed by weekly records of the child's handwriting. Eventually, the involuntary movements subside completely but some of the patients are left with residual cardiac damage.

*Treatment.* There is no specific treatment and steroids are of no value. Sedation with phenobarbitone or, if this is ineffective, chlorpromazine should be given during the active stage. The side of the bed may require padding to prevent damage to the child. If an ambulance journey is necessary the child must be well sedated before starting, otherwise the movements are likely to become much worse during the trip. Children nursed in hospital should be in a room of their own rather than in a noisy ward. A sensible mother can often nurse her child more satisfactorily at home. Bed rest should be continued until choreic movements have stopped, though if these persist it is worth trying active re-education in co-ordinated muscle movements, provided there is no evidence of rheumatic activity.

In view of the risk of cardiac damage, all patients should receive long-term prophylactic penicillin as prescribed for rheumatic fever (p. 653).

A long period of convalescence is necessary before returning to school since many children relapse once they are faced again with the stresses of school life, particularly as they are often conscientious, intelligent children who are worried by the amount of work they have missed while ill. To reduce this the child should be given tuition in hospital or at home as soon as he is fit enough; mild sedation on first return to school may be helpful.

### Rheumatoid arthritis

It has been suggested that this condition should be called 'rheumatoid disease'; such a change in terminology would be advantageous since the disease affects many other systems as well as the joints. Moreover, the joints may not be involved at the onset; it may even be several weeks or months before they show any changes. The aetiology is unknown and is unrelated to a preceding streptococcal infection. There has been no fall in incidence as in rheumatic fever. The disease affects patients from infancy to middle age; Still's disease is no more than an acute form of rheumatoid arthritis in children.

The onset is usually acute so that the exact day may be known. Fever is severe and may be high and swinging. In the early days the pain in the joints may be both generalized and fleeting from joint to joint, but it then settles in the wrists, hands, knees, elbows and ankles. These become painful and swollen with overlying shiny skin. A characteristic spindle-shaped swelling of the fingers develops from involvement of the interphalangeal joints. In some cases the cervical spine is affected. The joints are usually symmetrically involved, but sometimes one joint only is affected at the onset; this may cause difficulty in diagnosis. Considerable deformity may occur, the abnormal appearance being exaggerated by the muscle wasting which develops. Some degree of lymphadenopathy is present in all cases and the spleen is often enlarged. Transient erythematous rashes, often resembling erythema annulare, are common. Iridocyclitis occurs in a few patients.

The course of the condition is one of relapses and remissions. In each relapse there is a recurrence of the fever, the child is miserable and obviously unwell, while the joints swell up again. In the remissions the joint swelling goes down but some degree of residual periarticular thickening and disability usually remains. If the effusion is large, the articular cartilage is protected so that there is less spasm and pain and an improved chance of eventual healing. In the dry type the cartilage is eroded so that adhesions form and contractures result.

In those patients in whom the joint signs develop late, there may be a period of many weeks in which the child is obviously ill with bouts of swinging fever and lymphadenopathy. The spleen is commonly enlarged and skin rashes may be seen in such patients.

A pronounced polymorphonuclear leucocytosis is almost invariable at the onset and a moderate degree of anaemia develops. The sedimentation rate is considerably raised and the Rose-Waaler test, which is based on the presence of non-specific agglutinins, may be positive. This test is more specific but less sensitive than the Latex test in detecting rheumatoid factor. The serum gammaglobulin and alpha-2-globulin are always raised. The antistreptolysin O titre is low. X-rays in the early stages show only soft tissue swelling and slight widening of the joint space from an effusion, but generalized osteoporosis develops rapidly.

*Complications.* Pericarditis is a serious and not very uncommon complication which may come on acutely or insidiously. Unlike its occurrence in rheumatic fever, it does not indicate severe cardiac involvement since it is usually isolated. Myocarditis and endocarditis are exceptionally rare in rheumatoid arthritis, though nodules are sometimes seen. Other rare complications are pleurisy and pneumonitis.

*Treatment.* In mild cases salicylates may be tried, though the response is never as dramatic as in rheumatic fever. Opinions differ on the place of steroids in therapy, though in severe cases the response is striking. Short-term results with steroids are good but long-term results are probably not improved. If only one or two joints are affected, intra-articular hydrocortisone may be of value, though in weight-bearing joints caution must be exercised with this form of treatment lest the relief of symptoms leads to excessive use of the joint and increased destruction. If systemic steroids are used, a careful watch must be kept on the vertebrae as these may collapse from osteoporosis. If osteoporosis develops, the steroids must be stopped, in which case the bones will recalcify and no permanent disability result.

The grave disadvantage of long-term steroid therapy is its suppression of growth. For this reason alternate day prednisolone or ACTH should be used. Every effort should be made to stop this therapy before the start of puberty in order not to suppress the puberty growth spurt. Gold therapy is an alternative form of treatment for those with severe active disease.

General measures to correct the anaemia and improve the general condition are required. The diet should be high in protein and calcium; vitamin supplements should be provided. Any infection present must be treated. Physiotherapy should be carried out in order to encourage active movements and prevent deformities but passive movements which cause pain are contra-indicated.

### Dermatomyositis

This is a rare inflammatory disease affecting the skin, subcutaneous tissues and muscle. The onset is insidious with fever, muscle tenderness, general weakness and misery. An erythematous rash commonly first develops over the bridge of the nose and around the eyes, later occurring anywhere on the trunk and limbs. In the early stages an oedematous swelling of the malar area is almost constant. An additional early sign is dilatation of the capillaries in the nail beds and gum margin so that these are visible to the naked eye. The affected muscle becomes firm and thickened, the overlying skin and subcutaneous tissues being bound down so that the whole area feels solid. The face develops a smooth expressionless appearance and the child may be unable to open the mouth fully.

The prognosis is extremely grave; in acute cases death may occur in a few weeks. In other cases the process seems gradually to burn itself out, the muscles becoming atrophic and contractures developing. Deposits of calcium may occur in the subcutaneous tissues.

*Treatment.* Steroids are the only hope but, although a few cases respond dramatically, the response in the majority is poor.

### Scleroderma

The borderline between this condition and dermatomyositis is ill-defined, and calcinosis may occur in both. The skin becomes thickened and indurated owing to the deposition of collagen fibres, eventually becoming atrophic so that contractures develop and the face becomes mask-like. The disease usually starts in the face, forearm and hands; it may remain confined to them or spread to the rest of the body. Similar fibrous lesions may develop in the oesophagus leading to its obstruction.

*Morphea* is a localized form of scleroderma which occurs in the form of a plaque or band. It is violet at first, then undergoing atrophy to become a yellowish depressed area which may persist or disappear.

### Disseminated lupus erythematosus

This disorder of collagen is characterized by the circulation of auto-anti-bodies which produce the typical lupus erythematosus (LE) cell found in the bone marrow. This cell is a polymorphonuclear leucocyte containing a metachromatic inclusion body which displaces the nucleus. It can be produced by incubating the patient's serum with his own or another individual's white cells. This test, which is used in the diagnosis of the disease, is known as the 'LE phenomenon' and is due to the antigenic factor present in the globulin fraction of the serum. The disorder can be induced by drugs, especially hydrallazine and some of the hydantoins, subsiding when they are removed.

The disease is far more common in females. The onset is gradual with fever, joint pains and a characteristic erythematous rash like the wings of a butterfly over the bridge of the nose and cheeks. The disease affects all organs so that polyarthritis, pericarditis, pleural effusions, nephritis and neurological manifestations may occur. There is also anaemia, leucopenia, thrombocytopenia and a raised serum globulin.

*Treatment.* Apart from the stopping of drugs in drug-induced cases, the only hopeful form of therapy is the use of steroids, but the response is variable.

### Polyarteritis nodosa

This is a rare disease in childhood, characterized by lesions in the arterial walls which are essentially a cellular necrosis with protein denaturation. The clinical effects result from ischaemia due to vascular thrombosis; they are therefore widespread and depend on the distribution of the lesions. Renal involvement is usual but the onset in many cases is with peripheral neuritis. Skin lesions are common, the heart may be affected and infarction of the mesenteric vessels gives rise to the picture of an acute abdomen. Polymorphonuclear leucocytosis is usual.

*Treatment.* The results of steroid therapy may be dramatic, but the response is variable as in disseminated lupus.

### Anaphylactoid purpura (Henoch-Schönlein purpura)

In this condition there is involvement of the skin, intestines, joints and kidneys, either singly or together. The similarity to rheumatic fever and acute nephritis, together with its occasional occurrence following a streptococcal infection, has suggested that it may be an allergic reaction to the infection. But the incidence after streptococcal infection is by no means as frequent as with the other two conditions and, whereas the antistreptolysin O titre is raised in over 80 per cent of cases of rheumatic fever and acute nephritis, such a frequency is not found in anaphylactoid purpura. Moreover, in acute post-streptococcal nephritis the C3 component of complement is depressed, whereas this is normal in anaphylactoid purpura.

Renal involvement may produce the clinical picture of acute nephritis, nephrosis or chronic nephritis. Renal biopsy shows proliferative glomerulo-nephritis ranging in severity from minor focal lesions to diffuse involvement,

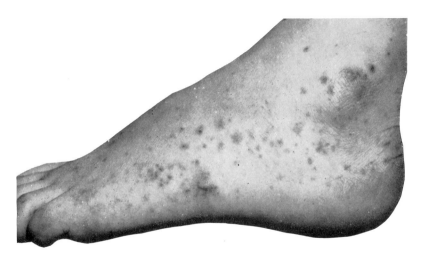

Fig. 139. Anaphylactoid purpura showing typical skin lesions. The deep red centre with lighter surround is visible.

including crescents; a minority of patients show minimal changes only (Meadow *et al.*, 1972).

It seems likely that the condition is a diffuse vascular disease caused by hypersensitivity to a variety of agents, of which the streptococccus is only one. Such an aetiology would explain the cases which have a clear-cut previous history of insect bites. The term 'anaphylactoid' is unfortunate since there is no connection with anaphylactic shock; it would have been better called 'allergic purpura'. Henoch described the intestinal and Schönlein the joint features, but these are both manifestations of the same disease.

*Clinical features.* The disease may occur at any age but is rare under 2 years. The rash is typical, starting as an itching urticarial eruption which changes to form pink maculo-papules which are usually a deeper red at the centre than at the periphery (Fig. 139). These lesions become progressively less raised and more dusky, so that by the following day the rash is composed of dusky red macules which do not fade on pressure and may coalesce to form large patches. The rash occurs predominantly on the buttocks, the lower back, and the extensor aspects of the arms and legs. A horizontal limit to the rash just above the buttocks is usually obvious.

Localized areas of soft tissue oedema may be found into which bleeding may occur. This may involve the testes so that the scrotum appears swollen and bruised.

The knees and ankles are the joints most commonly affected, though these are usually only slightly swollen, this being due to periarticular oedema rather than an effusion. Intestinal involvement causes abdominal pain from submucosal haemorrhages which may cause intestinal bleeding, sometimes leading to an intussusception. Occasionally, at laparotomy, an area of intestine is found to be scarlet and oedematous, possibly from vasospasm secondary to arteriolar damage.

Renal involvement probably occurs in most cases though in only about half the patients are there urinary changes. In the less affected patients there is proteinuria, microscopic haematuria and casts. In severe cases the clinical picture is that of acute nephritis or nephrosis, either of which may lead to chronic nephritis.

*Diagnosis.* This is difficult if the abdominal and joint symptoms occur before the rash but once the rash has appeared the diagnosis is easy. Differentiation from thrombocytopenic purpura is made by the finding of a normal platelet count; Hess's tourniquet test is usually negative.

*Course.* The condition is very liable to relapse, so that for several weeks crops of the typical maculo-papules appear and gradually fade. With each new crop there may be a recurrence of the abdominal and joint symptoms. Recurrences seldom occur after three months of freedom. The prognosis depends on the severity of the renal lesion. It used to be thought that renal involvement carried a high mortality rate but it is surprising to what an extent recovery is possible. This is probably related to the focal variation in the kidneys.

*Treatment.* Early ambulation does not affect the incidence of recurrence, therefore the child can be allowed up when he feels like it, provided this does not cause increased oedema of the feet. The management of renal complications is the same as for glomerulonephritis (p. 382). Steroid therapy is disappointing but should be tried in severe cases; it does not appear to affect the rash or the course of the renal disease but it may dramatically relieve the abdominal pain as well as improving the general condition.

# BIBLIOGRAPHY

ALEXANDER W.D. & SMITH G. (1962) Disadvantageous circulatory effects of salicylate in rheumatic fever. *Lancet*, **1**, 768.

ANSELL B.M. & BYWATERS E.G.L. (1963) Rheumatoid arthritis (Still's disease). *Pediat. Clin. N. Amer.*, **10**, 921.

ARON A.M., FREEMAN J.M. & CARTER S. (1965) Natural history of Sydenham's chorea: review of the literature and long-term evaluation with emphasis on cardiac sequelae. *Amer. J. Med.*, **38**, 83.

BYWATERS E.G.L. (1965) Rheumatic fever and rheumatoid arthritis. *Brit. med. J.*, **1**, 1655.

FEINSTEIN A.R. & AREVALO A.C. (1964) Manifestations and treatment of congestive heart failure in young patients with rheumatic heart disease. *Pediatrics*, **33**, 661.

ILLINGWORTH R.S., LORBER J., HOLT K.S. & RENDLE-SHORT J. (1957) Acute rheumatic fever in children. A comparison of six forms of treatment in 200 cases. *Lancet*, **2**, 653.

LAURIN C.A. & FAVREAU J.C. (1963) Rheumatoid disease in children. *Canad. med. Ass. J.*, **89**, 288.

LIETMAN P.S. & BYWATERS E.G.L. (1963) Pericarditis in juvenile rheumatoid arthritis. *Pediatrics*, **32**, 855.

MEADOW S.R., GLASGOW E.F., WHITE R.H.R., MONCRIEFF M.W., CAMERON J.S. & OGG C.S. (1972) Schönlein-Henoch nephritis. *Quart. J. Med.*, **41**, 241.

RHEUMATIC FEVER STUDY GROUP (1965) A comparison of short-term, intensive prednisone and acetylsalicylic acid therapy in the treatment of acute rheumatic fever. *New Engl. J. Med.*, **272**, 63.

SCHLESINGER B.E., FORSYTH C.C., WHITE R.H.R., SMELLIE J.M. & STROUD C.E. (1961) Observations on the clinical course and treatment of 100 cases of Still's disease. *Arch. Dis. Childh.*, **36**, 65.

VERNIER R.L., WORTHEN H.G., PETERSEN R.D., COLLE E. & GOOD R.A. (1961) Anaphylactoid purpura. *Pediatrics*, **27**, 181.

# CHAPTER 24

# DISEASES OF THE SKIN

## Impetigo contagiosa

This is seen in older children, particularly in those attending school; it is due to infection with the streptococcus or staphylococcus. Any area may be involved but lesions occur particularly on exposed sites such as the face, scalp and hands. They are multiple, starting as minute red macules which progress to form small vesicles; these rupture producing the typical lesions which consist of brown crusts on an erythematous base. Healing begins in the centre, producing circinate lesions that may be mistaken for ringworm. However, in ringworm the edge consists of numerous small vesicles or pustules (Fig. 142), whereas the circinate lesion of impetigo is made up of one large vesicle only.

The condition is highly contagious, any abrasion in a patient with impetigo being certain to produce a fresh lesion at that site. Impetigo frequently complicates other skin conditions, such as scabies, pediculosis, papular urticaria, insect bites, seborrhoeic dermatitis and the lesions of herpes simplex which occur round the edge of the mouth. The discharging ear from otitis media may be complicated by impetigo of the pinna.

*Treatment.* Impetigo spreads rapidly in a school so that affected children should be isolated, have their own towels and use separate baths. Infected crusts should be removed with saline or cetrimide lotion. If there is gross crusting a starch poultice will effectively clean the whole area.

An antibiotic ointment should be applied, its choice being determined by a number of principles which apply to the treatment of skin infections generally. Cultures for bacterial sensitivity should be set up before starting treatment. No antibiotic should be used locally which might later be required systemically since resistant organisms could be produced. Penicillin, streptomycin and sulphonamides should never be used locally since skin sensitivity to these drugs is especially liable to develop.

For the treatment of impetigo, chlortetracycline ointment is almost always effective against coccal infections. Other local antibiotics in use include bacitracin, framycetin and polymyxin. In areas such as the West Indies where acute nephritis following streptococcal impetiginized scabies is common (p. 382), systemic penicillin therapy should be given routinely. In other areas the results of bacterial swabs can be awaited.

BULLOUS IMPETIGO

In Great Britain this condition is seen only during the neonatal period when it is sometimes incorrectly called pemphigus neonatorum (see p. 112); in

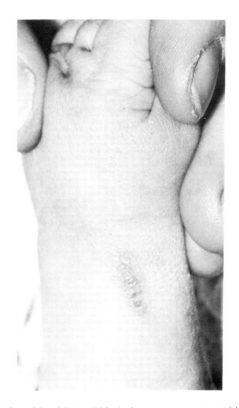

FIG. 140. Fetal sucking blister. This lesion was present at birth and for several days the baby continually sucked the area on the radial aspect of the left wrist.

tropical countries it may occur at any age. It is usually due to the staphylococcus. The lesions occur anywhere, but particularly in the axillae and groins, and consist of large flaccid bullae containing pus and a supernatant clear serum. These rupture easily leaving large raw areas; they do not form crusts to the same extent as impetigo contagiosa. Systemic penicillin and local chlortetracycline should be given pending the results of bacterial cultures.

FETAL SUCKING BLISTER

A bullous or vesicular lesion present at birth could be regarded as alarming if its simple aetiology were not appreciated. A considerable number of babies *in utero* suck the radial aspect of their forearm, wrist or hand so vigorously that at birth a localized area of vesicles on an erythematous base is present (Fig. 140). These babies commonly have an insatiable appetite for the skin of their own arms and hands (Murphy & Langley, 1963).

## Folliculitis and furunculosis

Folliculitis is a superficial infection of the hair follicle which, if neglected, gives rise to a number of similar lesions or goes on to form a furuncle or boil in which the infection is at the base of the hair follicle. Alternatively, the infection may start in the depths of the follicle as a boil. Staphylococci are the usual infecting organisms, the lesions occurring most often at sites of abrasions; consequently, they are especially found at the back of the neck and on the buttocks. Acne vulgaris and those skin disorders already mentioned which may be complicated by impetigo, may equally be complicated by boils. They are extremely painful during the stage of formation but, once they discharge their pus and the pressure is reduced, pain is relieved. Boils seldom occur singly because of the ease with which neighbouring hair follicles are infected with the same staphylococci. In recurrent cases the urine should be checked for sugar to exclude diabetes.

*Treatment.* Folliculitis is best treated with 1 per cent gentian violet provided the paint is acceptable to the patient. A boil will heal itself and treatment makes little difference to the time this takes though it can reduce pain and prevent spread. Stretching adhesive tape across a developing boil splints the skin, thereby reducing movement and consequent pain. Non-stick antibiotic dressings may help by reducing spread to nearby skin. For the same reason the skin should be kept clean with spirit. On no account should the boil be squeezed. In recurrent and resistant cases, systemic antibiotic therapy should be used and ultra-violet light treatment is of value.

## Hordeolum (stye)

This condition is due to folliculitis developing in the hair follicle of an eyelash and is usually due to *Staphlococcus aureus*. It may occur in association with seborrhoea of the scalp and this must be treated if recurrent styes are to be prevented (see p. 672).

## Napkin rashes

A rash in the napkin area, involving the genitalia, buttocks and inner aspects of the thighs is extremely common owing to the skin remaining in contact with urine and stool. The commonest cause is an ammonia dermatitis (see below). Additional factors are: infrequent napkin changing; the wearing of plastic pants which prevent evaporation; and the use of detergents instead of a pure soap to wash the napkins.

### AMMONIA DERMATITIS

Liberation of ammonia results from the action of bacteria in the stools, such as *Micrococcus urease*, which have the capacity to split the urea in the urine. This action takes place when stools and urine are left for long together. It occurs more easily if the stools are alkaline, as in the baby on cow's milk, whereas the breast-fed infant, whose stools are usually acid, is less liable to the problem.

The ammonia causes a chemical burn of the skin so that in severe acute cases the whole of the napkin area is red and moist. As this becomes chronic, the skin comes to feel like paper, being thick and wrinkled from lichenification and loss of elasticity. Peeling then occurs, particularly at the edges. In less severe cases there are isolated bluish-red papulo-vesicular lesions which soon break down to form shallow ulcers (Fig. 141). Their distribution is determined by where the urine lies, so that it is predominantly periurethral, involving the external genitalia, suprapubic region, inner aspects of thighs and sometimes the natal cleft. In circumcised boys the unprotected glans is involved, so that a meatal ulcer is common (p. 394).

The mother will commonly state that the urine smells strong. She may complain that it causes her eyes to water when she changes the napkins.

*Treatment.* This involves meticulous attention to detail. Wet napkins must not be allowed to remain in contact with the skin, frequent changing being required. Whenever possible the napkin area should be left exposed to the air, the child only lying on the napkin. The area is thoroughly washed with a pure soap whenever soiled. Plastic pants should be banned.

Urea-splitting organisms flourish in an alkaline medium, therefore the area should be treated with a mild acid. In the past, boric acid was used but unfortunately, fatal cases of boric poisoning have occurred when boric powder has been liberally applied to a large raw area on the buttocks. For this reason the use of boric acid in any form should be discontinued. In its place benzalkonium chloride, one of the quaternary ammonium compounds, should be used. The napkins are soaked for half an hour in a 1 in 80 solution (Roccal) after being thoroughly rinsed, since its germicidal action is reduced by the presence of soap. The same substance can be used locally as an ointment (Drapolene). As an alternative solution for the rinse, a weak solution of vinegar can be used, one ounce of vinegar being mixed with one gallon of water.

If benzalkonium chloride is not available, zinc and castor oil ointment will often be effective, provided the other measures are carried out. The skin must be protected from contact with urine. This can also be achieved by the application of gentian violet or egg-white. The use of egg white has the advantage of simplicity and treatment can start immediately, assuming there is an egg in the house. The white of an egg is whisked and then painted on

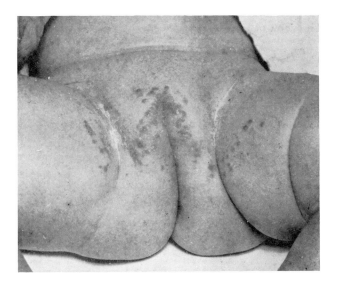

FIG. 141. Ammonia dermatitis. The lesions are papulo-vesicular, some having broken down to form shallow ulcers. The distribution is periurethral rather than perianal, indicating its urinary origin.

to the skin with cotton wool or directly with clean fingers. The skin is allowed to dry, a second coating then being applied so that a protective layer of albumen forms over the skin.

PERI-ANAL EXCORIATION

This is common following a period of loose motions in any baby. It occurs particularly during the first month of life if babies are put on cow's milk. It can be prevented by the application of a barrier cream when cow's milk feeding is instituted.

When a baby has oral thrush (p. 115) the stool contains the fungus. This can cause a napkin rash consisting of discrete oval erythematous macules, usually confined to the perianal area. The diagnosis can be confirmed by microscopic examination of scrapings. The lesions respond to local 1 per cent aqueous gentian violet which should be tried in all doubtful cases.

A seborrhoeic napkin rash is extensive and of a brownish-red colour. The diagnosis is made by the presence of other seborrhoeic lesions on the scalp, around the ears or in the axillae (p. 672). The area should be left exposed to the air and hydrocortisone ointment applied.

### Miliaria rubra (heat rash, prickly heat)

This condition, due to excessive heat, is very common in infants. In the tropics, where it frequently occurs, all ages are affected. The lesions consist of minute, itching, erythematous papules and vesicles situated at the openings of the sweat glands. They are therefore found particularly on the face, neck, shoulders and chest where the sweat glands are concentrated.

The contents of the vesicles may be crystalline from retention of sweat in the sweat duct; these are sometimes termed *sudamina*. They should be differentiated from *milia* which are yellowish-white opalescent spots seen particularly on the nose in many normal babies. These are due to blockage of the openings of the sebaceous glands and have nothing to do with the sweat; there is no associated inflammation, the lesions disappearing without treatment.

*Heat rash* is an ill-defined term which sometimes refers to miliaria rubra and at other times to intertrigo occurring mainly in the flexures.

*Treatment.* The child should be kept cool and dry, excessive clothing being removed. No wool should be used next to the skin; some cases are also sensitive to nylon which in any case is too hot for use in the tropics. When itching is severe a shower or bath will provide immediate relief. A dusting powder containing zinc oxide and starch, or calamine lotion should be applied. Ascorbic acid has been found to be successful in the treatment and the prevention of prickly heat (Hindson, 1968).

### Papular urticaria (lichen urticatus)

An extremely common condition in children of all ages, but especially seen between the ages of 6 months and 3 years. The lesions consist of red blotches or white weals, with a central papule sometimes surmounted by a vesicle. They are found mainly on the trunk and limbs; they cause intense itching so that they have often been scratched and secondarily impetiginized. The blotches or weals last a few hours only but the papules persist for longer.

*Aetiology.* The condition occurs particularly during the summer; both heat and the eating of fresh fruit may be causative factors. But flea bites and contact sensitivity to flea protein without being bitten are the major causes. The fleas involved are those of cat, dog and bird rather than of the human variety (Bolam & Burtt, 1956).

*Treatment.* The possibility of fleas should be investigated in all cases, any infected animal being treated with a dusting powder containing Gamma Benzene Hexachloride. This substance has superseded Dicophane (DDT) owing to its risk of poisoning. For the child, calamine lotion is the most soothing local preparation; he should be given the bottle of lotion so as to be able to dab it on whenever he feels the urge to scratch. Antihistamines by mouth are sometimes effective and always worth a trial. The lesions may become secondarily impetiginized and should then be treated in the same way as impetigo (see p. 663).

### Infantile eczema

This is an allergic condition, there often being a family history of allergy, particularly eczema or asthma. It is more common in boys and starts about the age of 3 months, always being worst in its first few weeks. The lesions commence on the cheeks and forehead as a bright red erythema which may rapidly become vesicular and weep. Rapid spread may occur to involve the flexor surfaces of the limbs or the whole body. There is intense irritation, so that the lesions become excoriated. After the acute onset there is a tendency for improvement, but the lesions may become chronic, persisting in the flexures as papular lichenified patches. Seborrhoea is often associated, in which case lesions are also present on the scalp and behind the ears. Infantile eczema is common among Negro babies in temperate climates, though rare in tropical climates; it appears to be associated with an increased incidence of seborrhoea when they live in a cool climate.

*Treatment.* Infantile eczema is much more common in babies fed on cow's milk rather than on breast milk so that a change from cow's milk to soybean milk may help. Contact with irritating clothes makes the condition worse, so that woollen clothes should not be worn; nylon may have a similar effect. As little clothing as possible should be worn since the skin should be kept cool.

The basis of management is to teach the mother how to keep the condition under control, explaining that eczema cannot be cured but that it can be kept down. She should be taught the basic principles of dermatology so that, within certain limits, she becomes the dermatologist. By this means, not only is the treatment of the skin more successful, but the mother is prevented from trying out the many remedies which will be recommended to her by friends. Moreover, it will no longer be necessary for her to return to the doctor for each relapse.

Standard dermatological practice is that a weeping surface requires a wet application, therefore a lotion is used. Once the lotion has dried the skin it is changed for a paste which is less greasy than an ointment and, since it contains powder, is able to absorb a limited amount of exuding fluid. Pastes should be applied thickly; they are followed by ointments which are greasy and should be well rubbed in, thus returning the skin to its normal soft state. These facts are explained to the mother who is given a lotion for the weeping areas and a paste for the dry areas. A suitable lotion is 1/1000 proflavine. A suitable paste contains tar and can be made up as follows:

| Liquor picis carb. | 1·5 ml |
|---|---|
| Arachis oil | 8 ml |
| Zinc paste | to 30 g |

She is instructed to dab the yellow lotion on to any weeping areas as often as possible. If these are extensive, a gauze dressing soaked in the lotion should be applied, this being kept moist by dropping further lotion on to it. Once the areas becomes dry she applies the white paste which will already be in use on dry lesions elsewhere. The paste should be cleaned off with liquid paraffin once a day and a fresh application made. Should a relapse occur in any area she returns to the yellow lotion for that area until it becomes dry again. On this regimen it is unusual for any area to weep for longer than 48 hours and the mother knows that she has the remedy at hand. She is much less anxious, she has the satisfaction of feeling that she is really treating her own child and she does not need to run to the doctor with every change in her child's condition.

When first seen, the patient's skin, particularly the scalp, is often covered by the previous applications which have become stuck to the weeping areas. In such a case the use of one starch poultice to clean up the whole area is most valuable before treatment is started.

In addition to local treatment, the mother is taught the principles of general management. The child must be prevented from scratching by being kept amused with toys, his attention being occupied as much as possible. He should never be left in a room on his own to amuse himself but be taken round the house by his mother as she does her housework. Finger nails must be kept short and arm splints applied if necessary. The most satisfactory arm splint is made by bandaging cardboard round the limb, since this still leaves the hands free for play.

Babies with lesions on the back of the head and neck have a habit of rolling their head on the pillow, causing severe excoriation. This can be prevented by the use of an old X-ray plate from which the emulsion has been cleaned. A hole is made at each corner so that a tape can be inserted; the plate is then tied to the bed. The corners of the plate should be rounded off and adhesive tape placed all round the edges as these are sharp.

Ung. emulsificans is useful as a soap substitute to avoid irritation. It can either be put into the bath or applied as a thin layer all over the child before getting in. Gentle sponging causes sufficient lather to remove dirt.

In the early stages, sedatives are necessary to reduce irritation. Chloral hydrate is suitable but large doses must be given to be effective. It is not unusual for a child of 6 months to require 300 mg or even 600 mg of chloral. Promethazine hydrochloride (Phenergan) is an antihistamine which is useful as a sedative; it is given in a dose of 1 mg/kg/day in three divided doses. Phenobarbitone 15–30 mg is another alternative. If large doses of sedative are required it is better to alternate the drug used in order to prevent a cumulative effect. Physical restraint in bed should not be needed.

Topical corticosteroids have not been mentioned first since, although they usually produce dramatic improvement when first used, their effect may be short-lived. It is preferable therefore to teach the mother the general management as outlined, keeping steroid ointments in reserve. Moreover, widespread and continued application of topical steroids can cause systemic side effects, particularly growth restriction and local atrophy. Percutaneous absorption of steroids occurs more readily in children than in adults (Feiwel, 1969). Fear of this by mothers and doctors may cause insufficient to be applied. Success with the tar paste is often related to the fact that the mother can be told to apply it very liberally.

One-half or one per cent hydrocortisone is a satisfactory local steroid for most cases. The fluorinated steroids, such as fluocinolone (Synalar) and betamethasone (Betnovate) may be more effective but carry a greater risk of side effects if used for long.

Children with eczema must not be vaccinated (p. 489).

### Seborrhoeic dermatitis

In young babies this condition is most commonly seen as a thick brown layer of crusts over the scalp, sometimes termed 'cradle cap'. It is often associated with inadequate washing of the head because mothers are frightened to do so, particularly near the anterior fontanelle. The crusts can sometimes be removed with olive oil or by washing the hair with a solution of sodium bicarbonate (one teaspoon to a pint of water). In resistant cases a coal tar preparation, such as Pragmatar, may be used. This contains tar in a water emulsifying base; it is applied as an ointment at night and as a shampoo in the morning. One per cent cetrimide solution is also effective in removing crusts; it must not be used with soap as this renders it inactive.

It has already been mentioned that some babies with infantile eczema have seborrhoea and in these the scalp may be as severely involved as the face; the ears are usually also affected. Treatment of the scalp is along the same lines as for eczema elsewhere on the body. Once the active phase has passed the scalp must be kept clear by regular shampooing.

In older children, seborrhoea is most commonly seen as 'dandruff' or 'scurf'. Spread can result from contact with the scales from the scalp. These fall first on to the eyelids, producing a pustular folliculitis of the eyelash follicles. This may lead to a hordeolum (stye, p. 665). Small crusts may be seen along the edge of the eyelid between the hairs; local treatment is ineffective until the primary cause in the scalp has been successfully treated. Local application of 1 per cent mercuric oxide eye ointment may then hasten the clearing of the crusts from the eyelids.

In addition to the eyelids, scurf falls on to the body and at the major points of contact may produce seborrhoeic dermatitis. These lesions are therefore seen especially on the face, shoulder blades, front of the chest and in the flexures. Acute seborrhoeic dermatitis of the body should be treated first with the tar paste (p. 670). Topical corticosteroids (see above) can be used if this fails. The same treatment can be tried for chronic lesions but, if unsuccessful, an ointment containing 2 per cent each of precipitated sulphur and salicylic acid should be used instead. In all cases of seborrhoeic dermatitis it is essential to get rid of scurf.

Scurf is treated by regular shampooing of the head, starting with three times a week and reducing to once a week. A spirit shampoo containing 3 per cent oil of cade is satisfactory or, alternatively, Pragmatar. A shampoo containing selenium sulphide is very effective but should be used only on isolated occasions as it is toxic if its use is regular and prolonged.

### Intertrigo

This is a problem in tropical countries. It occurs in the flexures, especially the groins, where the skin is red and may be weeping. Lesions in the groin must be differentiated from tinea cruris (see p. 679).

*Treatment.* Only very mild soothing applications such as calamine lotion should be used; in resistant cases steroid ointment is indicated. Once cured, meticulous attention must be paid to hygiene in order to prevent a relapse. Baths should be taken frequently, the flexures being carefully dried and a dusting powder applied.

### Urticaria neonatorum

This is an extremely common transitory condition affecting babies in the first 2–3 days of life. It bears no relationship to the ordinary form of urticaria described below. The lesions consist of pink weals with or without a white centre. Some of the lesions may be white spots only, looking like a pustule. But they are smaller and harder than the usual pustule and they disappear in a few hours, only to reappear elsewhere on the body.

The condition occurs more often in full-term than in preterm infants. Although often referred to as a heat rash there is no good evidence for this. Its cause is unknown. Possibly it is a reaction of the skin to the change from the intrauterine fluid environment to an air environment after birth. No treatment is required but mothers must be told why this is unnecessary because they are very worried by these spots.

### Urticaria (nettle-rash)

This is an allergic condition in which intensely irritating weals appear, similar to those produced by the sting of a nettle. The weals may remain discrete but if extensive they coalesce to involve large areas of the body. The cause is most often an item of food, such as fruit or shellfish, to which the child is sensitive, but it may be due to drugs, especially aspirin, or serum. It can be caused also by insect bites and is sometimes the result of an emotional disturbance. The condition can be caused by scabies and this possibility should always be investigated. It may be impossible to determine the cause.

*Treatment.* The child should be given a bowl of calamine lotion so that he can dab this on as often as he wishes. Antihistamine drugs should be tried and, if unsuccessful, ephedrine 15–30 mg may help.

### Angioneurotic oedema

This condition is comparable to urticaria, but the reaction is localized and severe swelling may occur. The lip or some other part of the face may be involved and sometimes the penis is affected. Occasionally, severe laryngeal oedema occurs. The cause is less easy to discover than with urticaria, usually none being found; the possibility of aspirin sensitivity should always be considered. The swelling seldom lasts longer than a few hours but in severe cases, particularly in those involving the larynx, steroid therapy should be employed.

### Acne vulgaris

This condition occurs at puberty, being more common in boys than in girls. It is due to an excessive output and overgrowth of the sebaceous glands, without corresponding hypertrophy of the ducts or hair follicles. Consequently, there is a 'bottle-neck' obstruction at the opening of the follicle which is increased still further by hyperkeratosis of the mouth of the follicle. Blockage of sebum occurs, producing the comedo or 'black-head' which is the primary lesion. The black is melanin, not ingrained dirt as used to be thought. The comedo causes chemical rather than bacterial inflammation, from excess fatty acids derived from the sebum. Secondary infection develops so that pustules and even boils form, resulting in scarring. The lesions are found particularly on the face, chest and over the shoulders, since the sebaceous glands are most numerous in these sites. Scurf is an additional factor. Those who are subject to acne always have a greasy skin.

*Treatment.* It is necessary to reduce the greasiness of the skin and clear the blocked sebaceous glands. The face should be washed in very hot water as often as possible; after each wash all obvious comedones should be removed with a comedo extractor (never the fingers). Calamine lotion with 3 per cent sulphur is then applied and, when dry, is rubbed well in. This lotion causes peeling of the skin and clearing of the follicles. It can be used during the day since, after being rubbed in, it is not obvious, in fact the patient will find that the slight colour from the lotion camouflages the lesions to some extent without making him look made up. Ultra-violet light increases the amount of desquamation; in severe cases the purchase of a home lamp is worth while. During its use the eyes should be protected by dark glasses. The scalp must be shampooed regularly to ensure that no scurf is allowed to accumulate.

Long-term tetracycline therapy is successful and acts mainly by reducing the level of fatty acids in the sebum. Diet in any form probably makes little difference although sweets and chocolate used to be regarded as harmful. X-ray therapy is dangerous and should not be used.

The patient is always extremely self-conscious of his spots, but he can be reassured that once the endocrine imbalance associated with puberty is passed, the lesions will disappear. He must be warned against squeezing the spots because the resultant scarring is permanent. Stress is a factor so that although greasy cosmetics make the condition worse it is better for a girl to use some cosmetics in order to lead a normal social life.

### Chilblain (erythema pernio)

These are due to arteriolar spasm in response to cold. The lesions occur on the extremities, consisting of painful and irritating red swellings, the surface of which may break down to form indolent fissures.

*Treatment.* The limbs must be kept warm and antipruritic ointment such as menthol, or mild rubefacients such as methyl salicylate may be applied locally.

### Alopecia areata

Children over the age of 5 years may quite suddenly develop a bald patch or even lose all their hair. The cause cannot usually be discovered but an acute emotional shock is sometimes a precipitating factor. The skin in the bald area is quite clean and smooth; stumps of hair like exclamation marks are visible at the edge. As long as these stumps are present the area is still increasing.

The condition must be differentiated from ringworm in which the bald patch is dirty grey and covered with fine scales. In ringworm the area is not completely devoid of hair, broken hairs being present which have lost their elasticity so that they do not rebound when bent over. The final differentiation is made by microscopic examination.

*Treatment.* Any possible emotional or infective cause must be eradicated. The most effective treatment is the intradermal injection of triamcinolone into the lesion. This usually causes regrowth of hair in 6 weeks (Beare, 1965).

## Psoriasis

Children are affected less often than adults but the condition may start in childhood. The acute lesions are small, dry, reddish-pink papules. In chronic cases large disc-like lesions are present, which are dry, slightly raised and covered with scales. These become silvery on scraping; when completely scraped off they leave minute bleeding points. The edge is well defined and there is seldom much irritation. The sites of election are the fronts of the knees and backs of the elbows, followed by the scalp, ears, chest and upper end of the natal cleft. Psoriasis is an occasional cause of a severe napkin rash in babies.

*Treatment.* In the acute stage calamine lotion is suitable. No strong application should be used as this may precipitate exfoliative dermatitis. In the chronic stage the best treatment is a combination of ultra-violet light and crude coal-tar working up to 4 per cent. The tar should be cleaned off while the patient is receiving the daily light treatment. Fluorinated steroid ointment is of use in the treatment of flexural psoriasis.

## Erythema multiforme

The cause of this condition is unknown but its behaviour suggests that it is a form of sensitivity reaction, possibly to the streptococcus. It is uncommon in young children. There is a seasonal incidence, the condition being seen most often during spring and autumn. In some patients the condition recurs annually. Systemic symptoms may precede or accompany the rash; they consist of malaise, fever and sore throat. Gastro-intestinal symptoms and joint pains may occur. The rash is symmetrical, starting as macular erythema, but every form of skin lesion may be seen. Sometimes a rainbow of concentric rings is produced, this variety being named *erythema iris*. The lesions particularly favour the backs of the hands and wrists; they have preferences for the extremities, tending to avoid the trunk. The eruption may occur in crops and, even if untreated, will disappear in 2–6 weeks, although it is always liable to recur.

*Treatment.* Any obvious infection should be treated; only mild and soothing applications should be used locally.

STEVENS-JOHNSON SYNDROME

This is a very severe form of erythema multiforme associated with involvement of the mucous membranes. The skin lesions are severe, vesicles and bullae being common. Lesions in the mouth are usual and there is often a grey or white membrane which leaves a bleeding ulcer when peeled off; vesicles and bullae may also be seen in the mouth. Conjunctivitis is common; often there is balanitis or vulvovaginitis. Pneumonitis sometimes accompanies the illness; its similarity to a virus pneumonia has suggested a virus origin for the whole disorder.

The condition has sometimes proved fatal, but a good response can be expected from steroid therapy; this should always be given, together with antibiotics.

## Pityriasis rosea

This is an acute self-limiting disease whose only importance lies in its differentiation from the infectious fevers of childhood. The first lesion is the 'herald patch' which precedes the main rash by about a week. It occurs especially over the lower ribs or anterior abdominal wall and is a red scaly macule which is larger than the subsequent lesions, being up to 4 cm in diameter. The rash itself consists of oval, rose-pink macules which start near the herald patch and spread all over the body; on the chest they have a tendency to arrange themselves with their long axes parallel to the underlying ribs. These lesions become buff-coloured and scaly before they disappear; the whole illness, which causes little constitutional upset, lasting 6–8 weeks. Itching is slight or absent and the mucous membranes are never involved.

*Treatment.* None is required.

## Ringworm

This is due to a number of different fungal infections which are highly infectious. Their lesions differ according to the type of fungus and the area of the body affected. The ringworm fungus lives on keratin, therefore it can affect only hair, skin and nails, never mucous membranes. It prefers an alkaline medium; hence it is commonly found in flexures and between the toes.

TINEA CAPITIS

Ringworm of the scalp is now more often due to *Microsporon canis*, which comes from animal sources, than to *M. audouini* which used to cause the majority of cases and is more infectious. This form of ringworm is confined to children. It causes one or more round or oval, bald patches which spread centrifugally and are sharply limited. The scalp is covered by dry and slightly adherent grey scales, the area being studded by broken hairs which are very friable and lack lustre. Diagnosis is confirmed by Wood's light, which causes the affected hairs to fluoresce, and by microscopy when spores are visible coating the hair.

*Treatment.* Griseofulvin, an antifungal antiobiotic, has revolutionized the treatment of this condition. This substance is selectively taken up by the newly formed keratin in the skin, hair and nails and, being a fungistatic agent, it prevents the further growth of the fungus in these sites; existing fungus is shed with the growth of these tissues. It is not toxic in the doses required for therapy, a week's course of 125 mg q.d.s. being usually sufficient. Although *M. canis* is less infective than *M. audouini*, the patients should be isolated from other children until fluorescence is no longer obtained with Wood's light; this usually takes about 3 weeks. Brushes, combs and towels belonging to the patient must be kept strictly away from other children and caps must not be shared.

### TINEA INTERDIGITALIS (EPIDERMOPHYTOSIS, ATHLETE'S FOOT)

This extremely common condition is due to an epidermophyton and is often the primary source of infection of tinea cruris and corporis. It is highly infectious, being spread by towels and in communal baths, so that it is an endemic problem in boarding schools. It is worst among white races in the tropics, seldom being seen in coloured races whose toes are more widely spaced since they less often wear shoes and socks.

Areas of white sodden skin with cracks and fissures appear between the toes, especially in the narrow cleft between the fourth, and fifth toes. The condition may spread directly to the skin of the foot, causing a papulo-vesicular eruption.

*Treatment.* Meticulous attention to hygiene is essential for cure and for the prevention of spread to others. The sodden skin between the toes should be removed by forceps each day and zinc undecylenate ointment applied. This substance should also be used in a dusting powder for the socks and shoes. Alternatively, Magenta Paint (Castellani's paint) can be used for local treatment. Treatment should always be continued for at least a week after the last sign of infection has disappeared in order to prevent a relapse. A clean pair of socks should be worn daily.

To cut short an outbreak in a school, attention must be paid to the bath-rooms, since the spread of infection is largely via the bathroom floor. The wearing of wooden clogs during shower baths reduces this contact and is of proven value (Jolly, 1948).

TINEA CIRCINATA (TINEA CORPOSIS)

This form of ringworm is most often due to infection with an epidermophyton, commonly spreading from athlete's foot originally caught from another patient. Microsporon and tricophyton infections may also cause tinea circinata, these having usually been acquired from animal sources.

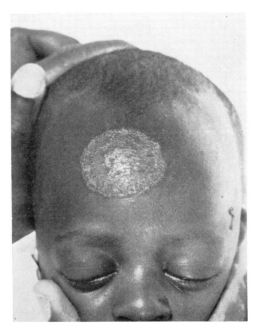

FIG. 142. Tinea circinata. Healing has taken place in the centre of the lesion, while active vesicles are visible at its edge.

The lesions, which are usually multiple, are circular and start as red, scaly areas which become covered with small vesicles. They grow centrifugally so that healing takes place in the centre while the active vesicles are present on the raised edge of the circle (Fig. 142). Diagnosis is confirmed by the finding of fungi in the scrapings.

*Treatment.* Benzoic acid compound ointment (Whitfield's ointment), which contains benzoic and salicylic acid, is usually effective. As an alternative, zinc undecylenate ointment may be used. Magenta Paint is remarkably effective but its bright colour limits its use. Griseofulvin should be kept for resistant cases, especially those due to *Tricophyton rubrum*.

This lesion is due to an epidermophyton infection and occurs on the inner aspect of the thighs, especially where the skin is in contact with the scrotum. It often extends into the natal cleft. The condition is very infectious and may have started as athlete's foot so that outbreaks sometimes occur in boarding schools. The lesion is similar to tinea circinata in that the growing edge of vesicles is at the periphery, but the moist warm site modifies it so that the central area remains inflamed though not vesicular, and may weep extensively. The rash is intensely irritating, excoriation making matters worse.

It must be emphasized that not every rash in the groin or between the toes is due to ringworm and, in hot climates particularly, a simple intertrigo is common. In intertrigo no vesicles are seen as in ringworm, the final diagnosis being made by microscopy. Treatment of intertrigo by antifungal agents leads to chronic dermatitis medicamentosa. It is equally important not to overtreat cases of ringworm, since the strong antifungal applications may lead to a sensitization dermatitis.

*Treatment.* In acute cases, only the mildest and most soothing applications should be used: calamine lotion with 1 per cent silver nitrate, or 1/10,000 potassium permanganate baths and compresses. When the acute stage has passed, a fungicidal ointment such as Whitfield's or zinc undecylenate can be used. Magenta Paint is particularly suitable for the tropics where sweating makes treatment with an ointment uncomfortable. The natal cleft should be treated in all cases, whether lesions are present or not, as spores may reside there, causing a relapse. Griseofulvin is used in resistant cases, but is unnecessary as a routine.

Ringworm of the nails is not common in children; it is usually due to *Tricophyton rubrum*. The nails become rough, opaque and friable, scales accumulating underneath. Diagnosis is confirmed by microscopy.

*Treatment.* This condition has been very resistant to treatment in the past, but griseofulvin is effective and should always be used.

## Granuloma annulare

This is a rare condition of unknown aetiology but it occurs more often in children than in adults. The lesions commonly appear on the hands and feet. These are nodules which group together to form a ring which is skin coloured and whose edge is raised. One or more rings may be present.

The condition must be differentiated from ringworm. Unlike ringworm it does not itch or scale. Skin scrapings should be examined for fungus in doubtful cases.

The lesions usually clear spontaneously in a few weeks; therefore the assessment of response to topical steroids or intralesional injections of triamcinolone, which are often used, is difficult.

### Scabies

This is due to infestation with *Sarcoptes scabei*, a mite which is just visible to the naked eye as a white speck. Transfer of infection is mainly by bodily contact and only to a slight extent from sleeping in infected bedding since the mite survives for only 24 hours away from the body. The female mite lays her eggs in one of her favourite creases, the eggs hatching into larvae in 3–7 days. The larvae scratch their way to the surface, then pass down the nearest hair follicle where they develop into adult mites. The lesions of scabies are therefore of two types: burrows containing adult female mites and their eggs; and a scattered follicular eruption containing the immature mites. The 'burrow' consists of a vesicle at the site of entrance and a linear elevation of the skin caused by the burrowing of the mite through the superficial layers of the skin.

The rash is extremely irritating, particularly at night when the mites are most active. Consequently, the lesions are usually excoriated and may well have become secondarily infected and impetiginized. Many of the burrows will have lost their roofs, but a thin line of dirt often marks their position. The sites of election are the webs of the fingers, palms, ulnar border of the hand, front of the wrist, medial aspect of the elbow, anterior axillary line, nipples, umbilicus, penis, natal cleft and the soles and webs of the feet. Lesions are not found in the scalp and the face is spared, except occasionally in infants who may be infected from their mother's breasts. An allergic reaction to the mite sometimes occurs in the form of urticaria, therefore the possibility of scabies should be remembered in all cases of urticaria.

Diagnosis is made from all other skin diseases by the very characteristic distribution and particularly by the lesions on the front of the wrists and the penis. It is confirmed by the finding of the mite just beyond the vesicle at the end of the burrow, using a needle and hand lens (provided by the auriscope).

*Treatment.* Benzyl benzoate is still a favourite preparation but it is sometimes irritating to children. Monosulphiram (Tetmosol) is an efficient alternative without this disadvantage. The child is given a hot bath using soap and gentle rubbing with a flannel in order to open up the burrows, the emulsion being then painted over the whole body and allowed to dry before applying a second layer. The application is repeated without a bath the next day. On the third day the patient is given a bath, afterwards dressing in clean clothing. All bedding and clothes must then be specially laundered using sufficient heat to kill all the mites. It is most important that all members of the family should be checked for scabies, treatment being given if necessary.

If there is severe secondary infection, this must be treated first. The risk of acute nephritis from secondary streptococcal infection is high in the West Indies (p. 382).

## Pediculosis (louse infestation)

### PEDICULUS CAPITIS

This is due to the head louse which causes intense irritation. It attaches its eggs to the hair as 'nits', which are small greyish-white lumps just visible to the naked eye. Secondary infection of the scalp lesions is common and is an important cause of impetigo of the scalp in children.

### PEDICULUS CORPORIS

This is due to the body louse which also causes extreme irritation. The louse lives in clothing, coming on to the body for feeding only, so that nothing but the scratch marks and the points of puncture where the insect has extracted blood, are visible. These are situated at points of close contact with clothing, especially the upper part of the back, sides of the trunk, anterior abdominal wall and the front and sides of the thighs. They are not seen on the face, hands and feet. Secondary infection is common.

### PEDICULUS PUBIS

This is caused by the crab louse which can attach itself to curly hair only; it therefore chooses the pubic and axillary hair and the eyebrows. It is seldom found in childhood.

*Treatment of Pediculosis.* A preparation containing Gamma Benzene Hexachloride should be used. This can be used as a shampoo for the hair, taking care to avoid the eyes, or as a cream or dusting powder for the body. The hair should not be washed for 24 hours after the application. It has superseded Dicophane (DDT) owing to the risk of poisoning with this substance.

## Molluscum contagiosum

This is caused by a virus and is contagious. The lesions are small papules with pearly-white umbilicated centres. The white centre can be squeezed out and is composed of degenerate cells. The lesions may occur anywhere, but particularly on the face and trunk.

*Treatment.* The cleanest method of treatment is to freeze the spot with ethyl chloride and then scoop it out with a curette. A simple home treatment is to dip the sharpened end of a match in iodine and insert this into the centre of each lesion once a day until it becomes red.

### Warts (verrucae)

These are epithelial growths due to a virus infection, which may occur anywhere, though they are most common on the hands and soles of the feet. They may be flat or raised; those on the soles (plantar wart) become pressed into the skin by the pressure of walking and may be very painful. Plantar warts are differentiated from simple corns by the fact that they contain blood vessels which are visible from the outside, whereas a corn has none.

All warts disappear in time—a few weeks or several years; 20–30 per cent disappear spontaneously, especially in children. Regression is partly due to an immune response but is also related to the limited life span of wart cells (Pyrhönen & Johansson, 1975). Patients on immunosuppressive drugs often develop intractable warts.

*Prevention.* Plantar warts are particularly transferred at swimming pools. Therefore, individuals with these warts should be barred from swimming pools unless they are wearing protective footwear (Plastsoks).

*Treatment.* In order to reduce the vast reservoir of wart virus all warts should be treated except in very young children. Treatment of these can be deferred for a few months in the hope of spontaneous cure but the warts should be covered with clear nail varnish to prevent spread.

Nightly formalin soaks for 6–8 weeks will cure 80 per cent of plantar warts up to 1 cm (Vickers, 1961). Formalin may cause painful fissuring between the toes but this can be prevented by the application of soft paraffin. The hyperkeratotic surface of the wart should be removed with a pumice stone or fine sand paper. Wart paints containing salicylic acid are an alternative to formalin.

Another method of treatment is freezing with carbon dioxide snow or liquid nitrogen. This is painful but very effective for all but plantar warts where the thickness of the keratin makes freezing difficult. Curettage under local anaesthesia is an alternative but injection into the sole of the foot is very painful.

### Kaposi's varicelliform eruption

This occurs as a complication of infantile eczema from secondary infection with herpes simplex or, occasionally, vaccinia. The history is so typical that it can be diagnosed by a description over the telephone. The mother of a child with eczema says that the skin has suddenly got worse and the rash 'seems to be spreading like wildfire'. Vesicles suddenly appear on the eczematous skin, multiplying with alarming rapidity and may spread to previously intact skin. These soon break, leaving small round shallow ulcers; only at the periphery of the area may the typical fresh lesions still be visible. The child becomes very toxic and febrile and may die.

*Treatment.* Idoxuridine is effective against the herpes virus and should be used in all cases where this is the cause. A wide-spectrum antibiotic should be used to reduce secondary infection. Strict isolation is required.

The risk of secondary herpetic infection in infantile eczema must always be remembered and it is preferable that nurses with a history of 'cold sores' should not nurse such patients.

## BIBLIOGRAPHY

BEARE M. (1965) Skin conditions of infancy and childhood. *Brit. med. J.*, **1**, 237.

BOLAM R.M. & BURTT E.T. (1956) Flea infestation as a cause of papular urticaria. *Brit. med. J.*, **1**, 1130.

FEIWEL M. (1969) Percutaneous absorption of topical steroids in children. *Brit. J. Derm.* **81**, Suppl. 4, 113.

HINDSON T.C. (1968) Ascorbic acid for prickly heat. *Lancet* **1**, 1347.

JOLLY H.R. (1948) Prevention of ringworm in the Tropics. *Brit. med. J.*, **1**, 726.

MURPHY W.F. & LANGLEY A.L. (1963) Common bullous lesions—presumably self inflicted—occurring *in utero* in the newborn infant. *Pediatrics*, **32**, 1099.

PYRHÖNEN S. & JOHANSSON E. (1975) Regression of warts. An immunological study. *Lancet*, **1**, 592.

VICKERS C.F.H. (1961) Treatment of plantar warts in children. *Brit. med. J.*, **2**, 743.

# CHAPTER 25

# DISORDERS INVOLVING MUSCLE

## INFANTILE HYPOTONIA ('THE FLOPPY INFANT')

The most common muscle disorders of infancy are those producing the syndrome of 'the floppy infant'. These range from hopeless cases in whom death can be anticipated at an early age, to those in whom improvement and eventual normality can be expected. The floppy infant may present at birth with paucity of movement or with hypotonia. Hypotonia is diagnosed by: bizarre postures; diminished resistance to passive movement; excessive range of joint movements. In later childhood the condition presents with delayed motor development.

To differentiate the causes two questions should be asked (Dubowitz, 1969):

1. Is this a paralysed child with incidental hypotonia?
2. Is this a hypotonic child without significant weakness?

The distinction is usually easy from observing whether the infant can raise an arm or leg against gravity. If this can be done the child is unlikely to be paralysed. This divides the cases into two groups:

*Paralytic.* The commonest type is infantile spinal muscular atrophy (Werdnig-Hoffmann disease). The congenital myopathies may be structural, such as central core disease, or metabolic when due to glycogen storage disease. Other neuromuscular disorders causing paralysis include the muscular dystrophies, myasthenia gravis, polymyositis and the myotonic syndrome. Muscle biopsy is the most useful investigation to differentiate this group.

*Non-paralytic.* Those associated with mental handicap form the largest component of this group. The remainder cover the whole range of paediatrics, hypotonia being an incidental feature of underlying disorders which are easily recognized.

The nomenclature in the past has been made difficult by the continued use of proper names to describe the conditions and it is preferable that these should be dropped. Three groups of patients will be considered:

1. Infantile spinal muscular atrophy (Werdnig-Hoffmann disease).
2. Symptomatic hypotonia.
3. Essential hypotonia ('Benign congenital hypotonia').

**Infantile spinal muscular atrophy (Werdnig-Hoffmann disease)**

This is the most serious and the most common cause of generalized infantile hypotonia. It is due to progressive degeneration of the anterior horn cells and may be present at birth or begin at any time during the first year of life. The condition is genetically determined, being inherited as an autosomal recessive characteristic. Although this is a neurological disorder, it is described here to make the subject of infantile hypotonia better understood.

The muscle paralysis reaches its maximum soon after the onset, but the course of the illness is progressively downhill with frequent bouts of pneumonia leading to death usually during the first year. The baby is so hypotonic that he seems to lie right in the mattress instead of on it, the limbs staying wherever they are put. The arms lie out on either side of the head and the legs take up the characteristic 'frog' position of abduction and external rotation at the hip. The proximal muscles are completely paralysed and wasted, and there is only minimal movement of the hands and feet. The tendon reflexes are absent. Fasciculation of the tongue may be present, its presence being diagnostic of the condition. Breathing is diaphragmatic only, so that it is very shallow, the lower chest being sucked in with each breath. When picked up, the child's head falls back and the lack of tone in the shoulder girdle causes him almost to slip through the hands when held round the chest. Despite all this the child is mentally alert, but the lack of chest movement, the feeble cough and the pooling of secretions in the pharynx from paralysis of the pharyngeal muscles, account for repeated lung infections. If the child survives to the second year, severe contractures develop. It is possible that some cases of arthrogryposis multiplex (p. 230) are due to this disorder, if paralysis started very early in intrauterine life.

Benign variants of the condition occasionally occur, permitting survival during infancy and even up to adolescence. In general, the later the onset the less severe the paralysis. However, the distribution of the paralysis in these cases whereby proximal muscles are most affected, legs worse than arms, and spinal muscles are involved remains the same as in the classic form of the disease.

Confirmation of the diagnosis is made by muscle biopsy. This shows atrophy of muscle fibres in groups, the characteristic of denervation. Soft tissue X-rays, to demonstrate the extreme degree of muscle atrophy, are sometimes helpful in those babies with so much fat that the true nature of the disease is obscured.

*Treatment.* No treatment is possible apart from the administration of antibiotics for each respiratory infection, thus prolonging life for only a short time. There are few more distressing diseases for both parent and doctor.

## Symptomatic hypotonia

A variety of different disorders may give rise to hypotonia in infancy. Some, such as mongolism, may be obvious from the start, but in others the cause is much less obvious.

### CENTRAL NERVOUS SYSTEM DISORDERS

Mentally handicapped children are likely to be hypotonic, this feature being seen in severe form in mongols. In the Prader-Willi syndrome (p. 453) of obesity, hypotonia, mental handicap and hypogonadism it is the hypotonia which is likely to be the first abnormality to be apparent.

All types of cerebral palsy may first present with hypotonia; only later may the involuntary movements of athetosis or the unsteadiness of ataxia develop so as to make a correct diagnosis possible. A few develop spasticity later, but this is more often present from the start; a small number of infants with hypotonia from cerebral palsy remain persistently as cases of flaccid diplegia. In such cases the reflexes are present and even brisk, despite the hypotonia, and the plantar responses are extensor. Intracranial birth inujry, particularly anoxia, causes hypotonia in young babies. Many of these children later show evidence of mental handicap or cerebral palsy, but a few with persistent hypotonia only, eventually make a complete recovery. Babies with one of the disorders affecting aminoacid, mucopolysaccharide or lipid metabolism (p. 568) may also present with hypotonia.

### NUTRITIONAL AND METABOLIC DISORDERS

Hypotonia is a feature of any acute illness and is seen also in malnourished infants. It also occurs in rickets, hypercalcaemia, renal tubular acidosis, coeliac disease and hypothyroidism.

### SKELETAL AND CONNECTIVE TISSUE DISORDERS

Hypotonia occurs in infants with osteogenesis imperfecta; it may be apparent before the occurrence of fractures has made the diagnosis obvious. Excessive mobility of the limbs, with some degree of hypotonia, is a feature of arachnodactyly, but the long fingers and toes should prevent any mistake being made.

*Congenital laxity of the ligaments* is a condition causing increased mobility of joints associated with hypotonia. The intelligence is normal and there is no loss of motor power. Some affected individuals become contortionists. The condition is inherited as a dominant trait.

## Essential hypotonia ('Benign congenital hypotonia')

This term has been applied to children with marked hypotonia without significant weakness who have a tendency to improve and no associated disease. It is a shrinking entity which will probably eventually disappear as newer techniques of investigation make diagnosis more precise. Some of the children who fit this category may have one of the non-progressive congenital myopathies which require specialized techniques for recognition of the muscle lesion.

## MYOPATHIES

In this group of disorders there is a primary degeneration of muscle. The diseases can be broadly separated into those with muscular dystrophy, where atrophy of the muscles is the principal feature, and those with myotonia, in which increased muscle tone and stiffness predominate.

### Muscular dystrophies

This is a group of heredofamilial disorders in which there is progressive weakness from atrophy of skeletal muscle. Different types are classified according to the muscle groups involved. The muscle fibres swell, then undergo hyaline degeneration, being replaced by connective tissue and fat. This connective tissue and fat may take up more space than the muscle it replaces, giving the limb the impression of being enlarged, hence the term 'pseudohypertrophy'.

#### PSEUDOHYPERTROPHIC MUSCULAR DYSTROPHY (DUCHENNE)

This form occurs almost entirely in boys, usually presenting during the first 5 years of life and transmitted as a sex-linked recessive character with a high mutation rate. Very rarely it occurs in females, being inherited as an autosomal recessive trait. The disease starts with symmetrical involvement of the pelvic girdle muscles and spreads up to the shoulder girdle. Pseudohypertrophy occurs mainly in the calf muscles, giving a false appearance of muscle strength. The child is first noticed to be waddling and then has difficulty in climbing up stairs, although coming down presents no problem. Weakness of the pelvic and spinal muscles leads to marked lordosis and difficulty in getting up from the ground. In order to do so he has to roll on to his side, then on to all fours and 'climb up his legs'. This mode of rising is not specific to pseudohypertrophic muscular dystrophy, although this is its commonest cause. It will occur in any condition where there is weakness of the pelvic girdle muscles and may be found in acute infective polyneuritis.

The disease progresses steadily and relatively rapidly, the child being usually unable to walk within 10 years of the onset. Deformities develop and death, usually from pneumonia, occurs during the late teens. Involvement of cardiac muscle by the dystrophic process is common and the majority show extensive ECG changes. Death from heart failure sometimes occurs.

Patients have an increased serum aldolase and serum creatine phosphokinase. The creatine phosphokinase is the more sensitive indicator, being elevated before the onset of the disorder. It can therefore be used diagnostically in newborn boys of affected families. Female carriers can also be identified by a raised serum creatine phosphokinase level but 30 per cent have normal levels. It may be possible to detect the carrier state from focal degenerative changes in a muscle biopsy and from minimal alterations in the electromyograph.

### FACIOSCAPULOHUMERAL MUSCULAR DYSTROPHY (LANDOUZY-DEJERINE)

This type may start at any time from early childhood to late adult life, occurring in both boys and girls. It is usually transmitted by an autosomal dominant gene, but occasionally by an autosomal recessive one. The muscles of the face and shoulder girdle are involved, the expression becoming like a mask. The eyes cannot be closed completely, the mouth droops so that the child looks as though he is pouting, and weakness prevents him from whistling when requested. Involvement of the shoulder girdle causes 'winging' of the scapula and the hand can be raised to the head only by swinging the arm round. Pseudohypertrophy is rare in this form of dystrophy.

Progression of the disease is very slow so that the disability is slight; most patients remain active to a normal age.

### LIMB GIRDLE MUSCULAR DYSTROPHY

This type usually starts in late childhood or shortly after puberty. It is usually transmitted as an autosomal recessive but occasionally as a dominant. Both the shoulder and pelvic girdle muscles are affected. The disease is slowly progressive so that the patient is usually unable to walk within 20–30 years of the onset.

*Treatment.* No specific treatment is available for muscular dystrophy but physiotherapy should be given. It is essential to keep the children on their feet since a period of bed rest leads to rapid deterioration in function. At the same time, over-exertion should be avoided since it appears to hasten muscle atrophy. Special attention should be paid to psychological management and to facilities for schooling.

### The myotonic syndrome

Myotonia congenita, paramyotonia and dystrophia myotonica are all varieties of a single disease process which may occur in a different form in members of the same family.

## MYOTONIA CONGENITA (THOMSEN'S DISEASE)

This disease occurs in boys and girls, its onset being at birth or shortly afterwards. It is usually transmitted as an autosomal dominant but sometimes as a recessive trait. Muscle stiffness resulting from myotonia is the presenting symptom and, once the muscle has contracted, it may remain so for half a minute. This characteristic can be demonstrated by tapping with a patellar hammer when a sustained muscle contraction occurs. With repetition of a movement the muscles seem to loosen up and become more normal, but they are always worse in cold weather. The lower limbs are most frequently involved and the affected muscles may hypertrophy. Stigmata of dystrophia myotonica may sometimes develop in later life. The expectation of life is not diminished.

## PARAMYOTONIA

This form of the syndrome is similar to myotonia congenita except that myotonia occurs only on exposure to cold.

## DYSTROPHIA MYOTONICA

This condition occurs most often in adults but may present in childhood as a cause of hypotonia. It is transmitted by an autosomal dominant gene or possibly by a group of recessive genes; other members of the family may show some or all of the manifestations of the disease. Weakness may be present in the face or limbs, the degree and distribution of the myotonia bearing no relation to the muscle weakness and wasting.

The lack of facial expression is striking, making the child look mentally handicapped. At the same time the patients are often of low intelligence. The electromyograph is diagnostic. Adults with the condition also show premature baldness, testicular atrophy and cataracts.

## MYASTHENIA GRAVIS

This disease results from a disturbance of transmission at the neuromuscular junction causing abnormal fatiguability of the voluntary muscles. Newer methods of staining have demonstrated abnormalities in the distal nerve fibres and the motor end plates. Although the disease is not common in children it probably occurs more often than is realized. Any muscle may be involved but the cranial nerves are usually the first to be affected, ptosis or dysphagia being common presenting symptoms. The disease then spreads to the trunk and limb muscles. Muscle strength is at its best in the early morning, becoming progressively more rapidly fatigued as the day draws on. A simple test for fatigue is to ask the child to grip the doctor's hand repeatedly. In children there is a greater tendency for the muscles to be symmetrically involved than in adults. The thymus may be enlarged on radiological examination.

The diagnosis is made by the dramatic improvement in muscle strength which occurs after the intramuscular injection of 1–2 mg edrophonium (Tensilon).

*Treatment.* Neostigmine acts for longer than edrophonium and is used in treatment. It works by depressing the activity of cholinesterase which normally destroys acetylcholine. Pyridostigmine is similar to neostigmine, but its action is slower and more prolonged, being therefore preferable. Maintenance therapy is usually required for life but spontaneous recovery sometimes occurs.

## BIBLIOGRAPHY

DODGE P.R., GAMSTORP I., BYERS R.K. & RUSSELL, P. (1965) Myotonic dystrophy in infancy and childhood. *Pediatrics*, **35**, 3.

DUBOWITZ V. (1969) The floppy infant. *Clinics in Developmental Medicine* No. 31. Spastics Society/Heinemann Medical, London.

WALTON J.N. (1960) The 'floppy' infant. *Cerebral Palsy Bull.*, **2**, 10.

WALTON J.N. (1964) Some diseases of muscle. *Lancet*, **1**, 447.

WALTON J.N. & NATTRASS F.J. (1954) On the classification, natural history and treatment of the myopathies. *Brain*, **77**, 169.

WOOLF A.L. (1960) Muscle biopsy in the diagnosis of the 'floppy baby': Infantile hypotonia. *Cerebral Palsy Bull.*, **2**, 19.

CHAPTER 26

# DISORDERS OF BONE AND JOINT

Many disorders affecting bones and joints are described in chapter 6 among the congenital malformations, while the rheumatic diseases are discussed in chapter 23.

## Bow legs

A certain amount of bowing of the legs is normal, particularly in the toddler age group. This is a physiological state which improves spontaneously from the age of 2 years, though it may persist until the fifth year. Normal bowing can become exaggerated if, during the early stages of walking, the infant has bulky layers of napkin between the legs; mothers should be warned against this.

Rickets (p. 557) must always be excluded, but is a rare cause.

## In-toeing (Pigeon toes)

It is common for young children to walk with their feet turned inwards. This usually results from medial femoral torsion which can be regarded as physiological during the first 5 years. In-toeing from this common cause must be differentiated from causes in the foot, especially metatarsus varus. Medial tibial torsion which may be associated with bow legs also causes in-toeing.

## Genu valgum (knock knees)

There should normally be about 2 cm of separation between the medial malleoli of the ankle when the patient is standing upright with the knees together. An increase in the space indicates genu valgum, being mainly seen in association with obesity. A reduction in weight is essential to correct the defect, being usually all that is required; if necessary, the inner side of the heel of the child's shoe can be raised by not more than 3 mm.

Rickets from lack of vitamin D or of renal origin is a rare cause of genu valgum.

## Pes planus (flat foot)

During the first year the foot looks flat owing to the normal pad of fat in the

691

sole obscuring the outline of the arch. During the first 5 years the foot, as indicated by the footprint, is always flat. The majority of feet believed to be flat in the early years are normal, or will become so during the first 7 years of life. The arch is restored in such children when standing on tiptoe and only if this is not so or there is pain in the foot, especially at the end of the day, is there any problem. In such patients the foot, though of normal appearance when not weight bearing, rolls into valgus on standing so that, viewed from behind, the navicular is unduly prominent on the inner side. There is excessive wear of the heel of the shoe on that side. For these patients an inside heel wedge of 5 mm should be applied to well-built shoes, or they may be given a shoe with a built-in inner raise.

The primary cause of postural flat feet in most cases is excessive mobility of the ligaments; for this reason foot exercises are probably of little value. But they do no harm and parents then feel that everything possible is being done.

A normal child does not require shoes until he begins to walk. These must be well fitting, particular attention being paid to see that the heel is gripped comfortably. Similar attention must be given to the socks which, if too small, cause crowding or clawing of the toes.

### Postural scoliosis

Lateral curvature of the spine is more often seen in girls from 10–15 years of age. The condition must be differentiated from structural scoliosis due to abnormalities of the vertebrae; this is achieved by asking the child to bend forward. A postural curve then disappears and there is no prominence of the posterior ribs on one side. The condition is occasionally due to inequality of the legs in which case equalizing the length, by placing an appropriately sized book under the shorter leg, will eliminate the scoliosis.

Postural scoliosis is not progressive, usually disappearing with exercises and attention to posture.

### Infantile idiopathic scoliosis

This condition is unassociated with any congenital abnormality of the vertebrae, although secondary changes may occur in them from the unequal stresses to which they are subjected. It presents during the first year of life and is often associated with plagiocephaly, rib cage moulding and pelvic tilting. Because of this, it is suggested that intrauterine moulding is an aetiological factor (Lloyd-Roberts & Pilcher, 1965). There is an unexplained increased incidence in boys. Complete spontaneous resolution occurs in the majority of cases.

### Transient synovitis of the hip ('observation hip')

This is a common condition in which the child develops pain in one hip associated with a limp. In some cases the pain is first felt in the knee although it is the hip which is at fault. It is much more frequent in boys than girls and occurs between the ages of 2 and 12 years. The child is not ill, is usually apyrexial, the only finding being painful limitation of hip movement. Internal rotation is most affected but there is also some limitation of external rotation and abduction. The hip X-ray is normal, as is the white cell count and the sedimentation rate. The pain disappears within a week leaving no sequelae.

The cause is unknown but the fact that it occurs more often in boys suggests that mild trauma is likely, though a clear history of trauma is usually lacking. For this reason the alternative title of 'observation hip' has been used to emphasize that the diagnosis is essentially one of exclusion; this title does not prejudge the aetiology or pathology (Monty, 1962). It is essential to exclude all forms of arthritis especially tuberculosis, Perthes's disease and slipped femoral epiphysis.

*Treatment.* No treatment should be given apart from bed rest. It is preferable that the leg should not be put on traction since fixing it only delays the natural spontaneous cure.

### Perthes's disease (pseudocoxalgia)

This is a common disorder of the hip affecting children between the ages of 3 and 10 years, with a peak incidence at 5 years. Boys are affected about four times more often than girls. The similarity in age and sex incidence with transient synovitis of the hip (see above) suggests a common aetiology but so far no definite relationship has been proved. Perthes's disease sometimes runs in families. The incidence of associated undescended testicle appears to be increased.

Pain in the hip is the presenting feature but is not severe and may well be intermittent. A limp is usually present, though it may not be easy to detect; the most useful early physical sign is loss of internal rotation. Some limitation of abduction is usually present.

In the early stages no radiographic changes may be seen. The first sign is an increase in the joint space and increased density of the epiphysis. This is followed by the typical flattening of the femoral head giving it a mushroom appearance. The cause of the condition is not known but it is believed to be due to avascular necrosis; this is likely in view of the slow development of flattening of the head.

*Diagnosis.* The condition must be differentiated from tuberculosis of the hip and from a slipped femoral epiphysis; it is more common than either of these. As a generalization, tuberculosis of the hip is seen particularly in children under 5 years of age, Perthes's disease in those aged 5 to 10 years and a slipped femoral epiphysis in those over 10 years old.

Hypothyroidism may cause epiphysial dysgenesis leading to flattening of the femoral head. The epiphysis is usually stippled but the radiological appearances of the two conditions may be identical. Hypothyroidism must be recognized by its associated features and, from an orthopaedic point of view, the retarded bone age is most helpful.

*Treatment*. Two very different methods of treatment are practised. There are those who treat the child by prolonged immobilization with traction until the head begins to reform, a process which takes very many months. On the other hand, some surgeons believe that the only essential is to prevent weight-bearing on the affected hip and, by using a patten-ended caliper, treat the child as an outpatient. Radiographic changes persist into adult life, although function is rarely affected at that age. The question, which still remains to be answered, is whether early non-weight bearing ambulation renders the child more liable to osteoarthritis of the hip in later life; probably this is rare but a long-term follow-up is required.

It is possible that new operative techniques using an osteotomy so that the head of the femur comes to be better contained within the acetabulum may shorten the period of immobilization.

The prognosis for boys is better than for girls. The younger the age of onset the better the results.

### Slipped femoral epiphysis

This condition occurs about the age of puberty and there may or may not be a history of trauma. It is bilateral in about 25 per cent of cases. The condition is more common in boys. The majority of patients are tall and growing rapidly; a smaller proportion are fat. Pain in the hip may come on suddenly or gradually; there is limitation of internal rotation and abduction. The leg is seen to be externally rotated on standing and when lying down.

X-rays show a widened and irregular epiphysial line which, if untreated, is followed by downward and backward displacement of the femur.

*Treatment*. Bed rest and traction are not recommended. Surgical techniques using pinning or osteotomy are used.

### Acute pyogenic arthritis

In the majority of cases this infection is due to a coagulase positive *Staphylococcus aureus*. A few cases are due to a haemolytic streptococcus, more particularly in infants; only in a small proportion of patients are other organisms responsible, such as meningococcus, pneumococcus and *Haemophilus influenzae*. The infection is usually blood borne although it may reach the joints by direct extension from osteomyelitis. This is particularly likely to occur in infants since in them the nutrient artery extends as far as the articular cartilage; after the first year it stops at the epiphysial plate which, by then, has formed a barrier (Fig. 143).

Older children complain of pain in the joint; this is inflamed and swollen from an effusion. In babies, the diagnosis is much less obvious and the condition must be sought in all infants with an undiagnosed infection. The natural puffiness of the limbs of many babies renders the swollen joint less obvious, the first indication being an apparent paralysis of the limb from pain.

Early diagnosis is essential since rapid destruction of the articular cartilage occurs. The growing epiphysis is very liable to be damaged or even absorbed, with subsequent deformity and shortening. All the pus should be aspirated from the joint and penicillin injected. These procedures should be carried out

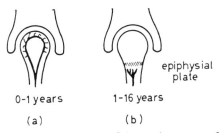

0-1 years     1-16 years

(a)       (b)

FIG. 143. Diagram showing the course of the nutrient artery of a long bone at different ages.
(a) In infancy the artery extends to the articular cartilage, permitting infection in the bone to reach the joint with ease.
(b) In older children the epiphysial plate intervenes, thus limiting the spread of infection.

at the same time since it is very difficult to find the joint cavity once it is no longer distended. If practical, the joint should be immobilized by traction, but in small babies this may prove impossible. Prolonged antibiotic therapy is required as for acute osteomyelitis (see below).

### Acute osteomyelitis (acute osteitis)

In this condition, as in acute pyogenic arthritis, the infecting organism is usually *Staphylococcus aureus*, though sometimes the streptococcus is found in young children. The organisms enter the bone via the nutrient artery, the primary site of the infection being the metaphysis. This site is often related to trauma which, although minimal, may have produced a small haematoma in the metaphysis. It is presumably for this reason that the bones of the lower limbs are involved much more frequently than those of the upper limbs.

Since there is no connection between the metaphysical and epiphysial vessels after the age of 1 year, the joint is not usually involved in children over that age and the growth mechanism is seldom damaged, although it may be overstimulated. In infants, as described above (Fig. 144), the joint is very likely to be involved and the epiphysis damaged. Rapid extension of the infection occurs through the cortex, causing necrosis and sequestrum formation; a subperiosteal abscess is likely to form in all cases in which treatment is not immediate.

In older children there is acute pain in the limb, a local area of tenderness being found in the bone; this produces the diagnostic sign of 'one-finger tenderness' (Neligan & Elderkin, 1965). The diagnosis in infants is much less obvious. The infection is extremely serious in the neonatal period when it may follow septicaemia resulting from pneumonia or gastroenteritis. In such young patients there is swelling of the limb but this may not be obvious so that at first it is realized only that the child has a severe general infection. The baby is extremely irritable, particularly when handled, refusing to use the affected limb ('pseudo-paralysis'). Unfortunately, there are no radiographic changes for about 10 days so that X-rays are of no help in diagnosis. The first X-ray sign is an area of rarefaction which is followed by periosteal new bone formation if the periosteum has been stripped by a subperiosteal abscess.

*Diagnosis.* The condition must be differentiated from a traumatic lesion, though this may have precipitated the development of osteomyelitis. Poliomyelitis raises difficulties if the child refuses to move the limb but, although the limb may be tender, it is seldom so acutely painful as in osteomyelitis and there is no swelling. A common error is to diagnose a primary infection of the subcutaneous tissues, but this condition is very unusual and in the majority of cases infection has spread from the bone.

*Treatment.* Cases seen within the first 24 hours may be treated with antibiotics alone but all others should be subjected to surgery. Early decompression of the periosteum reduces the risk of sequestrum formation from vascular thrombosis. If a subperiosteal abscess is present, it is usually unnecessary to drill the bone unless it is felt that drainage is inadequate. If no pus is present when the periosteum is incised, a number of drill holes should be made. Extensive exposure of the bone, as practised before the days of antibiotics, is no longer necessary. Splinting is used only when it seems likely to ease the pain or when required to immobilize a joint suspected of infection.

Blood cultures are usually positive in the early stages and should always be carried out to determine whether the correct antibiotic is being given. Pus obtained at aspiration should also be cultured and the sensitivities determined. In view of the risk that the infection is due to a penicillin resistant staphylococcus, it is a wise precaution to start treatment with sodium methicillin which is not affected by the penicillinase produced by such organisms. The drug must be given intramuscularly. Once the organism has been isolated and, provided it is sensitive to penicillin G, a change should be made. Penicillin must be given in very large doses (one mega unit every 4–6 hours is not excessive), and continued until the temperature is normal. Penicillin is then given in smaller dosage for at least a further month. If the child is anaemic a blood transfusion should be given.

Despite the great improvement in the management of acute ostomyelitis, chronic cases remain as serious a problem as ever due to the difficulty in eradicating the infection from dead bone. If this problem is to be prevented, early and thorough treatment of the acute case is essential.

### Osteomyelitis of the maxilla

This infection, occurring in infants, is not uncommon though the correct diagnosis is often missed. The manner in which the infection enters the maxilla is still uncertain. It may be blood borne or it may come from the maxillary sinus; alternatively, it may arise in the dental sac of the first deciduous molar.

The onset is sudden, the child soon becoming acutely ill with a swollen eye. The eyelids become oedematous and inflamed and the eye itself proptosed. The alveolus and the palate on the same side may also become swollen and pus appears in the nostril on the affected side only. Pus may also point externally near the eye or from the alveolus, the tooth being forced down by the pressure of the pus. There is swelling and induration of the cheek.

*Diagnosis.* The diagnostic error is to regard the condition as being due to an eye infection; many of the patients are sent first to eye specialists. The condition must also be differentiated from acute ethmoiditis; this gives a similar appearance as far as the eye is concerned but does not involve the cheek or palate.

*Treatment.* In addition to antibiotic therapy, the maxilla should be drained through the nose by puncturing the lateral nasal wall under the inferior turbinate. A tube can be left in position so that irrigation and local antibiotic instillation can be carried out. No incision should be made in the alveolus as this would damage the developing teeth; incisions around the eye should be avoided as they leave unsightly scars (Cavanagh, 1960).

### Infantile cortical hyperostosis (Caffey's disease)

This is a disease of unknown aetiology affecting infants, in which periosteal new bone formation occurs in one or more bones. The signs most often appear about the age of 10 weeks, although they may be present at birth. The onset is usually abrupt with fever, irritability and the appearance of one or more painful swollen areas under normal skin. Much of this enlargement is due to swelling of the soft tissues overlying the affected bone. The mandible is the most frequent bone to be involved, but any of the long bones and also the scapula, clavicle and ribs may be affected. Fresh lesions may develop after the child is first seen and recurrences occasionally occur. The X-ray appearances are very striking and new bone formation may extend along the whole shaft, though rarely beyond the metaphysis.

The lesions respond to steroid therapy but, since they are known to disappear slowly on their own, such treatment should be reserved for those with large swellings and severe symptoms. By the age of 3 years there is usually no trace left. Of great aetiological interest is the fact that a number of families have been reported in whom more than one member has been affected, so that there is the possibility of a genetic basis for the condition (Buskirk *et al.*, 1961).

*Diagnosis.* The condition is somewhat similar to syphilitic osteitis but there are no other manifestations of that disease. Hypervitaminosis A has produced a similar radiological picture but the patients are over the age of 1 year when the condition develops. Isolated involvement of the scapula has been mistaken for a sarcoma by those who have not previously met the condition. Scurvy is sometimes considered but, although periosteal new bone formation occurs during healing of the subperiosteal haematomata, such changes will not be present when the patient is first seen as they are in this condition. Moreover, there are none of the epiphysial changes seen in scurvy, nor the bleeding and other manifestations of the disease.

The condition must be differentiated from the 'Battered baby syndrome' (p. 705).

### Osteogenic sarcoma

This tumour affects older children and young adults, occurring more often in boys than girls (Larsson & Lorentzon, 1974). Its most common sites are the lower end of the femur or the upper end of the humerus or tibia. A painful swelling develops, the X-ray showing bone destruction and new bone formation. The typical picture is that of the 'sun-ray' appearance from new bone formation but this is not constant.

Histological examination shows atypical mesenchymal cells and an intercellular substance composed of various combinations of fibrous, hyaline, cartilaginous, myxomatous, osteoid and osseous tissues.

*Treatment.* The only hope is immediate amputation and irradiation but even so the prognosis is very poor. Metastases commonly occur into the lungs.

### Ewing's sarcoma

This tumour has the same age and sex distribution as the oesteogenic sarcoma and has a predilection for the same bones, but the shaft is more often involved than the end of the bone. Unlike the osteogenic sarcoma this tumour may metastasize to bone. The symptoms are similar but the X-ray appearance shows rarefaction of the shaft from bone destruction and surrounding sclerosis. Typically there is an 'onion-skin' appearance from periosteal new bone formation round the outside of the tumour, though this is not always present.

The histological appearance is that of a round cell sarcoma. The tumour does not form bone; in fact there is no intercellular substance so that the appearance is very different from the osteogenic sarcoma.

*Diagnosis.* Both these tumours are liable to be mistaken for osteomyelitis, this possibility being greater with the Ewing's tumour, since fever and leucocytosis often accompany the condition.

*Treatment.* The tumour usually responds dramatically to radiotherapy in the first place but, even if this is combined with surgery, the ultimate prognosis is still very bad. Cytotoxic chemotherapy is of value.

## BIBLIOGRAPHY

BUSKIRK F.W. van, TAMPAS J.P. & PETERSON O.S. (1961) Infantile cortical hyperostosis. An inquiry into its familial aspects. *Amer. J. Roentgenol.*, **85**, 613.

CAVANAGH F. (1960) Osteomyelitis of the superior maxilla in infants. *Brit. med. J.*, **1**, 468.

LARSSON S-E. & LORENTZON R. (1974) The incidence of malignant primary bone tumours in relation to age, sex and site. A study of Osteogenic Sarcoma, Chondrosarcoma and Ewing's Sarcoma diagnosed in Sweden from 1958 to 1968. *J. Bone Jt Surg.*, **56B**, 534.

LLOYD-ROBERTS G.C. & PILCHER M.F. (1965) Structural idiopathic scoliosis in infancy. *J. Bone Jt Surg.*, **47B**, 520.

MONTY C.P. (1962) Prognosis of 'observation hip' in children. *Arch. Dis. Childh.*, **37**, 539.

NELIGAN G.A. & ELDERKIN F.M. (1965) Treatment of acute haematogenous osteitis assessed in a consecutive series of selected cases. *Brit. med. J.*, **1**, 1349.

# CHAPTER 27

# ACCIDENTS AND POISONING

Whereas the incidence of disease in children is steadily decreasing, the number of accidents is steadily increasing. More children die from accidents than from any other single cause. But, in addition to deaths, there are many more children who sustain non-fatal injuries, many of which leave the child disabled.

All children are 'accident prone' but those who have already sustained one accident have a greater than average liability. This is not because they are especially accident prone but because their environment offers more opportunities for accidents. More accidents occur in the home than on the roads, and relatively few occur in school. The occurrence of one accident is the signal for redoubled efforts in preventive education for that family. Parents who have made one mistake are more likely to be making others. The causes in the home are parental carelessness and ignorance, combined with a lack of instruction and supervision of the children.

The greatest risk lies with the under-5 age group, boys being more susceptible than girls after the age of 1 year. Overcrowding increases the risk of accidents. The lack of outside play facilities with modern housing, especially flats, is a further reason for the increased number of accidents in the home. They also occur more often when the home routine is altered, such as when moving house, during decorating or when there has been a death in the home. Staying in other people's houses increases the dangers because the usual safety precautions for children may be lacking. Elderly relatives often leave dangerous medicines lying around. These and many other situations are associated with increased parental tension so that supervision of the children is less efficient.

Whenever a child is seen because of an accident a detailed history must be taken to determine its cause and to prevent future accidents. Has this child had other accidents and what caused them? Has he attended hospital for any other reasons? Has he ever been admitted to hospital; if so, what was the reason and did the experience have any harmful effect on him? How is he getting on at school and how much has he been absent? A quick history of the dynamics of the family must be obtained, including some information about the other children and whether they have had accidents. All this information is required to avoid overlooking a situation of child abuse (p. 705) as well as to prevent further accidents.

When an accident occurs in the home, the general practitioner or health visitor should go round the house with the parents, looking for possible danger points. Apart from such special visits they should always be looking for such risks whenever they visit a home. This direct instruction is more valuable than posters which are often ignored. The kitchen is the most dangerous room in the house and must be made safe. Knives and other potentially lethal instruments should not be left lying around.

*Fires*. All open fires must be protected by a guard, this being fixed to the wall. Electric fires should also be fixed to the wall. In England it is illegal for an electric fire to be sold unless equipped with a guard. Unfortunately however, these guards are often removed in the home. No matches should be left lying about. Gas taps should be left in a position in which they cannot be turned on by children. Drip-feed portable oil burners are particularly liable to cause fires.

*Clothes*. Long loose fitting clothing is always a danger; therefore, pyjamas should be worn in preference to nightdresses. All children's clothing should be made of flame-resistant fabrics.

*Electric points*. Three-point plugs should be supplied and, when not in use, should be protected by an unused plug.

*Saucepans*. No handles should be left protruding over the edge of the cooker where they can be grabbed by a toddler. Preferably, no saucepan with a long handle should be used; if used, the handle should be turned inwards. The only exception is if the cooker is fitted with a special rack into which the handles fit so that they cannot be moved from below.

*Teapots* should not be left on the table where they can be reached by a toddler.

*Tablecloths* should be turned in, rather than left hanging over the edge where they can be pulled down, together with the hot fluids. A washable top is preferable to a tablecloth.

*Feed bottles* should never be left propped up against the pillow for the baby to suck, since he is liable to vomit and inhale the vomitus.

*Stair rods* must be carefully secured since, if loose, they can cause falls down the stairs. A gate should be fixed at the top and bottom of the staircase if there are toddlers in the house. Quite young children can be taught how to go down the stairs backwards, this being safer than a gate.

*Upstairs windows* should always have guards. These guards should be placed so that the child's head cannot get stuck between the bars. They should be vertical so that they cannot be used as a climbing frame. An alternative safety method is to insert a screw so that limited opening only of the window is possible.

*Pillows.* Babies should not have pillows, owing to the possibility of suffocation. However, the risk of asphyxia from this cause is much less than previously believed; the majority of babies found dead in cots and thought to have died from suffocation have actually died from a fulminating infection, usually pneumonia (see Cot deaths, p. 367).

*Plastic bags* should not be brought into the homes of young children since they may draw them over their heads and then suffocate.

*Fireworks* should never be carried in trouser pockets since they are liable to explode when the child goes near a bonfire, causing appalling burns of the genitalia.

*Baths* for babies must not be too hot. The temperature should be tested by the mother's elbow before the baby is put in. Since the bottom of a bath retains heat, cold water must be put in first. If hot water is used first the bath may burn the child even though the temperature of the water is correct.

*Peanuts.* These should be barred from all children under the age of about 5 years. Fragments are very liable to be inhaled causing bronchial obstruction which is made worse by the local irritant effect of their arachis oil content (p. 362).

## HEAD INJURIES

These are extremely common in childhood, about half being due to road traffic accidents. In infancy the commonest cause is the battered baby syndrome (see below).

The immediate first aid measures are to secure an adequate airway and to stop bleeding. Moving the child from the site of the accident must be done with care, remembering the possibility of an associated injury to the spine.

Assessment of the severity of the head injury requires first a detailed history of the accident and the duration of any loss of consciousness. The level of consciousness should be determined. The pupils are examined for size and their response to light. A pupil which is progressively dilating and losing its light reaction indicates impaired function of the third nerve from expanding intracranial pressure on the same side. As the pressure increases, both sides become similarly affected. Bilaterally fixed dilated pupils are of grave prognostic significance. The examination of the child then determines the presence of focal neurological signs and whether there are injuries to other parts of the body. Deterioration is shown by fixed dilated pupils, slowing of the pulse, increase in the pulse pressure, increase or decrease in the respiratory rate (especially Cheyne-Stokes respiration) and the development of paresis.

*Treatment.* Many of the children will have sustained mild concussion only. These can often be observed at home as well, if not better, than in hospital. Vomiting can be a serious symptom and is usually an indication for admission to hospital. The children should be allowed up as soon as they feel like it and most will seldom want to stay in bed for more than one day. The finding of an uncomplicated linear fracture of the vault of the skull on X-ray makes no difference to the management.

### Compound and depressed fractures of the skull

A compound fracture should be explored without delay in order to stop any bleeding and to undertake usual wound toilet. Bone fragments are elevated, removed and autoclaved before being replaced. Torn dura is closed, using a fascial graft if there is a defect.

Depressed fractures which are not compound should be elevated in order to prevent underlying brain damage. Occasionally, a depressed fracture is not diagnosed for several days until a parent feels the dip in the bone after the initial swelling of the scalp has subsided. If the child is well, without neurological deficit, and the X-ray shows minimal depression only without bony spicules, elevation is not required.

## EXTRADURAL HAEMATOMA

In adults the occurrence of an extradural haematoma from a head injury is well recognized, but its frequency in children, especially infants, is not sufficiently appreciated. The signs usually differ from those classically described in the adult where an immediate brief loss of consciousness is followed by a lucid interval before the second loss of consciousness. The majority of children become stuporose some time after the injury, without any preceding loss of consciousness. Drowsiness and disorientation are the essential symptoms but the condition should be suspected before then if there is evidence of compression, shown by headache, vomiting or restlessness.

Bruising or oedema of the scalp are important signs, the scalp being shaved for complete examination. The swelling often overlies a fracture of the skull, most often of the temporal bone. Dilatation of the pupil and an extensor plantar response on the side of the lesion are common but do not occur in all cases. These signs may be followed by the development of hemiparesis on the opposite side, but children tend to pass directly from the stage of unequal pupils into a state of decerebrate rigidity.

Although bleeding from the middle meningeal artery is an important source of haemorrhage, it is not the only one. In fact in children an extradural haemorrhage may more often result from rupture of the thin-walled veins of the dura. In infants the amount of blood lost may be sufficient of itself to cause acute shock.

In all cases of suspected extradural haemorrhage an exploratory operation is essential.


## SUBDURAL HAEMATOMA

Trauma at any stage is liable to cause a subdural haematoma. It used to be diagnosed most often in infants following intracranial birth injury but is now much commoner as part of the battered baby syndrome (p. 705). The old concept of a spontaneous subdural haematoma at the age of about 6 months is a myth. The haematoma is often bilateral.

The subdural haematoma results from tearing of the numerous thin-walled draining veins which run from the cortex through the arachnoid to reach the venous sinuses of the dura. As the haematoma grows it is likely that further veins are torn. Bleeding continues until the raised intracranial pressure prevents further blood leak. The blood remains fluid though the reason for this is not clear. It is suggested that the haematoma clots and then becomes walled off by a membrane of invading connective tissue inside which the clot is broken down and liquefied. Since the membrane is semipermeable, fluid can be drawn across the membrane as a result of osmotic action. This is certainly possible though some cases develop this subdural effusion without membrane formation and so early after the injury that it is long before a clot could have broken down (Till, 1968).

Whatever the mechanism of this effusion of fluid into the subdural space, additional to the original collection of blood, the facts are that it is likely to increase in size. The fluid may be pure blood in the early stages, later becoming brown or yellow. This causes compression of the brain and progressive enlargement of the head.

The onset is usually insidious, the baby becoming irritable and failing to thrive. Vomiting is the commonest symptom. Convulsions are not uncommon and in some children are the presenting symptom. The anterior fontanelle is tense. Retinal and subhyaloid haemorrhages are an important and common diagnostic finding. Papilloedema occurs less often.

Diagnosis is made by subdural taps; both sides must be explored. When performing a subdural tap the skin should first be slid to one side. By this means, at the end of the procedure, the puncture hole in the skin is no longer opposite the hole in the dura, thereby preventing leakage. This investigation must be routine in all cases of suspected hydrocephalus since it is the only way in which the two conditions can be differentiated, although they may co-exist. If enlargement of the head is the reason for the tap and no effusion is found, ventriculography should be performed in order to determine whether hydrocephalus is its cause.

*Treatment.* Daily subdural taps should be carried out to reduce the pressure on the brain, though not more than 20 ml should be removed at any one time because of the dangerous effects of sudden changes in pressure. After the first tap the fluid removed should be replaced by half its equivalent of air. X-ray studies using this bubble of air can then determine the size of the effusion.

The condition is self-curing, in most cases, by means of daily taps. Occasionally, with a large effusion, it may be necessary to drain the fluid into the pleural space for a time by a subdural–pleural shunt operation. The more traumatic operation of craniotomy and removal of membranes is no longer recommended.

## CHILD ABUSE

### (Non-accidental injury; the battered baby syndrome)

Physical battering, although the most dramatic and best known form of child abuse, is only one end of the spectrum of the disorder. At the other end lie those children who are passively battered by being emotionally starved of affection. The problem has reached enormous prominence in recent years because it is so widespread and may have such tragic results for the child concerned and for the whole family. Child abuse has existed for generations but the increasing frequency with which it is now recognized is probably due to an actual increase, as well as to a greater awareness, of the problem.

The injury to the child, whether physical or emotional, is almost always caused by the parents. At least 90 per cent of those who batter their children do so because they were insufficiently mothered as children. 'Mothering' has nothing to do with mothercraft, which is the technical aspect of baby care, such as bathing, changing and feeding. It is the ability to give the baby loving attention 24 hours every day without feeling resentful or expecting something in return. It includes fathers, though with a different emphasis, and is included in 'parenting'. The ability to 'mother' is acquired from normal mothering experiences as a very young child; its failure leads to the 'cycle of deprivation', whereby harsh childhood experiences are repeated in the next generation.

Mothers are more liable to abuse babies whereas fathers are more likely to harm older children. The normal response of a mother to her crying baby is to comfort him by cuddling. Every mother feels exasperated by her baby's cries at times; the normal reaction when these cries become intolerable is to leave the baby crying for a time and go to another room to make herself a cup of tea or to have a smoke. The pathological response of the unmothered mother is to feel she must make her baby stop crying. This may cause her to shake or smack him and at its worst to kill the baby.

Such a mother does not hate her baby in the usually accepted sense of the word but the baby's demanding cries evoke responses which relate to her own childhood experiences. They make her feel inadequate as though her baby's cries are accusing her of not being able to make him happy. The baby represents herself as a baby and reminds her of her own unhappy childhood, whereas she expected the baby to supply her with the warmth of feeling which she had never received as a child. Parents who were strictly disciplined as children expect their children to conform and to behave properly. Fear of 'spoiling' the child is often strong.

Child abuse affects parents from every social class and of all levels of intellect. The only reason for the apparently larger numbers from the poorer social classes is their inability to be able to get away from their babies because of overcrowding, and they cannot afford the substitute care provided by nannies. In the old days, grandmothers were more often available; it is the loss of this support together with the increasing anxieties of modern life which, in part, account for the increase in the problem. Mothers who batter are very frightened of being left alone with their babies. They are exquisitely sensitive of loss of support from the environment and they cannot stand criticism because it makes them feel rejected. Pregnancy heightens their problems and increases their liability to batter. Marital disharmony is a common factor.

These deprived parents are not mentally ill. A very small proportion of battering parents are psychopathic and there are some who communicate by bashing—either verbally or physically—with everyone they meet.

Bonding between a mother and her new baby is not automatic. It is particularly liable to fail if the two are separated for any length of time, for example because the baby is in a special care unit. The same happens with animals separated from their young. This explains the higher incidence of battering in low birth weight babies and in those delivered by Caesarean section. It emphasizes the need for such mothers to be allowed to handle their babies even if the baby is in an incubator.

Mothers should be warned that 'instant love' for the newborn baby is often a myth. It takes many mothers time to fall in love with their babies just as it does with future husbands. Mothers who find they do not immediately love their babies often suffer guilt feelings because they have never been told that this is a common experience.

The reaction of the infant or toddler to repeated physical abuse may be one of 'frozen watchfulness'—he moves very little and just stares out of his un-smiling face. To survive he may undergo role reversal, whereby he mothers his mother, patting her knee and trying to make her happy. With his strict father he becomes excessively obedient in order to avoid his father's punishments. Some children who lack mothering become precocious in order to mother themselves or become the overactive demanding child whose needs cannot be met by his parents.

*Diagnosis.* It should be possible to make the correct diagnosis on the first occasion the child is brought to the doctor rather than waiting for several injuries to occur. The diagnosis must be considered for every injury to a young child. Probably 10–15 per cent of accidents to children under 2 years old are due to battering.

Parents who batter do not hide their children from doctors but they do not give an accurate history. It is the discrepancies in the history which give the diagnosis: the baby of 2 weeks who is stated to have bruised his cheek by banging it on the side of the cot; the spiral fracture of the humerus which is described as being due to a fall when this type of fracture can only result from the arm being twisted. Often a denial of the actual cause is based on a wish that it never happened—sometimes true amnesia occurs. A second vital point in the history is that there is commonly a delay of a day or more between the time of the injury and the visit to the doctor. The possibility of child abuse should be particularly considered in children brought in during the night. The mother's agitation is often out of proportion to the signs in the child and strange parental behaviour may lead them to leave the child before the admission procedure has been completed.

When the child is examined he is likely to be found bruised or to show other signs on the skin. Sometimes the injury fits a cigarette burn or where a sharp stone ring has been bored into the skin. The shape of an adult human bite may be apparent. The fraenum of the tongue in a baby may be torn or the lips or gum margins bruised because the bottle or fist has been rammed into his mouth to stop him crying.

X-ray changes have been over-emphasized so that their absence has led to a failure to make the diagnosis. The changes which may be found and which require the whole skeleton to be filmed are evidence of new or old fractures, epiphyseal fractures or displacements and periosteal new bone formation. Films should be repeated in 2 weeks since recent injury may not show until callus or periosteal new bone formation occurs.

Of great importance are retinal or subhyaloid haemorrhages resulting from shaking the baby. There may be clinical features of a subdural haematoma (p. 704). Blood dyscrasia must be excluded.

No child can thrive unless it is mothered. This passive battering is by far the commonest cause of 'failure to thrive' in young children, accounting for at least 20 per cent of such cases.

In coming to a diagnosis the doctor should not try to be a detective. There is no need to try to discover which parent caused the injury because the other parent is also always involved—by collusion. Sometimes the injury has been caused by another child in this disturbed family. What is helpful is to learn what the mother feels about her baby's crying—does it worry her and does her baby make her feel angry?

Doctors find the diagnosis difficult to make because it is so unpleasant and difficult to imagine that any parent could do such things to a child. Moreover, this difficulty may be increased by not knowing what to do once the diagnosis has been made.

*Treatment*. Whenever battering is suspected the child must immediately be moved to a place of safety, preferably a hospital for complete physical and general diagnosis. The fact that a child with 'failure to thrive' starts to thrive in hospital without any physical treatment confirms the diagnosis. It is the next step which is the problem since returning the child to his home will lead to a recurrence of battering if the parents have not responded to psychotherapy. What is really required is for someone to mother the mother. This has been undertaken successfully with foster grandparents (parent aides), (Kempe & Helfer, 1972). These are people who have successfully mothered their own family. Mothering the mother enables her to begin to be able to mother her own child. On no account must the foster grandparent pick up or show love to the baby, otherwise she will make the mother feel her inadequacy still more. Group therapy for battering parents has also proved successful.

These mothers must be encouraged to decide when the strain becomes too much and for them to know at which hospital or nursery they can leave the baby at this point. This approach has often not been sufficiently encouraged in the past because doctors and others have been obsessed by the possibility of a mother abandoning her baby. Providing a mother with somewhere to leave her child reduces the risk of her abandoning her baby as well as the chance of battering.

A different problem is when to call the police. Legally they should be involved in all cases involving 'wilful' assault. Ideally the doctors and the police should work closely together, but this will happen only when the police do not feel forced to take over and prosecute the parent in conflict with the doctor.

Some parents will never be safe with the child they have battered. For these a complete and permanent separation may be the only answer. We permit divorce when two individuals no longer love each other and we must consider a similar situation if parents and child can no longer live together safely. No child should be where he or she is not wanted (Freud, 1974).

*Prevention*. The major advance will come when mothers who are liable to batter their babies are identified and helped before the baby is born. This can be achieved by intensive work during the antenatal period. Taking a complete family history on the first antenatal visit will uncover many at risk. Those coming from a broken home are at increased risk, especially if the break occurred before the girl was 11 years old (Frommer & O'Shea, 1973). Women demanding a termination who present themselves late in pregnancy and women who are refused a termination are an important group; similarly women who fail to attend the antenatal clinic.

Women who do not want to be pregnant must be identified. They may be obvious from the way they dress, attempting to hide the pregnancy. It is important to gauge the woman's feelings when she first learns she is pregnant and to assess the changes in them as pregnancy proceeds.

It is usual for a mother to have two possible names for her unborn baby when she starts labour even though she may change the name when the baby is born. Lack of any names or a name for one sex only is easily discovered and is an additional sign of possible future problems.

Once the baby has been born a great deal can be learnt from the way the mother handles her baby. Is she able to cuddle him or does she hold him at arms length?

It is important to recognize that one child only in a family may be battered but that, whatever the situation, the whole family is in need of help. This will require the mobilization of many services, especially the Social Services. Successful treatment not only requires an end to abuse of the child at risk but also the prevention of recurrence in future children. Removal from the family of a child at risk, without adequate on-going therapy, results in the rapid replacement of the lost child by a new baby who is at grave risk of the same fate.

## BURNS

A high proportion of burnt children come from disturbed homes. There are similarities with the battered baby syndrome (see above) but also some very important differences (Martin, 1970). Whereas the mother of a battered child projects her hate and her aggressive feelings into her child who is then felt to be totally bad, the mother of the burnt child has mixed feelings for her child and normally maintains a protective front, having occasional lapses only.

Parents of burnt children are able to give an accurate history of the accident —unlike those who batter their child. They also feel marked guilt which helps to preserve a virtuous front; this is needed because the child is not all bad. This guilt wards off conscious recognition of destructive impulses but also punishes the mothers for having them. Recurrent burns are uncommon, in contradistinction to the child who is battered.

In order to be in a position to help the child, a psychiatric assessment of the family should be undertaken as early as possible. This is necessary since the burns themselves cause serious emotional problems from shock and the length of treatment, as well as from disfigurement.

The severity of the burn can be graded by the percentage of the body involved. If less than 50 per cent of the surface is burnt the child should survive; children can survive burns of up to 75 per cent. A more useful grading is between partial and full thickness (epidermis and dermic). If a pin prick can be felt it is a partial thickness burn and the skin will regenerate. Full thickness burns require grafting. Infection can convert partial thickness into full thickness.

*Treatment.* The immediate first aid measure is to immerse the burnt part in cold water. This reduces pain and cleans the skin but is only effective if undertaken within 5 minutes. The burn should not be touched and no dressing is required if there are no blisters. If blisters are present a dressing may be needed. A clean handkerchief bandaged lightly in position is a useful emergency measure.

There is no single standard method of treatment. Exposure allows for ease of observation, unimpeded movements and excretion. The eschar inhibits bacterial growth, provided it remains dry, though dermal drying delays epithelialization which requires moisture. Heat loss is a disadvantage and the frequent turning which is required is painful.

An alternative treatment is the use of 0·5 per cent silver nitrate compresses which reduce bacterial colonization. The dressing relieves pain and reduces the distress of the child and his parents caused by seeing the burnt part. There is less heat loss, while the moisture aids epithelialization provided bacterial growth is kept down.

Immediate skin grafting is a third method of treatment. If the graft takes, the results are speedy and successful but there is a higher mortality. All burnt children should be isolated to reduce the risk of infection.

Particular attention must be paid to acid–base control. Most children with burns involving 10 per cent or more of the body's surface require intravenous fluid therapy; this should be started as early as possible. Water, electrolytes and colloid are lost from the circulation in the fluid exuding from the burnt surface. Six per cent dextran is a valuable intravenous fluid to correct the electrolyte balance, having an osmotic pressure roughly equivalent to plasma, the alternative fluid for use. In severe cases no oral fluids should be given for the first 24 hours, since this will make the child vomit more than his intake. Moistened gauze may be given to suck and, after the first day, the child should be given oral fluids containing a high percentage of protein, owing to the great loss of protein from the burnt surface.

## POISONS

The risk of poisoning from drugs and household chemicals is very great. The most common drugs are aspirin, barbiturates and iron. The commonest household chemicals are paraffin, turpentine, disinfectants and cleaning agents. Boys are more commonly affected than girls, the maximum incidence being 1–3 years of age. About fifty children die from this cause every year in England and Wales.

Although there are many aspects of prevention, basically it is a matter of making these substances inaccessible to the children by ensuring that they are always in locked cupboards. However, the major cause of accidental poisoning is disturbed family relationships. The hazard must, of course, be reduced in all homes but the remarkable fact is that children from undisturbed families have few accidents even when the risk is high. Sobel (1970) found that accidental poisoning in children bore no relationship to home safety as measured by the quantity, toxicity, and availability of poisonous substances in the homes of the children he studied. On the other hand, it was intimately associated with parental psychopathology and disturbed family relationships.

Parental ignorance accounts for part of the problem, there being many who have no idea of the dangers to children of household paraffin or iron tablets. Not only should these substances be in locked cupboards but they should be clearly marked 'keep away from children' to remind mothers of the risks. Parents should never take pills in front of their children as this increases the chance that the child will later try them for himself.

Drugs should not be made attractive so that children mistake them for sweets, nor should the parents refer to them as 'sweets' when they are prescribed, as this may lead the child to help himself on some future occasion. Ideally, all dangerous drugs should be dispensed in separate cellophane strips, but this increases their expense.

In cases of accidental poisoning it is essential that the doctor treating the child should know what poison he is treating. As far as possible the names of drugs should be given on the containers and household materials should state their contents.

### General Treatment of Poisoning

The treatment of a child who has swallowed a poison is always an emergency. It consists of three approaches:

1. REMOVAL OF THE POISON

The child should be made to vomit. This may be achieved by putting a finger down the throat or by giving an emetic or by a combination of both. Suitable emetics for home use are a strong solution of salt or a solution of powdered mustard.

Ipecacuanha syrup is now preferred to gastric lavage (Reid, 1970), being quicker, safer, more effective and less frightening. The usual dose is 15 ml followed by 200 ml water. A further 15 ml should be given after 20 minutes if no vomiting has occurred. It should not be given to unconscious patients but gastric lavage is also not without risks in such children.

There are important exceptions to the use of emesis and lavage: if a corrosive poison has been taken, the oesophagus may be perforated by the tube; if household paraffin (kerosene) has been taken, some of the paraffin may be aspirated into the lungs during the procedures, causing a lipoid pneumonia.

It must be emphasized that these measures and the rush to hospital are very frightening for the child. This fear is an additional argument to use to parents when attempting to persuade them to lock up their drugs and poisonous chemicals.

Whenever possible, blood levels of the ingested poison should be measured in order to assess the severity of poisoning and the efficacy of treatment. The significance of the level relates to the time of ingestion. Forced alkaline diuresis increases the rate at which certain drugs are eliminated from the body. This is mainly of use in salicylate and phenobarbitone poisoning. It is not of value with other barbiturates because these are more protein-bound and are more widely distributed in the body, resulting in a lower plasma concentration.

### 2. ADMINISTRATION OF AN ANTIDOTE

These are of two types: chemical agents which, by direct combination, make the poison harmless or unabsorbable; and agents which counteract the action of the poison after it has been absorbed. Not every poison has an antidote but a poison-control centre to which a doctor can telephone for advice is of the greatest value. Apart from chemical agents, exchange transfusion and haemodialysis are useful methods for the removal of certain poisons from the circulation.

### 3. SUPPORTIVE THERAPY

The type of therapy depends on the poison involved. Those that depress the nervous system (CNS) should be counteracted by the administration of a stimulant. Those that stimulate the CNS should be counteracted by a depressant. Respiratory failure should be treated by artificial respiration and the giving of respiratory stimulants. Patients who are shocked should receive the general measures to alleviate shock. Vomiting may cause electrolyte imbalance which is corrected by parenteral fluid therapy. Electrolyte therapy is also required in cases with renal damage or in cases where disturbances of respiration have caused electrolyte imbalance. Temperature recordings should be frequent so that hypothermia and hyperthermia can be dealt with appropriately. In some cases the risk of secondary infection is increased so that prophylactic antibiotics should be given. Pain must be relieved by analgesics.

### Salicylate poisoning

Owing to its easy availability in many homes, aspirin is the most common drug to be accidentally ingested by children. The physical and laboratory findings show a considerable similarity to diabetic coma. The first change is a respiratory alkalosis resulting from the direct stimulant action of the salicylate on the respiratory centre. This lasts 6–8 hours only, being followed by a metabolic acidosis which is due to interference with carbohydrate metabolism, renal dysfunction and the acidity of the salicylate. Hyperpyrexia results from the action of salicylates in increasing heat production. When therapeutic doses of salicylates are used, this action is counteracted by increased heat loss through sweating, hence the therapeutic action of salicylates in lowering the temperature. But in salicylate poisoning the depletion of body fluid by excessive sweating, overbreathing, vomiting and diarrhoea makes further sweating impossible so that hyperpyrexia occurs as well as dehydration. Ketosis results from the increased rate of fat catabolism and the disturbance of carbohydrate metabolism, the latter also causing hyperglycaemia and glycosuria. Hypernatraemia and hypokalaemia develop in severe cases. Salicylates also cause hypoprothrombinaemia, leading to bleeding.

The earliest clinical feature is overbreathing, this being associated with vomiting and diarrhoea. Sweating occurs at first but stops once dehydration develops. The child becomes pale and collapsed, haemorrhages may occur, finally there being loss of consciousness followed by death.

The urinary findings are important. The ingestion of salicylates can cause a positive test for reducing substances because of their conjugation with glycine or glucuronic acid, or because there is an increased excretion of ascorbic acid which also causes the test to be positive. True glycosuria may also occur. Ketosis leads to the presence of acetone and diacetic acid in the urine. Diacetic acid gives a burgundy colour with ferric chloride, but it must be remembered that salicylates by themselves give a falsely positive ferric chloride test, the colour change being a violet or deep purple. To determine whether a positive test is due to salicylates the urine should be acidified and boiled. This causes the diacetic acid to be volatilized so that a repeat ferric chloride test is negative unless salicylates are present. Quantitative methods are available for the estimation of the level of salicylates in urine and plasma.

*Diagnosis.* The similarity of the clinical and biochemical features to diabetic coma is striking. Differentiation requires an accurate history, either of salicylate administration or of previous polyuria and thirst suggesting the onset of diabetes.

*Treatment.* Salicylates are retained in the stomach for a long time, therefore vomiting should be induced immediately, even if it is some hours since the salicylate was taken. The vomit should be tested with ferric chloride for the presence of salicylate.

Sodium bicarbonate should be given intravenously since this promotes the renal excretion of salicylate (Summitt & Etteldorf, 1964). The use of intravenous bicarbonate has been criticized on the grounds that the early respiratory alkalosis may still be present, but there is evidence that the degree of alkalosis is insufficient to contraindicate its use and results are better when it is given. Full biochemical control is necessary, additional potassium being required once dehydration has been corrected. Vitamin K should be given to counteract hypoprothrombinaemia.

If the child is unconscious, additional methods to remove the salicylate should be used, such as renal dialysis. If this is not available, an exchange transfusion or peritoneal dialysis should be performed.

### Barbiturate poisoning

This is common in children though fortunately they do not usually obtain a fatal dose. In mild cases there is drowsiness only. In more severe cases the patient is in light coma from which he can be aroused by vigorous manual stimulation; nystagmus and dysarthria occur and respirations are shallow. In the most severe cases the child is in deep coma associated with shock; respirations and reflexes are depressed.

*Treatment.* In mild cases the child should be kept awake by talking and manual stimulation. Amphetamine can be used as a stimulant but it is preferable to allow mild cases to recover without further drug therapy. In severe cases symptomatic treatment and the maintenance of respiratory function is the basis of management. Blood or plasma is given for shock, the child being kept warm but not overheated; the foot of the bed should be raised. A tracheostomy is usually necessary to permit adequate suction of the respiratory passages and for artificial respiration with a positive pressure respirator. If available, renal dialysis should be used to increase the elimination of the drug; failing this an exchange transfusion or peritoneal dialysis should be performed. All severe cases should receive prophylactic antibiotic therapy and a close watch kept on the urinary output. If acute renal failure develops, indicated by oliguria, treatment should be given as discussed on p. 387.

The risks accompanying the use of analeptic drugs has led to strong views as to whether or not they should be given; at most they should be administered only to severe cases. Bemegride is a powerful analeptic, though not a specific barbiturate antagonist as originally believed. It is available as a 0·5 per cent solution (5 mg per ml) for intravenous injection, the dose being 0·6 mg per kg. Amiphenazole is a powerful respiratory stimulant; it can be used in combination with bemegride in a dose of 0·2 mg per kg intravenously.

## Iron poisoning

The source is almost always the iron tablets which are freely given out to expectant mothers, often with no warning of their potential danger to children. Many of the tablets are highly coloured and look like sweets.

The immediate effect of the iron is its corrosive action on the gastric mucosa which may be sufficient to perforate the stomach. Vomiting is followed very rapidly by profound shock and coma. The child may then appear to improve for a few hours before symptoms from cerebral and hepatic damage appear. These are indicated by renewed restlessness, collapse, convulsions and coma. Jaundice may appear and there is biochemical evidence of a metabolic acidosis. If the child survives, pyloric stenosis may develop from scarring.

If death occurs in the acute phase, oedema and ulceration of the stomach are found, associated with a characteristic brown staining of the mucous membrane. The liver is always affected, a striking periportal necrosis occurring from the direct toxic action of the metal.

*Treatment.* The immediate first aid measure which the mother should be instructed to do is to push a finger down the child's throat in order to make him vomit. In hospital, vomiting is induced by ipecacuanha. Following this, 50 ml sodium dihydrogen phosphate or sodium bicarbonate are introduced into the stomach by mouth or tube.

Desferrioxamine (Desferal), a specific iron chelating agent, is then given intravenously, intramuscularly or by mouth. If this drug is not available, calcium disodium edathamil (EDTA), a less powerful chelating agent, can be used intravenously. Iron chelate causes the urine to be plumb coloured. This is helpful in deciding for how long the chelating agent should be given.

The acidosis must be corrected by the administration of bicarbonate or 1/6 molar sodium lactate intravenously. A blood transfusion may be necessary to compensate for the loss of blood.

The iron tablets are radiopaque so that a plain film of the abdomen will show whether they have all been removed by the washout.

## Paraffin (kerosene) poisoning

The accidental ingestion of household paraffin is particularly liable to occur since it is so often stored in old fruit juice bottles. Moreover, many parents are unaware of its danger; much more propaganda regarding this is required. In some developing countries there is the additional problem that kerosene is used as a 'medicine' for various ailments.

The kerosene causes acute gastric symptoms but the greatest danger is from its inhalation which occurs during vomiting, causing a lipoid pneumonia. For this reason the stomach should not be washed out nor vomiting induced since the risk of lipoid pneumonia is thereby increased.

### Chronic lead poisoning

In childhood the commonest cause of lead poisoning is the ingestion of flakes of paint containing lead. A common history is that the father has repainted the cot with a cheap paint containing lead. Poisoning may also result from the chewing of lead soldiers. Yellow and orange crayons contain lead chromate and are a further source of lead. Outbreaks of lead poisoning have occurred from the burning of old car batteries with subsequent accidental ingestion of the ash which contains a high content of lead, rather than the inhalation of fumes.

The earliest symptoms are irritability, pallor, colic, vomiting and constipation, often associated with pica. These may continue for some weeks before their seriousness is realized and the dramatic development of lead encephalopathy may be the occasion when the doctor is first called. This complication, resulting from acute cerebral oedema, is particularly liable to occur in young children. Severe vomiting is followed by convulsions, coma and death. Peripheral nerve palsies and a lead line on the gums are uncommon in children.

Laboratory studies show a moderate anaemia and there may be punctate basophilia. Glycosuria may occur and red cells are sometimes present in the urine; aminoaciduria also occurs, all these features resulting from tubular damage. There may be an excess of coproporphyrins in the urine. Lead is deposited in the growing ends of bone where it may be seen as a dense line on X-ray. Radiopaque material may be visible within the intestine.

The most valuable test is the blood lead level; a reading of over 40 $\mu$g per 100 ml is very suggestive of lead poisoning. Punctate basophilia and an excess of urinary coproporphyrins may both be negative so that a blood lead level is essential in all suspicious cases. There is also an increased urinary and faecal excretion of lead. In cases of lead encephalopathy the cerebrospinal fluid shows a rise of protein, and the cells may be increased.

*Diagnosis.* Vomiting as an early symptom has resulted in a mistaken diagnosis of 'cyclical vomiting' in some cases. Others present as anaemia of unknown cause. Glycosuria has caused a mistaken diagnosis of diabetes but being renal in origin, resulting from tubular damage, the blood sugar is normal. Lead encephalopathy is liable to be ascribed to encephalitis. In all children a history of pica is the most suggestive evidence in favour of lead poisoning; specific enquiry about pica should be made in all children with an obscure illness, particularly those with unexplained anaemia, convulsions or abdominal pain.

Florid cases of lead poisoning are now becoming uncommon with the reduction in the use of lead paint. Interest is now centred on lead pollution in the atmosphere and in water, from factories and other sources, and whether lower levels of blood lead can account for mental handicap, hyperactivity and other forms of neuropsychological dysfunction. Landrigan *et al.* (1975) in a study of symptom-free children living near a lead-emitting smelter found a lower age-adjusted performance IQ and a slower performance in a finger–wrist tapping test in the children with a blood lead above 40 $\mu$g per 100 ml compared with those whose level was below 40. Beattie *et al.* (1975) found a higher water-lead content in the homes of a group of mentally handicapped children compared with a group of normal children. David *et al.* (1972) concluded that there was an association between hyperactivity and raised blood-lead levels. They regard any lead elevation above 24·5 $\mu$g per 100 ml as dangerous.

*Treatment.* The use of the chelating agent calcium disodium edathamil (EDTA) has proved to be a great advance in therapy. Originally it was always given intravenously, this often proving difficult; the results with intramuscular therapy have been as satisfactory. Unfortunately, its action in lead encephalopathy is often delayed for up to 48 hours and cerebral symptoms may be exacerbated during this time. Dexamethasone and mannitol may be needed for up to 24 hours before the administration of EDTA in order to reduce the raised intracranial pressure.

Penicillamine is a drug which increases the excretion of lead and is an important additional form of therapy.

*Prognosis.* Apart from the immediate risk of death from lead encephalopathy (probably 25 per cent of such cases die) there is a serious risk of mental handicap if the child survives. It is hoped that the use of EDTA and penicillamine will reduce the incidence of this complication. Other sequelae are convulsions, blindness and speech defect.

### 'Native medicines'

In developing countries there is a greater risk of accidental injury from native medicines. Eyes may be injured and even blinded by the instillation of herbal remedies given to rouse a child from coma. Cow's urine in which tobacco leaves have been steeped is commonly used in W. Nigeria.

Aspiration pneumonia results from pouring such remedies into the throat of an unconscious child and the 'medicines' themselves may be poisoned. The cow's urine preparation mentioned above can cause hypoglycaemia.

Peritonitis may be caused by enemata containing pepper, ginger or other chemicals. Scarifications and incisions may lead to tetanus and septicaemia. The feet may be burnt when the legs of an unconscious child are immersed in hot water in an attempt to rouse him. The feet of such a child are sometimes placed near a fire causing severe burns of the soles.

### Pink disease (acrodynia)

The inclusion of pink disease in a chapter on poisons might be questioned, but its virtual disappearance from England since the removal of teething powders containing mercury, together with the evidence of mercury as an aetiological agent, renders this the most logical place for its discussion. Although teething powders have been the most important source of mercury, a few cases have been due to mercurial ointment. Mercury has been found in the urine in the majority of cases but it is probable that the symptoms result from an idiosyncrasy to the drug as well as to an overdosage.

*Clinical features.* The majority of patients are aged between 6 months and 2 years. The onset is insidious, a healthy cheerful baby being transformed into the most miserable irritable child one is ever likely to meet. Feeds are refused and extreme muscular hypotonia develops so that if the child has already started to walk, he goes off his feet and the tendon reflexes are lost. The hands, feet and other extremities, such as the ears and nose, become cold and pink from excessive arteriolar vasoconstriction associated with capillary dilatation. Profuse sweating occurs so that the extremities feel clammy and are intensely irritating. The child, if unchecked, will spend all day rubbing his hands and feet together in an attempt to allay the irritation, this only exaggerating the tendency to desquamation. Photophobia is intense, causing the child to adopt a characteristic posture in bed in which he burrows his head into the pillow in order to avoid the light.

### BIBLIOGRAPHY

BALOH R.W. (1973) The effects of chronic increased lead absorption on the nervous system. A review article. *Bull. Los Angeles Neurologic. Soc.*, **38,** 91.

BEATTIE A.D., MOORE M.R., GOLDBERG A., FINLAYSON M.J.W., GRAHAM J.F., MACKIE E.M., MAIN J.C., McLAREN D.A., MURDOCH R.M. & STEWART G.T. (1975) Role of chronic low-level lead exposure in the aetiology of mental retardation. *Lancet,* **1,** 499.

CAFFEY J. (1957) Some traumatic lesions in growing bones other than fractures and dislocations: clinical and radiological features. *Brit. J. Radiol.*, **30,** 225.

DAVID O., CLARK J. & VOELLER K. (1972) Lead and hyperactivity. *Lancet,* **2,** 1972.

FISCHER D.S., PARKMAN R. & FINCH S.C. (1971) Acute iron poisoning in children. The problem of appropriate therapy. *J.A.M.A.*, **218,** 1179.

FREUD A. (1974) Personal communication.

FROMMER E.A. & O'SHEA G. (1973) Antenatal identification of women liable to have problems in managing their infants. *Brit. J. Psychiat.*, **123,** 149.

HENDERSON F., VIETTI T.J. & BROWN E.B. (1963) Desferrioxamine in the treatment of acute toxic reaction to ferrous gluconate. *J. Amer. med. Ass.*, **186,** 1139.

JOLLY H. & FORREST T.R.W. (1958) Accidental poisoning in childhood. An experimental approach to the prevention of poisoning by tablets. *Lancet*, **1,** 1308.

KEMPE C.H. & HELFER R.E. (1972) In *Helping the Battered Child and his Family*. Ed. Kempe C.H. & Helfer R.E. Lippincott, Philadelphia.

LANDRIGAN P.J., WHITWORTH R.H., BALOH R.W., STAEHLING N.W., BARTHEL W.F. & ROSENBLUM B.F. (1975) *Lancet*, **1,** 708.

MARTIN H.L. (1970) Antecedents of burns and scalds in children. *Brit. J. med. Psychol.*, **43,** 39.

REID D.H.S. (1970) Treatment of the poisoned child. *Arch. Dis. Childh.*, **45,** 428.

SEGAR W.E. & HOLLIDAY M.A. (1958) Physiologic abnormalities of salicylate intoxication. *New Engl. J. Med.*, **259,** 1191.

SOBEL R. (1970) The psychiatric implications of accidental poisoning in childhood. *Ped. Clin. N.A.*, **17,** 653.

SUMMITT R.L. & ETTELDORF J.N. (1964) Salicylate intoxication in children—experience with peritoneal dialysis and alkalinization of the urine. *J. Pediat.*, **64,** 803.

TILL K. (1968) Subdural haematoma and effusion in infancy. *Brit. med. J.*, **3,** 400.

TSCHELTER P.N. (1963) Salicylism. *Amer. J. Dis. Child.*, **106,** 334.

WHITTEN C.F., KESAREE N.M. & GOODWIN J.F. (1961) Managing salicylate poisoning in children. *Amer. J. Dis. Child.*, **101,** 178.

CHAPTER 28

# ELECTROLYTE DISORDERS AND FLUID THERAPY

Children present a special problem with regard to fluid therapy since very large relative losses of fluid occur more rapidly than with adults. The water content of their bodies is relatively higher than that of adults, being highest of all in newborn infants in whom it comprises up to 80 per cent of the body weight. This relative excess of fluid is reciprocal with a diminution in the amount of fat. Despite this difference in the amount of body water, the electrolyte concentration of intracellular and extracellular fluids is similar in infants and adults.

The problems of management are made worse because their circulation is more easily overloaded, therefore intravenous fluids must be used with even greater caution than in adults. Since changes occur more rapidly in babies than in adults, a serious clinical state, which in an adult might take days to build up, may in a baby take only a matter of hours.

### Disturbances of acid–base balance

The pH of the extracellular fluid is normally maintained between 7·32 and 7·45; the normal $pCO_2$ is 35–55. The principal buffer mechanism responsible for maintaining normality is, in the short term, the bicarbonate–carbonic acid system. The amount of carbonic acid present is directly proportional to the $pCO_2$; therefore, changes in blood pH are reflected in the bicarbonate/ $pCO_2$ ratio and vice versa.* In the long term, the kidney is almost wholly responsible for acid–base homeostasis by its ability to excrete excesses of either hydrogen ions $H^+$ ('acid') or base, such as bicarbonate or phosphate.

Any change, actual or potential, in blood pH caused by a shift in $pCO_2$ is called 'respiratory'. All other changes in blood pH are called 'metabolic'. These metabolic changes are manifest, either directly or indirectly, by alterations in bicarbonate concentration. A disturbance of acid–base balance in which there is a *decrease* in the bicarbonate/$pCO_2$ ratio (i.e. in pH) is called 'acidosis'. An *increase* in the bicarbonate/$pCO_2$ ratio is called

* The relation between these parameters is expressed by pH $=$ constant $+$ log (bicarbonate mEq per litre/$pCO_2$ mm Hg).

720

'alkalosis'* Acidosis results from a rise in $pCO_2$ or a fall in bicarbonate or a combination of both. Alkalosis results from a fall in $pCO_2$, or a rise in bicarbonate or a combination of both.

*Respiratory acidosis* results from a rising $pCO_2$ due either to increased $CO_2$ production or respiratory failure.

*Respiratory alkalosis* results from a falling $pCO_2$ due to excessive ventilation. This occurs from voluntary or mechanically induced overbreathing and during excessive stimulation of the respiratory centre by nervous and chemical disorders such as anoxia, febrile states and the early stages of salicylate poisoning (see p. 713).

*Metabolic acidosis* is accompanied by a fall in bicarbonate concentration. This may be due to excessive external loss of bicarbonate and other bases as in diarrhoea, or due to an excessive internal 'consumption' of bicarbonate by excess hydrogen ions ($H^+ + HCO_3^- \rightarrow CO_2 + H_2O$). These excess hydrogen ions arise from either the metabolic overproduction of strong acids, or the inability to excrete the normal production of acid, or the ingestion of exogenous acids. Overproduction of keto-acids ('ketone bodies')—$\beta$-hydroxy-butyric and acetoacetic—occurs in uncontrolled diabetes mellitus and, to a much lesser extent, in starvation; lactic acid may accumulate in hypoxic states. Underexcretion of acid occurs in uraemia from any cause; it may also result from a specific renal tubular defect, as in renal tubular acidosis (p. 563). Toxic doses of salicylic acid may produce a metabolic acidosis (see p. 713).

*Metabolic alkalosis* is accompanied by a rise in bicarbonate concentration. This may be due to an excessive internal 'production' of bicarbonate or the ingestion of excessive bicarbonate. External losses of hydrogen ions ($H^+$) in acid gastric juice due to vomiting result in an increase of bicarbonate by internal 'production'; this is a reversal of the situation described under metabolic acidosis, viz. $CO_2 + H_2O \rightarrow H^+$ (lost in gastric juice) $+ HCO_3^-$. Vomiting as a cause of metabolic alkalosis occurs particularly from pyloric stenosis.

Hydrogen ions ($H^+$) may also be lost from the extracellular fluid space into the intracellular compartment in a situation of total body potassium deficiency. Hydrogen ions replace the lost potassium ions in the cell, causing an intracellular acidosis. However, the resultant net loss of hydrogen ions from the extracellular fluid causes an extracellular ('hypokalaemic') alkalosis in the face of this intracellular acidosis. In addition to potassium loss causing a

* Sometimes the terms 'acidosis' and 'alkalosis' are used to refer to the direction of actual or potential changes in blood pH. In that case the terms 'acidaemia' and 'alkalaemia' are used to denote situations in which the pH is actually below or above the normal range, respectively.

metabolic alkalosis, potassium deficiency is common to almost all states of chronic metabolic alkalosis.

Homeostatic mechanisms operate towards keeping the ratio constant: the response to a primary metabolic acidosis is a secondary (compensatory) respiratory alkalosis and vice versa. Similarly, the response to a primary respiratory acidosis is a secondary metabolic alkalosis and vice versa. According to the degree of effectiveness of the secondary response in restoring the ratio (and therefore the blood pH) to normal, the primary disturbance may be fully or, more usually, partially compensated. Respiratory compensation for metabolic alkalosis is always incomplete. Secondary respiratory changes occur rapidly by means of increased or decreased ventilation but secondary metabolic responses, which are mediated by the kidney, are slower, taking several hours.

### Clinical features of electrolyte and fluid disturbances

The limitations of electrolyte studies in the assessment of these patients is apparent. Moreover, not every hospital has facilities for all these investigations and in any case they may take a long time. Urgent cases must be treated without waiting for the results. Clinical assessment is therefore of prime importance, close attention also being paid to the weight, temperature and to the intake and output of fluids; the mother should always be asked the time since the child last passed urine.

Dehydration is the feature of the serious case. It causes sunken eyes, depressed anterior fontanelle, dryness of the mouth and loss of skin elasticity. When testing this elasticity, the skin over the ribs should be used rather than the abdominal skin which can give fallacious results: a marasmic baby may have loose abdominal skin from loss of weight rather than loss of fluid; lack of potassium can cause abdominal distension (see below) with consequent stretching of the skin.

The relative loss of sodium and water is seldom the same as their proportions in the extracellular fluid. Consequently, isotonic dehydration is rare. It is necessary, therefore, to differentiate hyponatraemic and hypernatraemic dehydration since their clinical management is totally different.

*Hyponatraemic dehydration* (salt deficit) occurs when the relative loss of sodium exceeds the loss of water; it is the commoner of the two types. Thirst is not a feature, the baby being limp and apathetic. Anorexia and vomiting are common. The skin is dry and inelastic. Convulsions may occur. In the most severe cases the infant is ashen grey and cold, lying with half open eyes in a state of shock; death frequently follows.

*Hypernatraemic dehydration* (water deficit) occurs when the relative loss of fluid exceeds the loss of sodium. It results from 3 situations particularly:

simple fluid depletion associated with inadequate replacement of excessive insensible loss in a feverish or comatose baby; excessive administration of sodium; mixed fluid and electrolyte loss when the loss of fluid predominates.

Thirst is very marked, the baby being restless, irritable and sometimes developing convulsions. The peripheral signs of dehydration are less marked than in hyponatraemic dehydration since the increased osmolality of the extracellular fluid causes a shift of water out of the cells into the extracellular compartment. The skin may therefore have a rubbery or doughy feel. The fluid lack commonly causes fever. Hypernatraemic states cause shrinking of the brain with meningeal congestion and vascular stasis which may lead to thrombosis. Cerebral thrombosis may leave the child mentally retarded and spastic. In general, the changes in hypernatraemic dehydration are more profound than those in hyponatraemic dehydration and peripheral circulatory failure often occurs despite a brief history. Acidosis is common.

*Acidosis* causes deep sighing respirations termed 'air hunger'. Acidotic patients are usually dehydrated and may be comatose.

*Alkalosis* causes few symptoms, dehydration being minimal. The respirations are shallow, the cry feeble and less frequent. The alkalotic baby, since he cries less often, may be mistakenly believed by his mother to have improved.

*Lack of potassium* causes flaccid muscular weakness; persistalsis is inhibited, leading to gaseous distension of the small intestine. In severe cases the full clinical picture of paralytic ileus is present. Changes in the electrocardiogram, resulting from low potassium, may be present; these comprise a lowered T wave and depression of the S-T segment.

*Vomiting* causes a loss of acid ($H^+$), sodium and potassium. The kidneys respond by excreting urine high in bicarbonate. When renal compensation fails the plasma bicarbonate rises; metabolic alkalosis ensues, frequently being associated with hypokalaemia.

*Diarrhoea* causes loss of an isotonic, alkaline solution, leading to dehydration and, in severe cases, shock. There is also a loss of potassium in the stools. Metabolic acidosis results from the following factors:

1. Loss of bicarbonate in the stools.
2. Dehydration causes diminished renal function from impairment of renal blood flow. An accumulation of acid metabolic products results.
3. The diminished intake of food causes glycogen depletion with consequent utilization of fat whose metabolism produces keto-acids.
4. Accumulation of lactic acid from generalized tissue anoxia.

Since severe vomiting alone produces alkalosis and severe diarrhoea alone produces acidosis, the acid/base state in the individual patient with these symptoms will depend on their relative proportions. In children with gastroenteritis diarrhoea usually predominates; consequently, such patients are usually acidotic.

In the management of electrolyte disorders the levels of sodium, potassium, bicarbonate, chloride, pH and urea should be estimated, though the limitations of such investigations must be understood. These levels, being obtained from the plasma, refer to the extracellular fluid alone; consequently, they give little information regarding absolute deficits or excesses of the substances measured. To do this they must be accompanied by an estimate, which is usually clinical, of the fluid volume state. Moreover, the values obtained give little information as to the state of the intracellular compartment which is three times greater than the extracellular compartment and differs considerably in its biochemical composition. For example, potassium is mainly intracellular and sodium extracellular. In this connection, the old concept that the cell membrane is relatively impermeable to these ions is incorrect; a constant exchange of sodium and potassium occurs across the cell membrane, the extracellular position of sodium resulting from active extrusion of this ion out of the cell by the 'sodium pump' mechanism.

A further limitation is that an electrolyte investigation determines only the biochemical state at one particular moment in the day whereas, for its proper understanding, a continuous picture of the electrolyte state is required. However, despite all these limitations, repeated electrolyte determinations give valuable assistance in judging the effects of treatment provided they are also accompanied by clinical assessment.

In the management of long-term problems it is also necessary, when planning replacement therapy, to estimate the total daily losses of electrolytes. For this, it is usually adequate to analyse only the urine, but if there is much loss of electrolytes in vomit or loose stools these fluids also should be analysed.

### Correction of fluid deficit

VOLUME REQUIRED

The normal infant's daily fluid requirements are:
   (a) Preterm baby for first 2 weeks—60 ml/kg on the first day, rising by 20 ml/kg each day until 150 ml/kg is reached.
   (b) Full-term baby for first 2 weeks—90 ml/kg on the first day, rising by 20 ml/kg daily until having 150 ml/kg.
   (c) Normal baby after age of 2 weeks—150 ml/kg.

A dehydrated baby requires additional fluid to his normal requirements in order to make up the deficit. This is calculated on a basis of $2\frac{1}{2}$ per cent of total body weight if mildly dehydrated and 5 per cent of body weight if moderately dehydrated. Severe dehydration may cause a deficit equivalent to 10 per cent of the body weight, but additional fluid replacement for such babies should start on a basis of 5 per cent and then be increased.

An extra quantity of fluid must be added to the above to take into account abnormal losses of water resulting from vomiting, diarrhoea or gastric aspiration.

RATE OF ADMINISTRATION OF INTRAVENOUS FLUIDS

To maintain normal fluid balance 6 ml/kg/hour is required. A dehydrated baby requires 20 ml/kg of normal saline by rapid injection followed by the remainder of the fluid deficit at a rate of 5–10 ml/kg/hour, aiming to replace the deficit in the first 4–6 hours. If there is persistent fluid loss from diarrhoea or gastric aspiration the rate may need to be continued at a maximum of 10 ml/kg. Great caution is needed when giving intravenous fluid as rapidly as this; if restlessness occurs the rate should be drastically reduced. In developing countries, supervision of the flow rate of drips may be by partially trained staff. Under these circumstances, in addition to prescribing the quantity of fluid required, a strip of adhesive tape should be stuck to the side of the bottle; on this should be marked the level the fluid must reach at specified times.

TREATMENT OF HYPERNATRAEMIC DEHYDRATION

Slow correction is essential since a rapid return of water to the brain cells causes cerebral oedema. Peripheral circulatory failure should be corrected by plasma or normal saline given at a rate of 20 ml/kg over 60 minutes. Further management is dependent on the underlying cause. 0·18 per cent saline and 4·3 per cent dextrose (i.e. 1/5 N saline in dextrose) is the solution used for maintenance, with added bicarbonate or lactate as required for the correction of acidosis. The rate of flow should not exceed 100 ml/kg for 24 hours and may thereafter be increased to 200 ml/kg /24 hours.

Hypocalcaemia and hypokalaemia should be corrected as soon as a satisfactory flow of urine has been established. Treatment should be monitored by serial estimations of plasma osmolality; the normal is 280–300 mOsm/l.

## Correction of sodium and glucose deficit

Sodium is the key to fluid therapy. Estimations based on chloride levels are unsatisfactory since variable factors affect the concentration of chloride ions in the extracellular fluid. Even when the most careful assessments of chloride deficiency are made, it is often found that once the baby is rehydrated the resultant chloride figure is lower than anticipated owing to the dilution effect following rehydration.

The first step is the replacement of sodium losses using normal saline. Thereafter the maintenance fluid—0·18 per cent saline and 4·3 per cent dextrose—is used. Glucose is required both for its calorie value and for the prevention of hypoglycaemia. 1 g glucose provides 4 calories; a baby requires a minimum of 40–60 calories per kg per day.

### Treatment of metabolic acidosis

Sodium bicarbonate or sodium lactate is the fluid used. Sodium lactate can be given intravenously and subcutaneously; sodium bicarbonate can be given intravenously but not subcutaneously.

For intravenous use bicarbonate is preferable to lactate since the actual substance deficient is being replaced. Lactate was used because bicarbonate was difficult to sterilize by heat, being destroyed with the liberation of $CO_2$. It has now been found that this can be prevented by sterilizing in an atmosphere of $CO_2$.

The quantity of bicarbonate required to correct the base deficit is calculated as follows:

mEq Sodium bicarbonate needed = Base deficit × Body weight in kg × 0·3

An 8·4 per cent solution of sodium bicarbonate provides 1 mEq bicarbonate per ml. It should be diluted before use. 50 ml of 8·4 per cent sodium bicarbonate added to 250 ml water provides a 1·4 per cent solution containing 50 mEq bicarbonate in 300 ml.

It is important to correct the deficit slowly in order to avoid sodium overload. In severe acidosis the initial calculation should be aimed to correct the bicarbonate to 15 mEq/l and the situation then rechecked. The pH should also be repeatedly checked.

If sodium lactate is used the quantity can be calculated on the basis that 4 ml/kg of M/6 sodium lactate will raise the plasma bicarbonate by 1 mEq/l.

### Treatment of metabolic alkalosis

Mild cases respond to normal saline since this provides an excess of $Cl^-$ ions in relation to $Na^+$ ions. If the base excess is greater than 5 mEq/l. and the pH more than 7·6, ammonium chloride should be given orally or intravenously.

The dose of ammonium chloride in mEq = Base excess × Body weight in kg × 0·3.

M/6 ammonium chloride (0·9 per cent solution) contains 167 mEq/l of each ion.

2 ml/kg M/6 ammonium chloride lowers the plasma bicarbonate by 1 mEq/l.

## Treatment of respiratory acidosis and alkalosis

Treatment must be directed at the cause of the respiratory problem. Respiratory acidosis may be due to acute airways obstruction as in asthma and respiratory distress syndrome. Ventilation may be necessary in addition to specific therapy.

Respiratory alkalosis results from overbreathing due, for example, to salicylate poisoning or emotional causes. Appropriate treatment for the underlying disorder must be given.

## Correction of potassium deficit

Potassium can be given safely only if the baby is rehydrated, the kidneys are functioning, and glucose administration has been started to ensure movement of potassium back into the cells. Oral potassium is much safer than intravenous potassium, excess of which can cause cardiac arrest. Potassium should therefore be given by mouth as soon as oral fluids are retained.

Oral K—1–2 g daily.

Intravenous K—not more than 3 mEq/kg/day. The fluid should contain not more than 40 mEq/litre.

For intravenous use the potassium can be given either as a concentrated solution (1 g potassium chloride contains 13 mEq potassium) which is added to the bottle of glucose-saline or as Darrow's solution (sodium 123 mEq, potassium 35 mEq, chloride 103 mEq, lactate 55 mEq, each per litre).

## Correction of calcium deficit

Acidosis causes mobilization of calcium from the skeleton with subsequent loss in the faeces and urine. In cases of gastroenteritis, when the diarrhoea ceases, calcium is rapidly redeposited in the bones leading to hypocalcaemia and, in severe cases, to tetany. The liability to hypocalcaemia is increased when the diarrhoea is prolonged and severe, or when nutrition is poor.

In cases of tetany up to 50 mg/kg of calcium gluconate can be given by slow intravenous drip. Ten per cent calcium gluconate contains 10 mg per ml; it must not be given at a rate faster than 1 ml per minute. A second observer should auscultate the apex beat and the injection must be stopped if the heart rate falls to 80 per minute. For maintenance therapy in cases of hypocalcaemia, 1 g calcium gluconate is given by mouth every 4–6 hours, together with 4000 units vitamin D daily. The vitamin D promotes the absorption of calcium from the upper intestinal tract.

## Protein

A normal baby's protein requirements are 2·5 g/kg/day. Babies on long term intravenous therapy require extra protein. This protein can be given as plasma, Trophysan, Aminosol or, if anaemic, as blood. One bottle of protein solution should be given for every two bottles of electrolyte fluid.

**Vitamins**

Babies on long term intravenous therapy should receive 1 mg of vitamin K daily and an intramuscular multivitamin preparation.

**Intravenous feeding**

Modern techniques and new preparations have made complete feeding possible by the intravenous route for prolonged periods (Harries, 1971). This may be required in cases of severe malabsorption, after extensive surgery involving the intestine in the newborn, in very low birth weight babies and in cases of renal failure.

Dehydration and acidosis must be corrected before the start of this treatment and frequent biochemical monitoring is required. The nutritional solutions used are aminoacid solutions (e.g. Vamin, Trophysan and Aminosol), fat emulsions (e.g. Intralipid), monosaccharides—either glucose or fructose—vitamins and minerals.

The risk of septicaemia is increased by the use of intravenous catheters, therefore all the peripheral veins should be used before resorting to the superior or inferior vena cava. This will require frequent changes of site since sclerosis of small veins soon occurs.

Abrupt termination of intravenous feeding may precipitate hypoglycaemia. Therefore, oral feeding should be reintroduced for several days before intravenous feeding is discontinued. Hypothermia may be a sign of severe hypoglycaemia.

**Fluid therapy if biochemical services are not available**

In developing countries, many hospitals will not have facilities for electrolyte estimations. Even where these facilities are available, intravenous fluids, if indicated, should be started immediately without waiting for results. The fluids given will depend on the clinical assessment: if there is gross clinical acidosis 150 ml of 8·4 per cent sodium bicarbonate can be given at the start; if the baby is dehydrated and salt depleted up to 10 ml/kg normal saline can be given. The solution chosen should be followed by an isotonic solution of glucose saline to correct the dehydration, preferably 0·18 per cent saline and 4·3 per cent dextrose (i.e. 1/5 N saline in dextrose).

**Routes of Administration**

This will depend on whether the baby is vomiting and on the degree of dehydration.

ORAL

This route should always be used if the baby will take by mouth and is not vomiting. If the baby refuses feeds but is not vomiting, the fluid can be given down an intragastric tube. If the baby is very dehydrated, even if not vomiting, intravenous fluids will be required in addition to intragastric. Moreover, in a very ill baby the fluid may not be absorbed from the intestine and there is the risk of inhalation of fluid vomited.

INTRAVENOUS

Whenever possible a 'stab' should be used in preference to a 'cut-down'. The rate of drip is dependent on the daily fluid requirements as given above but, in a very dehydrated baby, as much as 300 ml of fluid may be run in first by fast drip.

SUBCUTANEOUS

Considerable quantities of fluid may be absorbed subcutaneously, particularly if given with hyaluronidase. However, a very dehydrated baby is unable to absorb fluid by this route which should therefore not be used in such cases. If possible, solutions containing glucose should be avoided because they are irritating and may cause necrosis.

INTRAPERITONEAL

This route has many advantages over the subcutaneous and probably can always be substituted for it. It can be carried out by semi-trained staff and does not require prolonged supervision since the total fluid can be given in 10 minutes. This fluid forms a depot from which it is steadily absorbed over the next few hours. No local anaesthetic is required. The fluid must be warmed to blood heat beforehand since the injection of a large quantity of cold fluid could lower the body temperature. The needle should be inserted just above the umbilicus or in the flanks, after checking the position of the liver and spleen in order to ensure that these are not perforated. The risk of perforation of the intestines is reduced by turning the drip full on after penetration of the skin, before going through the peritoneum. In this way the intestines are pushed away from the needle by the force of flow of the fluid.

## BIBLIOGRAPHY

HARRIES J.T. (1971) Intravenous feeding in infants. *Arch. Dis. Childh.*, **46**, 855.
HARRIS F. (1972) *Paediatric fluid therapy*. Blackwell Scientific Publications, Oxford.
KING M. (1966) Ed. *Medical care in developing countries*. Oxford University Press, Nairobi.
WOOD B.S.B. (1974) Ed. *A paediatric vade-mecum*. 8th edition, Lloyd-Luke, London.

CHAPTER 29

# PAEDIATRIC DOSAGE GUIDE

The doses given are those for children except where the adult dose is stated; in that case the dose for a child is calculated as a percentage based on age, using the table below. For fuller details the reader is referred to *The Paediatric Prescriber* by Pincus Catzel, 4th Edition, published by Blackwell Scientific Publications Ltd.

The percentage method is particularly useful with new drugs. However, since the dose calculated by this method sometimes works out to be excessive for young infants, the dose based on weight is more often used in this guide.

| Age | Percentage of adult dose |
|---|---|
| Birth | 10 |
| 2 months | 15 |
| 4 months | 20 |
| 12 months | 25 |
| 18 months | 30 |
| 3 years | $33\frac{1}{3}$ |
| 5 years | 40 |
| 7 years | 50 |
| 10 years | 60 |
| 11 years | 70 |
| 12 years | 75 |
| 14 years | 80 |
| 16 years | 90 |
| 20 years | 100 |

*Acetylsalicylic acid*

Analgesic 10–15 mg/kg per dose.
Rheumatic fever 120 mg/kg daily. Maximum 8 g daily.

*Adrenaline*

1:1000 solution. In status asthmaticus 0·1 ml/kg/dose can be given sub-cutaneously to a maximum of 0·5 ml at a rate of 0·6 ml per minute.

*Amodiaquine hydrochloride* (Camoquin)

Available as tablets containing amodiaquine hydrochloride equivalent to 200 mg amodiaquine base.

Basic adult dose.
> In acute malaria: 600 mg orally, then 400 mg daily for 2 days.
> For malarial prophylaxis: 400 mg orally once weekly.

*Aminophylline*

> 3 mg/kg/dose given orally, intramuscularly (i.m.) or intravenously (i.v.)
> Suppositories 3–6 mg/kg.

*Amphetamine.* 5–20 mg/kg/day in three divided doses.

*Atropine sulphate.* 0·01 mg/kg/dose given subcutaneously. Maximum dose
0·4 mg. Can be repeated every 4–6 hours.

*Bephenium hydroxynaphthoate* (Alcopar)

> For hookworm.
> > Under 2 years: 2·5 g in single dose.
> > Two years and over: 5 g.

*Blood* for anaemia

$$\frac{80 \text{ ml/kg} \times \text{percentage deficiency of Hb.}}{100}$$

(6 ml/kg raises Hb by 1 g per cent.)

*Calcium gluconate*

> In tetany: up to 50 mg/kg i.v. slowly.
> Maintenance therapy: 1 g orally every 4–6 hours, plus 4000 units vitamin
> D daily to promote intestinal absorption of calcium.
> Five per cent calcium gluconate contains 50 mg/ml.

*Cephalosporins*

> Cephaloridine 30–50 mg/kg/day
> > i.m. or i.v. given in three divided doses.
>
> Cephalothin 30–50 mg/kg/day i.v. given in four divided doses. Is less
> nephrotoxic than cephaloridine.
> Cephalexin 25–100 mg/kg/day orally. Is slightly less active than cephalori-
> dine.

*Chloral hydrate*

> 25–50 mg/kg. Maximum 1 g.

*Chloramphenicol*

> Newborn and preterm babies: 25 mg/kg/day in four divided doses before
> meals.

Full-term babies aged 1–4 weeks: 50/mg/kg/day in four divided doses before meals.

Children: 75–100 mg/kg/day in four divided doses before meals. This dose for children should be checked against the maximum adult dose of 250–500 mg q.d.s. to ensure this is not exceeded.

These are maximum doses and must never be exceeded. A course of treatment should be for 5 days only to avoid the risk of agranulocytosis and aplastic anaemia. For the same reason, courses should not be repeated. Beware the grey baby syndrome (p. 110).

*Chlorothiazide*

40 mg/kg/day.

*Chloroquine*

*Chloroquine sulphate* (Nivaquin)

Available in tablets of 200 mg (150 mg chloroquine base).

As syrup (4 ml contains 75 mg base).

In 1 ml ampoules (30 mg base) for i.v.i. or i.m.i.

*Chloroquine phosphate* (Avloclor)

Available in tablets of 250 mg (155 mg base).

In 10 ml ampoules (400 mg base) for i.v.i. or i.m.i.

Acute malaria: oral 25 mg base/kg stat, then 12·5 mg/kg daily for 3 days. i.m. or i.v. 5 mg base/kg *maximum*.

Suppressive therapy: Basic adult dose 300 mg once weekly.

Suppressive therapy must commence 2 weeks before entering a malarious district and continue for 4 weeks after leaving the area.

*Chlorpromazine* (Largactil)

1 mg/kg/day.

*Colistin sulphate* (Colomycin)

50,000 units/kg/day intramuscularly in three divided doses.

*Corticotrophin* (ACTH). Use percentage method; adult dose 10–25 u i.m. 6 hourly, or 10–20 u i.v. over 6–24 hours.

*Co-trimoxazole* (Septrin)

A combination of trimethoprim and sulphamethoxazole in the ratio of 1:5. Dose (in terms of trimethoprim) 2 mg/kg/day.

*Deoxycortone*

Use percentage method.

Basic adult dose in crisis 5–20 mg i.m.
Maintenance 1–7 mg i.m. daily.

*Diazepam* (Valium)
Oral: 0·12–0·8 mg/kg/day in four divided doses.
Intramuscular or intravenous: 0·2 mg/kg.

*Digoxin*
Oral digitalizing dose: 0·08 mg/kg/day in four divided doses.
Maintenance dose: usually 0·02 mg/kg/day in four divided doses.

*Diphenhydramine hydrochloride* (Benadryl)
4 mg/kg/day by mouth in three divided doses.
Maximum dose 50 mg t.d.s.

*Ephedrine*
Small babies 8 mg.
For all other children 15 mg.
In asthma this should be given 4 hourly for the first 24 hours then t.d.s.
until bronchospasm ceases.
Nasal drops: $\frac{1}{2}$ per cent ephedrine in normal saline.

*Erythromycin*
20 mg/kg/day orally in four divided doses.

*Ethosuximide* (Zarontin)
20–50 mg/kg/day

*Folic acid*
15–20 mg daily by mouth or intramuscularly.
Maintenance 2·5–10 mg daily.

*Frusemide* (Lasix)
Oral: 1–3 mg/kg
Intramuscular or intravenous: 0·5–1·5 mg/kg.

*Gentamicin*
2·5 mg/kg/day given intramuscularly in three divided doses.

*Hydrochlorothiazide*
4 mg/kg/day.

*Hyoscine hydrobromide*

0·015 mg/kg as a single dose for premedication.

*Iron*

The required dose should be calculated as elemental iron, 6 mg/kg/day.
Ferrous sulphate contains 20 per cent elemental iron.
Therapeutic dose 20 mg/kg/day.
Prophylactic dose 10 mg/kg/day.
Mist. ferrous sulph. pro Inf. (BNF) contains 60 mg ferrous sulphate in 4 ml.
Sytron: a cherry flavoured preparation containing sodium ironedetate equivalent to 55 mg of iron in 10 ml.
Iron dextran (Imferon), an intramuscular preparation, contains 50 mg/ml. The total amount to be given is determined by the following formula: the iron deficiency in mg = weight (in kg) × 0·6 × percentage Hb deficient. Not more than 2 ml is given daily by intramuscular injection.

*Isoniazid* (INH)

20 mg/kg/day.
Maximum 400 mg daily.

*Isoprenaline* (Neo-epinine)

0·2 mg/kg sublingually.

*Kanamycin*

15 mg/kg/day given intramuscularly in two divided doses.

*Magnesium hydroxide mixture* (Cream of magnesia)

Up to 1 year: 4 ml.
1–5 years: 8 ml.

*Magnesium sulphate*. To reduce cerebral oedema.

Basic adult dose.
Intravenous: 10–25 ml of 10 per cent solution given slowly.
Intramuscular: 10 ml of 25 per cent solution given deeply.
Antidote: 10 ml of 10 per cent calcium gluconate which should be available to be given intravenously if cardiac depression occurs.

*Methandienone* (Dianobol)

0·04 mg/kg/day.

*Metronidazole* (Flagyl)

Basic adult dose: 200 mg t.d.s. for 3 days.

*Morphine sulphate.* Used in cardiac failure

Up to 0·2 mg/kg.
Maximum 10 mg.

*Nalorphine* (Lethidrone). Antagonist to morphine and pethidine for newborn babies.

0·25 mg i.v. or 0·5 mg i.m.

*Neomycin*

50 mg/kg/day by mouth in four divided doses.

*Nitrofurantoin* (Furadantin)

For urinary infections: 2·5 mg/kg/day.

*Novobiocin* (Albamycin)

15–30 mg/kg/day by mouth in four divided doses.

*Para-amino-salicylic acid* (PAS)

200 mg/kg/day.
Maximum 12 g daily.

*Paracetamol*

25 mg/kg.

*Paraldehyde*

Oral, rectal, intramuscular or intravenous (slowly) 0·2 ml/kg/dose. When given rectally it is added to twice its volume of olive oil or liquid paraffin and given as a retention enema.

Paraldehyde must be fresh and cannot be given with a plastic syringe. It is very painful when given intramuscularly.

*Paramethadione* (Paradione)

20–45 mg/kg/day in two to three divided doses.
Maximum 3 G at 12 years.

*Penicillin*

*Benzylpenicillin* (Penicillin G). Must be given parenterally since it is destroyed by gastric acid. 250,000 units i.m., q.d.s.

*Long acting penicillin.* Procaine penicillin G. 300,000 units i.m. once daily.

*Acid stable (oral) penicillin.* Phenoxymethylpenicillin (Penicillin V) 15–30 mg/kg/day.

*Penicillinase-stable penicillins.* The major use of these preparations is in the treatment of penicillin-resistant staphylococcal infection since they are less effective than penicillin G against other bacteria.

*Methicillin.* 100 mg/kg/day by intramuscular injection only in four divided doses.

*Cloxacillin.* 50 mg/kg/day oral, i.m. or i.v. in four divided doses.

*Flucloxacillin.* 25 mg/kg/day oral, i.m. or i.v. in four divided doses. This preparation is better absorbed from the gut than cloxacillin and is therefore preferable for oral use.

*Broad spectrum penicillins*

*Ampicillin.* 50–100 mg/kg/day oral, i.m. or i.v. in four divided doses. This preparation is particularly liable to cause rashes.

*Amoxycillin.* 20 mg/kg/day oral, i.m. or i.v. in four divided doses. This preparation is better absorbed than ampicillin and is therefore preferred.

'*Tailor-made*' *penicillins*

*Carbenicillin*—designed to destroy *pseudomonas pyocyaneus* but is also effective against gram-negative bacilli. 200 mg/kg/day i.m. or i.v. in four divided doses.

*Pentobarbitone* (Nembutal)

2–5 mg/kg.

*Pethidine hydrochloride*

1 mg/kg/dose orally or i.m.
Maximum 75 mg.

*Phenobarbitone*

2–3 mg/kg every 6–8 hours.
Maintenance 15–30 mg b.d.

*Phenytoin sodium* (Epanutin)

5 mg/kg/day.
Prolonged treatment with phenytoin leads to ataxia and gingival hyperplasia. The risk of gingival hyperplasia is reduced by good dental hygiene.

*Piperazine.* Given as Pripsen (piperazine phosphate and senna)

3–12 months: 5 g.

1–5 years: 7·5 g.

6 years and over: 10 g.

Dose should be repeated 2 weeks later to destroy those parasites which have hatched since the first dose.

*Primidone* (Mysoline)

5–20 mg/kg/day. Should be introduced slowly but later the dose can be doubled.

*Proguanil* (Paludrine)

Less then 5 years: 25 mg daily.

5–10 years: 50 mg daily.

Over 10 years: 100 mg daily.

*Promethazine hydrochloride* (Phenergan)

1 mg/kg/day.

*Pyrimethamine* (Daraprim)

Less than 5 years: 6·25 mg once weekly.

5–10 years: 12·5 mg once weekly.

Over 10 years: 25 mg once weekly.

*Quinalbarbitone* (Seconal)

5 mg/kg.

*Quinidine.* For paroxysmal tachycardia

100–200 mg every 2–8 hours, increasing daily until tachycardia ceases or toxic effects develop. For maintenance therapy give the effective dose 3–4 times daily for several months.

*Reserpine*

Basic adult dose: i.m. or i.v. 2·5–5 mg slowly.

Repeat in 12 hours if necessary.

*Salbutamol* (Ventolin)

2–6 years: 1–2 mg, 3–4 times daily.

6–12 years: 2 mg, 3–4 times daily.

*Spironolactone.* Aldosterone antagonist. Used in combination with chloro-thiazide.

Basic adult dose: 100 mg q.d.s. by mouth.

*Steroids*

Dose must be adjusted according to the response of the patient.

Usual equivalent doses of corticosteroids:

| | |
|---|---|
| Cortisone | 25 mg. |
| Hydrocortisone | 20 mg. |
| Prednisone and prednisolone | 5 mg. |
| Methylprednisolone | 4 mg. |
| Dexamethasone | 0·75 mg. |
| Betamethasone | 0·75 mg. |

*Prednisolone.* For routine oral steroid therapy. Use percentage method; adult dose 5–60 mg daily. Same dose can be given intramuscularly if there is vomiting. For i.v. or i.m. use in acute adrenal failure 25 mg may be given.

*Streptomycin sulphate.* 40 mg/kg/day. Overdosage causes prolonged coma. The dose can be given once daily for tuberculosis, except during the neonatal period, when it lasts only 9–12 hours. For all non-tuberculous infections it should be given every 6 hours as for penicillin with which it would usually be combined.

*Sulphadimidine* (Sulphamezathine)

125 mg/kg/day in four divided doses.

*Sulthiame* (Ospolot)

10–15 mg/kg/day in three divided doses.

*Tetracycline*

20–40 mg/kg/day in four divided doses.

*Thiopentone* (Pentothal)

20–40 mg/kg rectally as a basal anaesthetic.

TABLE 9. Equivalent Celsius and Fahrenheit temperature readings.

| Temperatures | | | | Temperatures | | | |
| --- | --- | --- | --- | --- | --- | --- | --- |
| °F | °C | °F | °C | °F | °C | °F | °C |
| 32 | 0·0 | 65 | 18·3 | 98 | 36·6 | 131 | 55·0 |
| 33 | 0·5 | 66 | 18·8 | 99 | 37·2 | 132 | 55·5 |
| 34 | 1·1 | 67 | 19·4 | 100 | 37·7 | 133 | 56·1 |
| 35 | 1·6 | 68 | 20·0 | 101 | 38·3 | 134 | 56·6 |
| 36 | 2·2 | 69 | 20·5 | 102 | 38·8 | 135 | 57·2 |
| 37 | 2·7 | 70 | 21·1 | 103 | 39·4 | 136 | 57·7 |
| 38 | 3·3 | 71 | 21·6 | 104 | 40·0 | 137 | 58·3 |
| 39 | 3·8 | 72 | 22·2 | 105 | 40·5 | 138 | 58·8 |
| 40 | 4·4 | 73 | 22·7 | 106 | 41·1 | 139 | 59·4 |
| 41 | 5·0 | 74 | 23·3 | 107 | 41·6 | 140 | 60·0 |
| 42 | 5·5 | 75 | 23·8 | 108 | 42·2 | 141 | 60·5 |
| 43 | 6·1 | 76 | 24·4 | 109 | 42·7 | 142 | 61·1 |
| 44 | 6·6 | 77 | 25·0 | 110 | 43·3 | 143 | 61·6 |
| 45 | 7·2 | 78 | 25·5 | 111 | 43·8 | 144 | 62·2 |
| 46 | 7·7 | 79 | 26·1 | 112 | 44·4 | 145 | 62·7 |
| 47 | 8·3 | 80 | 26·6 | 113 | 45·0 | 146 | 63·3 |
| 48 | 8·8 | 81 | 27·2 | 114 | 45·5 | 147 | 63·8 |
| 49 | 9·4 | 82 | 27·7 | 115 | 46·1 | 148 | 64·4 |
| 50 | 10·0 | 83 | 28·3 | 116 | 46·6 | 149 | 65·0 |
| 51 | 10·5 | 84 | 28·8 | 117 | 47·2 | 150 | 65·5 |
| 52 | 11·1 | 85 | 29·4 | 118 | 47·7 | 151 | 66·1 |
| 53 | 11·6 | 86 | 30·0 | 119 | 48·3 | 152 | 66·6 |
| 54 | 12·2 | 87 | 30·5 | 120 | 48·8 | 153 | 67·2 |
| 55 | 12·7 | 88 | 31·1 | 121 | 49·4 | 154 | 67·7 |
| 56 | 13·3 | 89 | 31·6 | 122 | 50·0 | 155 | 68·3 |
| 57 | 13·8 | 90 | 32·2 | 123 | 50·5 | 156 | 68·8 |
| 58 | 14·4 | 91 | 32·7 | 124 | 51·1 | 157 | 69·4 |
| 59 | 15·0 | 92 | 33·3 | 125 | 51·6 | 158 | 70·0 |
| 60 | 15·5 | 93 | 33·8 | 126 | 52·2 | 159 | 70·5 |
| 61 | 16·1 | 94 | 34·4 | 127 | 52·7 | 160 | 71·1 |
| 62 | 16·6 | 95 | 35·0 | 128 | 53·3 | 161 | 71·6 |
| 63 | 17·2 | 96 | 35·5 | 129 | 53·8 | 162 | 72·2 |
| 64 | 17·7 | 97 | 36·1 | 130 | 54·4 | 163 | 72·7 |

TABLE 10. Boys' height.

*Cross-sectional-type standards for supine length (up to 2) and height attained.*

| Age (yr) | Centiles (cm) | | | | | | |
|---|---|---|---|---|---|---|---|
| | 3rd | 10th | 25th | 50th | 75th | 90th | 97th |
| 0·08 | 50·2 | 51·4 | 52·7 | 54·0 | 55·4 | 56·6 | 57·8 |
| 0·25 | 56·6 | 57·9 | 59·2 | 60·7 | 62·1 | 63·4 | 64·7 |
| 0·50 | 63·8 | 65·2 | 66·6 | 68·2 | 69·7 | 71·2 | 72·6 |
| 0·75 | 67·9 | 69·4 | 71·0 | 72·7 | 74·4 | 75·9 | 77·4 |
| 1·00 | 71·2 | 72·8 | 74·5 | 76·3 | 78·1 | 79·7 | 81·4 |
| 1·25 | 74·0 | 75·7 | 77·4 | 79·4 | 81·3 | 83·0 | 84·7 |
| 1·50 | 76·5 | 78·3 | 80·1 | 82·1 | 84·2 | 86·0 | 87·8 |
| 1·75 | 78·7 | 80·6 | 82·5 | 84·6 | 86·7 | 88·7 | 90·5 |
| 2·00 | 80·7 | 82·7 | 84·7 | 86·9 | 89·1 | 91·1 | 93·1 |
| 2·0 | 79·7 | 81·7 | 83·7 | 85·9 | 88·1 | 90·1 | 92·1 |
| 2·5 | 83·5 | 85·6 | 87·8 | 90·2 | 92·6 | 94·8 | 96·9 |
| 3·0 | 87·0 | 89·3 | 91·6 | 94·2 | 96·8 | 99·1 | 101·4 |
| 3·5 | 90·4 | 92·8 | 95·3 | 98·0 | 100·8 | 103·2 | 105·7 |
| 4·0 | 93·5 | 96·1 | 98·7 | 101·6 | 104·5 | 107·1 | 109·7 |
| 4·5 | 96·5 | 99·2 | 102·0 | 105·0 | 108·1 | 110·8 | 113·5 |
| 5·0 | 99·4 | 102·2 | 105·1 | 108·3 | 111·5 | 114·4 | 177·2 |
| 5·5 | 102·2 | 105·2 | 108·2 | 111·5 | 114·8 | 117·8 | 120·8 |
| 6·0 | 104·9 | 108·0 | 111·1 | 114·6 | 118·1 | 121·2 | 124·3 |
| 6·5 | 107·6 | 110·8 | 114·0 | 117·6 | 121·2 | 124·4 | 127·6 |
| 7·0 | 110·3 | 113·5 | 116·8 | 120·5 | 124·2 | 127·5 | 130·8 |
| 7·5 | 112·9 | 116·2 | 119·6 | 123·4 | 127·2 | 130·6 | 133·9 |
| 8·0 | 115·4 | 118·8 | 122·3 | 126·2 | 130·0 | 133·5 | 137·0 |
| 8·5 | 117·9 | 121·4 | 125·0 | 128·9 | 132·9 | 136·4 | 139·9 |
| 9·0 | 120·4 | 124·0 | 127·6 | 131·6 | 135·7 | 139·3 | 142·9 |
| 9·5 | 122·8 | 126·5 | 130·2 | 134·3 | 138·4 | 142·1 | 145·8 |
| 10·0 | 125·1 | 128·8 | 132·6 | 136·8 | 141·0 | 144·8 | 148·5 |
| 10·5 | 127·2 | 131·0 | 135·0 | 139·3 | 143·6 | 147·6 | 151·4 |
| 11·0 | 129·4 | 133·3 | 137·4 | 141·9 | 146·4 | 150·4 | 154·4 |
| 11·5 | 131·7 | 135·8 | 140·0 | 144·7 | 149·4 | 153·6 | 157·8 |
| 12·0 | 133·7 | 138·0 | 142·4 | 147·0 | 152·2 | 156·6 | 160·9 |
| 12·5 | 136·3 | 140·7 | 145·3 | 150·3 | 155·4 | 159·9 | 164·4 |
| 13·0 | 138·7 | 143·4 | 148·2 | 153·4 | 158·7 | 163·5 | 168·2 |
| 13·5 | 141·5 | 146·4 | 151·3 | 156·8 | 162·3 | 167·2 | 172·0 |
| 14·0 | 145·0 | 150·0 | 155·0 | 160·7 | 166·3 | 171·3 | 176·2 |
| 14·5 | 148·4 | 153·4 | 158·4 | 164·0 | 169·6 | 174·6 | 179·6 |
| 15·0 | 152·3 | 157·1 | 161·9 | 167·3 | 172·7 | 177·6 | 182·4 |
| 15·5 | 155·9 | 160·4 | 165·0 | 170·1 | 175·2 | 179·8 | 184·3 |
| 16·0 | 158·9 | 163·1 | 167·4 | 172·2 | 177·0 | 181·3 | 185·5 |
| 16·5 | 160·7 | 164·8 | 168·9 | 173·5 | 178·0 | 182·1 | 186·2 |
| 17·0 | 161·7 | 165·7 | 169·8 | 174·3 | 178·8 | 182·8 | 186·8 |
| 17·5 | 162·0 | 166·0 | 170·0 | 174·5 | 179·0 | 183·0 | 187·0 |
| 18·0 | 162·2 | 166·2 | 170·2 | 174·7 | 179·2 | 183·2 | 187·2 |

TABLE 11. Girls' height.

*Cross-sectional-type standards for supine length (up to 2) and height attained.*

| Age (yr) | Centiles (cm) | | | | | | |
| --- | --- | --- | --- | --- | --- | --- | --- |
| | 3rd | 10th | 25th | 50th | 75th | 90th | 97th |
| 0·08 | 49·2 | 50·4 | 51·6 | 53·0 | 54·4 | 55·6 | 56·8 |
| 0·25 | 54·9 | 56·2 | 57·5 | 59·0 | 60·5 | 61·8 | 63·1 |
| 0·50 | 61·1 | 62·5 | 63·9 | 65·5 | 67·1 | 68·5 | 69·9 |
| 0·75 | 65·5 | 67·0 | 68·6 | 70·2 | 72·0 | 73·5 | 74·9 |
| 1·00 | 69·1 | 70·8 | 72·4 | 74·2 | 76·0 | 77·7 | 79·3 |
| 1·25 | 72·2 | 73·9 | 75·7 | 77·6 | 79·5 | 81·2 | 82·9 |
| 1·50 | 74·9 | 76·7 | 78·5 | 80·5 | 82·6 | 84·4 | 86·2 |
| 1·75 | 77·2 | 79·1 | 81·1 | 83·2 | 85·3 | 87·2 | 89·1 |
| 2·00 | 79·4 | 81·3 | 83·4 | 85·6 | 87·8 | 89·8 | 91·8 |
| 2·0 | 78·4 | 80·3 | 82·4 | 84·6 | 86·8 | 88·8 | 90·8 |
| 2·5 | 82·2 | 84·3 | 86·5 | 88·9 | 91·3 | 93·5 | 95·6 |
| 3·0 | 85·7 | 88·1 | 90·4 | 93·0 | 95·6 | 97·9 | 100·2 |
| 3·5 | 89·2 | 91·6 | 94·1 | 96·8 | 99·6 | 102·0 | 104·5 |
| 4·0 | 92·3 | 94·9 | 97·5 | 100·4 | 103·3 | 105·9 | 108·5 |
| 4·5 | 95·4 | 98·1 | 100·8 | 103·8 | 106·9 | 109·7 | 112·4 |
| 5·0 | 98·2 | 101·1 | 104·0 | 107·2 | 110·3 | 113·2 | 116·1 |
| 5·5 | 101·0 | 104·0 | 107·0 | 110·3 | 113·7 | 116·7 | 119·6 |
| 6·0 | 103·8 | 106·8 | 110·0 | 113·4 | 116·9 | 120·0 | 123·1 |
| 6·5 | 106·4 | 109·6 | 112·8 | 116·4 | 120·0 | 123·2 | 126·4 |
| 7·0 | 109·1 | 112·4 | 115·7 | 119·3 | 123·0 | 126·3 | 129·6 |
| 7·5 | 111·7 | 115·0 | 118·4 | 122·2 | 126·0 | 129·4 | 132·8 |
| 8·0 | 114·2 | 117·6 | 121·1 | 125·0 | 128·9 | 132·4 | 135·8 |
| 8·5 | 116·7 | 120·3 | 123·8 | 127·8 | 131·8 | 135·3 | 138·8 |
| 9·0 | 119·3 | 122·9 | 126·6 | 130·6 | 134·6 | 138·3 | 141·9 |
| 9·5 | 121·9 | 125·6 | 129·3 | 133·5 | 137·6 | 141·3 | 145·0 |
| 10·0 | 124·5 | 128·3 | 132·1 | 136·4 | 140·6 | 144·5 | 148·3 |
| 10·5 | 127·1 | 131·1 | 135·0 | 139·5 | 143·9 | 147·9 | 151·8 |
| 11·0 | 129·5 | 133·7 | 138·0 | 142·7 | 147·4 | 151·6 | 155·8 |
| 11·5 | 132·0 | 136·5 | 141·0 | 146·1 | 151·1 | 155·6 | 160·1 |
| 12·0 | 135·0 | 139·6 | 144·2 | 149·3 | 154·4 | 159·1 | 163·6 |
| 12·5 | 139·0 | 143·3 | 147·7 | 152·5 | 157·4 | 161·8 | 166·1 |
| 13·0 | 142·6 | 146·7 | 150·9 | 155·5 | 160·2 | 164·4 | 168·5 |
| 13·5 | 145·4 | 149·4 | 153·4 | 157·9 | 162·3 | 166·3 | 170·3 |
| 14·0 | 147·6 | 151·4 | 155·3 | 159·6 | 163·9 | 167·8 | 171·6 |
| 14·5 | 149·4 | 153·1 | 156·9 | 161·1 | 164·3 | 169·0 | 172·7 |
| 15·0 | 150·3 | 153·9 | 157·6 | 171·7 | 165·8 | 169·5 | 173·2 |
| 15·5 | 150·6 | 154·2 | 157·9 | 162·0 | 166·1 | 169·7 | 173·4 |
| 16·0 | 150·9 | 154·5 | 158·2 | 162·2 | 166·2 | 169·9 | 173·5 |

TABLE 12. Boys' weight.

*Cross-sectional-type standards for weight attained.*

| Age (yr) | Centiles (kg) | | | | | | |
|---|---|---|---|---|---|---|---|
| | 3rd | 10th | 25th | 50th | 75th | 90th | 97th |
| 0·00 | 2·50 | 2·80 | 3·10 | 3·50 | 3·80 | 4·10 | 4·40 |
| 0·25 | 4·65 | 5·01 | 5·43 | 5·93 | 6·45 | 6·99 | 7·43 |
| 0·50 | 6·38 | 6·80 | 7·32 | 7·90 | 8·58 | 9·20 | 9·90 |
| 0·75 | 7·48 | 7·98 | 8·55 | 9·20 | 9·95 | 10·63 | 11·45 |
| 1·00 | 8·3 | 8·8 | 9·5 | 10·2 | 11·0 | 11·7 | 12·6 |
| 1·25 | 8·9 | 9·6 | 10·2 | 11·0 | 11·8 | 12·6 | 13·5 |
| 1·50 | 9·4 | 10·1 | 10·7 | 11·6 | 12·5 | 13·3 | 14·3 |
| 1·75 | 9·8 | 10·5 | 11·12 | 12·2 | 13·1 | 13·9 | 14·9 |
| 2·00 | 10·2 | 11·0 | 11·8 | 12·7 | 13·7 | 14·6 | 15·6 |
| 2·25 | 10·5 | 11·4 | 12·2 | 13·2 | 14·2 | 15·1 | 16·2 |
| 2·50 | 10·9 | 11·9 | 12·7 | 13·7 | 14·8 | 15·8 | 16·9 |
| 2·75 | 11·2 | 12·2 | 13·1 | 14·2 | 15·3 | 16·3 | 17·4 |
| 3·0 | 11·6 | 12·7 | 13·6 | 14·7 | 15·8 | 16·9 | 18·0 |
| 3·5 | 12·3 | 13·4 | 14·5 | 15·6 | 16·8 | 18·0 | 19·2 |
| 4·0 | 13·0 | 14·3 | 15·3 | 16·6 | 17·9 | 19·1 | 20·4 |
| 4·5 | 13·7 | 15·0 | 16·1 | 17·5 | 19·0 | 20·2 | 21·8 |
| 5·0 | 14·4 | 15·7 | 16·9 | 18·5 | 20·0 | 21·5 | 23·2 |
| 5·5 | 15·1 | 16·5 | 17·7 | 19·5 | 21·2 | 22·8 | 24·8 |
| 6·0 | 15·9 | 17·3 | 18·6 | 20·5 | 22·4 | 24·0 | 26·5 |
| 6·5 | 16·6 | 18·1 | 19·5 | 21·5 | 23·6 | 25·4 | 28·3 |
| 7·0 | 17·4 | 19·0 | 20·6 | 22·6 | 24·9 | 26·9 | 30·3 |
| 7·5 | 18·2 | 19·9 | 21·6 | 23·7 | 26·1 | 28·4 | 32·3 |
| 8·0 | 19·1 | 20·9 | 22·7 | 25·0 | 27·5 | 30·0 | 34·4 |
| 8·5 | 20·0 | 21·9 | 23·9 | 26·2 | 28·9 | 31·6 | 36·5 |
| 9·0 | 21·0 | 22·9 | 25·0 | 27·5 | 30·3 | 33·4 | 38·8 |
| 9·5 | 21·9 | 24·0 | 26·2 | 28·9 | 31·9 | 35·3 | 41·0 |
| 10·0 | 23·0 | 25·2 | 27·5 | 30·3 | 33·6 | 37·3 | 43·3 |
| 10·5 | 24·0 | 26·3 | 28·7 | 31·9 | 35·6 | 39·7 | 46·3 |
| 11·0 | 24·9 | 27·4 | 30·1 | 33·6 | 33·7 | 42·6 | 49·5 |
| 11·5 | 26·0 | 28·6 | 31·6 | 35·5 | 40·2 | 45·4 | 53·3 |
| 12·0 | 27·1 | 29·9 | 33·2 | 37·7 | 42·7 | 49·0 | 57·2 |
| 12·5 | 28·1 | 31·3 | 35·0 | 40·0 | 35·7 | 52·5 | 61·0 |
| 13·0 | 29·6 | 33·0 | 37·1 | 42·6 | 49·0 | 56·0 | 64·4 |
| 13·5 | 31·2 | 35·1 | 39·7 | 45·5 | 52·2 | 59·4 | 67·8 |
| 14·0 | 33·3 | 37·7 | 42·6 | 48·8 | 55·4 | 62·5 | 70·9 |
| 14·5 | 36·0 | 40·6 | 45·7 | 51·9 | 58·4 | 65·4 | 73·7 |
| 15·0 | 39·0 | 43·7 | 48·7 | 54·7 | 60·9 | 68·0 | 75·9 |
| 15·5 | 42·7 | 47·0 | 51·7 | 57·4 | 63·0 | 70·1 | 77·5 |
| 16·0 | 45·7 | 49·6 | 54·1 | 59·6 | 65·0 | 71·7 | 78·6 |
| 16·5 | 47·5 | 51·3 | 55·6 | 61·0 | 66·2 | 72·8 | 79·5 |
| 17·0 | 48·6 | 52·3 | 56·6 | 61·9 | 67·1 | 73·6 | 80·2 |
| 18·0 | 50·0 | 53·5 | 57·8 | 63·0 | 68·0 | 74·5 | 81·0 |
| 19·0 | 50·4 | 53·7 | 58·1 | 63·3 | 68·3 | 75·0 | 81·6 |

TABLE 13. Girls' weight.

*Cross-sectional-type standards for weight attained.*

| Age (yr) | Centiles (kg) | | | | | | |
|---|---|---|---|---|---|---|---|
| | 3rd | 10th | 25th | 50th | 75th | 90th | 97th |
| 0·00 | 2·55 | 2·85 | 3·15 | 3·40 | 3·65 | 3·95 | 4·35 |
| 0·25 | 4·36 | 4·81 | 5·18 | 5·56 | 6·02 | 6·41 | 6·90 |
| 0·50 | 5·89 | 6·44 | 6·90 | 7·39 | 7·99 | 8·49 | 9·08 |
| 0·75 | 6·99 | 7·58 | 8·13 | 8·72 | 9·42 | 10·02 | 10·64 |
| 1·00 | 7·8 | 8·4 | 9·0 | 9·7 | 10·5 | 11·2 | 11·8 |
| 1·25 | 8·3 | 9·0 | 9·6 | 10·4 | 11·3 | 12·0 | 12·7 |
| 1·50 | 8·9 | 9·5 | 10·2 | 11·1 | 12·0 | 12·8 | 13·5 |
| 1·75 | 9·3 | 10·0 | 10·8 | 11·7 | 12·6 | 13·5 | 14·3 |
| 2·00 | 9·7 | 10·4 | 11·3 | 12·2 | 13·2 | 14·1 | 14·9 |
| 2·25 | 10·0 | 10·8 | 11·7 | 12·7 | 13·7 | 14·6 | 15·5 |
| 2·50 | 10·5 | 11·3 | 12·2 | 13·3 | 14·3 | 15·3 | 16·3 |
| 2·75 | 10·9 | 11·8 | 12·7 | 13·7 | 14·8 | 15·8 | 16·9 |
| 3·0 | 11·4 | 12·3 | 13·2 | 14·3 | 15·3 | 16·4 | 17·6 |
| 3·5 | 12·2 | 13·2 | 14·2 | 15·2 | 16·3 | 17·6 | 18·9 |
| 4·0 | 13·1 | 14·1 | 15·2 | 16·3 | 77·5 | 18·8 | 20·3 |
| 4·5 | 13·8 | 15·0 | 16·1 | 17·2 | 18·6 | 20·1 | 21·8 |
| 5·0 | 14·6 | 15·9 | 17·0 | 18·3 | 19·8 | 21·4 | 23·3 |
| 5·5 | 15·4 | 16·7 | 18·0 | 19·3 | 20·9 | 22·9 | 25·0 |
| 6·0 | 16·2 | 17·6 | 18·9 | 20·4 | 22·2 | 24·4 | 26·8 |
| 6·5 | 17·0 | 18·4 | 19·8 | 21·5 | 23·5 | 26·0 | 28·5 |
| 7·0 | 17·8 | 19·2 | 20·8 | 22·6 | 25·0 | 27·7 | 30·6 |
| 7·5 | 18·6 | 20·1 | 21·9 | 23·8 | 26·4 | 29·3 | 32·6 |
| 8·0 | 19·4 | 21·0 | 22·9 | 25·1 | 28·0 | 31·2 | 35·0 |
| 8·5 | 20·2 | 21·9 | 24·0 | 26·4 | 29·5 | 33·2 | 37·7 |
| 9·0 | 21·0 | 23·0 | 25·2 | 27·7 | 31·4 | 35·4 | 40·6 |
| 9·5 | 21·8 | 24·0 | 26·4 | 29·3 | 33·4 | 38·0 | 43·8 |
| 10·0 | 22·7 | 25·1 | 27·7 | 31·1 | 35·7 | 41·0 | 47·7 |
| 10·5 | 23·6 | 26·4 | 29·2 | 33·0 | 38·3 | 44·1 | 51·7 |
| 11·0 | 24·7 | 27·8 | 31·0 | 35·2 | 41·0 | 47·7 | 55·7 |
| 11·5 | 26·2 | 29·6 | 33·2 | 37·7 | 43·7 | 51·2 | 59·6 |
| 12·0 | 27·8 | 31·6 | 35·5 | 40·5 | 46·7 | 54·7 | 63·3 |
| 12·5 | 29·7 | 33·9 | 38·0 | 43·1 | 49·5 | 57·6 | 66·5 |
| 13·0 | 32·0 | 36·3 | 40·7 | 45·8 | 52·3 | 60·0 | 69·3 |
| 13·5 | 34·5 | 38·7 | 43·3 | 48·6 | 54·8 | 62·3 | 71·1 |
| 14·0 | 37·0 | 41·2 | 45·5 | 51·0 | 57·0 | 63·9 | 72·3 |
| 14·5 | 39·5 | 43·3 | 47·4 | 52·9 | 58·6 | 65·3 | 73·2 |
| 15·0 | 41·7 | 45·1 | 49·0 | 54·4 | 59·8 | 66·3 | 73·7 |
| 15·5 | 43·5 | 46·6 | 50·2 | 55·2 | 60·6 | 67·1 | 74·1 |
| 16·0 | 44·6 | 47·6 | 51·0 | 55·8 | 61·1 | 67·5 | 74·5 |
| 17·0 | 45·7 | 48·6 | 51·9 | 56·4 | 61·6 | 67·9 | 74·9 |
| 18·0 | 46·0 | 48·8 | 52·1 | 56·6 | 61·8 | 68·0 | 75·0 |
| 19·0 | 46·1 | 48·9 | 52·2 | 56·7 | 61·9 | 68·1 | 75·1 |

Tables 10–13 are taken from Tanner, J.M., Whitehouse R.H. & Takaishi M. (1966). Standards from birth to maturity for height, weight, height velocity and weight velocity: British children, 1965. *Arch. Dis. Childh.*, **41**, 613.

TABLE 14. Head circumference for boys and girls during the first seven years of life.

| Age | Boys | | | Girls | | |
|---|---|---|---|---|---|---|
| | Number | Mean (cm) | S.D. | Number | Mean (cm) | S.D. |
| 1 month | 295 | 37·3 | ±1·54 | 282 | 36·5 | ±1·41 |
| 3 months | 229 | 40·7 | ±1·43 | 230 | 39·8 | ±1·39 |
| 6 months | 275 | 43·6 | ±1·45 | 262 | 42·5 | ±1·42 |
| 9 months | 247 | 45·7 | ±1·40 | 259 | 44·6 | ±1·41 |
| 1 year | 289 | 46·8 | ±1·40 | 275 | 45·6 | ±1·22 |
| 1½ years | 255 | 47·9 | ±1·40 | 255 | 47·0 | ±1·30 |
| 2 years | 264 | 48·1 | ±1·47 | 260 | 48·0 | ±1·32 |
| 2½ years | 219 | 49·8 | ±1·39 | 221 | 48·8 | ±1·35 |
| 3 years | 216 | 50·4 | ±1·35 | 227 | 49·5 | ±1·35 |
| 3½ years | 226 | 51·0 | ±1·40 | 222 | 50·1 | ±1·45 |
| 4 years | 233 | 51·2 | ±1·41 | 229 | 50·7 | ±1·46 |
| 4½ years | 220 | 51·6 | ±1·45 | 217 | 51·0 | ±1·48 |
| 5 years | 224 | 51·8 | ±1·47 | 225 | 51·2 | ±1·40 |
| 7 years | 187 | 52·7 | ±1·48 | 194 | 52·2 | ±1·37 |

Table 14 is taken from Westropp C.K. & Barber C.R. (1956). Growth of the skull in young children. Part I. Standards of head circumference. *J. Neurol. Neurosurg. Psychiat.* **19,** 52.

# INDEX

Heavy type indicates main entry. Italic type is used for illustrations.

Encephalopathy
lead 717
risk after pertussis immunization 484
Encopresis **468**
emotional causes 305, 306
Endocardial fibroelastosis **375**
Endocarditis **372**
bacterial 190, **373**
clinical features 373
prognosis 374
prophylaxis 374
in rheumatoid arthritis 657
treatment 374
Endocrine glands, diseases *621*
Endometrial bleeding 46
Endomyocardial fibrosis **375**
*Entamoeba histolytica* 302
Enteric fever (typhoid, paratyphoid) **510**
*Enterobius vermicularis* **324**
Enuresis **466**
electric buzzer 468
treatment 466
use of drugs 468
Enzymes, duodenal, in cystic fibrosis 167, 170
*see also* Specific names
Eosinophilia 86
in hydatid disease 328
and roundworms 325
in schistosomiasis 329
in trichiniasis 328
Eosinophilic granuloma **617–619**
Epanutin, dosage 736
Ephedrine
dosage 733
in serous otitis media (glue ear) 338
Epicanthic fold 199, 219
Epidermal inclusion cyst 149
Epidermolysis bullosa **210**
dystrophic form 210
simple form 210
Epidermophytosis 677
Epididymo-orchitis
organisms causing 646
diagnosis from torsion of testicle 646
Epiglottitis, acute **336**
Epilepsy
idiopathic 414, *415*
fever 416
grand mal **416**
diagnosis 417
management of attack 419
prevention 418
treatment 418
general management 420

infantile spasms (lighting fits) 421
myoclonus 416
petit mal **420**
EEG 421, *422*, 423
hyperventilation 421
myoclonic 421
psychological factors 416
temporal lobe 416
intracranial injury 96, 101
in low birth weight infants 70
Epiloia *see* Sclerosis, tuberose
Epiphyses
slipped femoral **694**
diagnosis from transient synovitis, hip 693
Epistaxis **332**
Epstein-Barr virus in acute infective polyneuritis 412
in glandular fever 500
Epstein's pearls 149
Erb's paralysis 105, *106*
treatment 106
Erythema
iris 675
multiforme 675
nodosum 518
pernio 674
in rheumatic carditis 651
Erythroblastosis fetalis *see* Haemolytic disease of the newborn
Erythrogenesis imperfecta 592
Erythromycin
dosage 733
Erythrophagocytosis 612
*Escherichia coli* 388
ampicillin-resistant 400
gastroenteritis 113, 299
and infant feeding 76
meningitis 113, 398, 400
neonatal 108
pneumonia 114
Eskimos, mongolian blue spot 208
Ethambutol 530
Ethionamide 530
Ethisterone, congenital malformations 143
Ethmoiditis, acute 333
Ethosuximide
dosage 733
in petit mal 421
Eumydrin 160, 161
Eunuchoidism **286**
pituitary 286
testicular 286
Evening colic 84
Ewing's sarcoma 698